Scully's Oral and Maxillofacial Medicine

THE BASIS OF DIAGNOSIS AND TREATMENT

4th Edition

Scully's Oral and Maxillofacial Medicine

THE BASIS OF DIAGNOSIS AND TREATMENT

Stephen Challacombe
PHD, FRCPATH, FDSRCS, FMEDSCI,
DSC (H.C.), FKC
Martin Rushton Professor of Oral Medicine,
Centre for Host-Microbiome Interactions, Faculty
of Dentistry, Oral and Craniofacial Sciences,
King's College London, Guys Hospital, London

Barbara Carey
BDS, MB BCH BAO BA, FDS(OM) RCSI, FFDRCSI
(ORAL MEDICINE), FHEA
Consultant in Oral Medicine
Guy's and St Thomas' NHS Foundation Trust, London

Jane Setterfield
BDS, DCH, DRCOG, FRCP, MD
Professor of Oral and Dermatological Medicine
Honorary Consultant
Centre for Host-Microbiome Interactions, Faculty
of Dentistry, Oral and Craniofacial Sciences,
King's College London
Department of Oral Medicine and St John's
Institute of Dermatology, Guy's and St Thomas'
NHS Foundation Trust, London

ELSEVIER

© 2023 Elsevier Limited. All rights reserved.

First edition 2004
Second edition 2008
Third edition 2013

The right of Stephen Challacombe, Barbara Carey and Jane Setterfield to be identified as authors of this work has been asserted by them in accordance with the Copyright, Designs and Patents Act 1988.

No part of this publication may be reproduced or transmitted in any form or by any means, electronic or mechanical, including photocopying, recording, and any information storage and retrieval system, without permission in writing from the publisher. Details on how to seek permission, further information about the Publisher's permissions policies and our arrangements with organizations such as the Copyright Clearance Centre and the Copyright Licensing Agency, can be found on our website: www.elsevier.com/permissions

This book and the individual contributions it contains are protected under copyright by the Publisher (other than as may be noted herein).

Notices

Practitioners and researchers must always rely on their own experience and knowledge in evaluating and using any information, methods, compounds or experiments described herein. Because of rapid advances in the medical sciences in particular, independent verification of diagnoses and drug dosages should be made. To the fullest extent of the law, no responsibility is assumed by Elsevier, authors, editors or contributors for any injury and/or damage to persons or property as a matter of products liability, negligence or otherwise, or from any use or operation of any methods, products, instructions, or ideas contained in the material herein.

ISBN: 978-0-7020-8011-1

Content Strategist: Alexandra Mortimer
Content Project Manager: Anand K Jha
Design: Patrick C Ferguson
Illustration Manager: Akshaya Mohan
Marketing Manager: Deborah Watkins

Printed in Replika Press, India.
Last digit is the print number: 9 8 7 6 5 4 3 2 1

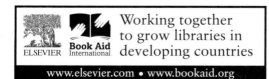

CONTENTS

v

PREFACE

We are pleased to have been invited to edit this fourth edition of one of the most popular textbooks in oral medicine. Professor Crispian Scully was an internationally known force in the development of oral medicine worldwide, and for his academic contributions at every level. This text has a particular place in the hearts and minds of students of oral medicine. Crispian Scully set out to deliver a book which was visual, practical, up to date and which summarised current thoughts on the diagnosis and, management. The third edition was laid out with each themed section in a different page colour for easy reference. We have tried to thoroughly update the book, yet be true to the basic concept of easy and enjoyable reading, with helpful summaries of each topic. Before the book was written, the publishers had the third edition peer reviewed and we have incorporated many of the changes suggested, adding in new material and leaving out some older material. We hope that the fourth edition of this highly successful book continues to offer readers with a systemized and objective approach to the practice of oral and maxillofacial medicine.

The book has been completely restructured with grouping of disorders into 7 themed section sections, with six new chapters not covered in the previous edition, combining of several of the short chapters in the third edition and with 30% of the figures being new or replacing older figures. Nevertheless, we have tried to remain true to the underlying principle of a visually attractive layout with as many examples of clinical conditions as allowed, yet with frequent text summaries of important diagnostic and management points. We have expanded sections on clinical features and management, including emerging therapies, as well as additional information on drug interactions and contraindications.

We have accepted that modern day students of oral medicine are unlikely to follow up long lists of references in textbooks. We have therefore included cardinal references only, particularly focussing on World Workshops of oral medicine reports, and Cochrane reviews of diagnosis and treatment of relevant conditions. It has become apparent to the world of oral medicine that outcomes of treatment both from the clinician's perspective and from the patient's perspective are now an essential part of the management of oral diseases. We have therefore included in this edition information on oral disease severity scores and patient reported outcomes which should be used for every patient.

This book presents a straightforward, accessible guide to the successful diagnosis and treatment of the most common and potentially serious disorders seen in oral medicine clinical practice. Maintaining a strong patient-centred approach throughout, the book also explores relevant systemic disorders and includes an updated recommended reading list. This clearly written book places a strong emphasis on practical issues and is beautifully illustrated with liberal use of tables, algorithms and clinical photographs.

Senior dental students, dental practitioners and trainees and practitioners in oral medicine, surgery and pathology in particular, will find this book to be both an excellent source of reference and a thoroughly practical guide for clinical diagnosis and contemporary non-surgical management of conditions affecting the oral and maxillofacial region.

We would like to thank Dr Parnyan Ashtari BDS, MPharm for her very helpful and important contributions to the chapters on drugs and drug reactions.

Thanks to Alison Taylor then of Elsevier, with whom the idea of this edition was nurtured and developed, to Anand K Jha of Elsevier, with whom we have had many interesting and useful conversations and the professional teams of copyeditors, typesetters and proofreaders who have all contributed to producing a revised text of which we hope that Crispian Scully would have been proud.

SJC, BC and JS, 2022

LEARNING OUTCOMES

"To study the phenomena of disease without books is to sail an uncharted sea, while to study books without patients is not to go to sea at all."
—Sir William Osler

This text will deal with oral and maxillofacial diseases and their medical management. It is intended that having read this book, the reader will be able to:

- Recognize the scope of oral and maxillofacial diseases and the importance of medical management in addition to the traditional dental focus of the discipline.
- Adopt a systematic approach to medical history taking that extends routine questions into certain relevant areas of enquiry that involve the body in general.
- Identify relevant follow-up questions that may further clarify the findings of the clinical examination and refocus the history.
- Examine patients and their oral lesions systematically and use the findings of specific features of the lesion and associated signs and symptoms, to start formulating differential diagnoses.
- Identify lesions and interpret the findings and develop a sense of the potential implications for the patient.
- Identify which sites may be affected by the presenting condition and what to look for at those sites.
- Understand the importance of recording disease severity for all conditions.
- Understand when clinical investigations are indicated, which are appropriate, and how to perform these investigations.
- Interpret the findings of routine clinical investigations (e.g. blood test results) and develop a sense of the potential implications for the patient.
- Identify a range of therapeutic options for the patient and understand the need for regular review and re-appraisal of the condition.
- Understand how treatment may impact, positively or negatively, upon the condition.
- Be able to record the clinical outcome of treatment using disease severity scoring.
- Advise the patient about the aetiology of oral lesions, and predisposing factors.
- Identify the need to refer for advice, investigations or treatment by dental, medical or surgical specialists.
- Recognize the importance of close liaison with colleagues in other disciplines, particularly imaging, medicine, pathology and surgery.

This book is dedicated to Professor Crispian Scully and to all those who enjoy the discipline of Oral Medicine. Professor Crispian Scully authored over 30 books in the field and his enthusiasm for every aspect of Oral Medicine increased awareness and understanding of the importance of the field internationally. Generations of students have benefited from his writings. Our editorship of this popular book fulfils a willing commitment to continue his work.

SECTION I

Fundamentals of Patient Management

Principles of Diagnosis: History

INTRODUCTION

Diagnosis means 'through knowledge' and entails acquisition of data about the patient and their complaint using the senses (HOTS):

- Hearing/listening
- Observing/seeing
- Touching/feeling
- Smelling (sometimes) (Fig. 1.1).

The purpose of making a diagnosis is to be able to offer the most:

- Appropriate, effective and safe treatment
- Be able to offer a more accurate prognosis.

Diagnosis is made by the clinical examination, which comprises the:

- history (anamnesis) — this offers the diagnosis in approximately 80% of cases
- physical examination
- supplemented by investigations in some cases (standard or special).

Each is based on a thorough, methodical routine. Diagnosis most importantly involves a careful history; the patient will often deliver the diagnosis from the history, although the findings from examination and investigations can be helpful, as can reference to the literature and Internet. To state the obvious, it is difficult to diagnose a condition that is unknown to the diagnostician; thus extensive reading of recent literature, clinical experience and discussion with colleagues are continually needed, as well as an enquiring mind. Continuing education is essential. Sometimes the diagnosis can be made by observing pathognomonic features (e.g. in dentinogenesis imperfecta, in which the abnormally translucent brownish teeth are characteristic).

There are some subtypes of diagnosis, including:

- Pathological diagnosis: provided from the pathology results but combined with history and examination to give the presumptive diagnosis.

- Provisional (working) diagnosis: the more usually made diagnosis. This is an initial diagnosis from which further investigations can be planned.
- Presumptive diagnosis: made after due consideration of all facts from the history, examination and investigations.
- Differential diagnosis: the process of making a list of possible diagnoses by considering the similarities and differences between similar conditions.
- Diagnosis by exclusion: identification of a disease by excluding all other possible causes.
- Diagnosis made on the results of response to treatment. For example, the pain of trigeminal neuralgia may be atypical, and the diagnosis can sometimes be confirmed only by a positive response to the drug carbamazepine.

COMMUNICATING WITH THE PATIENT

Patients' attitudes to healthcare, the benefits and risks from examination, investigations and treatment and the extent to which they find adverse effects tolerable can differ markedly from assumptions of the clinicians. Effective healthcare communication incorporates not only medical and dental information but also sensitive discussion of the patients' emotional and social wellbeing, always being culturally sensitive and tailoring to the patient's ability to understand.

Patients have personal wishes, needs and concerns that demand the understanding and respect of the clinician. Involving patients as full partners in decisions about their treatment leads to better health outcomes. Healthcare should:

- provide respectful care
- meet the patient's personal, cultural and religious needs
- educate and inform on relevant health issues
- facilitate patients making their own choices
- respect those choices.

Communicating requires time, patience and expertise: language can be a huge barrier. One of the most obvious ways to

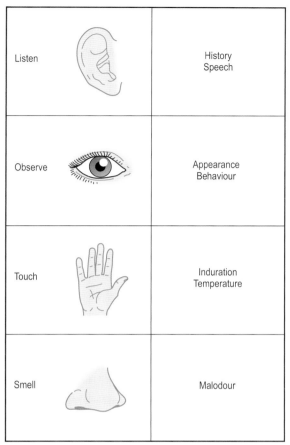

Listen		History Speech
Observe		Appearance Behaviour
Touch		Induration Temperature
Smell		Malodour

Fig. 1.1 The senses in diagnosis.

assist communication is to have material available in relevant different languages which is easily readable and understood.

Patient interviews are an opportunity to listen and ascertain the patient's feelings and concerns about healthcare and to explore what beliefs and practices are important to them. The clinician should use 'LEAPS':

- **L**isten
- **E**mpathise
- **A**sk
- **P**araphrase
- **S**ummarise.

The clinician should thereby endeavour to elicit the:
- patient's main problems
- patient's perceptions of their problems
- physical, emotional and social impact of their problems.

They should tailor information to what the patient wants to know, always checking patient understanding.
- Elicit the patient's reaction to information given.
- Determine how much the patient wants to participate in decision-making.
- Discuss management options.
- Greetings can 'make' or 'break' the professional relationship, especially if the patient is older and/or from a different culture. Key points to remember include to:
  - smile

- speak clearly and directly, making eye contact as appropriate
- greet using 'Good morning' or 'Good afternoon', or the greeting appropriate to their culture
- never use the first name alone, except when requested. Ask the patient what they prefer to be called, but as a default and at the initial greeting, use their title and surname
- say a few words to put the patient at ease
- explain who you are and what you do, what is happening and what will happen
- sensitively check whether the patient understands the conversation
- be careful about touching
- encourage the patient to establish a professional relationship.

For many people from non—Anglo-Saxon cultures, the customary greeting is a gesture other than the handshake. In addition, some may be uncomfortable shaking hands with a person of the opposite gender. Unless you are certain of their culture or religion, it is better to greet a patient with a handshake, seeing first if the person offers their hand, and then say 'Good morning/afternoon' and use their title followed by their last name.

Communication can thus be achieved through:
- active listening
- empathy
- appropriately using open questions
- frequently summarising
- clarifying where needed
- clearly explaining concepts
- checking patient's understanding
- checking patient's compliance with management recommendations.

Specific skills such as questioning styles, active listening, providing information and avoiding negative communication behaviours (e.g. inappropriate affect, the inappropriate use of closed questions or offering premature advice/reassurance) are crucial to success.

Avoid also the use of:
- technical terms and expressions
- abbreviations
- professional jargon
- abstract concepts
- colloquialisms
- idiomatic expressions
- slang
- metaphors
- euphemisms
- stereotype figures or symbols.

Breaking Bad News

Give any bad or unpleasant news tactfully and slowly, maintain confidentiality and check with the patient exactly who can be told about their condition, when and what they can be told.

A key healthcare professional (HCP) should be identified whom the patient can contact for further information and act as an advocate. Most important is verbal interaction, but alternative information sources (e.g. written leaflets, computer systems, DVDs) can help.

HISTORY TAKING

The first contact with the patient is crucial to success, and there should be a courteous approach to the patient with a professional introduction and every effort to establish communication, rapport and trust, and make the patient feel the focus of the clinician's interest. History taking is part of the initial communication between the dentist and patient. It is important to adopt a professional appearance and manner, and introduce oneself clearly and courteously. The clinician should enquire early on as to the main complaint and relevant social aspects such as occupation. The patient will know if you care, well before they care if you know.

The clinician should encourage the patient to tell the story in their own words, and use methodical questioning to elucidate further details.

Perhaps not surprisingly, many patients are apprehensive when confronted by a clinician, and therefore they may be easily disturbed if, for example, the clinician appears indifferent or unsympathetic. This can result in barriers to effective communication, which will simply hinder the clinician.

Due cognisance must also always be taken of the age, cultural background, understanding and intelligence of the patient when taking the history. It is the clinician's responsibility to elicit an accurate history; if that necessitates finding an interpreter, for example, then the clinician must arrange this. The ability to take a comprehensive and relevant medical history is fundamental to being a competent clinician.

The history is best given in the patient's own words, although the clinician often needs to guide the patient and may use protocols to ensure collection of all relevant points. It is imperative to be clear as to the patient's main complaint and ascertain key clinical features such as date of onset, duration, severity, whether constant or intermittent, previous treatments and whether there has been a response to any. Sometimes there may be several complaints. Do not assume that they are all interlinked, and take a detailed history for each. Determine how much each complaint bothers the patient. It is pointless in giving treatment for a complaint where the patient only needed reassurance about the diagnosis and which did not bother him or her.

It is important to cover the following areas:
- general information (name, date of birth, gender, ethnic origin, place of residence, occupation)
- presenting complaint(s)
- history of each of the present complaints
- past medical history
- dental history
- family history
- social and cultural history including lifestyle habits (e.g. use of tobacco, alcohol, betel)
- patient expectations.

By the end of the history, the clinician should have an idea of the patient's concerns, have assessed the patient's current problems and also have drawn up a provisional or differential diagnosis.

PRESENTING COMPLAINT

The history taking commences by identifying the current complaint(s) (e.g. 'sore mouth'). The 'history of the present complaint' is then taken (for each if there are more than one).

HISTORY OF THE PRESENT COMPLAINT

This should cover aspects relevant to the particular main complaint, such as:
- date of onset
- duration
- location(s)
- aggravating and relieving factors
- investigations thus far
- treatment already received and their perceived effectiveness.

'Leading questions' (i.e. those which suggest the answer) should be avoided. 'Open questions', which do not suggest an answer, are preferred. The history should be directed by the complaint, and in most oral medicine patients, it is important to establish whether there are cutaneous, gastrointestinal, genital, ocular or joint problems or a history of fever. Some patients bring descriptions or diagrams (Fig. 1.2). Then a series of relevant questions should elicit the 'past or relevant medical history'.

PAST OR RELEVANT MEDICAL HISTORY

The medical history should be taken to elicit all matters relevant to the:
- diagnosis
- treatment
- prognosis.

As a double check on the verbal history, the use of pre-printed, standardised, self-administered questionnaires may be helpful and may encourage more truthful responses to sensitive questions (Table 1.1).

There are a number of ways to take a good medical history, but all good clinicians have a systematic approach, from the history of the current complaints, then going through the body systems, current and past therapies for other medical complaints and previous illnesses.

The history should uncover, for example, medical history relevant to:
- Previous episodes of similar or related complaints.
- Other complaints that may be relevant. For example, in patients with mucosal disorders, it is important to ascertain whether there have been lesions affecting other mucosae (ocular or anogenital) or skin, hair or nails, gastrointestinal complaints or fever.
- Important to include are:
  - General symptoms, such as fever or weight loss.
  - Relevant symptoms related to body systems, such as:
    - nervous system (e.g. sensory loss)

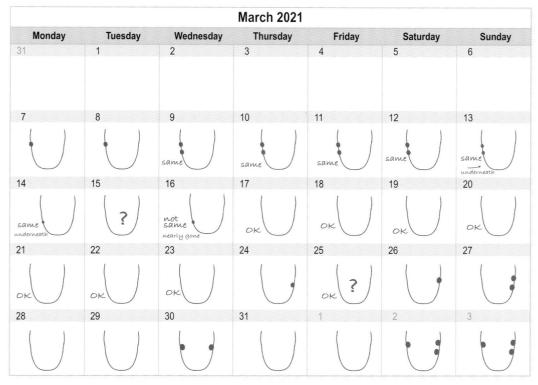

Fig. 1.2 Diary provided by patient showing recurrent tongue lesions.

TABLE 1.1	Systematic Recording of Relevant Medical History		
System	**Specific Problems**	**No**	**Yes**
CVS	Heart disease, hypertension, angina, syncope		
	Cardiac surgery, endocarditis		
	Bleeding disorder, anticoagulants, anaemia		
RS	Asthma, bronchitis, TB, other chest disease, smoker		
SKIN	Rashes, eczema, lichen planus, pemphigus, pemphigoid		
GU	Renal, urinary tract or sexually shared disease		
	Pregnancy, menstrual problems		
GI/Liver	Coeliac disease, Crohn disease		
	Ulcerative colitis		
	Hepatitis, other liver disease, jaundice		
CNS	CVE, multiple (disseminated) sclerosis, other neurological disease		
	Psychiatric problems, drug or alcohol abuse		
	Sight or hearing problems		
LMS	Bone, muscle or joint disease		
Endocrine	Diabetes, thyroid, other endocrine disease		
Allergy	Allergies — e.g. latex, aspirin, penicillin, plasters (Band-Aid)		
Drugs	Current or recent drugs/medical treatment		
Others	Previous operations, GA or serious illness		
	Other conditions (including congenital anomalies)		
	Family medical history		
	Born, residence or travel abroad		
	Pets		
	Infections (e.g. human immunodeficiency virus)		

CNS, Central nervous system; *CVS*, cardiovascular system; *GI*, gastrointestinal system; *GU*, genitourinary system; *LMS*, locomotor system; *RS*, respiratory system.

- respiratory system (e.g. cough)
- gastrointestinal disorders that may be associated with oral ulcers and other lesions
- skin lesions (solitary or rashes), itch or discolourations, which are common symptoms of skin disease, and there are sometimes oral lesions
- ocular problems or visual disturbance
- anogenital lesions, such as ulcers or warts
- psychiatric disorders, such as anxiety, depression and eating disorders, and drug abuse are relevant to orofacial conditions.
- Medical or surgical consultations, investigations and treatments, including radiotherapy.
- Current prescribed drugs (including self-medications and alternative medicines) because these may cause oral complaints or influence management. The British National Formulary (BNF) or equivalent is often indispensable because patients commonly misspell or do not know the names of drugs they are taking. Even though patients may have indicated drugs for specific conditions, it is always appropriate to ask separately about drug history.
- Complementary medicine and associated over-the-counter medicines.
- Previous illnesses.
- Hospitalisations and previous consultations.
- Operations.

- General anaesthetics.
- Specific medical problems that may influence operative procedures, particularly:
  - Allergies
  - bleeding tendency
  - cardiorespiratory problems
  - drug therapy such as anticoagulants or corticosteroids
  - endocrine disorders — especially diabetes
  - infectious diseases.

Patients may also carry formal warnings of certain conditions relevant to dental care. These may be written cards, smart cards (there are two kinds — memory cards and microprocessor cards) or MedicAlert-type bracelets or necklaces. These types of MedicAlert warning devices are recommended to be carried by anyone with:

- allergies to any drug or agent with the potential for causing a serious reaction
- chronic health problems, which might necessitate emergency treatment of a specific nature, such as diabetes, epilepsy, glaucoma or malignant hyperthermia
- the need to take regular medication, prosthesis, implants and conditions which might lead to difficulty in diagnosis during emergency care (e.g. long-term anticoagulants or long-term systemic corticosteroids).

Some patients bring quite precise written information which can be helpful (Fig. 1.3).

The Harley Street Clinic	Cystourethroscopy & Transurethral Prostatectomy OPERATION 08.02.2010
Clementine Churchill Hospital	Cystoscopy, ureteroscopic manipulation of calculus Insertion of Ureteric JJ Stent OPERATION 22.02.2014
Clementine Churchill Hospital	Removal of Ureteric JJ Stent 04.03.2014
Northwick Park Hospital	Lithotripsy ureteric calculus OPERATION 10.03.2014
The Harley Street Clinic	Cystourethroscopy Bladder biopsy & cystodiathermy urethral dilatation Excision left epididymal cyst OPERATION 16.05.2015
King Edward VII Hospital	Cystoscopy OPERATION 07.03.2016
The London Clinic	Laparoscopic cholecystectomy OPERATION 31.08.2016
King Edward VII Hospital	Cystoscopy OPERATION 09.06.2016
The London Clinic	Haemorrhoidectomy and sigmoidoscopy OPERATION 7.05.2020
Wimpole Street	Re: Blood pressure and Heart. Myocardial perfusion scan 18.10.2021
Princess Grace Hospital, Harley Street, London	Repair of right inguinal hernia using an open mesh technique. OPERATION 13.11.2021

Fig. 1.3 Part of medical history provided by patient: 7 hospitals, 9 operations and at least 15 procedures in 12 years!

A Medical History ABC

The medical history of dental patients should be directed to elicit any relevant systemic disease. For example, this may be achieved by an ABC:

- **Allergies or anaemia:** allergies can be a contraindication to use of materials such as latex. Anaemia: a reduction in haemoglobin level below the normal for age and gender can:
- be a contraindication to general anaesthesia
  - cause oral complications (i.e. candidosis, sore mouth, burning tongue, glossitis, ulcers, angular stomatitis).
- **Bleeding tendency:** a hazard to any surgical procedure, including some injections, and a contraindication to aspirin and some other nonsteroidal antiinflammatory drugs (NSAIDs).
- **Cardiorespiratory disease:** this may be a contraindication to general anaesthesia. Patients with various cardiac lesions are predisposed to develop endocarditis, which may be precipitated as a consequence of the bacteraemia associated with some forms of dental treatment. Cardiac patients may have a bleeding tendency because of anticoagulants. Oral lesions may be seen — such as calcium channel blocker–induced gingival swelling, or oral ulceration with nicorandil. NSAIDs and itraconazole are contraindicated in severe cardiac failure.
- **Drug use, allergies, recreational or abuse:** these may cause orofacial lesions or dryness, give an indication about underlying pathology or influence dental procedures or drug use. Drug allergies are a contraindication to the use of the responsible or related drugs. Drug abuse may give rise to behavioural problems and a risk of cross-infection. Corticosteroids absorbed systemically produce adrenocortical suppression. Such patients may not respond adequately to the stress of trauma, operation or infection, and stress may produce adrenal crisis and collapse.
- **Endocrine disease.**
  - Diabetes may cause:
    - the danger of hypoglycaemia if meals are interfered with
    - oral complications such as sialosis, dry mouth and periodontal breakdown.
  - Hyperparathyroidism may cause:
    - jaw radiolucencies/rarefaction
    - loss of lamina dura
    - giant cell granulomas (central)
    - hypercalcaemia and hyposalivation.
- **Fits and faints:** epilepsy and other causes of unconsciousness should be elicited before embarking on any procedures. Oral lesions may be seen, such as phenytoin-induced gingival swelling.
- **Gastrointestinal disorders** are relevant mainly because of possible vomiting with general anaesthesia, and possible oral manifestations.
- **Hospital admissions, attendances and operations:** this information often helps fill in gaps in the medical history and may be relevant if, for example, the patient has had a previous halothane anaesthetic or has had radiotherapy. Successful prior surgery in the absence of any serious post-operative haemorrhage also suggests the absence of any inherited bleeding tendency.

- **Infections:** the possibility of transmission of infection to patients or staff is ever present:
  - blood-borne infections: hepatitis B virus (HBV) and hepatitis C virus (HCV) and human immunodeficiency virus (HIV) are the main agents of concern
  - respiratory infections: current or very recent respiratory infections, such as coronaviruses, or tuberculosis, may be transmissible and a contraindication to general anaesthesia
  - sexually shared infections: imprecise diagnosis or empirical treatment serves only to spread these infections, as contact tracing is normally undertaken only on proven cases of sexually transmitted (venereal) disease.
- **Jaundice and liver disease:** these are important because of the associated bleeding tendency, drug intolerance and possible viral hepatitis and oral carcinoma.
- **Kidney disease:** this may cause a bleeding tendency and impaired drug excretion. The other main problems are in relation to the immunosuppression created following a kidney transplant, liability to neoplasia and gingival swelling from ciclosporin.
- **Likelihood of pregnancy:** because of the danger of abortion or teratogenicity, it is important during pregnancy, particularly the first trimester, to avoid or minimise exposure to drugs, radiography and infections. Pregnancy can influence some conditions such as recurrent aphthous stomatitis, pyogenic granulomas and Behçet syndrome and may produce gingivitis or epulides.
- **Malignant disease,** including those on radiotherapy or chemotherapy (where oral lesions may occur): malignant disease may underlie some oral complaints, such as pain or sensory changes, and can result in significant morbidity and even mortality. Oral complications are very common after cancer therapies.
- **Neuropsychiatric conditions:**
  - Mental health: there are many oral problems, and drug therapy may produce oral conditions, such as dry mouth.
  - Down syndrome: there are many oral problems, and cervical spine involvement may predispose to spinal cord damage during general anaesthesia.
- **Other relevant conditions:** every condition which is elicited from the medical history should be checked for relevance, but the following can be highly relevant, even though rare in most populations:
  - glucose-6-phosphate dehydrogenase deficiency is a contraindication to some drugs
  - hereditary angioedema: any dental trauma may result in oedema and a hazard to the airway
  - malignant hyperthermia (malignant hyperpyrexia): various general anaesthetics and other agents may be contraindicated
  - Primary generalised nodal osteoarthritis (PGNO) can be associated with hyposalivation and sialadenitis
  - porphyria: intravenous barbiturates, metronidazole and other agents may be contraindicated
  - suxamethonium sensitivity: suxamethonium is contraindicated.
- **Prosthesis and transplant patients:** patients after transplants may be at risk from infection, neoplasms and

iatrogenic problems, such as bleeding, gingival swelling or graft-versus-host disease (Chapter 34). Patients with transplants are also liable to present a number of complications to dental treatment — in particular the need for a corticosteroid cover, a liability to infection and a bleeding tendency.

There is no good evidence for infection of prosthetic joints arising from oral sepsis. However, if the orthopaedic surgeon wishes an antimicrobial cover, the dentist must consider the medicolegal implications. The complications of infection of ventriculoatrial valves are so serious that it may be reasonable to give an antimicrobial cover, if the responsible neurosurgeon so advises.

Patients with cardiac pacemakers and similar devices may be in danger in relation to the use of equipment which can interfere, such as magnetic resonance imaging (MRI), diathermy and electrosurgery.

- **Rheumatoid arthritis**: Sjögren syndrome is commonly associated with rheumatoid arthritis (RA), which can be part of the diagnosis. Cervical spine involvement may predispose to spinal cord damage if the neck is flexed during general anaesthesia.

DENTAL HISTORY

The dental history will give an idea of the:
- regularity of attendance for dental care
- attitude to dental professionals and to treatment
- recent relevant dental problems
- recent restorative treatment.

FAMILY HISTORY

This may reveal familial outbreaks of diseases such as contagious infections (e.g. hand, foot and mouth; tuberculosis) and hereditary problems, such as amelogenesis imperfecta, haemophilia or hereditary angioedema, and familial conditions, such as recurrent aphthous stomatitis or diabetes. Some

TABLE 1.2 Clinical Signs and Symptoms Which May Reflect Potentially Serious or Life-Threatening Connotations

Features	Comments
Abnormal blood vessels supplying a lump	May be malignancy
Actinic cheilitis (solar elastosis)	Potentially malignant
Angioedema	Potentially lethal through airway obstruction
Behçet syndrome	May cause thromboses of dural sinuses or vena cavae
Cancer	Potentially lethal
Dysphagia	May be malignancy
Erythema multiforme	Potentially lethal if Stevens–Johnson syndrome or toxic epidermal necrolysis (TEN)
Facial palsy	May be malignancy or cerebrovascular event
Extraction socket not healing	May be malignancy
Headache (see Chapter 45)	Severe and first time could indicate malignant hypertension, a tumour, abscess, haematoma. meningitis, metastases, giant cell arteritis or subarachnoid haemorrhage.
Human immunodeficiency virus (HIV) infection	Potentially serious but no longer lethal due to effectiveness of antiretroviral therapy
Indurated lesion	Firm infiltration beneath the mucosa may be malignant
Lesion fixed to deeper tissues	To deeper tissues or to overlying skin or mucosa may be malignant
Leukoplakia	Potentially malignant
Lichen planus	Potentially malignant
Lump	Especially if hard may be malignant
Lymph node enlargement	Especially if there is hardness in a lymph node or fixation. Enlarged cervical nodes in a patient with oral carcinoma may be caused by infection, reactive hyperplasia secondary to the tumour, or metastatic disease. Occasionally, a 'positive' lymph node is detected in the absence of any obvious primary tumour
Lymphoma	Potentially lethal
Numbness	May be malignancy
Pain	May be malignancy
Pemphigus	Used to be potentially lethal, but can be well controlled by therapy
Red lesion	Erythroplasia or erythroplakia may be malignant or potentially malignant
Red/white mixed lesion	Erythroleukoplakia may be malignant or potentially malignant
Submucous fibrosis	Potentially malignant
Syphilis	Used to be potentially lethal, but can be well controlled by therapy
Tooth mobility	Can be very rarely caused by malignancy
Tuberculosis (TB)	Potentially lethal
Ulcer	If persistent, with fissuring or raised exophytic margins may be malignant or chronic infection
Weight loss	May be malignancy or infection such as HIV or TB
White lesion, especially if irregular surface	Verrucous leukoplakia may be malignant or potentially malignant

diseases are more prevalent in certain ethnic groups (e.g. pemphigus in Jews and Asians; Behçet syndrome in people from Asia or the Mediterranean area).

SOCIAL AND CULTURAL HISTORY

The social history may reveal:
- whether the patient has a family or a partner — and the degree of support that can be anticipated
- information about the patient's attitudes to treatment (e.g. some patients may refuse operation, others may decline medication)
- information about the patient's residence, which can suggest the socioeconomic circumstances of the patient
- information about contacts with pets and other animals, which may be relevant to some infectious diseases, such as cat-scratch disease or toxoplasmosis
- whether the patient has travelled overseas, which may be relevant to some infectious diseases, such as tuberculosis, tropical diseases such as Leishmaniasis and deep mycoses such as histoplasmosis
- the patient's sexual history, which may be relevant to some infectious diseases, such as HIV, herpes simplex virus (HSV), human papillomavirus (HPV), hepatitis A virus (HAV), HBV, and HCV
- any occupational problems, which may be relevant to some disease, and access to care
- relevant habits (tobacco, alcohol, betel and recreational drug use) — for example, tobacco use underlies several oral diseases, including periodontal disease and cancer
- relevant hobbies, such as swimming in pools that may cause tooth erosion or scuba diving that may underlie temporomandibular pain

- information about the patient's culture and diet — may lead, for example, to vitamin deficiencies and glossitis or angular cheilitis (as in vitamin B_{12} deficiency in vegans)
- information about stress; several orofacial complaints are stress related or modulated by stress.

Standardised forms will help with the recording of data, the relevance of which can sometimes be surprising (see Table 1.1).

Patient expectations can only be assessed by polite enquiry. Each patient is an individual with their own specific thoughts and beliefs. Some cultures have medical understanding quite separate from that of Westernised medicine.

PROGNOSIS

Prognosis (from the Greek — literally, fore-knowing, foreseeing) is a medical term to describe the likely outcome of an illness. A number of conditions and lesions seen in oral medicine, especially cancer and pemphigus, can have potentially serious prognoses (Table 1.2), whilst others have potential to become malignant (e.g. leucoplakia). It is crucial that the appropriate information is clearly and compassionately communicated with the patient.

RECOMMENDED READING

Maguire P., Pitceathly C., 2002. Key communication skills and how to acquire them. BMJ. 325, 697−700.
Glick M., 2019. The relevance of oral health. J. Am. Dent. Assoc. 159 (8), 637−638.

2

Principles of Diagnosis: Examination

It is wise for clinicians to make themselves thoroughly aware of the wide variation in normal appearances of all sites of mucosa, which can be related to age, gender and racial origin. 'Until you appreciate the range of normal, you will be unable to detect the abnormal'.

John Hunter 1764

INTRODUCTION

The clinical examination of the patient should start as the patient enters the clinic and is greeted by the clinician. The history and clinical examination are designed to put the clinician in a position to make a provisional diagnosis or a differential diagnosis. Special tests or investigations may be required to confirm or refine this diagnosis or elicit other conditions. Physical disabilities, such as those affecting gait, and learning disability are often immediately evident as the patient is first seen, and blindness, deafness or speech and language disorders may be obvious. You should also be able to assess the patient's mood and general wellbeing, but, if in any doubt, ask for advice. Other disorders, such as mental problems, may become apparent at any stage. The patient should be carefully observed and listened to during history taking and examination; speech and language can offer a great deal of information about the medical and mental state. Some patients bring written material that can be helpful (e.g. an accurate list of their illnesses and/or medications), and increasingly patients use the Internet and come with printouts. Others may bring less meaningful drawings or histories. All these factors can help to build a picture of the patient and their condition. As a general rule, if you think a patient looks ill, they probably are.

Always remember that the patient has the right to refuse all or part of the examination, investigations or treatment. A patient has the right under common law to give or withhold consent to medical examination or treatment. This is one of the basic principles of healthcare. Patients are entitled to receive sufficient information in a way they can understand about the proposed investigations or treatments, the possible alternatives and any substantial risk or risks, which may be special in kind or magnitude or special to the patient, so that they can make a balanced judgment.

GENERAL EXAMINATION

Medical problems may manifest in the fully clothed patient with abnormal appearance or behaviour, pupil size, conscious level, movements, posture, breathing, speech, facial colour, sweating or wasting. General examination may sometimes include the recording of body weight and the 'vital signs' of conscious state, temperature, pulse, blood pressure and respiration. The dentist must be prepared to interpret the more common and significant changes evident in the clothed patient.

Vital Signs

Vital signs include conscious state, temperature, pulse, blood pressure and respiration:

- The conscious state: any decrease in this must be taken seriously, causes ranging from drug use to head injury. The **AVPU** scale (alert, verbal, pain, unresponsive) is a system by which a health care professional can measure and record a patient's level of consciousness.
- The temperature: the temperature is traditionally taken with a thermometer, but temperature-sensitive strips and sensors are now widely available. The normal body temperatures are: oral 36.6°C; rectal or ear (tympanic membrane) 37.4°C and axillary 36.5°C. Body temperature is usually slightly higher in the evenings. In most adults, an oral temperature greater than 37.8°C or a rectal or ear temperature greater than 38.3°C is considered a fever (pyrexia). A child has a fever when ear temperature is 38°C or higher.
- The pulse: this can be measured manually or automatically (Fig. 2.1). The pulse can be recorded from any artery but in particular from the following sites:
  - the radial artery, on the thumb side of the flexor surface of the wrist

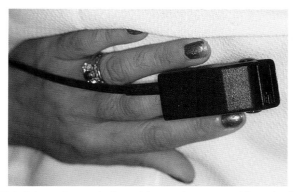

Fig. 2.1 Pulse oximeter (nail varnish must be removed from the finger tested).

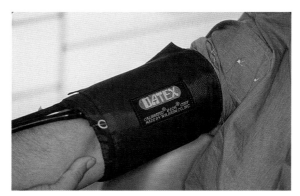

Fig. 2.2 Sphygmomanometer.

- the carotid artery, just anterior to the mid-third of the sternomastoid muscle
- the superficial temporal artery, just in front of the ear.

Pulse rates at rest in health are approximately as follows:
- infants, 140 beats/min
- adults, 60 to 80 beats/min.

Pulse rate is increased in:
- exercise
- anxiety or fear
- fever
- some cardiac disorders
- hyperthyroidism and other disorders.

The rhythm should be regular; if not, ask a physician for advice. The character and volume vary in certain disease states and require a physician's advice.

- The blood pressure: this can be measured with a sphygmomanometer (Fig. 2.2) or one of a variety of machines. With a sphygmomanometer the procedure is as follows: seat the patient; place the sphygmomanometer cuff on the right upper arm, with approximately 3 cm of skin visible at the antecubital fossa; palpate the radial pulse; inflate the cuff to approximately 200 to 250 mmHg or until the radial pulse is no longer palpable; deflate the cuff slowly while listening with the stethoscope over the brachial artery on the skin of

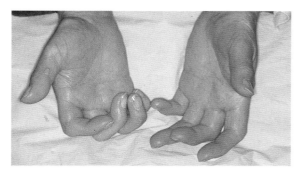

Fig. 2.3 Raynaud syndrome in scleroderma.

the inside arm below the cuff; record the systolic pressure as the pressure when the first tapping sounds appear; deflate the cuff further until the tapping sounds become muffled (diastolic pressure); repeat; record the blood pressure as systolic/diastolic pressures (normal values approximately 120/80 mmHg, but these increase with age).

Respiration

The normal reference range for respiration in an adult is 12 to 20 breaths/min.

Other Signs

- Weight: weight loss is seen mainly in starvation, malnutrition, eating disorders, cancer (termed cachexia), human immunodeficiency virus (HIV) disease (termed 'slim disease'), malabsorption and tuberculosis and may be extreme as in emaciation. Obesity is usually due to excessive food intake and insufficient exercise.
- Hands: conditions such as arthritis (mainly rheumatoid or osteoarthritis) (Figs. 2.3 and 2.4) and Raynaud phenomenon (Chapter 56; Fig. 2.3), which is seen in many connective tissue diseases, may be obvious. Note the temperature of the hands (cold in Raynauds). Disability, such as in cerebral palsy, may be obvious (Fig. 2.5).
- Movement: asymmetrical gait may indicate arthritis of hips or knees (osteo or rheumatoid).
- Feet: hallux valgus of big toes may indicate osteoarthritis and is associated with dry mouth
- Skin: lesions, such as rashes — particularly blisters (seen mainly in skin diseases, infections and drug reactions), pigmentation (seen in various ethnic groups, Addison disease and as a result of some drug therapy).
- Skin appendages: nail changes, such as koilonychia (spoon-shaped nails) — seen in iron deficiency anaemia, hair changes, such as alopecia, and finger clubbing (Fig. 2.6), seen mainly in cardiac or respiratory disorders. Nail beds may reveal the anxious nature of the nail-biting person (Fig. 2.7).

Extraoral Head and Neck Examination

The face should be examined for lesions (Table 2.1) and features such as:

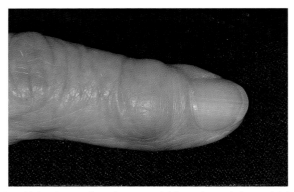

Fig. 2.4 Heberden nodes of osteoarthritis on interphalangeal joints of first and second fingers.

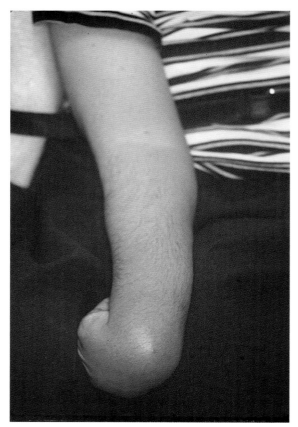

Fig. 2.5 Cerebral palsy.

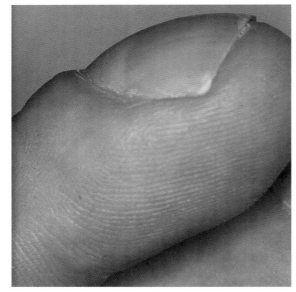

Fig. 2.6 Clubbing.

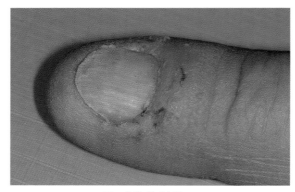

Fig. 2.7 Nail biting.

- asymmetry
- swellings (seen in inflammatory and neoplastic disorders in particular)
- pallor (seen mainly in the conjunctivae or skin creases in anaemia)
- rash, such as the malar rash in systemic lupus erythematosus. Malar erythema may indicate mitral valve stenosis
- erythema, seen mainly on the face in an embarrassed or angry patient, or fever (sweating or warm hands), and then usually indicative of infection.

Eyes should be assessed for visual acuity and examined for features such as:
- redness, seen in trauma, eye diseases or Sjögren syndrome
- scarring, seen in trauma, infection or pemphigoid
- jaundice, seen mainly in the sclerae in liver disease
- exophthalmos (protruding eyes), seen mainly in Graves thyrotoxicosis
- corneal arcus which may be seen in hypercholesterolaemia. A thin, whitish circle around the iris can be a normal finding in old people and then termed arcus senilis.

Inspection of the neck, looking particularly for swellings or sinuses, should be followed by careful palpation of all cervical lymph nodes and salivary and thyroid glands, searching for swelling or tenderness. The neck is best examined by observing the patient from the front, noting any obvious asymmetry or swelling, then standing behind the seated patient to palpate the lymph nodes (Fig. 2.8). Systematically, each region needs to be examined lightly with the pulps of the fingers, trying to roll the **lymph nodes** against harder underlying structures. Lymph

TABLE 2.1   The Commoner Descriptive Terms Applied to Lesions

Term	Meaning
Atrophy	Loss of tissue with increased translucency, unless sclerosis is associated
Bullae	Visible accumulations of fluid within or beneath the epithelium, >0.5 cm in diameter (i.e. a blister)
Cyst	Closed cavity or sac (normal or abnormal) with an epithelial, endothelial or membranous lining and containing fluid or semisolid material
Ecchymosis	Macular area of haemorrhage >2 cm in diameter (bruise)
Erosion	Localised loss/thinning of epithelium which usually heals without scarring; can follow a blister
Erythema	Redness of the mucosa produced by atrophy, inflammation, vascular congestion or increased perfusion
Exfoliation	The splitting off of the epithelial keratin in scales or sheets
Fibrosis	The formation of excessive fibrous tissue
Fissure	Any linear gap or slit in the skin or mucosa
Gangrene	Death of tissue, usually due to loss of blood supply
Haematoma	A localised tumour-like collection of blood
Keloid	A tough heaped-up scar that rises above the rest of the skin, is irregularly shaped and tends to enlarge progressively
Macule	A circumscribed alteration in colour or texture of the mucosa
Nodule	A solid mass in the mucosa or skin which can be observed as an elevation or can be palpated; it is >0.5 cm in diameter
Papule	A circumscribed palpable elevation <0.5 cm in diameter
Petechia (pl. petechiae)	A punctate haemorrhagic spot approximately 1—2 mm in diameter
Plaque	An elevated area of mucosa >0.5 cm in diameter
Pustule	A visible accumulation of free pus
Scar	Replacement by fibrous tissue of another tissue that has been destroyed by injury or disease An *atrophic* scar is thin and wrinkled A *hypertrophic* scar is elevated with excessive growth of fibrous tissue A *cribriform* scar is perforated with multiple small pits
Sclerosis	Diffuse or circumscribed induration of the submucosal and/or subcutaneous tissues
Tumour	Literally a swelling The term is used to imply enlargement of the tissues by normal or pathological material or cells that form a mass The term should be used with care, as many patients believe it implies a malignancy with a poor prognosis
Ulcer	A breach of the epithelium, often with loss of underlying tissues, produced by sloughing of necrotic tissue
Vegetation	A growth of pathological tissue consisting of multiple closely set papillary masses
Vesicle	Small (<0.5 cm in diameter) visible accumulation of fluid within or beneath the epithelium (i.e. small blister)
Wheal	A transient area of mucosal or skin oedema, white, compressible and usually evanescent (AKA urticaria)

from the superficial tissue of the head and neck generally drains first to groups of superficially placed lymph nodes, then to the deep cervical lymph nodes (Figs. 2.9—2.12 and Table 2.2).

- Parotid, mastoid and occipital lymph nodes can be palpated simultaneously using both hands.
- Superficial cervical lymph nodes are examined with lighter fingers because they can only be compressed against the softer sternomastoid muscle.
- Submental lymph nodes are examined by tipping the patient's head forward and rolling the lymph nodes against the inner aspect of the mandible. (Fig. 2.12d)

Submandibular lymph nodes are examined in the same way, with the patient's head tipped to the side which is being examined. Differentiation needs to be made between the submandibular salivary gland and submandibular lymph glands. Bimanual examination using one hand beneath the mandible to palpate extraorally and with the other index finger in the floor of the mouth may help.

- The deep cervical lymph nodes which project anterior or posterior to the sternomastoid muscle can be palpated.

The jugulodigastric lymph node in particular should be specifically examined, as this is the most common lymph node involved in tonsillar infections and oral cancer.

- The supraclavicular region should be examined at the same time as the rest of the neck; lymph nodes here may extend up into the posterior triangle of the neck on the scalene muscles, behind the sternomastoid.
- Parapharyngeal and tracheal lymph nodes can be compressed lightly against the trachea.

Some information can be gained by the texture and nature of the lymphadenopathy. Tenderness and swelling should be documented. Lymph nodes that are tender may be inflammatory (lymphadenitis). Consistency should be noted. Nodes that are increasing in size and are hard, or fixed to adjacent tissues may be malignant.

Both anterior and posterior cervical nodes should be examined, (Fig. 2.12b) and if systemic disease is a possibility, then other nodes, liver and spleen should also be examined. Generalised lymphadenopathy with or without enlargement of other

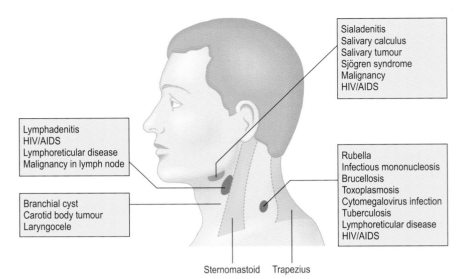

Sialadenitis
Salivary calculus
Salivary tumour
Sjögren syndrome
Malignancy
HIV/AIDS

Lymphadenitis
HIV/AIDS
Lymphoreticular disease
Malignancy in lymph node

Branchial cyst
Carotid body tumour
Laryngocele

Rubella
Infectious mononucleosis
Brucellosis
Toxoplasmosis
Cytomegalovirus infection
Tuberculosis
Lymphoreticular disease
HIV/AIDS

Sternomastoid   Trapezius

Fig. 2.8 Some causes of neck swelling.

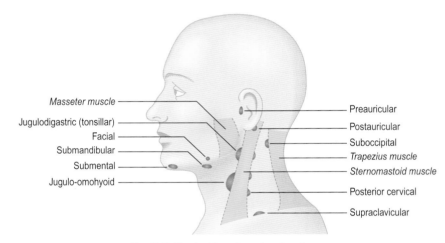

Masseter muscle
Jugulodigastric (tonsillar)
Facial
Submandibular
Submental
Jugulo-omohyoid

Preauricular
Postauricular
Suboccipital
Trapezius muscle
Sternomastoid muscle
Posterior cervical
Supraclavicular

Fig. 2.9 Cervical lymph nodes: locations.

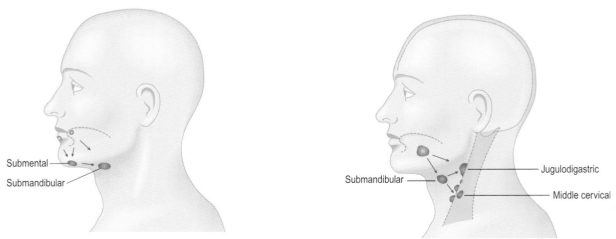

Submental
Submandibular

Fig. 2.10 Submental and submandibular lymph node drainage.

Submandibular

Jugulodigastric
Middle cervical

Fig. 2.11 Submandibular and deep cervical lymph node drainage.

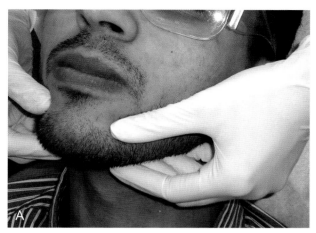

Fig. 2.12 Extra oral examination.

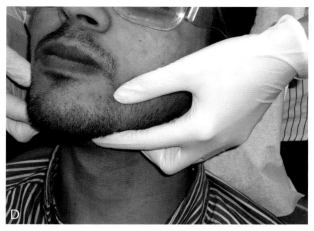

Fig. 2.12d

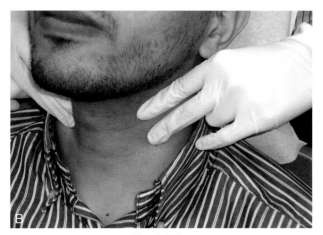

Fig. 2.12b

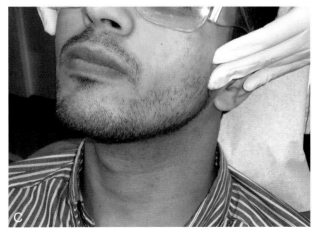

Fig. 2.12c

lymphoid tissue, such as liver and spleen (hepatosplenomegaly), suggests a systemic cause.

The temporomandibular joints (TMJs) and muscles of mastication should be examined and palpated (Fig. 2.12C). Although disorders that affect the TMJ often appear to be

TABLE 2.2 Cervical Lymph Nodes and Their Main Drainage Areas

Area	Draining Lymph Nodes
Scalp, temporal region	Superficial parotid (pre-auricular)
Scalp, posterior region	Occipital
Scalp, parietal region	Mastoid
Ear, external	Superficial cervical over upper part of sterno-mastoid muscle
Ear, middle	Parotid
Over angle of mandible	Superficial cervical over upper part of sterno-mastoid muscle
Medial part of frontal region, medial eyelids, skin of nose	Submandibular
Lateral part of frontal region, lateral part of eyelids	Parotid
Cheek	Submandibular
Upper lip	Submandibular
Lower lip	Submental
Lower lip, lateral part	Submandibular
Mandibular gingivae	Submandibular
Maxillary teeth	Deep cervical
Maxillary gingivae	Deep cervical
Tongue tip	Submental
Tongue, anterior two-thirds	Submandibular, some midline cross-over of lymphatic drainage
Tongue, posterior third	Deep cervical
Tongue ventrum	Deep cervical
Floor of mouth	Submandibular
Palate, hard	Deep cervical
Palate, soft	Retropharyngeal and deep cervical
Tonsil	Jugulodigastric

unilateral, the joint should not be viewed in isolation, but always considered along with its opposite joint, as part of the stomatognathic system. Some practitioners palpate using a pressure algometer to standardise the force used, and undertake range-of-movement (ROM) measurements. The area should be examined by inspecting:

- Facial symmetry, for evidence of enlarged masseter muscles (masseteric hypertrophy) suggestive of clenching or bruxism. A bruxchecker can help confirm bruxism.
- Mandibular opening and closing paths, noting any noises or deviations.
- Mandibular opening extent, measuring the interincisal distance at maximum mouth opening.
- Lateral excursions, measuring the amount achievable.
- Joint noises, by listening (a stethoscope placed over the joint can help).
- Both condyles, by palpating them, via the external auditory meatus, to detect tenderness posteriorly, and by using a single finger placed over the joints in front of the ears, to detect pain, abnormal movements or clicking within the joint.
- Masticatory muscles on both sides, noting tenderness or hypertrophy:
  - Masseters, by intraoral—extraoral compression between finger and thumb. Palpate the masseter bimanually by placing a finger of one hand intraorally and the index and middle fingers of the other hand on the cheek over the masseter over the lower mandibular ramus.
  - Temporalis, by direct palpation of the temporal region and by asking the patient to clench the teeth. Palpate the insertion of the temporalis tendon intraorally along the anterior border of the ascending mandibular ramus.
  - Lateral pterygoid (lower head), by placing a little finger up behind the maxillary tuberosity (tenderness is the 'pterygoid sign'). Examine it indirectly by asking the patient to open the jaw against resistance and to move the jaw to one side while applying a gentle resistance force.
  - Medial pterygoid muscle, intraorally lingually to the mandibular ramus.
- The dentition and occlusion. This may require monitoring of study models on a semi or fully adjustable articulator. Note particularly missing premolars or molars, and attrition.
  - The mucosa. Note particularly occlusal lines and scalloping of the tongue margins, which may indicate bruxism and tongue pressure.

Examine the jaws. There is a wide normal individual variation in morphology of the face. Most individuals have facial asymmetry but of a degree that cannot be regarded as abnormal. Maxillary, mandibular or zygomatic deformities or lumps may be more reliably confirmed by inspection from above (maxillae/zygomas) or behind (mandible). The jaws should be palpated to detect swelling or tenderness. Maxillary air sinuses can be examined by palpation for tenderness over the maxillary antrum, which may indicate sinus infection. Transillumination or endoscopy can be helpful.

The major salivary glands should be inspected and palpated (parotids and submandibulars) for:

- symmetry
- evidence of enlargement
- pain or tenderness
- evidence of salivary flow from salivary ducts
- saliva appearance
- evidence of oral dryness (The clinical oral dryness score (CODS) can be used and examines 10 sites/parameters in the mouth including mirror sticking to mucosa or tongue, no salivary pooling in the floor of mouth, loss of architecture of gingivae, depapillation of the tongue and uncleared food or epithelial debris). (See Chapter 20: Dry Mouth). Hyposalivation can be confirmed by sialometry (salivary flow rate).

Salivary glands are palpated in the following way:

- Parotid glands are palpated by using fingers placed over the glands in front of the ears, to detect pain or swelling. Early enlargement of the parotid gland is characterised by outward deflection of the lower part of the ear lobe, which is best observed by looking at the patient from behind. This sign may allow distinction from simple obesity. Swelling of the parotid sometimes causes trismus. Swellings may affect the whole or part of a gland, or tenderness may be elicited. The parotid duct (Stensen duct) is most readily palpated with the jaws clenched firmly because it runs horizontally across the upper masseter, where it can be gently rolled; the duct opens at a papilla on the buccal mucosa opposite the upper molars.
- The submandibular gland is best palpated bimanually with a finger of one hand in the floor of the mouth lingual to the lower molar teeth, and a finger of the other hand placed over the submandibular triangle. The submandibular duct (Wharton duct) runs anteromedially across the floor of the mouth to open at the side of the lingual fraenum.

Examine the cranial nerves (Table 2.3). In particular, facial movement should be tested and facial sensation determined. Facial symmetry is best seen as the patient is talking. Movement of the mouth as the patient speaks is important, especially when they allow themselves the luxury of some emotional expression. Examination of the upper face (around the eyes and forehead) is carried out in the following way:

- If the patient is asked to close their eyes, any paralysis (palsy) may become obvious, with the affected eyelid failing to close and the globe turning up so that only the white of the eye is showing (Bell sign).
- Weakness of orbicularis oculi muscles with sufficient strength to close the eye can be compared with the normal side by asking the patient to close the eyes tight and observing the degree of force required to part the eyelids.
- If the patient is asked to wrinkle the forehead, weakness can be detected by the difference between the two sides. Weakness might reflect an upper motor neuron lesion (central) or lower motor neuron lesion (peripheral).

The lower face (around the mouth) is best examined by asking the patient to:

- smile
- bare the teeth or purse the lips

TABLE 2.3 Cranial Nerve Nomenclature and Examination

	Cranial Nerve		Findings in Lesions	Examination
I	Olfactory	Sensory	Impaired sense of smell for common odours (do not use ammonia)	Ask patient to identify smell (e.g. coffee/perfume)
II	Optic	Sensory	Visual acuity reduced using Snellen types ± ophthalmoscopy: nystagmus Visual fields by confrontation impaired Pupil responses may be impaired	Assess vision in each eye
III	Oculomotor	Motor	Diplopia; strabismus; eye looks down and laterally ('down and out') Eye movements impaired Ptosis (drooping eyelid) Pupil dilated Pupil reactions: direct reflex impaired, but consensual reflex intact	Check pupil constriction, eye movement
IV	Trochlear	Motor	Diplopia, particularly on looking down Strabismus (squint) No ptosis Pupil normal and normal reactivity	Assess ability to look downwards and inwards
V	Trigeminal	Both	Reduced sensation over face ± corneal reflex impaired ± taste sensation impaired Motor power of masticatory muscles reduced, with weakness on opening jaw; jaw jerk impaired Muscle wasting	Motor: assess patient's ability to clench jaw. Sensory: assess facial response to touch
VI	Abducens	Motor	Diplopia (double vision) Strabismus Lateral eye movements impaired to affected side	Check lateral deviation of eye
VII	Facial	Both	Impaired motor power of facial muscles on smiling, blowing out cheeks, showing teeth, etc. Corneal reflex reduced ± taste sensation impaired	Motor: assess ability to smile, frown, symmetry Sensory: check taste on anterior 2/3 of tongue
VIII	Vestibulocochlear	Sensory	Impaired hearing (tuning fork at 256 Hz) Impaired balance ± nystagmus ± tinnitus	Check balance, hearing
IX	Glosso pharyngeal	Both	Reduced gag reflex Deviation of uvula Reduced taste sensation Voice may have nasal tone	Motor: ask patient to swallow. Check gag reflex. Sensory: check taste on posterior 1/3 tongue
X	Vagus	Both	Reduced gag reflex Voice may be impaired	Check symmetry of soft palate and uvula
XI	Accessory	Motor	Motor power of trapezius and sternomastoid reduced	Ask patient to shrug shoulder against resistance
XII	Hypoglossal	Motor	Motor power of tongue impaired, with abnormal speech ± fasciculation, wasting, ipsilateral deviation on protrusion	Ask patient to stick out tongue

- blow out the cheeks or whistle.

The cranial nerves can be examined further:

- Facial sensation: progressive lesions affecting the sensory part of the trigeminal nerve initially result in a diminishing response to light touch (cotton wool or air spray) and pin-prick (gently pricking the skin with a sterile pin or needle without drawing blood), and later there is complete anaesthesia.
- The corneal reflex: this depends on the integrity of the trigeminal and facial nerves, either of which, if defective, will give a negative response. This is tested by gently touching the cornea with a wisp of cotton wool twisted to a point. Normally, this procedure causes a blink, but, if the cornea is anaesthetic (or if there is facial palsy), no blink follows,

provided that the patient does not actually see the cotton wool. If the patient complains of complete facial or hemifacial anaesthesia, but the corneal reflex is retained or there is apparent anaesthesia over the angle of the mandible (an area not innervated by the trigeminal nerve), then the symptoms are probably functional (non-organic).

Intraoral Examination

Most oral diseases have a local cause and can be recognised fairly readily. Even those that are life-threatening, such as oral cancer in particular, can be detected at an exceedingly early stage. However, even now, oral cancer is sometimes overlooked at examination, and the delay between the onset of symptoms of oral cancer and the institution of definitive treatment still often exceeds 6 months. The same story applies to pemphigus — another potentially lethal disease that presents in the mouth. Any lesion persisting for more than 3 weeks should be taken seriously.

Many systemic diseases, particularly infections and diseases of the blood, gastrointestinal tract and skin, also cause oral signs or symptoms that may constitute the main complaint, particularly, for example, in some patients with pemphigoid, HIV, leukopenia or leukaemia.

Therefore, the examination should be conducted in a systematic fashion to ensure that all areas are included. If the patient wears any removable prostheses or appliances, these should be removed in the first instance, although it may be necessary later to replace the appliance to assess its fit, function and relationship to any lesion.

Complete visualisation with a good source of light is essential (Fig. 2.13); magnifying loupes or microscope help enormously. All mucosal surfaces should be examined, starting away from the location of any known lesions or the focus of complaint, and lesions recorded on a diagram (Fig. 2.14). There have been many attempts to improve the visualisation of mucosal lesions, including the use of toluidine blue vital dye and fluorescence, where a light source is used to enhance the visualisation or to identify the optimal site for biopsy. These have not yet proven to be superior to conventional visual examination in terms of specificity or sensitivity. A review of currently available products showed insufficient evidence (Table 2.4). However, conventional oral examination remains the gold standard.

The lips should first be inspected. The labial mucosa, buccal mucosa, floor of the mouth and ventrum of the tongue, dorsal surface of the tongue, hard and soft palates, gingivae and teeth should then be examined in sequence (Box 2.1):

- Lips: features, such as cyanosis, are seen mainly in the lips in cardiac or respiratory disease; angular cheilitis is seen mainly in oral candidosis or iron or vitamin deficiencies. Many adults have a few yellowish pinhead-sized papules

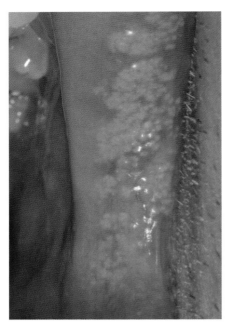

Fig 2.14 Sebaceous glands in lips: Fordyce spots.

in the vermilion border (particularly of the upper lip) and at the commissures; these are usually ectopic sebaceous glands (Fordyce spots) and may be numerous, especially as age advances (see Fig. 2.14). Endogenous pigmentation may be present in those of African or Caribbean origin (Fig. 2.15)

- **Labial mucosa** normally appears moist with a fairly prominent vascular arcade. Examination is facilitated if the mouth is gently closed at this stage, so that the lips can then be everted to examine the mucosa. In the lower lip, the many minor salivary glands, which are often exuding mucus, are easily visible. Therefore, the lips feel slightly nodular and the labial arteries are readily felt.
- Cheek **(buccal) mucosa** is readily inspected if the mouth is held half open. The vascular pattern and minor salivary glands so prominent in the labial mucosa are not obvious in the buccal mucosa, but Fordyce spots may be conspicuous, particularly near the commissures and retromolar regions in adults, and there may be a faint horizontal white line where the teeth meet (linea alba). Place the surface of a dental mirror against the buccal mucosa; it should slide and lift off easily, but, if it adheres to the mucosa, then there may be hyposalivation.
- The floor of the mouth and the ventrum of the tongue are best examined by asking the patient to push the tongue first into the palate and then into each cheek in turn. This raises for inspection the floor of the mouth — an area where tumours may start (the coffin or graveyard area of the mouth). Its posterior part is the most difficult area to examine well and one where lesions are most easily missed. During this part of the examination the quantity and consistency of saliva should be assessed. Examine for the pooling of saliva in the floor of the mouth; normally there is a pool of saliva.

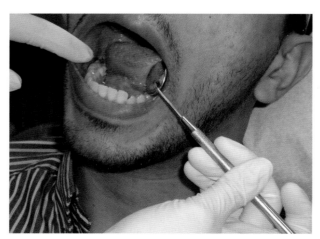

Fig. 2.13 Mouth examination.

TABLE 2.4 Summary of Adjunct Methods for Earlier Detection of Potentially Sinister Lesions

Basis	Product	Sensitivity/Specificity	Comment
Vital dye	Toluidine blue (TB) (tolonium chloride)	High sensitivity 93%—97% for identifying oral squamous cell carcinomas and moderate specificity 73%—92%	Many studies had methodological flaws
Light-based detection systems	Chemiluminescence	High sensitivity (77%—100%), but low specificity. Combination with TB may have better specificity and positive predictive value	Few reliable studies have appeared. More studies awaited, especially for precancer
	Tissue fluorescence imaging (VELscope®)	High sensitivity 97%—100% and high specificity 94%—100%	Promising
Exfoliative cytology	Brush biopsy	Moderate sensitivity for detection of abnormal cells 52%—100% and specificity 29%—100%	Scalpel biopsy usually preferred

BOX 2.1 The More Commonly Used Tooth Notations

Palmer
Permanent dentition

Upper

87654321 | 12345678

Right | Left

87654321 | 12345678

Lower

Deciduous dentition (anonymous classification)

EDCBA | ABCDE
EDCBA | ABCDE

Universal
Permanent dentition

    1 2 3 4 5 6 7 8 | 9 10 11 12 13 14 15 16
32 31 30 29 28 27 26 25 | 24 23 22 21 20 19 18 17

Deciduous dentition

A B C D E | F G H I J
T S R Q P | O N M L K

Fédération Dentaire Internationale (two-digit)

Permanent dentition

18 17 16 15 14 13 12 11 | 21 22 23 24 25 26 27 28
48 47 46 45 44 43 42 41 | 31 32 33 34 35 36 37 38

Deciduous dentition

55 54 53 52 51 | 61 62 63 64 65
85 84 83 82 81 | 71 72 73 74 75

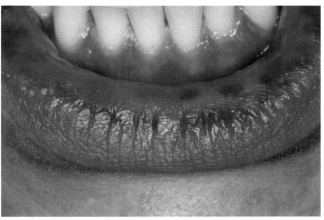

Fig 2.15 Natural pigmentation of lips.

filiform but relatively few fungiform papillae. Behind the circumvallate papillae, the tongue contains several large lymphoid masses (lingual tonsil) and the foliate papillae lie on the lateral borders posteriorly. These are often mistaken for tumours. The tongue may be fissured (scrotal), but this is a developmental anomaly. A healthy child's tongue is rarely coated, but a mild coating is not uncommon in healthy adults. The voluntary tongue movements and sense of taste should be formally tested (Chapter 18). Abnormalities of tongue movement (neurological or muscular disease) may be obvious from dysarthria (abnormal speech) or involuntary movements, and any fibrillation or wasting should be noted. Hypoglossal palsy may lead to deviation of the tongue towards the affected side on protrusion.

- The palate and fauces consist of an anterior hard palate and posterior soft palate, and the tonsillar area and oropharynx. The mucosa of the hard palate is firmly bound down as a mucoperiosteum (similar to the gingivae) and with no obvious vascular arcades. Ridges (rugae) are present anteriorly on either side of the incisive papilla that overlies the incisive foramen. Bony lumps in the posterior centre of the vault of the hard palate are usually tori (torus palatinus). Patients may complain of a lump distal to the upper molars that they think is an unerupted tooth, but the pterygoid hamulus or tuberosity is usually responsible for this complaint. The soft palate and fauces may show a faint

- The dorsum of the tongue is best inspected by protrusion, when it can be held with gauze. The anterior two-thirds is embryologically and anatomically distinct from the posterior third and separated by a dozen or so large circumvallate papillae. The anterior two-thirds is coated with many

vascular arcade. Just posterior to the junction with the hard palate is a conglomeration of minor salivary glands. This region is often also yellowish. The palate should be inspected and movements examined when the patient says 'Aah'. This depresses the dorsum of the tongue, and using a mirror, this also permits inspection of the posterior tongue, tonsils and oropharynx and can even offer a glimpse of the larynx. Glossopharyngeal palsy may lead to uvula deviation to the contralateral side. Bifid uvula may signify a submucous cleft palate.

- Gingivae in health are firm, pale pink, with a stippled surface, and have sharp gingival papillae reaching up between the adjacent teeth to the tooth contact point. Look for gingival deformity, redness, swelling or bleeding on gently probing the gingival margin. The 'keratinised' attached gingivae (pale pink) is normally clearly demarcated from the non-keratinised alveolar mucosa (vascular) that runs into the vestibule or sulcus. Bands of tissue, which may contain muscle attachments, run centrally from the labial mucosa onto the alveolar mucosa and from the buccal mucosa in the premolar region onto the alveolar mucosa (fraenae).

- Teeth: the dentition should be checked to make sure that the expected complement of teeth is present for the patient's age. Extra teeth (supernumerary teeth) or deficiency of teeth (partial loss — hypodontia or oligodontia — or complete loss (anodontia)) can be features of many syndromes, but teeth are far more frequently missing because they are unerupted, impacted or lost as a result of caries or periodontal disease. The teeth should be fully examined for signs of disease, either malformations, such as hypoplasia or abnormal colour, or acquired disorders such as dental caries, staining, tooth surface loss or fractures. The occlusion of the teeth should also be checked; it may show attrition or may be disturbed, as in some jaw fractures or dislocation of the mandibular condyles.

Oral Disease Scoring Systems

These are now available for many oral mucosal diseases where the presence and severity of disease at each of 17 oral sites is summated to give a severity score (Fig. 2.16). The efficacy of

treatment can be assessed by scoring the condition again after treatment. Disease severity scoring systems are tools which can help clinicians assess both the severity of the objective clinical findings as well as the subjective features of the disease, including its impact on patients' lives. There are three essential aspects that are important in defining 'the intensity of the disease': (a) clinical score measuring the level of inflammation, area and specific clinical features (e.g. ulceration); (b) subjective reporting of pain that disease is inflicting; and (c) a questionnaire relating to how the condition affects patients' functioning and their lives (i.e. oral health—related quality of life (OHRQoL)). There are now several validated and universally used tools for oral diseases which should be used at every patient visit.

ORAL DISEASE SEVERITY SCORING

The benefits of a scoring system for mucosal disease severity are that:

- they can indicate the severity of disease,
- they are needed to indicate the efficacy of any treatments,
- they may distinguish between or reveal subgroups of activity,
- they may assist in deciding to implement or withhold treatment,
- they are a routine clinical audit tool which can also be used for research.

Any such oral disease scoring systems (ODSSs) must be objective and reproducible, they should be easy to use and they should be widely applicable. Fortunately, such ODSS have been created and validated and in use for recurrent aphthous ulceration, OLP, pemphigus, mucous membrane pemphigoid, orofacial granulomatosis and dry mouth assessment.

Oral Disease Severity Score for OLP

The ODSS is a comprehensive oral scoring system previously validated for OLP and bullous diseases (Fig. 2.17). In the ODSS, the oral cavity is divided into 17 sites. These sites include outer and inner lips, buccal mucosae, soft and hard palates, oropharynx, floor of mouth and the gingivae in sextants.

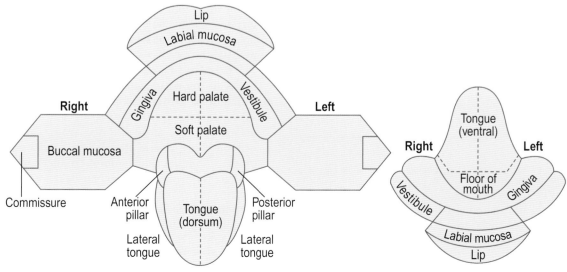

Fig. 2.16 Mouth chart.

Oral disease severity score

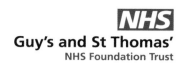

Guy's and St Thomas'
NHS Foundation Trust

Date:			Consultant:	

Name:			M / F:	
Hospital no.			Diagnosis:	
DoB:			Management:	

Site	Site	Activity		Pain
Upper lip (1)				0
Lower lip (1)				
R Buccal mucosa (1 or 2)				1
L Buccal mucosa (1 or 2)				
Gingivae (1 each segment)				2
Lower R				
Lower central				3
Lower L				
Upper R				4
Upper central				
Upper L				5
Dorsum of tongue (1 or 2)				
R Ventral tongue (1)				6
L Ventral tongue (1)				
Floor of mouth (1 or 2)				7
Hard palate (1 or 2)				
Soft palate (1 or 2)				8
Oropharynx (1 or 2)				
Total				9
				10

TOTAL SCORE	

Site score
  0 if no lesion
Buccal mucosa
  1 if less than 50% of area affected
  2 if greater than 50% of area affected
Dorsum of tongue, floor of mouth, hard or soft palate or oropharynx
  1 unilateral
  2 bilateral

Activity score
  0 normal / white patch
  1 mild erythema / white patch in PV
  2 marked erythema
  3 ulceration

Pain score
Analogue scale from 0 (no discomfort) – 10 (unbearable / most severe pain imaginable) that they
have encountered with this condition as an average in the preceding week.

(Continued)

Fig. 2.17 Oral disease severity scoring for site and activity elements for OLP. The oral disease scoring systems for an individual patient visit is the sum of sites, activity at each site and a pain score. Site score = 1 for each site affected, 2 for large sites. Activity score = ranges from 0 to 3 at each site. Pain = average pain over last week from 0 (no discomfort) to 10 (unbearable/the most severe pain imaginable). (Reproduced with permission from Challacombe, S.J., McParland, H., Proctor, G., et al., 2018. How cross-disciplinary research has increased our understanding of oral mucosal diseases. In: Meurman, J.H. (Ed.), Translational Oral Health Research. Springer International, Berlin, pp. 1–12.)

Chronic oral mucosal disease questionnaire-15 (COMDQ-15)

Instructions: Please answer the following questions by ticking one of the following boxes for each.

Physical discomfort	Not at all	Slightly	Moderately	Considerably	Extremely
How much do certain *types of food/drink* cause you discomfort (spicy food, acidic food)?	0	1	2	3	4
How much do certain *food textures* cause you discomfort (rough food, crusty food)?	0	1	2	3	4
How much does the *temperature of certain foods/drinks* cause you discomfort?	0	1	2	3	4
How much does your oral condition lead to discomfort when *carrying out your daily oral hygiene routine* (brushing, flossing, mouthwash usage)?	0	1	2	3	4
How much do you feel you *need medication to* help you with activities of daily life (talking, eating etc.)?	0	1	2	3	4
Medication and treatment					
How concerned are you about the possible *side effects of the medications* used to treat your oral condition?	0	1	2	3	4
How much does it frustrate you that there is *no single standard medication* to be used in your oral condition?	0	1	2	3	4
How much does *the use of the medication limit* you in your *everyday life* (routine / the way you apply or take your medications)?	0	1	2	3	4
Social and emotional					
How much does your oral condition get you *down*?	0	1	2	3	4
How much does your oral condition cause you *anxiety*?	0	1	2	3	4
How much does the *unpredictability* of your oral condition bother you?	0	1	2	3	4
How much does your oral condition make you *pessimistic about the future*?	0	1	2	3	4
How much does your oral condition *disrupt social activities* in your life (social gatherings, eating out parties)?	0	1	2	3	4
Patient support					
How satisfied are you with the *level of support and understanding* shown to you by *family* regarding this oral condition?	4	3	2	1	0
How satisfied are you with the *level of support and understanding* shown to you by *friends/work colleagues* regarding your oral condition?	4	3	2	1	0

Fig. 2.18 Chronic Oral Mucosal Diseases Questionnaire-15. (Reproduced from Wiriyakijja, P., Porter, S., Fedele, S., et al 2020. Development and validation of a short version of chronic oral mucosal disease questionnaire (COMDQ-15). J. Oral. Pathol. Med. 49 (1), 55–62. doi:10.1111/jop.12964.)

Site score: Each site receives a score of one if disease is present, with larger sites such as the buccal mucosa, tongue and palate being doubled if greater than 50% area is involved or if lesions are bilateral.

An *activity score* between 0 and 3 is assigned to describe the severity of disease at each site; for example, no activity = 0 (keratosis only), mild inflammation (erythema or healing areas) = 1, marked erythema = 2 and ulceration = 3. If the site score is 2 (i.e. affecting >50%), the activity score is doubled.

A *pain score* (subjective score provided by patient between 0 and 10) is then added to provide the *total score*. The theoretical maximum total score is 106; however, greater than 95% of patients have scores in the range from 0 to 60, representing a clinical range from remission to severe disease. The ODSS takes an average of 90 seconds to complete.

OLP is the most common oral mucosa disease, affecting approximately 1% to 2% of the adult population at any one time but can also present in a wide variety of clinical appearances. The ODSS or any scoring system needs to be able to embrace this wide variety of appearances. Different clinical phenotypes appear to be relatively consistent over many years and clinical photographs form an additional tool for recording outcomes.

Oral Health—Related Quality of Life

OHRQoL is assessed by using validated questionnaires that measure a patient's oral health self-perception of their capability for daily activities. The Oral Health Impact Profile (OHIP)-14 is a widely accepted tool in the form of a questionnaire showing good sensitivity to any improvement of OHRQoL in relation to clinical improvement (e.g. due to treatment).

Patients respond to 15 questions (Fig. 2.18) by selecting one of the answers from a 5-point scale (from 'not at all' to 'extremely'). Scores are then added and may range from 0 to 60.

RECOMMENDED READING

Carrasco-Labra, A., et al. (Eds.), 2020. How to Use Evidence-Based Dental Practices to Improve Your Clinical Decision-Making. ADA Publishing, Chicago, IL.

Escudier, M., Ahmed, N., Shirlaw, P., et al., 2007. A scoring system for mucosal disease severity with special reference to oral lichen planus. Br. J. Dermatol. 57 (4), 765—770.

Glick, M., Williams, D.M., Kleinman, D.V., Vujicic, M., Watt, R.G., Weyant, R.J., 2016. A new definition for oral health developed by the FDI World Dental Federation Opens the Door to a Universal Definition of Oral Health. J. Am. Dent. Assoc. 147 (12), 915—917.

Tappuni, A.R., Kovacevic, T., Shirlaw, P.J., Challacombe, S.J., 2013. Clinical assessment of disease severity in recurrent aphthous stomatitis. J. Oral. Pathol. Med. 42 (8), 635—641.

Watt, R.G., Serban, S., 2020. Multimorbidity: a challenge and opportunity for the dental profession. BDJ 229 (5), 282—286.

3

Principles of Diagnosis: Investigations

It is a truism that 'Accurate diagnosis is the only true cornerstone on which rational treatment can be built'.

C Noyek

The principle is thus to perform the necessary investigations to enable a specific diagnosis to be made.

INFORMED CONSENT

Following history taking and examination, investigations may be required to help make or confirm the diagnosis and to be able to offer a prognosis. Investigations should not be undertaken without first obtaining informed consent.

It is the professional duty of dental clinicians to help patients understand their condition. Patients commonly complain that they have been ill-informed about their diagnosis, investigations and the results of these. This may be because they have been informed but did not understand the significance. Patients should always be involved in the decision-making about their management. Patients are increasingly well-informed: some attend with specific questions and a few have detailed dossiers and seek special investigations. Careful discussion with the patient is the best approach. Other ways to help are by:

- Writing important points down for the patient for them to take away.
- Using patient information sheets.
- Offering guidance to other sources of information, such as written material and websites of oral medicine societies (e.g. European Association of Oral Medicine, British & Irish Society of oral Medicine) or those of the disease from which they suffer (e.g. Sjögren syndrome).
- Arranging contact with other patients with the same problems, either through patient self-help groups or individually. Self-help groups are now available for patients with chronic

serious conditions, such as cancer, pemphigus, trigeminal neuralgia, Behçet syndrome or Sjögren syndrome.

- Explaining the condition, diagnosis, investigations, management and prognosis to someone who can act as an advocate. This could be the patient's parent, partner, friend or relative. This should only be done if appropriate and only with the patient's express consent.

Consent is implied for taking a history and performing relevant clinical examinations. However, this does not apply to investigations; the clinician must clearly explain the:

- nature of investigation
- potential benefits
- possible adverse effects
- problems and disadvantages of not carrying out the investigations.

These points must be explained clearly to the patient, in a way that can be readily understood. Routine urinalysis, for example, is usually accepted as part of medical and insurance examinations though some patients question its use in dentistry. For other procedures, informed consent should always first be obtained, particularly where there could be adverse effects, such as pain, bleeding, infection, scarring or loss of sensation after a biopsy.

Verbal informed consent is adequate for non-invasive procedures, but for invasive or risky procedures, signed, witnessed and written informed consent should be obtained. Remember that patients are free to decline any or all investigations should they so wish, but it is wise for the clinician to clearly record that decision in writing in the case records. A patient has the right under common law to give or withhold consent to medical examination of treatment. This is one of the basic principles of healthcare. Patients are entitled to receive sufficient information in a way they can understand about the proposed treatments, the possible alternatives and any substantial risk or risks which may be special in kind or magnitude or special to the patient, so that they can make a balanced judgement, remember also that patients are entitled to change their minds and to withdraw consent.

INVESTIGATIONS

Following history taking and examination, investigations may be required to help make or confirm the diagnosis and prognosis, or sometimes simply to exclude some diagnoses in order to reassure the patient (and partner, family or clinician). An inadequate investigation could lead to a:
- misdiagnosis
- missed diagnosis
- complaint of bad practice
- legal action.
  However, superfluous investigations may be:
- liable to engender undue anxiety on the part of the patient, partner or relatives
- time-consuming
- expensive
- occasionally associated with adverse effects, or even dangerous.
  The following points should be borne in mind with regard to any form of investigation:
- The first principle must be to do no harm.
- Informed consent is required.
- Only an operator adequately skilled in a procedure should perform it.
- Surgical procedures are invasive, and this includes venepuncture and biopsy; an oral biopsy is rarely a pleasant procedure.

This chapter discusses a number of common investigations: others appear elsewhere in the book.

All bodily fluids and tissues are potentially infectious. Barrier precautions must, therefore, always be employed in order to prevent transmission of infection to patients or staff during investigations involving body fluids or tissues.

These procedures can often be carried out in general practice but, for a number of reasons, the dental professional may elect to refer to a specialist. The same applies to other investigations, particularly where there are issues when medical experience or a medical or specialist opinion could be helpful if not essential.

Blood Testing

Details of the various blood tests commonly used are shown in Table 3.1. During venepuncture, remember:

- The antecubital fossa is most commonly used since veins here are usually large and easily seen. Veins at other sites, such as the dorsum of the hand or the cephalic vein, can be difficult to identify and venepuncture can be painful there.
- Blood is withdrawn automatically into a vacutainer. If a syringe is used, withdraw slowly, making sure that there is no air in the syringe. A too rapid removal of blood may cause haemolysis.
- If the specimen tube contains an anticoagulant, ensure mixing by gently rolling the tube.
- Carefully dispose of the needle in the sharps container.
- Label the blood collection tubes with the patient's name, hospital or clinic number, date and time, etc.
- Complete and sign the appropriate request forms and give date, relevant clinical data, patient's name and number, etc.

Urinalysis

This is routinely performed with 'dip-sticks'. It may reveal:
- glycosuria: which may suggest diabetes mellitus
- ketonuria: which may be a sign of diabetic ketoacidosis or starvation
- bilirubin or urobilinogen: which may indicate hepatobiliary disorders
- proteinuria: which may be due to menstruation, or indicate renal, urinary tract or cardiac disease
- haematuria: which may be due to menstruation or indicate renal or urinary tract disease.

Saliva Testing

The most common use of saliva is for assessing volume or infections. Spitting or drooling into sterile universal containers is the preferred procedure, and if for xerostomia, then for a timed period. This may reveal:
- hyposalivation (less than 0.15 mL/min)
- candidiasis on culture
- bacterial infections on culture
- positive coronavirus or other viruses on lateral flow testing
- hypersalivation (rare).

A diagnosis of hyposalivation may be confirmed by assessing clinical oral dryness using a validated CODS scale (see Chapter 20).

Skin Testing

Absorption of many substances through the intact skin is poor and variable, but direct application to the surface of the skin is used for patch testing. The epidermal barrier may be overcome either by removing it or by introducing the material directly with a needle into the dermis (intradermal injections). A positive test is typically a weal and flare and may be taken as one which is significantly greater than the control. Assessment of what is significant is sometimes difficult. Resuscitation equipment and 1 in 1000 epinephrine (adrenaline) must be at hand to cope with any untoward allergic reactions.

The following techniques for skin testing are most commonly used:

TABLE 3.1   Blood Tests in Common Use

Test	Blood Sample Required	Comments
Full blood count (FBC)	5 mL anticoagulated with dry potassium edetate (EDTA) and received in the haematology laboratory within 24 h	The laboratory investigation is most frequently requested because anaemia and changes in the white blood cell count occur so commonly. Cells are usually counted and sized in automatic blood cell counters Folate can be assayed on this sample Blood film can be prepared from the same sample if indicated, for visual inspection of blood cells
Erythrocyte sedimentation rate (ESR), C-reactive protein (CRP) or plasma viscosity (PV)	As above	ESR raised in any inflammation and anaemias. CRP raised in infections and inflammation, PV increases if the concentration of certain globulins is increased, or a fall in the albumin level
Coagulation screen	5 mL anticoagulated with liquid sodium citrate and received in the haematology laboratory within 4 h or within 24 h for warfarin control by the prothrombin time or international normalised ratio (INR)	Required to diagnose coagulation disorders
Ferritin, iron, transferrin, folate and vitamin B_{12} (cobalamin) levels	10 mL added to a plain tube and received in the haematology laboratory within 24 h	Useful in the diagnosis of anaemias due to deficiencies
Blood grouping and cross-matching	10 mL added to a plain tube and received in the haematology laboratory within 4 h	Required prior to blood cell transfusion or major surgery
Blood glucose	Special tube (sodium fluoride)	Used to diagnose hypoglycaemia or hyperglycaemia, which is often due to diabetes mellitus
Serum urea, creatinine and electrolyte levels	Plain tube (no anticoagulant)	Used to diagnose renal failure (raised urea and creatinine levels) and electrolyte disturbance
Serum liver function tests include bilirubin, aspartate aminotransferase, alanine aminotransferase, alkaline phosphatase, albumin and globulin	10 mL added to a plain tube	Useful in the diagnosis of jaundice, liver and biliary tract disorders
Serum calcium, phosphate and alkaline phosphatase	10 mL added to a plain tube	Useful in the diagnosis of metabolic bone disease in particular
Serology	10 mL added to a plain tube	Useful for assay of various disease-specific antibodies
Thiopurine methyltransferase (TPMT)	10 mL added to a plain tube	Essential before prescribing azathioprine

Patch Tests

Patch tests are usually carried out on the back or the forearm and are used to detect contact allergy of the delayed hypersensitivity type. A battery of test allergens (European Standard Contact Dermatitis Testing Series) is often used. Patch testing is usually carried out with Finn chambers on Scanpor, a non-woven adhesive skin-friendly tape that contains no colophony. Results are usually read at 48 to 72 hours and again up to 1 week but can also be read at 0.5 hours to detect contact urticaria. At times, patch testing may usefully be combined with scratch testing (see below).

Intradermal Injections

A test solution must always be compared with a control solution (e.g. sterile saline) injected in a comparable site at the same time. The back and the flexor aspects of the forearms are most conveniently used. The injections are made into the superficial layer of the dermis through a fine-bore (26G or 27G) needle with its bevel pointing upwards. The quantity of which may be conveniently injected varies from 0.01 to 0.1 mL. Precise measurement of smaller quantities is difficult and requires syringes with especially well-fitting plungers and a micrometre screw gauge. For routine clinical purposes, an approximation is sufficient, either 0.05 mL or the amount, which just causes a visible wheal (0.01 to 0.02 mL).

Prick Test

This is a modification of the intradermal injection. A small quantity of the test solution is placed on the skin and a prick is made through it with a sharp needle. This should be superficial and not sufficient to draw blood. The size of the weal and flare is measured after 15 minutes. This test gives reproducible results and is convenient for routine allergy testing. Because of the discrepancy in quantities injected, the testing solutions are made up of different strengths for prick testing and intradermal testing. The intradermal injections of prick test solutions may be dangerous.

Modified Prick Test

Here a drop of the test solution is placed on the skin. A needle is then inserted very superficially and almost horizontally into the skin and lifted to raise a tiny tent of the epidermis. This test is slightly more sensitive than the ordinary prick test but gives no more reproducible results.

Scratch Test

The scratch test resembles the prick test. A linear scratch about 1 cm long, but not sufficient to draw blood, is made through the epidermis. This test gives less reproducible results than the prick test.

The optimal time for reading intradermal reactions varies with the pharmacological agent or the type of immunological reaction. Most such tests are read at either 15 to 20 minutes or at 48 hours, but it may be important to read the tests at other times (e.g. at 4 to 12 hours or after 4 days).

Biopsy

A biopsy is the removal of a small piece of tissue from the living body for the purpose of diagnosis by microscopic examination. It is often indicated in order to confirm or make a precise diagnosis, especially in the case of mucosal lesions, when a specimen for immunostaining is often also called for.

Indications for biopsy include (Table 3.2):
- lesions that have neoplastic or premalignant features or are enlarging
- persistent lesions that are of uncertain aetiology
- persistent lesions that are failing to respond to treatment
- confirmation of the clinical diagnosis
- lesions that are causing the patient extreme concern.

Biopsy Precautions

Ensure that comprehensive medical history is completed and if the patient is on:
- anticoagulants: warfarin requires an up-to-date international normalised ratio (INR) of less than 4 within 36 hours of biopsy
- corticosteroids: if 10 mg or above for greater than 3 months, may require supplementary 100 mg hydrocortisone before procedure
- immunocompromised: if neutropenic (neutrophils <1.5) requires broad-spectrum antibiotic prophylaxis such as 3 g ampicillin orally at least one hour before the procedure (or co-amoxiclav 2 g i.v. 30 minutes).

Biopsy Technique

Tissue may be obtained by two main methods: techniques not requiring anaesthesia (e.g. exfoliative cytology and brush biopsy) and techniques requiring local anaesthesia (analgesia). Those requiring local anaesthesia are largely employed, and include:
- scalpel or tissue punch — incisional biopsy
- scalpel, diathermy or laser cutting — excisional biopsy
- curettage
- needle biopsy, which requires a larger bore needle such as:
  - cutting biopsy using a 14 G Tru-Cut needle
  - fine-needle aspiration biopsy (FNA or FNAB) using a 22 G or 25 G standard disposable needle
  - ultrasound-guided fine-needle aspiration cytology (US-FNAC).

Fig. 3.1 shows the equipment required. In the case of suspected potentially malignant or malignant mucosal lesions, it can be difficult to decide exactly which is the part of the lesion that is best biopsied. The most significant information can be gained from red mucosal areas (erythroplasia) rather than

TABLE 3.2 Main Indications for Biopsy

Indication	Examples
Lesions that have neoplastic or premalignant features or are enlarging	Actinic cheilitis Erythroplakia Leukoplakia Lichen planus Focal pigmented lesions Lumps
Persistent lesions of uncertain aetiology	Soft or hard tissue
Persistent lesions failing to respond to treatment	Ulcers or lesions, such as some radiolucent or radio-opaque bone lesions
Persistent focal lesions involving the gingival/periodontium	Lumps, ulcers or non-healing extraction sockets
Confirmation of clinical diagnosis	Labial salivary gland biopsy to confirm Sjögren syndrome
Lesions causing the patient extreme concern	Patients may prefer biopsy or excision biopsy of a persistent red, white or pigmented lesion or lump

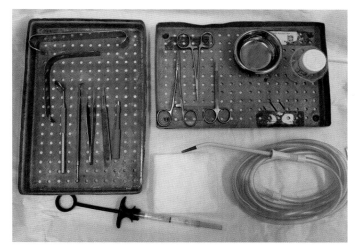

Fig. 3.1 Biopsy trays, containing biopsy instruments: retractors, mirrors, tissue forceps, biopsy punch, etc. Second tray: sutures, suture forceps, scissors, pot with fixative, etc. Local anaesthetic syringe, suction tubing.

white areas (leukoplakia) and it can sometimes be helpful to stain the mucosa before biopsy with toluidine blue dye (vital staining), which is taken up by nuclei and stains pathological areas mainly, causing suspect mucosal areas to stain blue. Usually, a single biopsy is taken, but multiple biopsies may be indicated where:

- additional investigations, such as immunostaining, are required
- malignant disease is suspected
- there are widespread leukoplakic or erythroplakic field changes (such biopsies may be termed 'mapping' biopsies).

Biopsy Procedure

Informed consent is mandatory for biopsy as for all operative procedures, particularly noting any possible adverse effects, such as post-operative pain, bleeding or loss of sensation. Care must be taken not to produce anxiety where it is not necessary; some patients equate biopsy with a diagnosis of cancer. Complete the request form with the:

- patient's full name
- patient's date of birth
- hospital number, if applicable
- date
- site of biopsy
- clinical résumé
- dates, and numbers, of all previous biopsies.
  The container must be labelled clearly with:
- patient's full name
- patient's date of birth
- number
- date
- specimen site.

Mucosal Biopsies

Mucosal biopsies are excisional (removal of the complete lesion) or incisional and taken with a scalpel or biopsy punch, or sometimes a diathermy or laser, usually under local analgesia. Excisional biopsy is preferred for small, isolated and probably benign lesions.

The biopsy should include lesional and normal tissue and should be large enough to handle and to provide adequate information about the lesion. In the case of ulcerated mucosal lesions, most histopathological information is gleaned from the peri-lesional tissue, since by definition most epithelium is lost from the ulcer itself. Where there are similar lesions affecting several sites, which is often the case for example in lichen planus, then it is often better to biopsy buccal mucosal lesions than gingival, palatal or tongue lesions. Gingival biopsies may damage the gingival architecture, a protective pack such as Coe-pak must be worn for a week or so, and the lesions may be complicated to interpret histologically since gingivitis is often superimposed. Palatal lesions similarly may need a dressing and can be painful after biopsy. The tongue is a very sensitive, vascular and mobile organ, and biopsies can lead to discomfort, some interference with function, and the constant movement

causes discomfort and may lead to sutures failing. In contrast, a biopsy from the buccal mucosa can be done virtually painlessly, with little post-operative swelling or discomfort, and sutures may not be needed — especially when a punch has been used. The punch has the advantages for incision biopsy that:

- the incision is controlled
- an adequate specimen is obtained (typically 4 mm or 6 mm in diameter)
- the patient is not disturbed by the sight of a scalpel
- suturing may not be required.

However, only a fairly small biopsy is obtained with the punch and, in some instances, epithelium may be sheared off — especially in vesiculobullous disorders. If a larger piece of tissue is needed, or the whole lesion is to be removed, the scalpel has advantages, particularly when the lesion is on the gingivae, especially lingually or other areas in which it is difficult to gain access with a punch or when mucosa is fragile (e.g. pemphigus). A number 15 blade is usually chosen.

To carry out a biopsy:

- Use a clinical biopsy checklist (Fig. 3.2).
- A local anaesthetic should be given.
- Ensure tissue representative of the lesion is obtained. In mucosal lesions, include some normal tissue as well as the lesion (biopsies of ulcers alone are inadequate) (Fig. 3.3).
  - Choose the site to enable suturing after scalpel biopsy (Fig. 3.4)
  - When a vesiculobullous disorder is suspected, include peri-ilesional tissue and use a scalpel or a punch, the latter is especially useful for gingival or multisite MMP (Fig. 3.5).
- Do not squeeze with forceps as this can cause crush artefacts. Sutures may be used to hold the tissue and also to mark specific areas of biopsy.
- Place the biopsy specimen onto a small piece of paper before immersing in fixative, as this prevents curling. Put small specimens for histological examination immediately into buffered formalin or another fixative in at least its own volume of fixative, preferably 10-fold more, and leave at room temperature ($20°C$). A further biopsy specimen (or half of a larger biopsy) should be placed in Michels medium or immediately snap-frozen ($-70°C$) if immunostaining or a frozen section is required. If the bacteriological examination is required, for example, in suspected tuberculosis, send a separate specimen without fixative.
- Suture if necessary, preferably using a fine needle and resorbable suture such as Vicryl 3/0 or Vicryl Rapide 4/0, which will not require the patient to re-attend for removal Non-resorbable sutures, such as silk, are also available. For very small lesions suture may not be needed, or a silver nitrate stick can be used for haemostasis (see Fig. 3.4).
- The use of an inverted suture technique means that there is no knot left in the mouth to irritate the patient.

Immunostaining and Immunofluorescence

Specimens for immunostaining should not be fixed in formalin but placed immediately in Michel's solution. If frozen sections

Patient label / identifier

Oral medicine biopsy safety checklist (LocSSIP)

NHS
Guy's and St Thomas'
NHS Foundation Trust

Adapted from WHO surgical safety checklist v1.12 updated 24/01/19

DATE and TIME:

Pre operation (Brief)

- Introduction of team & roles
- Concerns relating to: Staff, equipment, planned surgery, emergency drugs, resuscitation equipment addressed

Pre operation (Sign in)

Sign in/time out/sign out/debrief should be read out loud by the assistant

Tick once checked

- Patient's full name and DOB
- Diagnosis, treatment plan and consent form present
- Medical history and allergies
- Relevant investigations reviewed
- Equipment present, functioning correctly and sterile
- Medical history checked
- Escort present (if required)
- Post-operative complications discussed

Pre operation (Sign in)

Biopsy site	Histo formalin	DIF Michel's

Pause (Time out)

VERBAL TIME OUT pause immediately prior to treatment

- Consent visible
- Correct site
- Equipment ready

Post operation (Sign out)

- Swab / gauze / sharps / instrument counts complete
- Procedure documented in clinical records
- Specimen label correct
- Appropriate follow-up arranged

Post operation (Debrief)

Any equipment issues / safety concerns that need to be addressed?   o Yes   o No

Any areas for improvement?   o Yes   o No

Comments

Operator	**Assistant**
Name:	Name:
GDC:	GDC:
Signature:	Signature:

Fig. 3.2 Biopsy checklist.

---

are required, biopsies must be handed immediately to laboratory staff for freezing, or immediately snap-frozen (on solid carbon dioxide or liquid nitrogen) and taken within an hour or so to the laboratory.

Direct immunofluorescence is a qualitative technique used to detect immune deposits (antibodies and/or complement) in the tissues. It is a one-stage technique, requiring patient lesional or perilesional tissue (see Fig. 3.3). Immunostaining usually uses a fluorescein stain, which fluoresces apple green under ultraviolet light, and is termed 'immunofluorescence'. It is useful in the diagnosis, particularly of vesiculobullous disorders, such as pemphigoid and pemphigus.

Indirect immunofluorescence is a qualitative and quantitative technique used to detect immune deposits (circulating antibodies and/or complement) in the serum. It is a two or more-stage technique requiring patient serum and animal tissue.

Oral Smears for Cytology

Cytology is rarely used but prepared in this way, smears will keep for up to 3 weeks:

- Take smears with a wooden or metal spatula, or dental plastic instrument.
- Spread smears evenly on the centres of two previously labelled glass slides.
- Fix smears immediately in industrial methylated spirit. Do not allow to dry in the air, as cellular detail is rapidly lost and artefacts develop.
- After 20 minutes of fixation, the smears can be left to dry in the air or left in fixative.

Lymph Node Biopsy

Lymph nodes should not be subjected to open biopsy if a malignant disease is suspected: FNAB or FNAC is better, or the biopsy deferred until the time of operation. A sentinel lymph node (SLN) is the first node(s) to which cancer is likely to spread from the primary cancer. To identify the SLN, the surgeon injects in the area of the primary tumour, a radionuclide or dye. The substance is identified in the SLN by scanning (radionuclide) or visual inspection (dye). Once located, the SLN is excised and examined histopathologically (this is SLN biopsy).

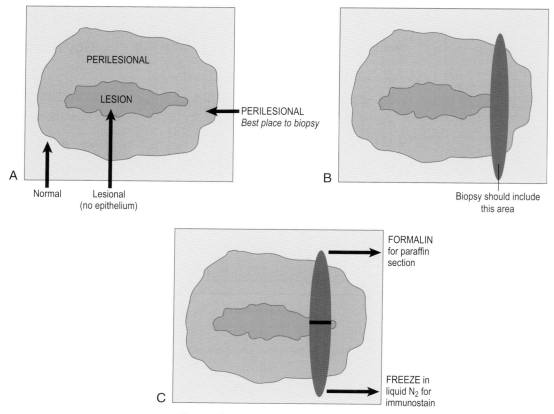

Fig. 3.3 Where to take a scalpel biopsy.

Labial Salivary Gland Biopsy

- Warn the patient of possible post-operative mild hypoaesthesia.
- Give the patient local analgesia.
- Make a linear mucosal incision about 5 to 8 mm long (to one side of the midline in the lower labial mucosa) or an x-shaped incision over the swelling, which overlies the salivary gland (Fig. 3.6).
- Excise at least four lobules of the salivary gland.
- Suture the wound if necessary.

Frozen Sections for Rapid Diagnosis

This procedure, in which the section is examined whilst the patient is still under anaesthesia, is useful in cases where malignancy is suspect and in resections, to check the resection margin for tumour infiltration and to assess whether the margins are tumour-free.

Communicate with the pathologist at the latest by the day before the operation. Specimens should be immediately snap-frozen (on solid carbon dioxide or liquid nitrogen) and taken immediately to the laboratory or collected by the pathology team. Telephone the laboratory when the specimen is on its way. Warn the pathologist about any tissue containing calcified material that could break the microtome. The results should be transmitted by the pathologist to the clinician direct.

Other Investigations

Tables 3.3–3.8 summarise the investigations of various sites.

Imaging Using Radiation

Because of the cumulative effect of radiation hazard, all investigations using x-rays must be justified by benefiting the patient. The clinician requesting the examination or investigation must be satisfied that each investigation is necessary and that the benefit outweighs the risk.

In the UK, the Ionising Radiation (Medical Exposure) Regulations (2000) (IR(ME)R2000) require exposure of patients to be 'as low as reasonably achievable' (ALARA).

Radiography

The request form for radiography should be completed and signed by the clinician or entered online and should include the following:

- Vital patient data: full name, address, date of birth, unit number, ward, clinic or outpatient department and specialist in charge.
- Details that facilitate correct investigations and accurate opinion:
  - investigations required (region to be examined and, where relevant, special investigation needed)
  - diagnostic problem
  - relevant clinical features
  - known diagnoses
  - previous relevant operations.
- Other information, for example, whether the patient is a walking or trolley case, whether there is an infectious risk, whether an urgent or routine report is required, the date, place and type of previous radiographs.

A protective lead apron having a lead equivalence of no less than 0.25 mm is worn by the patient only where the primary x-ray beam can strike the pelvis, such as in vertex-occlusal radiography, and a neck shield is indicated if the thyroid is to be exposed.

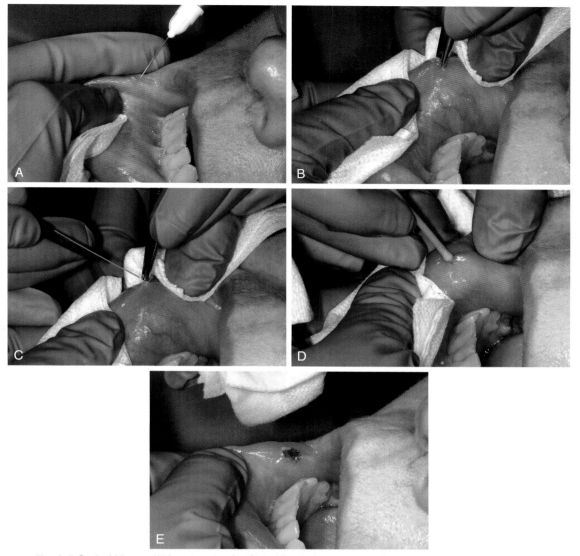

Fig. 3.4 Scalpel biopsy. (A) Local analgesia; (B) holding lesion (a polyp); (C) removing lesion; (D) cauterising with silver nitrate and (E) completion.

A particular problem arises during pregnancy, because of the hazard to the foetus. Enquiry as to pregnancy must always be made (risk of foetal irradiation) before performing radiography or other imaging procedures that involve radiation exposure by the primary beam to the abdomen and pelvis. Although most dental radiography does not constitute a risk, the clinician should always ascertain whether a woman is pregnant before requesting a radiograph and the investigation required should be discussed with the patient, who may wish to defer it until after pregnancy.

Note whether the patient:
- is of child-bearing potential
- is taking the contraceptive pill
- has had a hysterectomy
- has been sterilised.

Restricting x-ray investigations with a relatively high gonad radiation risk on women of child-bearing age to the 10 days following the start of a menstrual period (the 10-day rule) has now fallen somewhat into disfavour.

Portable X-Rays

- The quality of portable films is rarely as good as that of corresponding films taken using non-portable equipment.
- The examination should take place in the ward only if there is an absolute contraindication to the patient being brought to the radiography department. If there is any doubt about the advisability of bringing the patient to the department, consult a radiologist.
- Theatre radiography is done only when its results are needed during the operation.

Plain Radiography

This is useful in the diagnosis of fractures, dislocations, bone and tooth disorders, joint disease and foreign bodies.

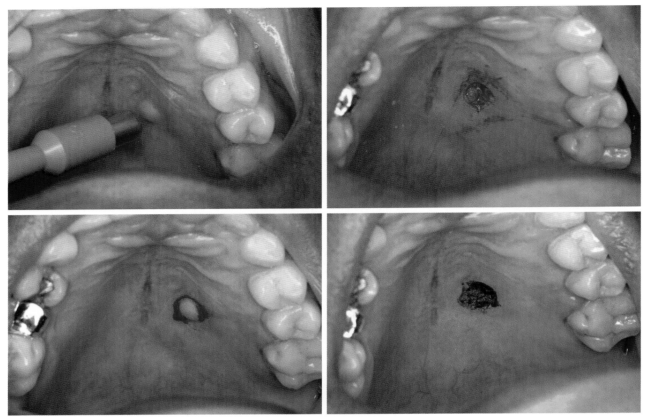

Fig. 3.5 Punch biopsy; the disc of tissue is removed with scissors or scalpel. (A) 5 mm punch and palatal lesion; (B) tissue around lesion having been cut; (C) base of the lesion removed by scalpel and (D) area cauterised. (Courtesy of Dr. H. McParland.)

Chest Radiography

The chest radiograph is valuable in investigating chest disease, heart disease (e.g. heart failure) and general medical problems, such as malaise, fever or weight loss (e.g. bronchial carcinoma, tuberculosis and other chest infections). Chest radiography to exclude latent TB and other pathologies is now part of the suggested protocols for immunosuppressant therapy.

Intra-Oral Radiography

- Periapical radiographs are useful for demonstrating pathology in the periapical region (abscess, granuloma, cyst, etc.) and the tooth root, periodontium and adjacent bone.
- Bitewing radiographs show both upper and lower premolar and molar teeth on one film, but do not show the tooth apex. They are useful for revealing approximal caries and demonstrating the alveolar crest.
- Occlusal films may be useful in assessing the facial and lingual cortices and adjacent areas such as the floor of the mouth and palate.

Dental Panoramic Tomography (DPT) (or Orthopantomography (OPTG))

This is valuable as a general survey and typically shows the antra and temporomandibular joints well. The radiation dose is considerably lower than a full mouth survey using periapical films, but it:

- lacks the detail obtained by other films, such as periapical radiography
- does not show detail in the anterior jaws
- does not show caries until this is advanced
- can result in ghost shadows and blurring
- examines only a slice of tissue.

Sialography

Sialography involves the instillation of radio-opaque contrast media into the salivary duct followed by oblique lateral and posteroanterior (PA) or rotated PA radiographs. Use of a sialogogue, such as lemon juice, to empty the gland gives an 'emptying film'. Sialography is not commonly used nowadays but can occasionally help to:

- detect ductal obstruction
- detect the rare cases of salivary aplasia
- assess patients with hyposalivation
- assess patients with salivary swelling.

Arthrography

The main indication is in suspected internal joint derangements but is rarely used and has been superseded by MRI. It involves the injection of radio-opaque contrast media (usually iohexol or iopamidol) into the lower space of the temporomandibular joint.

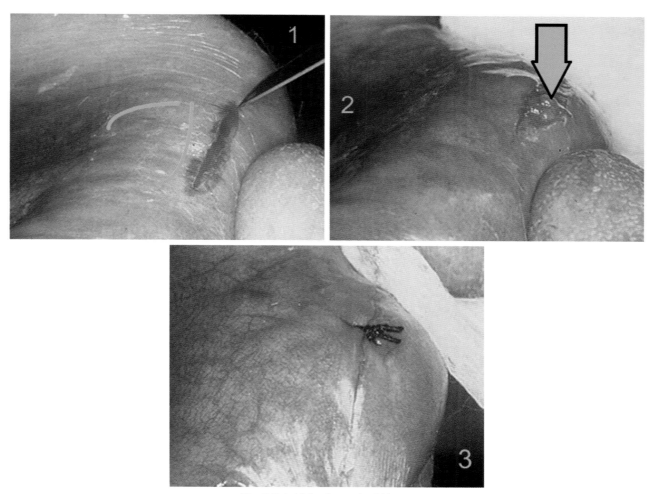

Fig. 3.6 Labial salivary gland biopsy

Angiography

Angiography involves the injection of radio-opaque contrast media into the arteries (arteriography) or veins (venography). The main indications include:
- diagnosis or delineation of vascular anomalies or tumours
- assessment of tumours in the deep lobe of the parotid gland
- assisting surgical procedures (e.g. microvascular surgery or embolisation).

Computed Axial Tomography (CAT or CT)

CT integrates information from multiple radiographic 'slices' into images of internal tissues (e.g. brain, orbit, sinuses, neck, salivary glands, tongue). It has considerable advantages for visualising complex head and neck anatomical areas inaccessible to conventional radiographs and is good for visualising hard tissue lesions especially. CT imaging of the head can provide images of bones, soft tissue and blood vessels and is:
- particularly useful for determining tumour spread, to exclude cranial base or intracranial pathology and planning surgery and implant placement
- expensive
- a fairly high radiation exposure (CT of the head can give the equivalent exposure to about 100 chest radiographs).

Cone-beam CT (CBCT) is a smaller, faster and safer modification of CT. Using a cone-shaped x-ray beam, the CBCT scanner size, scanning time and radiation dosage are all reduced; the time needed for a CBCT scan is typically under one minute and the radiation dosage is up to a hundred times less than that of a regular CT. CBCT is thus increasingly used to image jaws and related structures.

Functional CT using positron emission tomography (PET), four-dimensional computed tomography (4D-CT) and single-photon emission computed tomography (SPECT) is increasingly used.

Scintiscanning (Radionuclide Scanning)

Radioactive pharmaceuticals with an affinity for specific organs or tissues can be detected and measured by a gamma camera.

Salivary Scintigraphy

Intravenous sodium pertechnetate is taken up by salivary (and thyroid) glands and secreted in saliva. Scintiscanning is not commonly used in salivary gland investigation but can sometimes help in the diagnosis of:
- Sjögren syndrome
- ductal obstruction
- salivary neoplasms
- salivary aplasia.

It may also help locate a lingual thyroid.

TABLE 3.3   Investigative Procedures in Diseases of the Jaws and Sinuses

Procedure	Advantages	Disadvantages	Remarks
Transillumination	Simple	—	Helpful to show a fluid level
Fibre-optic nasendoscopy	Simple; good visualisation	Skill needed	Useful to examine nasal passages, pharynx and larynx
Radiography	Reveals much data not obvious on clinical examination	Specialised techniques may be difficult	Upper occlusal radiography is useful for detecting cysts Other radiographic views may fail to show cysts, since if the antrum is large with outpouchings into the alveolar process and zygomatic bone, may look similar to cysts Occipitomental radiography (Waters) views of the skull taken at 15 and 30 degrees, are the best radiographs for viewing the antra These views can show an opaque antrum, a fluid level or fractures
Computed tomography (CAT, CT, CBCT), MRI	Reveal data often not seen on clinical or conventional radio-graphic examination MRI uses no radiation	Expensive and not univer-sally available Interpretation requires additional training	Demonstrates both hard and soft tissues and give spatial relationships CBCT or coronal CAT of the antrum can be useful for showing the extent of a neoplasm, particularly in the posterior and superior maxilla CAT and MRI are useful particularly in detecting the extent of spread of a malignant neoplasm and have the great advantage of demonstrating the posterior maxilla, the intratemporal fossa, the floor of the orbit and the nasoeth-moidal sinuses — sites not readily seen by other imaging
Aspiration	Simple	May introduce infection	May show the presence of haemangioma The protein content of cyst fluid may be of diagnostic value (protein levels lower than 4 g/100 mL in keratocysts)
Bone biopsy	Definitive	Invasive	Invasive
Bone scan	Surveys all skeleton	Those of any radionuclide procedure	May reveal pathology (e.g. metastases or osteomyelitis)

CT, Computed tomography; *CBCT*, Cone-beam computer tomography; *MRI*, magnetic resonance imaging.

TABLE 3.4   Investigative Procedures in Temporomandibular Joint Disease

Procedure	Advantages	Disadvantages
Radiography	Simple Can reveal much pathology	Radiation exposure
CAT scan, CBCT	Can provide excellent information	Expensive Radiation exposure
Arthrography (double-contrast)	Provides excellent information	Danger of introducing infection Painful
MRI	Provides excellent information without exposure to ionising radiation	Non-invasive Expensive and not universally available
Arthroscopy	Minimally invasive Good visualisation	Requires anaesthesia Technically demanding

CAT, Computed axial tomography; *CBCT*, Cone-beam computer tomography.

Bone Scans

Intravenous technetium methylene diphosphonate is taken up by osteoblasts, and bone scans can be useful in:

- assessing condylar or coronoid hyperplasia
- detecting metastases
- detecting bone invasion
- determining the activity of bone disease
- determining the degree of osteoporosis.

Dual-Energy X-Ray Absorptiometry

The current standard of bone mineral density (BMD) assessment is dual-energy x-ray absorptiometry (DEXA) and is based upon a person's BMD T-score at the femoral neck and lumbar spine. For the degenerative spine, CT densitometry of the spine is equal to or superior to DEXA for assessing vertebral fracture risk. Both are helpful in assessing the impact of long-term systemic steroids.

TABLE 3.5 Investigative Procedures in Salivary Gland Disease

Procedure	Advantages	Disadvantages and Comments
Sialometry[a] (salivary flow rates)	Simple rapid useful procedure which may confirm or refute hyposalivation	Somewhat imprecise Wide range of normal values Commonly used
Blood tests	Simple and useful to reveal systemic disease (e.g. rheumatoid arthritis or Sjögren syndrome)	Will not usually reflect local disease of salivary glands
MRI	Useful for investigating space-occupying lesions and suspected malignancy, or infections	Expensive, not universally available, but no irradiation
Ultrasound	Useful, inexpensive, non-invasive and often helpful diagnostically	Increasingly used. Helpful in Sjögren syndrome
Plain radiography	Lower occlusal and oblique lateral or OPT may show submandibular calculi Soft PA film may show parotid calculi	Calculi may not be radio-opaque Sialography may be needed
CT, CBCT	Useful to investigate salivary duct obstruction, infections or abscesses	Not universally available; high radiation dose
Sialendoscopy	Useful to investigate salivary duct obstruction	Not universally available
Sialochemistry	Research investigation; rarely helpful clinically	Salivary composition varies with many factors Far less useful than blood and other tests Rarely used
Sialography	Useful to eliminate gross structural damage, calculi or stenoses	Time-consuming and somewhat insensitive. May cause pain or, occasionally, sialadenitis[b] Uses x-rays Less commonly used
Salivary gland biopsy	LSG biopsy is simple and may reflect changes in other salivary (and exocrine) glands. Major gland biopsy and FNAC may be useful	Biopsies are invasive Major gland biopsy can result in facial palsy or salivary fistula and thus uncommonly used
Scintigraphy and radiosialometry	Measures uptake of radionuclide[c] (radiosialometry more quantitative) High uptake (hotspots) may reveal tumours	Expensive and with hazards associated with the use of radionuclides Taken up by thyroid gland; rare instances of thyroid damage Rarely used

CAT, Computed axial tomography; *CBCT*, Cone-beam computer tomography; *FNAC*, fine-needle aspiration cytology; *LSG*, Labial gland; *MRI*, magnetic resonance imaging; *OPT*, orthopantomography.

[a]Unstimulated whole salivary flow rates are usually used; flow rates less than 0.15 mL/min are low. Alternatively, stimulate parotid salivary flow with 1 mL 10% citric acid on to tongue; flow rates less than 0.5 mL/min/gland may signify reduced salivary function. Alternatively, pilocarpine 2.5 mg i.v. may be used, but is contraindicated in cardiac patients or those with hypertension.
[b]Combined sialography with CAT scanning may be useful in the diagnosis and localisation of salivary gland lesions, particularly parotid neoplasms.
[c]Usually technetium pertechnetate.

Positron Emission Tomography

PET can produce maps of tissue metabolic activity based either on blood flow or glucose utilisation and is increasingly used to detect second primary tumours and metastases (see Chapter 53).

Non-Radiation Imaging
Magnetic Resonance Imaging

MRI depends on the distribution of protons (hydrogen nuclei) in tissues and their effect on a magnetic field and does not involve ionising radiation. The MRI signal has two components:
- $T1$, in which the proton is spinning under the magnetic influence and radiofrequency to return to the original value (spin-lattice or longitudinal relaxation time). T_1-weighted scans are a standard basic scan, in particular, differentiating fat from water — with water darker and fat brighter. T_1-weighted images cause fat like the myelin in brain white matter to appear bright (light grey); grey matter appears grey, cerebrospinal fluid (CSF) appears black.

- $T2$, which depends on the gradual dephasing of the protons in the transverse or transaxial plane (spin–spin, or transverse relaxation times). T_2-weighted scans show fat darker, and water lighter. Brain white matter appears dark grey, grey matter appears grey and CSF appears white.

The advantages of MRI are that it is:
- especially good for visualising soft tissues and lesions
- useful for imaging the temporomandibular joint
- good for revealing bone invasion.

The disadvantages of MRI are that it is:
- not good for imaging bone
- fraught with producing image artefacts where metal objects are present (dental metal restorations, implants, orthodontic and other metal-containing appliances, bone plates, metallic foreign bodies, joint prostheses, etc.)
- expensive.

Contraindications to the use of MRI include the presence of ferromagnetic implanted devices in the brain or eye, such as

TABLE 3.6 Investigative Procedures in Oral Mucosal Disease

Procedure	Advantages	Disadvantages	Remarks
Biopsy	Gives definitive diagnosis in many instances	Invasive	Mucosal biopsies should be submitted for histopathological and often direct immunofluorescence examinations if a vesiculobullous disorder is suspected
Bacteriological smear and culture	Simple clinical procedure	Isolation of organisms does not necessarily imply causal relation with the disease under investigation Some organisms are non-cultivable	Anaerobic techniques may be indicated especially in oral lesions in the immunocompromised host Nucleic acid studies increasingly used
Fungal smear and culture	Simple clinical procedures	As above	Candida hyphae suggest Candida species are pathogenic Raised salivary counts indicate infection
Viral culture	Simple sensitive clinical procedure Often gives diagnosis more rapidly than does serology	May require special facilities and may only give the retrospective diagnosis	False-negative results possible Indicated in some acute ulcerative or bullous lesions Serology should also be undertaken Nucleic acid studies increasingly used
Microbial DNA studies	PCR or NAAT now often used	May require special facilities	Rapid and specific results Increasingly used
Haematological screen, haemoglobin red cell and white cell indices	Simple clinical procedure	Prevalence rate may not be high	Essential to exclude systemic causes of oral disease, especially in ulcers, glossitis or angular stomatitis
Serology	Demonstration of a rise in titre-specific antibodies between acute and convalescent serum may be diagnostically useful Specific tests available (e.g. HIV antibodies)	Serum autoantibodies may not mean disease Serum autoantibodies may be undetected in pemphigoid Diagnosis of viral infections is retrospective	Essential in suspected HIV and other infections, connective tissue disease, autoimmune or other immunological disorders

HIV, human immune deficiency viruses; *NAAT*, nucleic acid amplification tests; *PCR*, Polymerase chain reaction.

nerve stimulators, cochlear implants or intracranial vascular clips. Metal objects outside the brain and eye are not a contraindication: cardiac valves, inferior vena cava filters, IUDs and metallic prostheses are safe unless there is doubt as to positional stability. However, cardiac pacemakers, insulin pumps, neurostimulators, cochlear implants, etc. may be de-programmed.

Thus, MRI gives sensitive images of the internal organs and tissues (e.g. brain or spine), but in the presence of metal, there may be artefacts.

Ultrasound Scanning

- 'Ultrasound' is a term that applies to sound waves with a frequency above the audible range of human hearing.
- Ultrasonography (US) (diagnostic sonography) is non-invasive, simple, inexpensive and very helpful in imaging soft tissues with virtually no contraindications and is thus increasingly used.
- US gives useful imaging of soft tissues (e.g. subcutaneous tissues, muscle, tendons, vessels) and internal organs (e.g. lymph nodes, thyroid or salivary glands) and foreign bodies. Ultrasound (Doppler) is also useful for investigating vascular disease. Colour Doppler ultrasound (CDUS) may be useful.
- Ultrasound is increasingly useful in the assessment of major salivary glands (Fig. 3.7)

- US diagnostically uses high-frequency sound waves (2 to 18 Hz) with wavelengths of 0.6 to 0.01 mm and involves no ionising radiation exposure. Sonographers use a hand-held probe (a transducer) placed directly on and moved over the area to be imaged. When the sound strikes the interface between media, the energy reflects as an echo, which may be displayed as a unidimensional wave image (an A-scan) or, when a sweeping beam is used, as a two-dimensional monochrome image (a B scan). There is abrupt impedance with calcified lesions, or foreign bodies, such as glass or metal.

Endoscopy

Endoscopy is typically performed with flexible fibre-optic endoscopes, under local analgesia, sometimes with conscious sedation or general anaesthesia. Relevant endoscopic procedures include:

- nasendoscopy
- oesophagoscopy
- bronchoscopy
- panendoscopy usually refers to triple endoscopy (nasendoscopy, oesophagoscopy and bronchoscopy)
- gastroscopy (the oesophagus, stomach and duodenum)
- sialoendoscopy
- colonoscopy.

TABLE 3.7 Imaging Available for Lesions in Different Locations

Location of Lesions	Plain Radiography	Other Imaging
Mandible	Rotational tomography Oblique lateral CT, CBCT	MRI Bone scan
Mandibular condyle	Reverse Towne Submentovertex CT, CBCT	MRI Bone scan
Temporomandibular joint	Rotational tomography Transcranial CT Transpharyngeal CT, CBCT	MRI Arthrography Bone scan
Maxilla	30 occipitomental CT, CBCT	MRI Bone scan
Paranasal sinuses	OM rotational tomography for maxillary antra Upper occlusal or lateral Submentovertex CT, CBCT	MRI Bone scan
Skull	PA skull rotational tomography 10 occipitomental Lateral skull CT	MRI Bone scan
Salivary glands	Oblique lateral Rotated PA CT	Ultrasound MRI Sialography Scintigraphy
Intra-oral	Rotational tomography CT, CBCT	Ultrasound MRI

CT, Computed tomography; *CBCT*, Cone-beam computer tomography; *MRI*, magnetic resonance imaging; *PA*, posteroanterior.

TABLE 3.8 Significance of the More Common Serum Autoantibodies

Autoantibody	Main Significance[a]
DNA antibodies (ds-DNA (*Crithidia luciliae*))	Systemic lupus erythematosus
Anti-topoisomerase 1 (Sc1-70)	Scleroderma
Anticentromere antibodies (ACA)	Scleroderma
Rheumatoid factor (RF)	Rheumatoid arthritis (RA) (sometimes systemic lupus erythematosus)
Robert (Ro), also known as soluble substance A antigen (SS-A)	Sjögren syndrome
Lane (La), also known as soluble substance B antigen (SS-B)	Sjögren syndrome only in presence of SS-B
Epithelial intercellular cement (desmoglein [Dsg]) Dsg3 in mucosal PV, Dsg1 in skin	Pemphigus
Epithelial basement membrane zone (e.g. BP180, integrin)	Pemphigoid[b]
Parietal cell antibody; intrinsic factor antibodies	Pernicious anaemia

[a]The presence of autoantibodies does not always indicate disease.
[b]Other immune-mediated subepithelial blistering diseases.

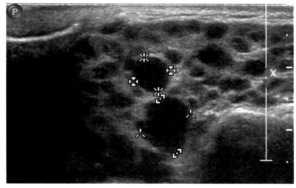

Fig. 3.7 Ultrasound scan of parotid gland in Sjögren syndrome demonstrating large non-vascular foci. (Courtesy of Dr. Jackie Brown.)

Risks from endoscopy include possible:

- infection
- bleeding
- punctured organs.

Bleeding may occur at the site of a biopsy or polyp removal. Typically minor, such bleeding may simply cease spontaneously or be controlled by cautery. Surgery is seldom necessary. Perforation, however, generally requires surgery, though some cases may be treated with antibiotics and intravenous fluids.

Thermography

An infrared camera detects areas of changed vascularity but has the disadvantage of needing the patient to be 'precooled'. It is rarely practical in clinical practice but sometimes used in clinical research.

Photography

This is exceedingly useful to record lesions, and support disease severity scoring. The advent of digital photography has considerably improved the quality.

INVESTIGATIONS OF SPECIFIC MEDICAL PROBLEMS RELEVANT IN ORAL MEDICINE

Allergies

Allergy is an abnormal immune response (usually a type I or type IV hypersensitivity response) to an antigen — a protein or allergen. Many allergies have a hereditary component, but the prevalence of allergies appears to be increasing and people who suffer allergies to one type of substance are more likely to suffer allergies to others. Common allergens are pollen, dust mites, mould, pet dander, nuts, shellfish, milk and egg proteins, and latex but, in many cases, the allergen cannot be reliably identified.

Diagnosis is based on clinical history and presentation including a family history of allergy; plus, skin-prick or patch testing to identify contact allergens (see above), or an elimination diet to identify food allergens.

Assays of serum IgE levels may indicate general atopic status and an assay of specific serum IgE antibodies (radioallergosorbent test [RAST]), if available, may confirm.

Anaemia

Deficiency of any of the vitamins and minerals essential for normal erythropoiesis (haematinics), including iron, copper, cobalt, vitamins A, B_{12}, B_6, C, E, folic acid, riboflavin and nicotinic acid, may be associated with defective erythropoiesis and eventually, a fall in haemoglobin (anaemia). Iron, vitamin B_{12} and folate are the haematinics for which deficiency states manifest most often clinically, sometimes even when haemoglobin levels are normal. Haematinics may be decreased due to dietary or gastrointestinal causes, or from increased losses (e.g. iron in chronic or severe haemorrhage).

Dietary sources of iron and B_{12} are largely animal, while folate is present in green vegetables. Vegans may lack B_{12}.

Normal gastric function is required for iron absorption (hydrochloric acid is needed) and for B_{12} absorption (intrinsic factor from gastric parietal cells is needed). These haematinics are absorbed in the small intestine, B_{12} mainly in the ileum. Diseases in those sites may cause deficiencies, as may some drugs.

Iron is stored in haemoglobin and B_{12} in the liver, but stores of folate are lacking. Thus, deficiencies take some months or years to manifest in patients with iron or B_{12} deficiencies.

Anaemia is caused mainly by:
- reduced erythropoiesis
- haemolysis
- haemorrhage.

The most common cause of anaemia in resource-rich groups is an iron deficiency caused by chronic haemorrhage (commonly menorrhagia). After a thorough history and examination, the following are required for the diagnosis of the extent and type of anaemia:
- haemoglobin concentration
- a full blood film (full blood count/full blood picture/complete blood count)
- red cell indices
- white cell count and differential
- levels of serum iron (ferritin), vitamin B_{12} and corrected whole blood folate.

Deficiency States and Anaemias

Once the type of deficiency or anaemia has been established, the cause must be found and treated.

In iron deficiency, unless it is clear that menorrhagia is the cause, the site of blood loss should be sought, usually in the gastrointestinal, or sometimes genitourinary, tract:
- Iron deficiency anaemia is usually microcytic (red cell mean corpuscular volume (MCV) is reduced) and managed by treatment of the cause, and oral iron supplements. Only rarely is blood transfusion necessary, usually when the haemoglobin is less than 9 g/dL and surgery is required urgently. Packed red cells should then be used in preference to blood.

- Folate or vitamin B_{12} deficiencies may result in a macrocytic (megaloblastic) anaemia (MCV raised).
- Folate deficiency is commonly dietary in origin. Treatment of folate deficiency is by treatment of the cause and with oral folic acid.
- Vitamin B_{12} deficiency is seen in vegans but otherwise is rarely dietary in origin; more commonly, it is caused by a gastrointestinal lesion or pernicious anaemia. Treatment is by treatment of the cause if possible and with vitamin B_{12}, usually by injection for life.
- Deficiencies of multiple haematinic factors, e.g. iron, folate and vitamin B_{12}, may well be caused by disease of the small intestine, such as coeliac disease (gluten-sensitive enteropathy).

Sickle Cell Anaemia

Sickle cell anaemia is the homozygous form of a hereditary condition affecting haemoglobin composition (sickle haemoglobin [HbS]) resulting in red blood cells adopting a sickle shape, especially in hypoxia. It is:
- found mainly in patients of African heritage and some originating from the Mediterranean countries and Asia
- a risk for general anaesthesia.

It is therefore important to rule out sickle cell anaemia in all black patients and record results to prevent unnecessary retesting:
- Check the medical history. In sickle cell anaemia, at low oxygen tensions (t45 mmHg), the erythrocytes become inelastic and sickle-shaped and then either 'sludge', blocking capillaries and causing infarcts (e.g. in bone and brain), or rupture, causing haemolytic anaemia.
- Do a full blood picture.
- Do a sickle screening blood test, such as a simple solubility test (e.g. the SickleDex test) which detects any HbS and is, therefore, positive both in patients with sickle cell anaemia and the sickle trait (see below).
- Further haematological examination, including haemoglobin electrophoresis, is theoretically required for confirmation. In practice, however, a positive solubility test with a low haemoglobin level can be taken as being diagnostic of sickle cell anaemia. A positive solubility test with a normal haemoglobin level may indicate the sickle cell trait (see below).

In the sickle trait, sickling occurs only at much lower oxygen tensions (<20 mmHg), which are unlikely to occur in normal clinical practice.

Bleeding Tendencies

A bleeding tendency can be caused mainly by a blood platelet defect (thrombocytopenia) or blood coagulation defect (anticoagulant drugs, haemophilia, von Willebrand disease). Screening tests typically include:
- platelet count
- function tests
- activated partial thromboplastin time (APTT)
- prothrombin time (PT) and INR — the ratio of the patient's PT to a control
- clotting factor assays.

Screening tests will eliminate two-thirds of suspected cases, and the remaining third will require more detailed tests to accurately define a diagnosis. Consult the haematologist immediately before undertaking other investigations; bleeding and clotting time assays are quite unsatisfactory, and special investigations may well be required, such as factor VIII clotting activity or related antigen assay.

Endocrine Disorders

Adrenocortical Function Testing

- Blood pressure: is low in hypoadrenocorticism (Addison disease), high in hyperadrenocorticism (Cushing disease).
- Plasma cortisol levels: the diurnal rhythm of plasma cortisol is a sensitive index of adrenal function; cortisol values are normally highest between 6.00 a.m. and 10.00 a.m. and lowest between midnight and 4.00 a.m. Samples taken at 8.00 a.m. and 4.00 p.m. should differ by at least 5 mg/100 mL. The sample taken at 8.00 a.m. should be 5 to 25 mg/100 mL. Plasma cortisol at 8.00 a.m. to 9.00 a.m. is often less than 6 mg/100 mL in hypoadrenocorticism. Diurnal variation in cortisol is lost in hyperadrenocorticism.
- Synacthen test (ACTH stimulation test): this is performed in the following way. Take blood at 8.00 a.m. to 9.00 a.m. for the plasma cortisol level; give 0.25 mg synacthen subcutaneously or intramuscularly; after 30 minutes, take a further blood sample for the cortisol level. Normally, synacthen results in a rise in cortisol levels to greater than 18 mg/100 mL. This rise is lost in hypoadrenocorticism (at an earlier stage in disease than the low cortisol level is found).
- Abdominal radiography: this may show calcified adrenals if tuberculosis is the cause of hypoadrenocorticism (but rarely used now).
- Serum autoantibodies: patients with Addison disease may have various circulating autoantibodies.
- Electrolytes: plasma potassium is raised, and sodium-reduced in Addison disease.

Diabetes

Diabetes is often detected at routine urinalysis by detecting glycosuria (and ketonuria), but there are other causes of glycosuria and ketonuria, and diabetics do not always have glycosuria. Diabetes is best diagnosed by testing for raised blood glucose above 11 mmol/L or fasting level over about 7 mmol/L usually establishes the diagnosis (plasma glucose levels are about 1 mmol/L higher). Haemoglobin A_{1c} (HbA$_{1c}$) is now the most popular and widely used biomarker for the diagnosis and monitoring of DM. HbA$_{1c}$ levels are directly related to blood glucose levels but have the advantage of less diurnal variation. Glucose tolerance testing is indicated only if blood sugar values are borderline. A widely accepted simplified glucose tolerance test (GTT) is as follows: give the patient 75 g glucose orally; assay blood glucose levels 2 hours later; a level greater than 11.1 mmol/L is diagnostic of diabetes; a level less than 11.1 mmol/L excludes diabetes.

Diabetic control is best by serial measurements of blood glucose levels throughout the day with a glucometer. Glycosylated haemoglobin or fructosamine are usually monitored regularly to assess longer-term control. Non-diabetics have up to 7% glycosylated haemoglobin: 7% to 9% represents good control, over 13% shows poor control in diabetes.

A small amount of ketonuria, as shown by an Acetest tablet test, is usually of no importance, but a strongly positive test, especially if confirmed by a positive ferric chloride reaction (Gerhardt's test), indicates a serious degree of ketosis. Confirmation is obtained by finding a low serum bicarbonate concentration.

Hyperparathyroidism

Blood for calcium levels should be collected early in the morning from a fasting patient and a tourniquet should not be used (venous stasis and a fall in pH alter calcium levels). The blood collection should be done along with serum for albumin assay (albumin levels influence calcium levels) and may need repeating several times to exclude hyperparathyroidism.

Granulomatous Disorders

Granulomatous disorders may present a difficult differential diagnosis, which can include Crohn disease, orofacial granulomatosis, sarcoidosis and tuberculosis. Investigations indicated may then include:
- lesional biopsy
- erythrocyte sedimentation rate (ESR) or C-reactive protein (CRP)
- serum angiotensin-converting enzyme (SACE)
- a tuberculin skin test
- interferon-gamma release assay from patient lymphocytes
- chest imaging
- gastrointestinal endoscopy, radiography and biopsy
- thiopurine methyltransferase or thiopurine S-methyltransferase (TPMT) if azathioprine immune suppressive therapy is being considered (see Chapter 4).

Immunodeficiency

Immune defects should be suspected if there are recurrent or persistent infections or other features such as neoplasms. Laboratory tests needed to confirm the diagnosis of immunodeficiency and to identify the type of disorder include:
- total white blood cell count, the percentages of each main type and CD4 count
- immunoglobulin levels. One in 300 people have a deficiency
- red blood cell count
- platelet count
- levels of complement proteins and C1 esterase inhibitor. Useful in angio-oedema
- Skin tests using candida or other antigens may be done if the immunodeficiency is thought to be due to a T-cell abnormality.

Inflammatory Diseases

- Glucose-6-phosphate dehydrogenase (G6PD) deficiency is an inborn error of metabolism that is predisposed to red blood cell breakdown, especially in the face of infection or inflammation
- Faecal calprotectin: elevated levels indicate the migration of neutrophils to the intestinal mucosa, which occurs during intestinal inflammation. May eliminate the need for invasive colonoscopy.
- Zinc: deficiency can manifest as non-specific oral ulceration or stomatitis, Rarely it can cause angular cheilitis or loss of taste

Sexually Shared Infections

Human Immunodeficiency Viruses

Diagnosis of acute human immunodeficiency viruses (HIV) disease is from other causes of glandular fever syndromes (Table 3.9) and diagnosis of HIV infection in any event includes:

- clinical features (see Chapter 53)
- lymphopenia
- a severe T-helper lymphocyte defect (reduced CD4$^+$ cells and CD4:CD8 ratio)
- ideally, HIV antibody *and* p24 antigen are tested simultaneously (after counselling)
- HIV-RNA quantitative assays (viral load tests)
- Confirmatory assays are then required to confirm HIV antibody and antigen/RNA.

Syphilis

Dark ground/darkfield (DGM) of a lesion may demonstrate *Treponema pallidum* in lesion exudate or lymph nodes but is not reliable for examining oral lesions where contamination with commensal treponemes is likely. Test material from oral lesions submitted on dry swabs using the polymerase chain reaction (PCR).

Serology is indicated; a *T. pallidum* enzyme immunoassay (EIA) which detects both IgG and IgM, is recommended. The *T. pallidum* particle assay (TPPA) is preferred to the *T. pallidum* haemagglutination assay (TPHA) and is used in combination with a cardiolipin antigen/reagin test such as VDRL (Venereal Disease Research Laboratory) or RPR (rapid plasma reagin) to maximise the detection of primary infections. An EIA IgM test should be performed in addition to these routine screening tests since IgM becomes detectable in the serum 2 to 3 weeks after infection and IgG 4 to 5 weeks after infection. An additional test, such as immunoblotting based on recombinant antigens or the fluorescent antibody absorbed (FTA-abs) test, can be used in the case of a discrepancy between the EIA and TPPA. An EIA for anti-treponemal IgM should be performed on all sera reactive in one or more of the screening tests. Quantitative VDRL/RPR tests should then be performed before therapy.

Always exclude other sexually shared infections.

Gonorrhoea

Gonococcal pharyngitis may be seen, particularly in men who have sex with men. Always exclude other sexually shared infections. Microscopy, a direct smear for Gram-staining (Gram-negative diplococci), while useful for other sites, is not suitable for oral or pharyngeal specimens where many other bacteria are present including Gram-negative cocci of other genera. Take a bacteriological swab from the area, for culture and sensitivities. Direct plating of the specimen and the use of transport swabs both give acceptable results. Transport swabs should be stored in the refrigerator at 4°C and transported to the laboratory as soon as possible, preferably within 48 hours. Tests that probe or amplify specific nucleic acid sequences (nucleic acid amplification tests (NAATs)) have the ability to detect small amounts of nucleic acid and can detect non-viable organisms. They may have increased sensitivity (>90%) compared with cultures (<60%) but cultures provide viable organisms for susceptibility testing.

Hepatitis Viruses B and C

Seroconversion for virus antibody may take 3 months so antibody tests may give false-negative results when a patient presents with acute hepatitis.

Hepatitis B virus (HBV) testing is for hepatitis B surface antigen (HB$_s$Ag) and IgM anti-HBc antibody. If HB$_s$Ag-positive, proceed to hepatitis B 'e' antigen (HB$_e$Ag) and antibody (HB$_e$Ab) testing. About one in five are HB$_e$Ag positive and at high risk of infectivity. Those who have HB$_s$Ag should later be screened again at 3 months, and again if still positive. Those positive at 9 months are 'chronic carriers'. Assays for anti-HBc and HB$_s$Ag in saliva samples have been used for surveillance and research but are not available for diagnostic use.

Hepatitis C virus (HCV) testing includes ELISA for serum anti-HCV or other immunoassays (e.g. chemiluminescence). Tests to confirm a positive result include a recombinant immunoblot assay (RIBA), using another ELISA, or proceeding directly to an assay for HCV-RNA by reverse-transcriptase

TABLE 3.9 Glandular Syndromes

Syndrome	Causal Agents	Investigations
Infectious mononucleosis (classic glandular fever)	Epstein–Barr virus (EBV)	Paul–Bunnell test (heterophile antibodies) EBV antibodies
EBV-negative glandular fever	Cytomegalovirus (CMV)	CMV antibodies
Acute HIV seroconversion	Human immune deficiency viruses (HIV)	HIV antibody and antigen T4 (CD4) cell depletion
Erythema subtilum	Human herpes 6 virus	HHV-6 antibodies
Toxoplasmosis	*Toxoplasma gondii*	Sabin–Feldman dye test — specific IgM antibodies
COVID-19	*SARS-CoV2*	Reverse-transcriptase polymerase chain reaction (RT-PCR) for antigen Lateral flow for antigen ELISA for antibodies

polymerase chain reaction (RT-PCR) or another genome amplification assay.

COMMUNICATING THE DIAGNOSIS

Communicating a diagnosis is the act of 'communicating to the individual (or his/her personal representative) a diagnosis identifying a disease or disorder as the cause of symptoms of the individual in circumstances in which it is reasonably foreseeable that the individual or his/her personal representative will rely on the diagnosis, including to decide whether to agree to any intervention recommended'.

Clinicians should reassure the patient where possible, and:
- Communicate assessment findings and ensure that the information is understood by the patient or appropriate substitute decision-maker.
- Communicate further information about their disease or diagnosis as appropriate, or if requested.
- Follow their ethical and professional responsibility to refer the patient to another appropriate HCP if this is likely to be in the patient's best interests.

COMMUNICATING RISK

People with high-risk behaviours such as tobacco, alcohol or recreational drug use should not only be encouraged to change these behaviours but also to understand the need for vigilance and follow-up. Personalised communications (especially when supported by written and visual materials) are the most effective in promoting screening uptake.

COMMUNICATING A DIAGNOSIS OF A POTENTIALLY LETHAL CONDITION

While a diagnosis of a potentially lethal condition may not be unexpected to the patient, it cannot fail to be distressing to them and their families. Patients tend to recall only a little of the information that they are given, and so at the initial diagnosis, the focus should be on stating the news and dealing with the initial emotional responses. Breaking bad news is difficult both for the patient and also the clinician, and the key principles are:
- Preparing: provide a conducive environment, making sure there is sufficient time, privacy and confidentiality as these factors are important, so minimise non-essential people in the room unless the patient needs or wants family, friends or an interpreter present.
- Communicating the news.
- State the news.
- Elicit the response of the patient or carer or family member.
- Deal tactfully with emotional responses.

Communicating bad news, especially across a language and/or cultural barrier can be difficult, time-consuming and frustrating. At the very least, most patients will feel intimidated. It is important, therefore, to (if relevant):
- ask the patient about their preferred language

- never assume agreement or fluency until you are sure from the patient feedback
- remember that even those with a good grasp of the language may well not understand medical or dental terminology. Explain as you proceed
- use direct eye contact, and speak slowly and clearly, using uncomplicated terminology, remembering also that some individuals have hearing impairment
- remember that head-nodding and smiles do not necessarily indicate understanding or agreement. Ask questions to ascertain understanding, not just enquiries with a 'yes' or 'no' answer. Silence can have many meanings and sometimes indicates a lack of agreement
- establish if there is a spokesperson for the patient and the patient's confidence in that person, and what the patient wishes the clinician to impart
- always offer the patient an opportunity to ask questions.

ENSURING FOLLOW-UP

- Arrange a follow-up meeting or discussion by telephone within 1 or 2 days.
- Arrange to meet the patient and carer or family member again.
- Discuss and review the situation with the healthcare team, both in terms of impact on them and whether communications could have been improved.

EXAMPLE OF A PATIENT INFORMATION SHEET

A Biopsy
- A biopsy is the taking of a small piece of tissue for microscopic examination.
- This is usually carried out after a local anaesthetic injection in the area, such as used for fillings.
- A biopsy is painless, though maybe a little sore when the injection wears off after a couple of hours.
- Stitches may be used.
- Stitches may be resorbable or need to be removed in the next week. It is usually not a problem if the stitches come out themselves earlier than 1 week.

Possible Complications
- bleeding: pressure for 5–10 min from a gauze swab will almost invariably stop the bleeding
- soreness or pain: paracetamol will usually control any discomfort; aspirin should not be used as it can cause bleeding
- swelling: this should subside spontaneously over 3–4 days
- bruising: this should clear spontaneously over 4–5 days.

There are usually no long-term consequences. Any scar is usually almost invisible, any discomfort goes quickly and any slight numbness recovers. Rarely there may be:
- altered sensation
- restricted mouth opening
- reactions to drugs
- allergies
- local infection.

If you are at all concerned, for advice kindly telephone ....

RECOMMENDED READING

Glick, M., 2006. Informed consent: a delicate balance. J. Am. Dent. Assoc. 137 (8), 1060–1064.

Ni Riordain, R., Meaney, S., McCreary, C., 2011. A patient-centered approach to developing a quality-of-life questionnaire for chronic oral mucosal diseases. Oral. Surg. Oral. Med. Oral. Pathol. Oral. Radiol. Endod. 111 (5), 578–586, 586.e1–586.e2.

Wiriyakijja, P., Porter, S., Fedele, S., et al., 2020. Meaningful improvement thresholds in measures of pain and quality of life in oral lichen planus. Oral. Dis. 26 (7), 1464–1473.

Principles of Treatment

Optimal treatment necessitates an accurate diagnosis (itself the result of history, examination and appropriate investigations), an assessment of disease severity and a review of responses to treatment. Our aim should be to treat every patient as we would wish our families, or ourselves, to be treated.

INTRODUCTION

Many of the conditions seen in oral and maxillofacial medicine practice have systemic manifestations, or they may be seen in patients with medical problems. It is crucial, therefore, always to collaborate closely with the medical and any other attendants in the care of the patient, as well as fully discussing issues with the patient. Clinical risk management concedes that there is an inherent risk in all healthcare processes including treatments. This must be discussed with the patient, and informed consent obtained. Risk management should be considered before starting, during and after treatment. Good communication skills are needed to allow clinicians to show empathy and to provide disclosure. Risk management after an adverse reaction includes skills in acknowledging bad outcomes or errors and the freedom to say 'sorry'.

Some patients have conditions that are amenable to care in a primary care setting, or shared care with a specialist, but those patients who have severe disease, multisystem disease or who require very sophisticated investigations, medications (see Chapter 5) or therapies are best managed by a specialist and often more than one medical/surgical specialist. Indeed, some orofacial conditions involve not only the mouth but also other mucosae (anogenital, ocular, pharyngeal, etc.), skin, other organs, mental health issues or complex hospital-based therapies such as medical oncology, and so multi-disciplinary teams can often offer optimal healthcare.

EVIDENCE-BASED MEDICINE AND TREATMENT

Few treatments available for patients with oral and maxillo-facial medical problems have yet been rigorously studied in the disorders in question. The evidence base that guides the use of therapeutic agents in these conditions is, therefore, very limited. Ethically, this presents a complex challenge. It is difficult to decline care for a patient on the basis that there is no evidence base. Rather, it is essential to offer treatment to patients, and this is clearly the case even where the evidence base is limited, but clinicians must be aware of the danger of inappropriate or over-treatment. There is thus a responsibility of every clinician in oral medicine to contribute to the evidence base of their treatment. The practical aspects can be assured by disease severity scoring before and after every treatment for every patient, and the wellbeing of each patient can be assessed before and after treatment by a quality-of-life assessment.

Oral Disease Severity Scoring

Until relatively recently, there had been a lack of any method to routinely assess disease severity and thus of quantifying responses to therapies. Fortunately, tools such as the Oral Disease Severity Score (ODSS), (see Chapter 2) have been created and validated for use in nearly all of the common oral mucosal diseases including recurrent aphthous stomatitis, lichen planus, pemphigus, mucous membrane pemphigoid, orofacial granulomatosis and for dry mouth assessment. They appear to be objective, reproducible, easy to use and widely applicable.

The benefits of a scoring system for mucosal disease severity are that they:
- can indicate the severity of disease
- are needed to indicate the efficacy of any treatments
- may distinguish between or reveal subgroups of activity
- may assist in deciding to implement or withhold treatment
- are a routine clinical audit tool that can also be used for research.

Quality of Life Assessment

Quality of life (QoL) is a concept encompassing many aspects, not only wealth, employment and housing, but also physical and mental health, recreation, leisure, and social belonging and in healthcare, QoL is often seen in terms of how it is negatively affected, on an individual level, in a chronic debilitating illness such as cancer. Health-related quality of life (HRQoL) is a subset of QoL, involving:
- physical functioning
- psychological functioning
- social interaction and disease
- treatment-related symptoms.

Just as the ODSS provides the clinician with a semi-objective measurement of disease responses to treatment, patient-reported outcome measures (PROMS) allow the patients to offer their own assessment of the success, or otherwise, of treatment. Applying one of the health-related questionnaires before and after treatment will provide a patient-based evidence of outcomes to supplement ODSS.

QoL can be assessed by interview or patient-completed 'instruments' (questionnaires) which include the:
- Visual Analogue Scale (VAS)
- Hospital Anxiety and Depression Scale (HADS)
- Short-form McGill Pain Questionnaire (SFMPQ)
- Health-related QoL Questionnaire (HRQoL)
- Oral Health Impact Profile (OHIP-14)
- Medical Outcome Study 36-Item Short-form (SF-36)
- Chronic Oral Mucosal Diseases Questionnaire (COMDQ)
- Behçet Syndrome Activity Score (BSAS)
- EULAR Sjögren's Syndrome Patient Reported Index (ESSPRI)

PSYCHOLOGICAL AND SOCIOLOGICAL ASPECTS OF TREATMENT

Treatment is much more than the simple use of a drug or the performance of a procedure; a holistic approach involving the whole psychology of the patient is important. Remember always that patients know whether the clinician cares, well before they care whether the clinician knows all the answers. Anxiety and depression are two common conditions to be addressed.

A range of questionnaire measures of anxiety exists. A particularly useful one is the Generalised Anxiety Disorder Assessment (GAD-7). The GAD-7 is easy and quick to complete and gives a score in the range of 0 to 21, with higher scores indicating higher levels of anxiety.

Many oral medicine patients have chronic conditions that can be difficult to live with and can be associated with distress and depression. These include pain, fatigue and altered facial appearance. It is estimated that at any one time, approximately 7% of the population will be experiencing marked symptoms of depression. The HADS is one of the most widely used tools to assess and monitor symptoms of anxiety and depression. The HADS questionnaire has seven items each for anxiety and depression subscales. Scoring for each item ranges from 0 to 3, with 3 representing the highest level of anxiety or depression. Scores range from 0 to 21. A total subscale score of greater than 8 points denotes symptoms of anxiety or depression. Another useful way of assessing depression is the Patient Health Questionnaire (PHQ-9), which assesses nine diagnostic features. It takes only a few minutes for the patient to self-complete. Scores range from 0 to 27, with higher scores indicating greater severity of depressive symptoms (and need for referral and possible Cognitive Behavioural Therapy).

Many orofacial conditions are chronic and have no cure, and for a few disorders, the prognosis is poor or, fortunately rarely, the condition may even be lethal. Therefore, compassion and patient education and participation are important. Empowering patients allows them to take control of their lives and decisions affecting their wellbeing. Such education and reassurance are always helpful; a supportive and understanding clinician is invariably welcomed by the patient, their partner and family.

It is thus important to:
- do no harm
- manage the patient as a whole, but in the context of their individual perceptions, aspirations, general health and social setting
- offer hope — not all conditions can be cured, but most can be controlled or at least ameliorated. General improvements in oral and systemic health also help control symptoms in several other orofacial disorders
- work with the patient and family and involve the patient in all decisions. Discuss the condition, diagnosis and possible therapies with the patient (and possibly partner and family, provided the patient consents)
- warn of possible consequences (good and bad) of treatment or no treatment

- obtain express informed consent before any invasive procedure
- offer advice on what patients themselves can do for their problems, including support from family, partners and friends, as well as care groups.

PROVIDING INFORMATION ABOUT TREATMENT

Information about financial issues and the impact of treatment on the ability to work, function physically, relationships and QoL, support from other bodies (e.g. alcohol, smoking or other drug support groups), disease support groups (e.g. cancer help groups or the pemphigus support groups, Sjögren Syndrome Society, etc.) or other information sources (e.g. patient information sheets, the internet) can be helpful. Many drugs used for oral conditions are used 'off-label' and this must be understood by, and agreed with, the patient (Chapter 5).

LIFESTYLE CHANGES

There is no doubt that certain lifestyle habits, such as the use of tobacco products, areca nut products, recreational drugs and alcoholic beverages, should be discouraged, especially in patients with oral mucosal diseases. Linkage of habits with an oral mucosal condition may provide an incentive to change. Indeed, sometimes, the cessation of these habits may lead to the resolution of the condition. Diet and/or oral hygiene may also benefit from improvement.

PREVENTIVE CARE

Dental Bacterial Plaque Control

Dental staff should ensure the patient has appropriate oral health education, and maintains particularly good oral hygiene since the limited evidence available suggests that good plaque control helps the resolution of some mucosal lesions as well as gingivitis.

The most important devices in oral hygiene are floss and a toothbrush; many are effective but:
- soft toothbrushes and silica-based toothpaste are the least abrasive
- powered toothbrushes may assist oral hygiene, especially in those with impaired manual dexterity
- interspace and other toothbrushes can access areas difficult to clean.

Toothpastes are available that offer tooth whitening, plaque control, desensitisation, calculus (tartar) control, tooth remineralisation and malodour control, and some combine all facets (Table 4.1).

Antiplaque mouthwashes are commonly used to reduce infection and minimise malodours, particularly if the patient is immunocompromised. Many mouthwashes have only a transient antiseptic activity (Table 4.2), but:
- Chlorhexidine digluconate is the most widely used antiplaque agent and is active, especially against Gram-negative rods,

it helps control plaque and periodontal disease and has some anticaries and antifungal activity. It has good substantivity (ability to bind to hard and soft tissues and be released over a long period) but binds tannins and thus can cause dental staining if the patient drinks coffee, tea or red wine. Rarely, it causes other adverse effects, including:
- overgrowth of enterobacteria (e.g. in leukaemic patients)
- mucosal desquamation
- hypersensitivity or anaphylaxis
- salivary gland pain or swelling.
- Triclosan is a chlorinated bisphenol with some substantivity and a broad spectrum of antibacterial activity, and a significant antiplaque effect, without staining the teeth.
- Cetyl pyridinium chloride is a newer mouthwash ingredient that has powerful anti-microbial activity, including anti-viral and is found in several commercial products
- Phenolics, such as Listerine, have some antiplaque effect and do not stain teeth, but have low substantivity.
- Oxygenating mouthwashes may have a place in the control of anaerobic infections, such as necrotising gingivitis.
- Sanguinarine is marketed for activity against bacterial plaque and malodour, but with low activity in these respects.

Caries Prevention

A diet of low cariogenicity is important (see below). Fluoride is also helpful for anti-cariogenic activity, especially useful for patients with hyposalivation (Table 4.3). Fluorides may be usefully applied in dental surgery, and daily at home (1% sodium fluoride gels or 0.4% stannous fluoride gels). Young children may need fluoride supplements if their water supply has a low fluoride content. Amorphous calcium phosphate (ACP) may also help. Chewing gum may stimulate salivation and help caries prevention and reduce malodour.

Diet

A healthy balanced diet is indicated to help the maintenance of oral health and resolution of oral conditions. In particular:
- Many mucosal lesions are aggravated by irritants, such as tobacco and alcohol, and these also decrease salivary flow and should thus be avoided.
- A softish diet, avoiding toast and potato crisps, spices and acids, such as in tomatoes and citric fruits and drinks, may be indicated whilst a patient has a sore mouth. Foods that can be eaten, however, include:
  - milk and other dairy products, low-fat only
  - cooked, canned or frozen vegetables
  - cooked or canned fruit with the skin and seeds removed, such as apple sauce or canned peaches
  - refined hot cereals, such as oatmeal and cream of wheat
  - lean, tender meats, such as poultry, whitefish and shellfish that are steamed, baked or grilled
  - pudding and custard
  - eggs.

TABLE 4.1   Active Principles in Toothpastes (Dentifrices)

Anticaries	Antibacterials	Anti-Hypersensitivity	Anti-Tartar	Whiteners	Anti-Malodour	Others
Amine fluorides	Chlorhexidine	Formaldehyde	Azocycloheptane diphosphonate	Benzalkonium chloride	Chlorhexidine	Enoxolone
Calcium phosphate	Fluorides	Potassium citrate	Gantrez acid (polyvinyl methyl ether and maleic acid copolymer)	Calcium carbonate	Triclosan	Essential oils
Calcium pyrophosphate	Hexetidine	Potassium chloride		Calcium phosphates	Zinc chloride	Keratin
Calcium trimetaphosphate	Hydrogen peroxide	Potassium nitrate		Carboxymethyl cellulose	Zinc citrate	Panthenol
Nicomethanol fluorhydrate	Plant extracts	Sodium citrate	Potassium pyrophosphate	Citroxaine		Permethol
Potassium fluoride	Potassium peroxydiphosphate	Sodium fluoride	Zinc chloride	Pentasodium triphosphate		Provitamin B_5
Sodium fluoride (NaF)	Sanguinarine	Stannous fluoride	Zinc citrate	Potassium tetra pyrophosphate		Tocopherol
1450–1500 ppm (<600 ppm in child paste)	Siliglycol	Strontium chloride hexahydrate		Sodium benzoate		Vitamin E
Sodium monofluorophosphate (Na_2FPO_3)	Sodium bicarbonate	Strontium fluoride		Sodium bicarbonate		
Stannous fluoride	Stannous pyrophosphate			Sodium tripolyphosphate		
Xylitol	Triclosan					
	Urea peroxide					
	Xylitol					
	Zinc chloride					
	Zinc citrate					
	Zinc trihydrate					

TABLE 4.2 Examples of Mouthwashes With Significant Antimicrobial Activity

Agent	Dose	Comments[a]
Chlorhexidine gluconate	0.12%—0.2% aqueous mouthwash, rinse for 1 min twice daily. Also 0.5%—1.0% gel or spray	A cationic chlorinated bisbiguanide with significant antiplaque, antiviral and antifungal activity and oral retention; traces can still be found in saliva after 24 h May stain teeth or tissues if the patient drinks tea, coffee or red wine
Triclosan	0.03% mouthwash, rinse for 1 min twice daily	A non-ionic chlorinated bisphenolic antiseptic with moderate antiplaque and antifungal activity, but less retention in the mouth than chlorhexidine More effective against plaque when with copolymer or zinc citrate
Povidone iodine	0.5%—1% mouthwash used twice daily	Significant antiplaque, antifungal and antiviral activity (including SARS-CoV2). Should be used for up to 2 weeks at a time. Avoid iodine sensitivity
Cetylpyridinium chloride	0.05% mouthwash used twice daily	A quaternary ammonium compound with antiplaque activity, but less than chlorhexidine. Significant antiviral activity (including SARS-CoV2) May stain teeth and cause an oral burning sensation
Hydrogen peroxide	1.5% mouthwash used twice daily up to 1 week	Several commercial preparations. Effervescent in contact with organic tissue. Antibacterial, especially anaerobes

[a]All occasionally may cause mucosal irritation.

TABLE 4.3 Example Regime for Caries Prevention

Eliminate Active Caries	Restorative Dental Care
Preventive measures	Patient education Dietary modification Fluorides: 1.23% acidulated fluoride or 2% neutral fluoride gels in 4-min tray applications 4 times daily over 4 weeks; or home fluoride applications by gels or rinses Amorphous calcium phosphate (ACP) Xylitol chewing gum; chew for 5 min 5 times daily Chlorhexidine mouthwashes; 0.2% used twice daily for 1 min
Examine at 6 monthly recall appointments	Reinforce preventive message Monitor restorations Monitor cariogenic micro-organisms (*Streptococcus mutans* testing)

TABLE 4.4 Topical Agents That May Help Reduce Pain From Mucosal Lesions

Agent	Use
Benzydamine hydrochloride	Rinse or spray every 1.5—3 h
Lidocaine	Topical solution or gel may ease pain
Carboxymethyl cellulose	Paste or powder used after meals to protect area
Benzocaine	Lozenges, sucked twice-hourly Spray 5% four hourly

In persons with dry mouth, pureed non-irritant foods and cool moist fruits, such as melon, are helpful, and patients should consider:
- Eating a soft, high protein moist diet.
- Substituting moist fish, eggs or cheese for red meat.
- Taking food and drinks lukewarm rather than hot.
- Soaking bread and/or rolls in milk or sauces.
- Eating moistened casseroles and meats with gravies, sauces, soups and stews.
- Blending food and drink.
- Eating yoghurt, fresh fruit, powdered milk, soy milk, rice milk.
- Eating fruit smoothies/slushies.
- Drinking milkshakes.
- Avoiding dry foods (bread, dry meat, pastries, toast and crackers, snack foods that are dry and salty).
- Avoiding citric foods, juices such as tomato, orange, grapefruit-based products and sauces.
- Avoiding fizzy sodas and sparkling water.
- Although vitamin and iron deficiencies are not common, supplements may be required if the diet is lacking.

Symptomatic Care

Specific therapies are not available for all conditions, and the best that can then be offered is the control of symptoms; this is called symptomatic treatment. Attention should be directed to relieving the following (Table 4.4):
- Pain and discomfort: antipyretics/analgesics, such as paracetamol, help relieve pain and a soft diet may help. In mucositis, potent analgesics such as opioids or buprenorphine may be indicated (see Chapters 5 and 41). Erosive or ulcerative lesions can be protected with muco-adhesives such as Orabase. Soft diet and topical agents, such as topical local anaesthetics (e.g. lidocaine) or 0.15% benzydamine mouth rinse or spray, may help symptomatically. Benzocaine is generally well tolerated and non-toxic when applied topically as recommended except in young children.
- Fever: paracetamol helps relieve fever and adequate fluid intake is important.
- Malodour (Chapter 17).
- Anxiety: patient information is an important aspect of management and goes a long way to relieve anxiety, but there may need to be reassurance, and sometimes recourse to mild anxiolytics, such as diazepam 2.5 mg or temazepam 5 mg.

Surgery

This can range from the simple excision of a lump such as a papilloma, to removal of a tooth, or resection of a malignant neoplasm. Referral to a surgeon may be indicated.

- All surgery is invasive.
- Scalpel, laser or electrosurgery are widely available.
- Only an operator adequately skilled in a procedure should perform it.

Other Less-Invasive or Non-Invasive Treatments

These include:
- cryotherapy
- soft laser therapy
- photodynamic therapy (PDT)
- appliances (e.g. splints, tissue conditioning).

DRUG TREATMENT AND INTERACTIONS

In the UK, registered dentists are legally entitled to prescribe from the entirety of the *British National Formulary* (BNF) and *BNF for Children* (BNFC), but within the National Health Service (NHS) dental prescribing is restricted to those drugs contained within the 'List of Dental Preparations' in the *Dental Practitioners Formulary* (DPF). The National Prescriptions Centre offers guidance (www.npc.co.uk).

The BNF, published by the British Medical Association and the Royal Pharmaceutical Society of Great Britain, includes the DPF and is a valuable source of information and advice on therapy. The BNF is revised twice yearly, and only the current issue should be consulted; it is available on the internet and as a mobile phone app. The BNFC is also available online or as part of the BNF app and can help with dose adjustments in children.

Drugs do not necessarily have predictable effects: patients vary in their responses by virtue of various intrinsic or extrinsic factors (Table 4.5).

Also, always remember the following:
- Avoid any drug if the patient is allergic or intolerant to it.
- Use the safest drugs; virtually all drugs can have some adverse effects.
- Use only drugs with which you are totally familiar and use their generic (non-proprietary) drug names.
- Check that the prescription is legible, the drug doses, contra-indications, interactions and adverse reactions.
- Warn the patient of and discuss possible adverse effects or interactions.
- Reduce drug doses for children, older patients and those suffering from liver or kidney disease.
- Consider the possibility of altered drug metabolism. For example:
- Han Chinese or other Asians with the HLA allele B*1502 may develop Stevens-Johnson syndrome (Chapter 29) and toxic epidermal necrolysis (Chapter 29) after exposure to carbamazepine or phenytoin
- Thiopurine methyltransferase or thiopurine S-methyltransferase (TPMT) is an enzyme that metabolises thiopurines such as

TABLE 4.5 Some Factors Influencing Drug Responses	
Intrinsic	**Extrinsic**
Genetic	Alcohol
Absorption	Climate
Distribution	Culture
Metabolism	Diet
Excretion	Drug compliance
Body weight	Smoking
Enzyme polymorphisms	Stress
Height	Sunlight exposure
Race	
Gender	
Physiological	
Body weight	
Age	
Cardiovascular function	
Diseases	
Height	
Renal function	
Liver function	

azathioprine and 6-mercaptopurine (6MP). Patients who may need these drugs should first have their TMPT activity assayed as patients with low activity (3% prevalence) or absent activity (prevalence 0.3%) are at a heightened risk of drug-induced bone marrow failure.

- The cytochrome P450 system of enzymes (CYP isoenzymes) in the gastrointestinal mucosa and liver metabolises many drugs, and various isoenzymes metabolise drugs by oxidation, typically reducing their effect. CYP isoenzymes may have different activities between individuals and ethnic groups; this increases, for example, the activity of some anxiolytics such as diazepam (up to 6% of Whites, but up to 23% of Asians are sensitive to diazepam). Antidepressants and analgesics may also be affected. Alcohol and smoking can affect CYP.
  - Some drugs, for example, erythromycin, inhibit CYP leading to the reduced ability to metabolise drugs, such as ciclosporin.
  - Grapefruit juice and Seville oranges contain flavonoids that can inhibit CYP and thus increase the activity of, for example, ciclosporin and some protease inhibitors.
  - Some over-the-counter (OTC) herbal preparations, such as St. John's Wort, can induce CYP; they can thus reduce the effect of protease inhibitors, antidepressants, warfarin, anticonvulsants and the contraceptive pill:
    - —CYP2C9 influences phenytoin and warfarin effects
    - —CYP2C19 effects diazepam and citalopram
    - —CYP2D6 effects codeine.
- Avoid drug use in pregnancy and breastfeeding, where possible.
- Avoid aspirin for children under 12 years of age, because of the risk of Reye syndrome (Chapter 54), for patients with cardiac failure, those with peptic ulcers, or those with

bleeding tendencies such as haemophilia or thrombocytopenia and in those taking anticoagulant drugs, since it exacerbates bleeding.

- Avoid NSAIDs in patients with cardiac failure, those with peptic ulcers, or those with bleeding tendencies such as haemophilia or thrombocytopenia and in those taking anticoagulant drugs, since they exacerbate bleeding.
- Avoid metronidazole, azole antifungals and some other antimicrobials in patients on warfarin, since they displace it from plasma proteins and increase bleeding.
- Avoid itraconazole in cardiac failure, as it can exacerbate it.
- Avoid tetracyclines in children under 8 years, pregnancy or breastfeeding, as they can cause tooth discolouration.
- Avoid macrolides (azithromycin, clarithromycin, erythromycin) in people with cardiac disease, as they can cause arrhythmias.
- Avoid intramuscular (i.m.) injections in patients with bleeding tendencies, such as haemophilia or thrombocytopenia, and in those taking anticoagulant drugs, as haematomas can result, and take care with surgery.
- Take care if surgery will involve bone in patients who have been on bisphosphonates, as osteochemonecrosis can result, or in patients who have been irradiated in the head and necks (osteoradionecrosis can arise).

Prescribing for Children

- Doses of all drugs are much lower for children than for adults; always check against the recommended dose per unit body weight and age.
- Some drugs are contraindicated (e.g. tetracyclines are contraindicated under the age of 7 to 8 years; also, aspirin is contraindicated in all children under 12 years old) (Table 4.6).
- Oral preparations are invariably preferable to injectable drugs.

Prescribing in Pregnancy and During Breastfeeding

Because of the danger of damage to the foetus, all drugs should be avoided in pregnancy, during breastfeeding, or where pregnancy is possible, unless their use is essential. In particular, avoid tetracyclines, which stain teeth, and retinoids and thalidomide, which are teratogenic. The prescriber, patient and pharmacy must comply with regulations in terms of thalidomide.

Prescribing for the Older Patient

- A number of drugs should be avoided for the older patient (Box 4.1), notably many drugs affecting the CNS and some NSAIDs.
- Lower drug doses are almost invariably indicated because even in apparently healthy older people, there are changes in body water: fat ratios, and reduced liver and kidney drug clearance, along with increased sensitivity to many drugs. Particular care should be taken when there is the possibility of renal or hepatic dysfunction; this will necessitate substantially reduced drug doses.
- Compliance may be poor.

TABLE 4.6 Drugs to Use With Caution or Avoid in Children

Drug to Avoid	Comments
Aspirin	May cause Reye syndrome in <12 years old
Benzocaine	Avoid in children <12 years old,
Ciprofloxacin	Musculoskeletal damage
Diazepam	Paradoxical reactions
Ibuprofen	Gastrointestinal bleeding; cardiac damage
Nasal decongestants	Tachyphylaxis
Promethazine	Paradoxical reactions in <2 years old
Sugar-containing medications	May cause caries/obesity
Tetracyclines	Tooth staining in <8 years old

BOX 4.1 Drugs to Avoid in Older Patients (Beers Criteria: Age, Other Medications, Comorbidities, etc.)

- Amitriptyline
- Benzodiazepines
- Chlorpheniramine
- Doxepin
- Imipramine
- Indometacin
- Meperidine
- Naproxen
- Piroxicam
- Pentazocine
- Promethazine
- Propoxyphene

Drugs and Food Absorption

Most oral drugs are best given with or after food. However, oral drugs that should be given at least 30 minutes before food, since their absorption is otherwise delayed, include:
- aspirin
- erythromycin
- paracetamol
- penicillins (including ampicillin and amoxicillin)
- rifampicin
- tetracyclines (except doxycycline).

Grapefruit juice disturbs the absorption and metabolism of some drugs and, therefore, should be avoided by persons taking:
- ciclosporin
- calcium channel blockers (e.g. nifedipine)
- terfenadine.

Prescribing in Different Cultures

Some key concerns for different groups of patients are set out in Table 4.7.

TABLE 4.7   Main Concerns About Drugs and Healthcare Products for Certain Demographic Groups of Patients

Groups	Main Concerns
Buddhist	Animal and genetically modified (GM) products
Catholics	GM derivatives and those developed by foetal experimentation
Jehovah's Witnesses	Not able to accept food and products that may contain blood or blood derivatives
Hindus	Gelatin-containing products, animal products and alcohol
Jains	Strict vegetarians but will not eat root vegetables. Some patients, particularly those who follow vegan or vegetarian diets, may object to the use of animals to meet the needs of humans
Muslims	Porcine and bovine derivatives, alcohol, non-Halal animal derivatives, E-numbers derived from porcine products, and emulsifiers derived from animals
Jews	Products derived not only from pork, but also from any animal that had not been slaughtered according to Jewish law (Kosher). Devout Jews may wish to avoid alcohol
Sikhs	Beef and its derivatives

Use of healthcare products and consumables produced through the exploitation of animals, if production has involved cruelty to animals or animal research, or exploitation of resource-poor or otherwise disadvantaged people may upset some people. From Scully, C., Wilson, N., 2005. Culturally Sensitive Oral Healthcare. Quintessence Publications, London.

Alcohol (ethanol) is used widely in pharmaceutical formulations as an antimicrobial preservative or as a solvent and may be unacceptable to Muslims and some other patients.

Gelatin is made of protein derived from animal bones, cartilage, tendons and other tissues, such as pigskin. The other most commonly used agents of animal derivation are insulin, heparin and haemostatic agents, such as blood coagulation factors and topical agents. Such products may be contraindicated for use on religious or cultural grounds.

Some artificial saliva preparations contain animal mucin, which may be unacceptable on religious grounds to some Muslims, Hindus, Jews and Rastafarians. Products containing carboxymethyl cellulose may then be preferred.

Most oral healthcare products are licensed only as 'cosmetics', which are less rigorously tested than pharmacological products, although they must still be labelled with all active and inactive ingredients. Toothpastes fall into this category. Some oral healthcare products are licensed as pharmacological products and because they must be labelled with all ingredients — active and inactive — this readily affords the opportunity to avoid certain religious and ethnic group restrictions. Some mouthwashes contain colourants or excipients that may be animal derivatives and many contain alcohol, which may raise objections on religious grounds, although the objections are not always well-founded, when the religious rules are consulted. Some toothpastes may contain 'glycerine', manufactured synthetically or derived from animal fat, and this may not be included in the ingredients. Oral healthcare products that might contain animal derivatives could include some:

- analgesics
- antimicrobials
- bone fillers
- colourants
- drug capsules
- emulsifiers
- haemostatic materials
- polishing (bristle) brushes
- prophylaxis pastes
- toothpastes
- waxes.

Adverse Reactions to Drugs

No drug should be used unless there are good indications since almost any drug may produce unwanted or unexpected adverse reactions (side-effects). Some produce oral adverse reactions. The true incidence of adverse drug reactions is often not known, and many adverse reactions are probably not, at present, recognised as drug related.

A full medical history should always be taken, and questions should be asked specifically about drug use (including OTC preparations) and adverse drug reactions, since the medical status may influence the choice of drugs used. G6PD deficiency must be excluded before using dapsone. TPMT must be assayed before azathioprine use. HLA-B1502 testing is necessary before carbamazepine use. Polypharmacy should be avoided, and practitioners should use only drugs with which they are familiar.

Patients should be warned if serious adverse reactions are liable to occur (e.g. systemic corticosteroids) and provided with the appropriate warning card to carry.

After injections, there is always a small chance that anaphylactic shock or a vasovagal attack may occur.

Oral Use of Drugs

The oral route is generally the preferred route for drug administration.

Subcutaneous Injection of Drugs

Subcutaneous injections can be given into a skin fold, pinched up over the anterior abdominal wall or anterior thigh with vertical insertion of a 25 G (orange hub) needle and are used for injection of drugs such as:

- insulin
- heparin
- opiate analgesics.

Intramuscular Injection of Drugs

This is used to obtain a more rapid effect than a subcutaneous injection, or where intravenous (i.v.) injection is impractical or carries a greater risk of anaphylactic or cardiac stimulant reaction. A 23 G (blue hub) needle is used. Intramuscular injection is used for:

- epinephrine (adrenaline) in the emergency treatment of anaphylactic shock or cardiac arrest
- glucagon, in the emergency treatment of hypoglycaemia
- antipsychotics (e.g. chlorpromazine, haloperidol) in the emergency treatment of acute psychoses
- midazolam or diazepam in the management of epileptic fit (buccal midazolam is superseding this)
- antimicrobials.
  Adverse effects of i.m. injections include the following:
- pain
- bruising, due to local haematoma formation. Intramuscular injections are contraindicated in patients with bleeding tendencies (e.g. haemophilia or induced by anticoagulant therapy)
- nerve damage, which may lead to paralysis, especially in bleeding disorders. This risk is minimised by using either the side of the thigh, or the upper, outer quadrant of the gluteus maximus muscle in the buttock or the deltoid muscle in the upper, outer arm
- collapse, usually due to a faint.
  Anaphylactic shock, especially after injections with antimicrobials, such as penicillin. The patient should be observed for 30 minutes after the injection, with facilities for resuscitation available.

Intravenous Injection of Drugs

Intravenous injection is used to achieve a rapid effect in emergencies, for example:

- epinephrine (adrenaline) in the management of cardiac arrest only
- diazepam in the management of status epilepticus
- heparin in the management of acute pulmonary embolism.
  Intravenous infusion through an indwelling catheter is used:
- when administration by other routes is not possible (e.g. blood transfusion, or fresh frozen plasma or coagulation factor concentrates)
- for hydration with i.v. fluids (e.g. saline or dextrose) when oral intake of fluids is not possible (e.g. unconsciousness or semiconsciousness, impaired swallowing [e.g. after stroke], vomiting, or fasting prior to surgery or other procedures)
- for antimicrobial treatment of severe infections or prophylaxis when using, for example, vancomycin.
  Veins preferred for i.v. injections are those in the antecubital fossa, the preferred sites for infusions are the forearm or dorsal hand veins (which allow joint mobility). Note that:
- following insertion of the needle (usually 21 G (green hub) or 23 G (blue hub)) or catheter, the fact that the needle is in a vein and not elsewhere should be confirmed by aspiration of blood and by the absence of local pain or swelling on injection or infusion of a small amount of the material to be administered
- Intravenous catheters should be taped in place, and sterile precautions (and rotation of catheter sites) observed to minimise the risk of local thrombosis and sepsis
- when prolonged IV access is required (e.g. in the treatment of endocarditis or malnutrition), a central venous catheter can be inserted (under fully sterile conditions) into the internal jugular or subclavian veins. Such Hickman lines (central catheters) are also useful in monitoring central venous pressure and fluid replacement in circulatory shock.
  The patient should be observed for 30 minutes after the injection, with facilities for resuscitation available.

Intralesional Injection of Drugs

In several chronic mucosal conditions, intralesional drugs may be given. Most commonly, 0.5 to 1 mL triamcinolone acetonide (available as 10 mg/mL and 40 mg/mL) is injected in divided doses beneath a chronic ulcer (e.g. ulcerative lichen planus) to aid healing. This can also be considered in the chronic lip swelling of orofacial granulomatosis.

REFERRAL TO A SPECIALIST

Referral may be indicated when the practitioner is faced with:
- a complicated or serious diagnosis (especially cancer, HIV infection, pemphigus, Behçet syndrome)
- a doubtful diagnosis
- a patient who has extraoral lesions or other indications of possible systemic disease
- a situation where investigations are required, but not possible or appropriate to carry out in general practice
- a situation where therapy may not be straightforward and may require potent agents
- a situation where drug use needs to be monitored with laboratory or other testing (e.g. for liver functional disturbances)
- a patient who needs access to an informed opinion or care outside normal working hours.
  Should a referral be required, it should always be in writing, giving a concise background to the referral (Fig. 4.1) including:
- patient's last name, first name(s), date of birth, full address and telephone, mobile phone, fax and e-mail where possible; primary care medical practitioner's name, address and telephone, fax and e-mail
- referring clinician's name, address, telephone, fax and e-mail
- referral urgency (real or perceived)
- reason for referral
- relevant history including duration or recurrences
- findings including site, size and nature
- provisional diagnosis
- treatment already offered and any response
- relevant medical, dental and social history
- any special needs such as transport or translator.

PATIENT REFERRAL FORM (to be completed by referring CLINICIAN)

1.   **PATIENT**

LAST Name: .... First Name(s) ....

Date of Birth: .... Address: ....

Postcode: ....

Telephone: (Home) .... (Work) ....

(Mobile) .... (Fax) ....

Gender: M/F .... Hospital No. (if known) ....

2.   **REFERRING CLINICIAN**

Name: .... Telephone No.: ....

Address: ....

.... Postcode: ....

Fax: .... E-mail: ....

3.   **REFERRAL**

Urgency with which you wish patient to be seen: if possible

Immediately ☐   within: 2 weeks ☐   within: 3 months ☐

Fig. 4.1 Patient referral form.

Patient's main complaint ....

Purpose of referral:.......................... for advice only ☐   for advice and care ☐

Comments ....

4.   HISTORY

Dental Specify... No ☐   Yes ☐

Medical: does the patient have

	No	Yes		No	Yes		No	Yes
Allergies			Bleeding tendency			Medication		
Heart problems			Diabetes			Any other problem		

Detail ....

Other (Specify)...

Please enclose other relevant information such as medication, radiographs, study casts, lab results
(if available)

....

Date: ....   Signature of Referer: ....

Fig. 4.1 cont'd

RECOMMENDED READING

Escudier, M., Ahmed, N., Shirlaw, P., et al., 2007. A scoring system for mucosal disease severity with special reference to oral lichen planus. Br. J. Dermatol. 157 (4), 765–770.

Ní Ríordáin, R., Shirlaw, P., Alajbeg, I., et al., 2015. World Workshop on Oral Medicine VI: Patient-reported outcome measures and oral mucosal disease: current status and future direction. Oral. Surg. Oral. Med. Oral. Pathol. Oral. Radiol. 120 (2), 152–160.e11.

Ormond, M., McParland, H., Donaldson, A.N.A., et al., 2018. An oral disease severity score validated for use in oral pemphigus vulgaris. Br. J. Dermatol. 179 (4), 872–881.

Osailan, S.M., Pramanik, R., Shirlaw, P., Proctor, G.B., Challacombe, S.J., 2012. Clinical assessment of oral dryness: development of a scoring system related to salivary flow and mucosal wetness. Oral. Surg. Oral. Med. Oral. Pathol. Oral. Radiol. 114 (5), 597–603.

Agents Used in the Management of Orofacial Diseases

INTRODUCTION

Three main areas of therapeutic intervention are treatment of orofacial mucosal diseases, the relief of pain, discomfort and anxiety, and the treatment of infections. In each area, assessment of response to the treatment given is mandatory. Where specific therapies are available, especially if evidence based, they should be used: for some conditions, the best that can be offered is symptomatic treatment — the control of symptoms, and in all cases, attention should be given to relieving pain, discomfort and anxiety.

Clinicians and patients must understand that many orofacial conditions are chronic and although they can be ameliorated, they cannot all be cured. Many mucosal conditions can only be controlled with continued immunomodulatory therapy. Often, the dose of drug used to control acute symptoms can then be reduced to a maintenance dose to maintain control.

Many of the agents used for the treatment of oral diseases are used 'off-label' — the practice of prescribing a drug for an unapproved indication or in an unapproved age group, unapproved dose or unapproved form of administration. Off-label use is very common in medicine and it is legal for a clinician to independently decide to prescribe a drug off-label, but it is illegal for the company to promote off-label uses to prescribers. The General Medical Council UK (GMC) supports medical practitioners to prescribe off-label or unlicensed drugs if no appropriate licensed drug is available or they are satisfied it is as safe and effective as the licensed alternative. The European Medicines Agency (EMA) states 'a medicine should be a treatment prescribed and dispensed with only the best interests of the patient in mind, and with the patient fully informed and involved in the decision-making process'. Unfortunately, many of the treatments used in oral medicine lack an evidence base to facilitate change from 'off-label' to 'on-label'. In any event, patients must always be consulted and consent to off-label use of drugs and records made of responses to treatment.

See http://www.eaasm.eu; http://www.ema.europa.eu; https://www.gov.uk/government/organisations/medicines-and-health care-products-regulatory-agency

There are three distinct areas involved in the management of oral mucosal diseases:

Section I Treatment of Mucosal Diseases
Section 2 Relieving Pain, Discomfort and Anxiety
Section 3 Treatment of Mucosal and Systemic Infections

SECTION I TREATMENT OF MUCOSAL DISEASES
TOPICAL ANTI-INFLAMMATORY AGENTS
Topical Corticosteroids (Table 5.1)

Glucocorticoids are used for immunosuppression. They may have a wide range of antiinflammatory actions, including to inhibit:

- pro-inflammatory cytokines produced by Th cells and macrophages:
  - tumour necrosis factor α (TNF-α)
  - interferon γ (IFN-γ)
  - interleukins (IL-1b, IL-6, IL-10, IL-12, IL-18).

transcription of immune genes such as IL-2 gene. IL-2 is the main cytokine necessary for development of T-cell immunologic memory (which depends upon the expansion of antigen-selected T-cell clones)

- inflammatory cell (neutrophil, macrophage and mast cell) emigration, chemotaxis, phagocytosis, respiratory burst and the release of various inflammatory mediators (lysosomal enzymes, cytokines, tissue plasminogen activator, chemokines, etc.) via annexin-1 (lipocortin-1), a 37 kDa member of the annexin superfamily of proteins (antiinflammatory) stimulated by glucocorticoids
- eicosanoid, prostaglandin and leukotriene production (via cyclooxygenase (COX) inhibition).

Topical corticosteroids (see Table 5.1) are useful in the management of many oral ulcerative conditions where there is no systemic involvement, such as recurrent aphthous stomatitis:

- These corticosteroids are used locally on a lesion as a spray, gel or cream, or as a mouthwash if there are extensive lesions: many are used off-label and this must be discussed with the patient.
- Gels and sprays are better than ointments, since the latter adhere poorly to the mucosa. Ointments when mixed with a carrier such as Orabase can be effective. However, creams can be bitter and are rarely used and gels can irritate.
- The corticosteroid needs to be in contact with the mucosa for some minutes for it to have any significant effect;

TABLE 5.1 Topical Steroid Preparations Used in Oral Medicine

Corticosteroid	Example	Use	Comments
Mild Potency			
Hydrocortisone oromucosal 2.5 mg tablets (mucoadhesive buccal tablets)	Corlan 2.5 mg 'pellets'	Dissolve in mouth close to ulcers every 6 h	Use at an early stage of ulceration in recurrent aphthous stomatitis. Useful in children
Fluocinolone acetonide 1:10 dilution (0.0025%)	(Synalar)	Apply to lesion	Adrenal suppression unlikely
Medium Potency			
Betamethasone soluble phosphate 0.5 mg tablets	Betnesol	Use as mouthwash	Adrenal suppression unlikely
Betamethasone valerate 0.1% cream	Betnovate	Apply to lesion	Adrenal suppression unlikely
Fluocinolone 0.025% cream	Synalar	Apply to lesion	Adrenal suppression unlikely
Triamcinolone acetonide 0.1% in carmellose gelatine paste	Adcortyl, Kenalog	Apply to lesion	Adheres best to dry mucosa; affords mechanical protection; of little benefit on tongue or palate. Unavailable in the UK
High Potency			
Beclometasone (beclomethasone) dipropionate spray 100 mL	Beclometasone dipropionate	Two puffs tds to lesions	Adrenal suppression possible
Budesonide spray 100 mL	Budesonide	Two puffs tds to lesion	Adrenal suppression possible
Fluocinonide 0.05% cream, gel or ointment	Metosyn	Apply to lesion	Adrenal suppression possible
Fluticasone propionate spray	Flixotide	One puff	Adrenal suppression possible
Fluticasone propionate 0.05% cream	Cutivate	Apply to lesion	Adrenal suppression possible
Very High (Super) Potency			
Betamethasone dipropionate 0.05% cream	Diprosone	Apply to lesion	Adrenal suppression possible
Clobetasol propionate 0.05% cream or ointment	Dermovate	Apply to lesion	Adrenal suppression possible
Prednisolone sodium phosphate 5 mg suppositories	Predsol	Dissolve slowly in mouth	Adrenal suppression possible

patients should, therefore, time its use for at least 3 minutes on each occasion.

- Patients should not eat or drink for 30 minutes after using the corticosteroid, in order to prolong contact with the lesion.
- The corticosteroid can usefully be applied in a silicone splint worn overnight for treatment of desquamative gingivitis.

Topical corticosteroids are the primary therapeutic agents used to treat ulcerative mucosal lesions which have an immunologically based aetiology (aphthae, erythema multiforme, lichen planus, pemphigoid). A mild potency agent such as hydrocortisone may be effective but more typically a medium potency corticosteroid such as betamethasone or a higher potency one such as fluocinonide or beclomethasone are required, moving to a super-potent topical corticosteroid, e.g. clobetasol, if the benefit is inadequate (see Table 5.1).

With many topical corticosteroids, there is little systemic absorption and thus no significant adrenocortical suppression, but it is difficult to predict the absorption — especially through atrophic and/or inflamed and ulcerated mucosae. In patients using potent corticosteroids for more than a month, it is prudent to add an antifungal, since candidosis may arise.

Drawbacks of the topical corticosteroids are that:
- there are few randomised controlled trials (RCTs)
- they are not uniformly effective
- occasionally candidosis is a complication
- they can damage collagen
- they are often not licensed for use in the mouth so must be used 'off-label'.

Topical Calcineurin Inhibitors

Calcineurin inhibitors act by binding to immunophilins (cyclophilin and macrophilin) and the resultant complexes inhibit calcineurin, which under normal circumstances induces the transcription of IL-2. These include (Table 5.2):
- Ciclosporin
- Tacrolimus
- Pimecrolimus.
  Used off-label, they can be:
- effective in oral ulcerative disorders
- more effective if used along with topical corticosteroids
- expensive.
  Tacrolimus is:
- available as 0.1% and 0.03% ointment

- liable to cause stinging for greater than 15 minutes (decreases on continued use)

only rarely associated with adverse effects, but the US Food and Drug Administration (FDA) in 2005 issued a public health advisory warning about possible carcinogenicity but there is currently no strong evidence of an increased rate of malignancy in treated patients.

INTRALESIONAL CORTICOSTEROIDS

These are occasionally useful in the management of chronic intractable local lesions, such as ulcerative lichen planus and orofacial granulomatosis (triamcinolone acetonide available as 10 mg/mL and 40 mg/m). Intra-articular corticosteroids are occasionally indicated where there is intractable pain from a non-infective arthropathy. Some examples include:
- prednisolone sodium phosphate, up to 22 mg
- methylprednisolone acetate, 4 to 80 mg
- triamcinolone acetonide, 2 to 3 mg
- triamcinolone hexacetonide, up to 5 mg.

SYSTEMIC THERAPIES

Immunomodulatory Agents

The aim of most immunomodulatory treatment is to suppress the damaging effects of autoimmunity and associated inflammation. However, immunosuppression can have a number of adverse effects (see Chapter 33). Adverse effects are associated mainly with systemic agents and thus topical immunomodulatory agents are the preference in the treatment of disease restricted to the oral cavity, mainly the corticosteroids.

Systemic Antiinflammatory Agents

Tetracyclines

Tetracyclines, distinct from their non-antimicrobial actions, have antiinflammatory actions, which include inhibition of:
- pro-inflammatory cytokines
- matrix metalloproteinases (MMPs), including collagenases MMP-1, MMP-8 and MMP-13
- prostaglandin synthesis
- nitric oxide release
- caspase activation (by minocycline).
  Adverse effects of tetracyclines can include:
- hyperpigmentation of teeth and bones

TABLE 5.2 **Alternative Topical Immunosuppressants (Calcineurin Inhibitors)**		
Drug	**Dose**	**Comments (see Table 5.17)**
Ciclosporin (Neoral or Sandimmune), used as mouthwashes or in an adhesive preparation	100–1500 mg/mL daily as a mouthwash; <50 mg/mL daily in an adhesive preparation	Adverse effects rare with topical applications
Tacrolimus (Protopic or Prograf)	0.1%–0.03% ointment	Adverse effects rare with topical applications; has 10–100-fold potency of ciclosporin; FDA advisory caution: related to cancer arising in lichen planus

- gastrointestinal discomfort
- nausea, anorexia
- photosensitivity
- hypersensitivity
- lupoid reactions

Tetracyclines are therefore contraindicated in:
- children under 8 years and in pregnant/nursing mothers
- liver disease
- lupus erythematosus
- myasthenia gravis
- porphyria.

Tetracycline absorption is inhibited by zinc, iron, milk and antacids.

Systemic Immunosuppressants

Systemic immunosuppressants are shown in Table 5.3. They are used especially in organ transplantation and in autoimmune disorders, but their adverse effects can be serious and may include the following:
- infections, especially with viruses, fungi and mycobacteria, such as tuberculosis
- lymphoproliferative disorders
- malignancies, such as lip carcinoma
- possible teratogenicity.

The main ones used in oral medicine practice are systemic steroids, azathioprine and mycophenolate mofetil (MMF), colchicine, pentoxifylline and dapsone (used primarily in mucous membrane pemphigoid).

Azathioprine

Azathioprine is an immunosuppressive acting mainly on T cells. It is a 6-mercaptopurine pro-drug, which blocks nucleotides and purine synthesis and works via 6-thioguanine to disrupt the making of RNA and DNA by cells. It is used alone or in combination with other immunosuppressive therapy to prevent rejection following organ transplantation, and to treat an array of autoimmune diseases, including rheumatoid arthritis, pemphigus, systemic lupus erythematosus, Behçet disease and other forms of vasculitis, autoimmune hepatitis, atopic dermatitis, myasthenia gravis. There is an increasing evidence base for their use in severe oral mucosal disease. It is also an important therapy and steroid-sparing agent for inflammatory bowel disease (such as Crohn disease and ulcerative colitis) and for multiple sclerosis.

Azathioprine should not be used before performing a thiopurine methyltransferase (TPMT) test since 1:400 people are homozygous negative for this enzyme which breaks down azathioprine and about 1:200 have low TPMT levels; do not use azathioprine if TPMT level is low. May take 2 to 3 months to have real effect. Macrocytosis is common and regular checking of FBC is essential during long-term treatment irrespective of TPMT status. Leukopenia is the most common adverse event, but anaemia and thrombocytopenia are also seen. May also cause nausea, hypersensitivity, susceptibility to infection, liver dysfunction, arrhythmias, hypotension, nephritis,

carcinogenicity. Absolute contraindications are hypersensitivity to azathioprine/6-MP; severe infections; severely impaired hepatic or bone marrow function; pancreatitis; live vaccines. Azathioprine can be used in pregnancy and lactation with caution (see BSR guidelines).

Interactions: allopurinol, cyclophosphamide, methotrexate, ciclosporin, co-trimoxazole, trimethoprim, clozapine, ribavirin and febuxostat (increase the myelotoxic effect), aspirin (bleeding), other immunosuppressants (increase the risk of infection), warfarin (reduced effect).

Mycophenolate Mofetil

Mycophenolate mofetil is a lymphocyte selective immunosuppressive agent which inhibits inosine monophosphate dehydrogenase (blocks guanosine nucleotide, purine and DNA synthesis). It thus inhibits de novo purine synthesis on which lymphocytes are critically dependent for their proliferation, whereas other cell types can use salvage pathways. MMF thereby prevents the proliferation of T cells, and the formation of antibodies by B cells. It is particularly useful in the treatment of autoimmune blistering diseases including bullous pemphigoid, mucous membrane pemphigoid, epidermolysis bullosa acquisita, paraneoplastic pemphigus, pemphigus foliaceus and pemphigus vulgaris.

Thalidomide

Thalidomide suppresses TNF-α synthesis and modulates interferon-gamma-producing CD3$^+$ cells. Originally used as a sedative, thalidomide was withdrawn in 1961 because of birth defects when given to pregnant women. Females given thalidomide must take effective contraceptive measures while taking thalidomide and for 3 months after finishing the tablets.

Thalidomide can be very effective in severe RAS nonresponsive to immunosuppression, Behçet and oral ulceration in HIV disease (see Table 5.3). It is widely used globally in the treatment of leprosy.

Peripheral neuropathy (which may be permanent) can occur during thalidomide treatment. Nerve conduction tests are needed before the start of treatment, and these should be repeated every 6 months. Nerve damage will recover on stopping the treatment in approximately 50% of cases. Thalidomide makes most people feel drowsy. It should be taken at night. Drowsiness persisting during the day makes it unsafe for patients to drive or operate machinery and may impair alertness and ability to think clearly. Alcohol must be avoided.

Colchicine

Colchicine, in the form of the autumn crocus (Colchicum autumnale), was used as early as 1500 BC to treat joint swelling. An alkaloid, Colchicine inhibits mitosis by binding to tubulin in microtubules, and thus depresses neutrophil motility and activity. It is a medication used to treat gout and Behçet disease. Other uses for colchicine include the prevention of pericarditis and familial Mediterranean fever. Adverse effects include

TABLE 5.3   Systemic Immunomodulatory Agents[a]

Agent	Dosage	Comments (see Table 5.17)
Prednisolone (give as enteric coated prednisolone with meals)	Initially 30—80 mg orally each day in divided doses, reducing as soon as possible to 10 mg/day	Limit dosage in hypertension and diabetes mellitus. May produce adrenal suppression. May cause weight gain, osteoporosis
Azathioprine	2—2.5 mg/kg daily (50—150 mg/day)	A 6-mercaptopurine pro-drug, which blocks nucleotides and DNA. Licenced for autoimmune bullous disorders, lupus, dermatomyositis
		Assay thiopurine methyltransferase (TPMT) first; do not use azathioprine if TPMT level is low. May take 2—3 months to have real effect. Macrocytosis and leukopenia are common and regular FBC essential irrespective of TPMT status. Anaemia and thrombocytopenia also seen. May also cause nausea, hypersensitivity, susceptibility to infection, liver dysfunction, arrhythmias, hypotension, nephritis and carcinogenicity. Absolute contraindications are: hypersensitivity to azathioprine/6-MP; severe infections; severely impaired hepatic or bone marrow function; pancreatitis; live vaccines; pregnancy; and lactation
		Interactions: allopurinol, cyclophosphamide, methotrexate, ciclosporin, co-trimoxazole, trimethoprim, clozapine, ribavirin (increase the myelotoxic effect), aspirin (bleeding), other immunosuppressants (increase the risk of infection), warfarin (reduced effect)
Mycophenolate mofetil	1000 mg once or twice daily. 250 mg capsules and 500 mg tablets. Oral suspension (1 g/5 mL) and 500 mg vials of MMF for i.v. injection. Mycophenolic acid 180 mg and 360 mg delayed release tablets.	Inhibits inosine monophosphate dehydrogenase (blocks guanosine nucleotide, purine and DNA synthesis) and thereby blocks T- and B-cell proliferation and leukocyte recruitment. May take several months to have real effect. More gastrointestinal, haematological effects (red cell aplasia) and infections than with azathioprine. No liver or kidney damage. Contraindicated in pregnancy
Colchicine	up to 500 ugm daily	An alkaloid, colchicine inhibits mitosis by binding to tubulin in microtubules, and thus depresses neutrophil motility and activity. Adverse effects include diarrhoea and myelotoxicity. Contraindicated in pregnancy, older patient, cardiac, renal or hepatic disease
Dapsone	1 mg/kg daily (usually 100—200 mg). Give also vitamin E 800 IU/day, and cimetidine	May take many months to have beneficial effect. Haemolysis, hypersensitivity. Interactions: trimethoprim and methotrexate (both increase the risk of haematological complications). Protect from sun exposure
Hydroxychloroquine	200—400 mg/day	May take 3—6 months to have effect. May cause retinal damage and visual impairment. May cause myelotoxicity. Contraindicated in patients with renal or hepatic disease
Pentoxifylline	400 mg twice daily	A xanthine derivative, a cyclic nucleotide phosphodiesterase inhibitor that improves blood flow through blood vessels, and inhibits pro-inflammatory cytokine (TNF) production, leukocyte—endothelial cell adhesion, chemokines and leukocyte—keratinocyte adhesion. Common adverse reactions are nausea, dysphagia and flushing. Contraindicated in cerebrovascular haemorrhage, myocardial infarction
Cyclophosphamide	1—2 mg/kg daily	Transformed by cytochrome p450 to active phosphoramide mustard and acrolein, which reacts with DNA. Leukopenia always — but reversible. Also causes cystitis. Small risk of cancer with prolonged use
Levamisole	50 mg 3 times daily for 3 days	Promotes leukocyte chemotaxis. May cause dizziness, taste disturbance, nausea, agranulocytosis
Tacrolimus	100 mg/kg daily	Used in transplants mainly. Contraindicated in pregnancy. May cause cardiomyopathy
Thalidomide	50—200 mg/day at night initially, then maintain on alternate-day therapy. Severe RAS and Behçet syndrome	Suppresses TNF-α synthesis. May take 2—3 months to have real effect. Females must take effective contraceptive measures while taking thalidomide and for 3 months after finishing the tablets. Peripheral neuropathy can occur. Nerve conduction tests are needed. Thalidomide makes most people feel drowsy and should be taken at night. Alcohol must be avoided. May predispose to venous or arterial thromboembolism, including myocardial infarction and CVEs. Thalidomide may also predispose to neutropenia; thrombocytopenia; syncope and bradycardia; and serious skin reactions, including Stevens—Johnson syndrome

[a]Many can increase liability to infection and, long term, possibly also neoplasia.

diarrhoea and myelotoxicity. Used widely in PAPFA syndrome and often in severe RAS. It is available as a generic medication in the United Kingdom.

Dapsone

Dapsone is an antibiotic commonly used in combination with rifampicin and clofazimine for the treatment of leprosy. Dapsone was first studied as an antibiotic in 1937. (https://en.wikipedia.org/wiki/Dapsone-cite_note-Zhu2001-4) Its use for leprosy began in 1945. It is on the World Health Organization's (WHO) List of Essential Medicines, the safest and most effective medicines needed in a health system. Dapsone is available both topically and by mouth, is available as a generic drug and is not very expensive.

Additionally, it has been used for acne, dermatitis herpetiformis and various other skin conditions including pemphigoid. It has been used widely for treatment of mucous membrane pemphigoid.

Severe side effects may include a decrease in blood cells, red blood cell breakdown especially in those with glucose-6-phosphate dehydrogenase deficiency (G-6-PD), or hypersensitivity. Common side effects include nausea and loss of appetite.

Pentoxifylline

A xanthine derivative, a cyclic nucleotide phosphodiesterase inhibitor that improves blood flow through blood vessels, and inhibits pro-inflammatory cytokine (TNF) production, leukocyte — endothelial cell adhesion, chemokines and leukocyte — keratinocyte adhesion. Its primary use in medicine is to reduce pain, cramping, numbness or weakness in the arms or legs which occurs due to intermittent claudication, a form of muscle pain resulting from peripheral artery diseases. Used in severe RAS and other ulcerative oral conditions.

Systemic Corticosteroids (see Table 5.3)

Indications

Systemic corticosteroids are often indicated for the management of:
- Bell palsy (in association with antivirals)
- giant cell arteritis
- pemphigus
- multisystem diseases, such as some lichen planus, erythema multiforme or pemphigoid
- severe or resistant recurrent aphthae or aphthous-like ulceration.

Adverse Effects

Systemic corticosteroids must always be used with caution because of potential adverse effects (Table 5.4), which may include, apart from those noted above:
- Adrenocortical suppression: this may occur after a course of greater than 3 weeks of systemic corticosteroids and may persist for 1 year or more. Adrenocortical suppression makes the patient liable to collapse if stressed, traumatised or having an infection, operation or general anaesthetic.
- Weight gain and mooning of the face: weight should be monitored. A diet low in salt, fats and calories helps control weight and prevent hypertension.
- Hypertension: the blood pressure must always be monitored.
- Precipitation of diabetes: the blood glucose must always be monitored.
- Cataract: ophthalmological monitoring is indicated.

TABLE 5.4 Summary of Potential Adverse Effects of Immunosuppressant and Antiinflammatory Agents

	Latency (weeks)	Pregnancy Risk (FDA)[a]	ADVERSE EFFECTS			
			Blood	Liver	Cancer	Main Others
Azathioprine	4–8	Low	+	+	+	Neuropathy
Ciclosporin	1–2	Low	−	+	+	Hypertension Nephrotoxic
Colchicine	2–4	Low	+	−	−	Blood neuromyopathy
Corticosteroids	1–2	Low	−	−	+/−	Osteoporosis Hypertension Weight
Cyclophosphamide	2–4	Yes	+	+	+ Bladder	Cystitis Leukaemia
Dapsone	50–100	Low	+	+	−	Idiosyncrasy
Hydroxychloroquine	>24	Low	−	+	+/−	Ocular toxicity, renal toxicity
Mycophenolate	8–12	Yes	+	+	+/−	Gastrointestinal

[a]FDA guidance against use in pregnancy, yes — there is positive evidence of human foetal risk based on adverse reaction data from investigational experience or studies in humans, but potential benefits may warrant use of the drug in pregnant women despite potential risks.

- Osteoporosis: patients on protracted courses should have bone densitometry monitoring and be given bisphosphonates and calcium.
- Avascular necrosis of the femoral head.
- Psychoses.

Patients should always be given a steroid card, warned of possible adverse reactions and warned of the need for an increase in the dose if ill or traumatised or having an operation. A baseline DEXA scan should be undertaken in those at risk and where therapy is prolonged. Gastric and bone protection should be prescribed concurrently.

Corticosteroid-Sparing Immunosuppressants

Because of possible adverse reactions of corticosteroids, drugs with alternative modes of action are used as alternatives or in combination with corticosteroids and are termed 'steroid-sparing' immunosuppressants. However, most of these drugs may have serious, adverse effects in addition to those noted above, and so they are used by specialists.

Of these steroid-sparing drugs (see Tables 5.3), most require monitoring for potential adverse effects (summarised in Table 5.4).

Biologics

Generated by recombinant biotechnology, biologic agents (BAs) target specific steps in pro-inflammatory pathways and are now widely used in the treatment of a variety of inflammatory immune-mediated and neoplastic conditions. The use of biological therapy in the management of inflammatory oral mucosal conditions is commonly off-label and rarely used by oral medicine specialists, especially as many need to be given intravenously in hospitals. The suffix indicates their origin from a biological source, e.g. plasma cells that include human (suffix 'mab'), humanised (suffix 'zumab') or chimeric (mouse–human; suffix 'ximab') monoclonal antibodies or variant fusion proteins (suffix 'cept').

Three broad classes exist (Table 5.5):
- lymphocyte modulators (e.g. rituximab [anti-CD20])

- TNF-α cytokine inhibitors include the monoclonals infliximab (Remicade), etanercept (Enbrel) and adalimumab (Humira)
- interleukin inhibitors such as ustekinumab (used in psoriasis and which inhibits IL-12/IL-23).

These agents have been used in a wide variety of diseases, including some oral conditions. BAs have been used in a variety of oral diseases including Behçet disease, severe RAS, bullous diseases, OLP, Crohn disease/OFG, Stevens–Johnson syndrome (SjS), cGvHD and in oral cancer therapy (see Table 5.5). By and large, bullous diseases and oral cancer are the oral disorders for which BAs are mostly used and an evidence base exists. Safety concerns are such that their use requires precautionary considerations, including screening for co-existing medical conditions and an appreciation of potential adverse effects.

Potential adverse effects of biologics may include:
- Infections: screening for mycobacterial infections with consideration of prophylactic anti-TB therapy if there is evidence of latent disease, and definitive treatment in active disease, and for risk factors for HBV, HCV and HIV infection should be performed prior to anti-TNF therapy. Other opportunistic bacterial and fungal infections are also more prevalent in patients receiving TNF-α inhibitors, most frequently histoplasmosis and invasive candidosis.
- Cardiac failure: potentiated with TNF-α blockade, so the agents should be used with caution and it would seem prudent to monitor cardiac function in patients receiving therapy, and discontinue treatment if cardiac function declines.
- Increased risk of malignancy: for non-melanoma skin cancer and possibly for melanoma and lymphoma.
- Pregnancy and paediatric considerations: there is a potential increased occurrence of congenital abnormalities with TNF-α inhibitors used in pregnancy.
- Adverse drug reactions: range from minor reactions at injection sites to hypersensitivity reactions and anaphylaxis, including some oral adverse effects (see Chapter 33)

TABLE 5.5		Biological Agents Relevant to Oral Medicine: Applications and Potential Oral Adverse Effects of Selected Agents			
Adalimumab	TNF-α	Crohn disease, rheumatoid arthritis, psoriasis	OFG, Behçet, RAS	OLP, EM, SCC, candidosis
Cetuximab	EGFR	Head and neck cancer	Oral SCC	Stomatitis, taste alteration, xerostomia
Etanercept	TNF-α	Crohn disease, rheumatoid arthritis, psoriasis, sarcoid	MMP, Behçet disease, RAS, SjS	Candidosis, EM, OLP, SCC?
Infliximab	TNF-α	Crohn disease, rheumatoid arthritis, psoriasis, sarcoid	OFG, cGVHD, Behçet disease, SjS	OLP, osteomyelitis, ulcers, parotitis, EM
Panitumumab	EGFR	Cancers	-	Mucositis
Rituximab	CD20	NHL, rheumatoid arthritis	PV, MMP, SjS	Candidosis

cGVHD, Chronic graft versus host disease; *EGFR*, epidermal growth factor receptor; *EM*, erythema multiforme; *IL*, interleukin; *MMP*, mucous membrane pemphigoid; *NHL*, non-Hodgkin lymphoma; *OFG*, orofacial granulomatosis, *OLP*, oral lichen planus; *PV*, pemphigus vulgaris; *RAS*, recurrent aphthous stomatitis, *SjS*, Stevens–Johnson syndrome.

Lymphocyte modulators carry similar adverse reactions and safety concerns, including the risk of progressive multifocal leukoencephalopathy (PML), which led to licence withdrawal of some by the FDA and EMA. Of this group, rituximab is licenced, but safety concerns include:

- infections
- immune toxicity
- severe infusion reactions
- tumour lysis syndrome with hyperkalaemia and acute renal failure and arrhythmias
- cardiac arrest
- lung toxicity.

Retinoids

The retinoids are a class of chemical compounds that are vitamers of vitamin A or are chemically related to it. Retinoids have found use in medicine where they regulate epithelial cell growth and are used particularly in the treatment of acne. Retinoids come in the form of topical treatments, which are applied directly to the skin, and oral capsules. Well-known retinoids include tretinoin, adapalene and isotretinoin. The oral form of isotretinoin is often known by the brand name of Roaccutane.

Tretinoin as a 0.1% cream or 0.01% gel, or acitretin (pro-drug of etretinate) 10 to 25 mg/day orally, may be of value in controlling lichen planus and have been used in leucoplakia with less success. Systemic retinoids, however, are teratogenic and may disturb liver function and blood lipids.

SECTION 2: RELIEVING PAIN, DISCOMFORT AND ANXIETY

ANALGESICS

Pain is the most important symptom suggestive of orofacial disease, but absence of pain does not exclude disease. There is considerable individual variation in response to pain, and the threshold is lowered by tiredness and psychogenic and other factors. It is important, therefore, where possible, to:

- identify and treat the cause of pain
- relieve factors that lower the pain threshold (fatigue, anxiety and depression)

- use analgesics (agents that relieve pain without causing loss of consciousness)
- avoid polypharmacy.
- try simple topical or oral analgesics before embarking on more potent or injectable preparations or opioids. Non-opioid analgesics act primarily at the periphery, do not produce tolerance or dependence, and do not alter the patient's perception; they are used for mild to moderate pain. Opioid analgesics act on the central nervous system (CNS) and alter the patient's perception; they are more often useful for severe pain. Pain control may require continued or intermittent medication.

Topical Analgesics

Topical analgesics are available as pain-relieving creams, lotions, rubs, gels and sprays. (Table 5.6). The three main types of topical analgesics apart from benzydamine (which has an antihistamine action) include:

- Local anaesthetics (mainly lidocaine, lidocaine—aprilocaine cream (EMLA) and benzocaine): benzocaine, however, can cause methaemoglobinaemia. Topical analgesics such as lidocaine may ease mucosal discomfort or joint-related pain (see Chapter 5).
- Rubefacients or counterirritants which act by counter-irritation: capsaicin, a preparation derived from peppers, and methylsalicylates, derived from willow bark and often combined with menthol; capsaicin can, by depleting substance P in sensory nerve endings, and by blocking conduction in type-C nociceptive fibres, be helpful in oral dysaesthesia and post-herpetic neuralgia.
- Nonsteroidal antiinflammatory agents which act by penetrating deep into tissues to inhibit cyclooxygenase (COX) enzymes responsible for development of inflammatory processes can be helpful in joint-related pain (see Chapter 41).

Systemic Analgesics

Systemic analgesics (Table 5.7) can reduce pain, in some cases, such as nonsteroidal antiinflammatory drugs (NSAIDs), through an eicosanoid-depressing, antiinflammatory action. The term 'eicosanoids' is used as a collective name for molecules derived from 20-carbon fatty acids — mainly the

TABLE 5.6 Topical Analgesics Use in Oral Mucosal Diseases

Nonsteroidal antiinflammatory: Benzydamine	0.15% (Oral rinse)	Swish for 1 min and spit out 15 mL/tid
Mucosal protectant: Sucralfate	Oral rinse 20%	Swish for 1 min and spit out 15 mL/qid
Mucosal protectant: Aloe vera gel	At 70%	0.5 mL/tid
Mucosal protectant: Chamomile	Gel 2%	Apply 0.5 mL/bid
Anaesthetic: Lidocaine	Gel 2%	Apply 3—5 times per day
Topical analgesic: Capsaicin	Cream 0.025%	Apply 2—3 times per day
Antimicrobial: Lactoperoxidase	Oral rinse (Biotene®)	Swish for 1 min and spit out 15 mL qid
Low-level laser therapy		As manufacturer's instructions
Benzodiazepine: Clonazepam	(Oral rinse)	1 mg/10 mL for 3 min and spit out tds
Benzodiazepine: Clonazepam	(Oral dissolving tablets 1 mg)	Suck 1 tab for 3 min and spit out tds or dissolve in 5 mL and swish
Calcineurin inhibitor: Cyclosporine	(Oral rinse) bid	2 mL for 45 s and spit out bid for two weeks and then reduce

TABLE 5.7	Some Systemic Analgesics Used in Oral Medicine	
Agent	**Adult Dosage**	**Comments (see Table 5.17)**
Nonsteroidal Antiinflammatory Drugs (NSAIDs)		
Ibuprofen	400 mg up to 4 times daily	Caution in asthma, peptic ulcer, bleeding tendency, breastfeeding, cardiac, renal and liver disease, pregnancy, older patient, aspirin hypersensitivity. May cause arrhythmias and cardiac infarction
Mefenamic acid	250–500 mg up to 3 times daily	Caution in asthma, peptic ulcer, bleeding tendency, breastfeeding, cardiac, renal and liver disease, pregnancy, older patient, aspirin hypersensitivity
Non-NSAIDs		
Paracetamol	500–1000 mg up to 6 times daily (maximum 4 g/day)	Caution in liver or renal disease; those on antiretrovirals
Opioids		
Codeine phosphate	10–60 mg up to 6 times daily orally (or 30 mg i.m.)	Contraindicated in liver disease, late pregnancy
Dihydrocodeine	30 mg up to 4 times daily (or 50 mg i.m.)	Contraindicated in children, hypothyroidism, asthma, renal disease

leukotrienes and prostanoids. Leukotrienes play an important role in inflammation, especially as part of the slow-reacting substance of anaphylaxis. Prostanoids (prostaglandins (PGs), prostacyclin, thromboxanes) mediate local symptoms of inflammation such as vasoconstriction or vasodilatation, coagulation, pain and fever. All prostanoids originate from prostaglandin H catalysed by the enzyme PGH2-synthase, which is a combination of a peroxidase and a COX.

COX catalyses the formation of prostaglandins and thromboxane from arachidonic acid (itself derived from cellular phospholipase A_2). Prostaglandins stimulate protective gastric mucin and bicarbonate but reduce gastric acid, renal excretion and blood platelet formation. Prostaglandins released via COX-2 act (among other things) as messenger molecules in inflammation.

Nonsteroidal Antiinflammatory Drugs

Most NSAIDs act as non-selective inhibitors of COX, inhibiting both the isoenzymes COX-1 and COX-2. NSAIDs, including aspirin, are useful analgesics, but can cause:

- further deterioration of cardiac function, if this is already impaired in cardiac failure
- peptic ulceration, especially in those over 75 years old or who have a history of peptic ulceration. Thus it is best to add a proton pump inhibitor, such as misoprostol. Ibuprofen appears to be the conventional NSAID with the lowest risk of gastrointestinal adverse effects but can produce thromboses, arrhythmias or myocardial infarction. COX-2 inhibitors, such as celecoxib, etoricoxib, valdecoxib and parecoxib, have fewer gastrointestinal effects, but may have serious cardiac adverse effects
- further deterioration of renal function, if this is already impaired
- a bleeding tendency, by interfering with platelet activity
- premature closure of the ductus arteriosus in pregnancy third trimester.

Aspirin

Aspirin has been in use longer than most other NSAIDs, and the efficacy and adverse effects are well recognised. Aspirin is a useful analgesic, but it can also cause:

- bleeding — irreversibly blocking the formation of thromboxane A_2 in platelets
- asthma
- fluid retention
- nausea, diarrhoea or tinnitus
- interference with a number of drugs, including antihypertensives, diuretics and methotrexate
- allergies
- Reye syndrome — a serious liver disease, in breastfeeding, by passing in milk to the child and in children under age 16 years (see Chapter 54)
- complications in mothers in late pregnancy.

Paracetamol

Paracetamol inhibits COX but, although it is sometimes grouped together with the NSAIDs, it lacks the adverse effects of NSAIDs, is not a true NSAID and lacks significant antiinflammatory properties. There is speculation that it acts through the inhibition of COX-3 isoform, or that it acts centrally. Generally speaking, paracetamol has few adverse effects, drug interactions or contraindications. Chronic pain requires regular analgesia (not just as 'required') however, and it is important not to overdose with paracetamol — which is hepatotoxic in high doses. In children, paracetamol can helpfully be given in sugar-free syrups.

Opioids and Narcotics

- Opioids are analgesics used for moderate to severe pain such as that from cancer or mucositis.
- Opioids are narcotics, controlled drugs and all are capable of causing addiction.

TABLE 5.8 Selected Antidepressants Used in Oral Medicine

Drug	Dose	Comments (see Table 5.17)
Amitriptyline	10–50 mg/day	Contraindications: recent myocardial infarction, arrhythmias, liver disease
Nortriptyline	10–50 mg/day	Contraindications as for amitriptyline
Dosulepin (dothiepin)	25 mg 3 times daily or 75 mg at night	
Doxepin	10–100 mg/day in divided doses	
Fluoxetine	20 mg/day	Caution with: epilepsy, pregnancy, cardiac, liver or kidney disease, allergy, mania
Venlafaxine	75 mg in morning	Contraindications: recent myocardial infarction, arrhythmias, liver disease

- Opioids may cause constipation, respiratory depression, nausea, drowsiness and urinary retention.

NON-ANALGESIC AGENTS

Non-analgesic agents, which may be effective in some types of pain, include, for example, antidepressants and anticonvulsants.

OTHER CNS-ACTIVE DRUGS

Antidepressants

Treatment of depression is by psychotherapy and medication. If there is any possibility of a suicide attempt, the patient must be seen by a psychiatrist as a matter of urgency. Antidepressants may, by altering brain neurotransmitters such as serotonin (5-hydroxytryptamine) and noradrenaline, control depression. Antidepressants (Table 5.8) can also be useful for the relief of some neuropathic pain, when they can have analgesic effect within 1 to 7 days (before they have any antidepressant effect) and at lower doses than needed for treatment of depression.

No antidepressant drug is perfect and all suffer from at least one of the following drawbacks:

- Delayed onset of action from 7 to 28 days. Although some improvements may be seen in the first few weeks, most antidepressant medications must be taken regularly for 3 to 4 weeks (in some cases, as many as 8 weeks) before the full therapeutic effect starts.
- Anticholinergic effects.
- Sedation.
- Agitation.
- Cardiotoxicity.
- Weight gain.

Patients often are tempted to stop antidepressant medication too soon but they should continue for *at least* 4 to 9 months to prevent recurrence. The natural history of most depression is of remission after 3 to 12 months.

There are many different classes of antidepressants from which to choose therapies but the main ones are:

1. Tricyclic antidepressants (TCAs): often effective but frequently producing anticholinergic adverse effects such as dry mouth. TCAs with balanced effects on serotonin and noradrenaline reuptake (e.g. amitriptyline, nortriptyline) may be more effective than those acting mainly on noradrenaline uptake (e.g. maprotiline). The most commonly used doses are Amitriptyline 10 to 50 mg/day and Nortriptyline 10 to 50 mg/day. Both may induce xerostomia, dizziness and drowsiness, blurred vision, weight gain, trouble urinating, headache, dysgeusia, constipation (see Table 5.8).

2. Selective serotonin reuptake inhibitors (SSRIs): newer antidepressants, with the advantage over older antidepressants of less severe antimuscarinic activity, weight gain or cardiac conduction effects. SSRIs generally have fewer adverse effects than tricyclics and do not interact with alcohol and are thus often preferred by both patients and practitioners. However, gastrointestinal effects are common and they can produce dry mouth and arrhythmias.

Antidepressants:

- Must be prescribed only in limited amounts, as there is a danger they may be used in a suicide attempt.
- May take up to 3 to 4 weeks before the antidepressant action takes place. Monitoring of plasma concentrations may be helpful in ensuring optimal dosage.
- Doses should be reduced for the older patient.
- Should not be withdrawn prematurely.
- Are usually contraindicated in patients with cardiac or liver disease.
- May have adverse effects, often via anticholinergic activity and thus cause:
  - hyposalivation, but the complaint of dry mouth may also be a manifestation of depression
  - epileptogenic effects (tricyclics and fluoxetine)
  - drowsiness
  - visual impairment
  - constipation and urinary retention.
- Antidepressants
  - may make it impossible for patients to drive vehicles, as they may suffer drowsiness and visual impairment
  - may interact with alcohol.
- Tricyclic antidepressants interact with antiarrhythmics, antiepileptics, antihistamines, antihypertensives, antipsychotics, apraclonidine, beta blockers, brimonidine, diuretics, the contraceptive pill, nefopam, norepinephrine (noradrenaline) and tramadol. However, neither tricyclic (TCAs) nor monoamine oxidase inhibitor (MAOIs) antidepressants significantly interact with adrenaline in dental local anaesthetic solutions.

TABLE 5.9 Drugs Used in the Management of Trigeminal Neuralgia

Drug	Dose	Comments (see Tables 5.18 and 5.19 and Chapter 43)
Baclofen	5 mg three times daily	Contraindicated in peptic ulceration and pregnancy. Common adverse effect of sedation. Avoid abrupt withdrawal
Carbamazepine	Prophylactic for trigeminal neuralgia — not analgesic. Initially 100 mg once or twice daily. Many patients need about 200 mg 8-hourly. Do not exceed 1800 mg daily	Contraindicated in Han Chinese or in patients with HLA-B1502, cardiac, renal and liver disease, glaucoma and pregnancy. Occasional dizziness, diplopia and blood dyscrasia, often with a rash and usually in the first 3 months of treatment. Interferes with contraceptive pill. Possible interactions with antimalarials, anticonvulsants, diltiazem, verapamil, gefitinib, diuretics, erythromycin, clarithromycin, dextropropoxyphene, fluconazole, miconazole, CNS depressants, cimetidine, isoniazid, lithium
Oxcarbazepine tablets	300 mg initially, then 1200—2400 mg/day	As for carbamazepine
Gabapentin	300 mg up to three times daily	Similar adverse effects to carbamazepine. Headache common. Contraindicated in psychiatric disease, renal disease, diabetes and pregnancy. Avoid sudden withdrawal
Phenytoin	150—300 mg daily	Contraindicated in Han Chinese or other patients with HLA-B1502, and in liver disease and pregnancy. Produces gingival swelling. Similar other adverse effects to carbamazepine. Avoid sudden withdrawal
Pregabalin	300—600 mg daily	Infection, ataxia, blurred vision, constipation, diplopia, dizziness, drowsiness, fatigue, headache
Lamotrigine	25—200 mg daily	Blurred vision, diplopia, ataxia, dizziness, drowsiness, dry mouth, headache

Anticonvulsants

Anticonvulsants are the standard treatment of idiopathic trigeminal neuralgia (Table 5.9). However, as these agents may cause blood dyscrasias or hepatic dysfunction, it is important to monitor full blood counts and liver function (see Chapter 33). The main agents used are Gabapentin 300 to 2400 mg/day, Pregabalin 150 to 300 mg/day and Lamotrigine 25 to 200 mg/day. All anticonvulsants have side effects which may include dizziness, drowsiness, sexual dysfunction, xerostomia, angioedema, gastrointestinal symptoms (nausea, vomiting, diarrhoea) and mood disturbances.

Hypnotics

- Pain, anxiety or depression may cause insomnia.
- Hypnotics may help sleep but should not be prescribed without forethought.
- Benzodiazepines such as temazepam 10 mg every night or Diazepam 6 to 15 mg/day are, in general, the preferred hypnotics, but are contraindicated in severe respiratory disorders and are also addictive. Benzodiazepines can also cause drowsiness, ataxia, palpitations, dysuria, xerostomia, diplopia, slurred speech and hypotension

- Hypnotics often potentiate alcohol and other CNS depressants and may impair judgement and dexterity.
- Hypnotics may be contraindicated in the older patient and in those with liver or respiratory disease.
- Barbiturates should not be used; barbiturates are addictive and are dangerous in overdose

Anxiolytics (Table 5.10)

- Identify and treat the cause of the patient's anxiety wherever possible.
- It is important to differentiate between agitated depression and simple anxiety; the treatment is different.
- Reassurance is often remarkably effective at calming the anxious patient but there are times when a mild anxiolytic, such as a benzodiazepine like diazepam 2 to 10 mg, or a non-benzodiazepine, such as buspirone 5 mg orally three times daily, or zopiclone 3.75 mg orally up to three times daily can be helpful.

TABLE 5.10 Anxiolytics Relevant in Oral Medicine

Drug	Dose	Comments (see Tables 5.9 and 5.10)
Clonazepam topical	0.5 mg/mL solution. 5 mL for 5 min 2—4 times a day. Spit out	Can be used in burning mouth syndrome
Diazepam	2—30 mg/day in divided doses	Benzodiazepines. Avoid in glaucoma. Use with caution in the older patient, care with alcohol, driving or operating machinery
Temazepam	5—10 mg at night	As for diazepam
Zopiclone	3.75 mg 2—3 times daily	Non-benzodiazepine. Avoid in respiratory or neuromuscular disease, liver disease, renal disease, pregnancy, breastfeeding. Use with caution in the older patient, care with alcohol, driving or operating machinery

- Numerous benzodiazepines are now available as anxiolytics. All may produce dependence (especially lorazepam) and there is often little to choose in terms of anxiolytic effect between the different drugs. Most cause unsteadiness and some confusion.
- Zopiclone (see Table 5.10), a benzodiazepine-like drug, was introduced and initially promoted as having less dependence and withdrawal than benzodiazepines, but is now known to be addictive.
- Beta blockers (e.g. propranolol) may be more useful if anxiety is causing tremor/palpitations.
- Drowsiness (particularly when used together with alcohol) and impaired judgement are common in patients taking anxiolytics, so patients must be warned of the dangers of driving, operating machinery or making important decisions.
- Doses of anxiolytics should be reduced for the older patient, since adverse effects, particularly sedation, are common.

SECTION 3 TREATMENT OF INFECTIONS
ANTIBACTERIAL THERAPY

Indications for the Use of Antibacterials

Confirmed Infections (together with appropriate surgical or other measures), such as:
- cervical fascial space infections
- osteomyelitis
- odontogenic infections in ill or toxic patients (e.g. if the patient is immunocompromised)
- acute ulcerative gingivitis
- specific infections, such as tuberculosis and syphilis.
  Antimicrobials should be used in some instances of surgical conditions if they do not respond to local measures:
- pericoronitis
- dental abscess
- dry socket (localised osteomyelitis).
  Antimicrobials should be used for prophylaxis:
- of infective endocarditis in at-risk patients having invasive oral procedures
- in cerebrospinal rhinorrhoea
- in most facial or compound skull fractures
- in major oral, maxillofacial and craniofacial surgery (e.g. osteotomies or tumour resection)
- in surgery involving bone in immunocompromised or debilitated patients
- in surgery involving bone in patients who have been taking bisphosphonates
- in surgery involving bone following radiotherapy to the jaws
- possibly in patients with hydrocephalus shunts having invasive oral procedures
- possibly in some patients with prosthetic joint replacements having invasive oral procedures, especially following rheumatoid arthritis.

Using Antibacterials

- The practitioner should attempt to obtain relevant specimens before commencing therapy.
- For most infections, a 5-day course of antibiotics is adequate.
- Antibiotic prescriptions should be reviewed at 48 hours and 5 days, and in the light of microbiology results.
- Most infections should be treated with a single antibiotic only. Exceptions include endocarditis prophylaxis, tuberculosis treatment and some infections in immunocompromised persons.
  Always enquire first about allergies and other contraindications.

Most Useful Antibacterials

- The bacteria which cause most odontogenic infections are usually sensitive to penicillins.
- Anaerobes have now been implicated in many odontogenic infections, and these often respond to penicillins or metronidazole.
- Amoxicillin 500 mg three times daily is effective, and produces high blood antimicrobial levels, with good patient compliance.
- Flucloxacillin 500 mg four times daily is also effective against many oral bacterial infections.
- If the patient is allergic, has had penicillin within the previous month (resistant bacteria) or has methicillin-resistant *Staphylococcus aureus* (MRSA), a different antimicrobial should be used.
- Drainage must be established if there is pus; antimicrobials will not remove pus.
- A sample of pus (as much as possible) should be sent for culture and sensitivities, but, if antimicrobials are indicated, they should be started immediately and in adequate doses.
- If a lesion fails to respond to an antimicrobial reconsider possible:
  - inadequacy of drainage
  - inappropriateness of the antimicrobial
  - inadequate antimicrobial dose
  - antimicrobial insensitivity of causal micro-organism, e.g. staphylococci are now frequently resistant to penicillin and some show multiple resistances (e.g. MRSA) when vancomycin is usually effective
  - patient non-compliance
  - local factors (e.g. foreign body)
  - unusual type of infection
  - impaired host defences (unusual and opportunistic infections are increasingly identified, particularly in the immunocompromised patient)
  - non-infective cause for the condition.

In serious, unusual or unresponsive cases of infection, consult the clinical microbiologist.

ANTIFUNGAL THERAPY

Antifungals (Table 5.11) are used:
- to treat oral or oropharyngeal fungal infections, but underlying predisposing factors should be corrected first
- until there is no evidence of residual clinical lesions or symptoms, and should be continued for at least 2 weeks more, to reduce the risk of recurrence
- topically often effectively and, importantly, they are without serious adverse effects apart from occasional drug interactions (e.g. topical miconazole can enhance the effect of warfarin) (see Table 5.11)
- systemically and though sometimes more effective against *Candida*, systemic use can be associated with adverse effects or drug interactions (Table 5.12).

Polyene Antifungal Agents

These include:
- **Nystatin** is antifungal by interfering with fungal cell membranes. It binds to ergosterol, an essential component of fungal cell membranes, disrupting the cell membrane and leading to potassium leakage and fungal inhibition. Nystatin, topically, used at least four times daily, 500,000 units for adults and 100,000 units for children. Higher doses may be required in immunocompromised patients. Compliance can be a problem because of the taste, but suspensions often overcome this disadvantage. Nystatin, if swallowed, may lead occasionally to gastrointestinal side effects, such as nausea, vomiting and diarrhoea.
- **Amphotericin** has a similar mode of action to nystatin and is also used four times daily locally as lozenges. It can be given intravenously for systemic candidosis, but there is

then a considerable risk of toxicity, which may manifest as fever, vomiting, and renal, bone marrow, cardiovascular and neurological toxicity.

Azole Antifungal Agents

Azoles are synthetic antifungals with broad-spectrum activity and are fungistatic, but are expensive and usually used mainly systemically, though miconazole in particular is often used topically. Liquid or suspension forms can also be used for topical effect (see Table 5.11). Azoles inhibit the fungal cytochrome P450-dependent enzymes, which are essential catalysts for the 14-demethylation of lanosterol in sterol biosynthesis, and, therefore, block the synthesis of ergosterol, the principal sterol in fungal cell membranes. One adverse effect of azoles, therefore, is the accumulation of precursors of ergosterol. Azoles include:
- imidazoles (clotrimazole, econazole, ketoconazole and miconazole)
- triazoles (fluconazole, itraconazole, voriconazole and posaconazole). Fluconazole, voriconazole and posaconazole are available as suspensions, and itraconazole as a liquid; preparations which may find favour for use in patients with dry mouths and for use as topical therapy.

The absorption of ketoconazole and itraconazole is dependent on gastric acid and so any drugs that increase gastric pH (e.g. H_2 antagonists, proton pump inhibitors), and antacids, metal ion-containing drugs (e.g. sucralfate) and vitamin supplements can decrease antifungal absorption. P-glycoprotein (P-gp) — a versatile drug transporter — functions as a 'detoxification' pump that expels drugs back into the intestinal lumen. P-gp also works in concert with the cytochrome P450 (CYP) 3A4 enzymes in intestine and liver where drug metabolites are produced for renal elimination.

Ketoconazole and itraconazole not only affect P-gp but are highly dependent upon metabolism through several CYP 450

TABLE 5.11	Topical Antifungal Agents Used in Oral Medicine	
Agent	**Dosage and Duration (continue for at least 48 h after lesions have cleared)[a]**	**Comments (see Table 5.17)[b]**
Topical		
Chlorhexidine	0.12%–0.2% mouth rinse twice daily	Tooth staining, especially if the patient drinks tea, coffee or red wine
Nystatin	100,000 IU/mL suspension 100,000 IU 6-hourly for at least 14–21 days[c]	Topical use — often no problems, but may cause unpleasant taste, nausea or gastrointestinal disturbance. Suspension contains sucrose
Fluconazole	Oral suspension 10 mg/mL 1 mL 4 times a day	Available topically but may be absorbed systemically. May interact with many drugs

Miconazole	Oral gel 20 mg/g. Apply qds for at least 7 days
	20 mg mucoadhesive buccal tablet, 25 mg/mL gel.
	   50 mg daily for at least 14–21 days[c]
	50 mg/g denture lacquer; apply weekly for at least
	   2 weeks. Not available in the USA
		Available topically but may be absorbed systemically. May interact with many drugs, including anticoagulants, antidiabetic drugs, ciclosporin, cisapride, midazolam, phenytoin, statins and terfenadine. May impair oral contraceptive. Avoid in pregnancy and porphyria

Clotrimazole	10 mg/mL solution 1 mL qds for up to 14 days	Local irritation or burning. Hypersensitivity reported
Posaconazole	Available as oral suspension[c] 200 mg/5 mL	Very expensive. Broad spectrum of activity against numerous yeasts and filamentous fungi. Interactions (see Table 5.13)

[a]Higher doses are used in HIV infection.
[b]Check pharmacopoeia for other contraindications, cautions and interactions.
[c]Do not take with food; swish around mouth and swallow; for additional topical effect, do not rinse mouth or eat or drink for 30 minutes.

TABLE 5.12   Main Systemic Antifungal Drugs

Systemic Tablets/Capsules

Drug	Dose	Notes
Fluconazole	50–200 mg/day capsules or suspension[a] 50 mg/5 mL for at least 14 days	Less toxic than ketoconazole. May interact with many drugs, including anticoagulants, statins, antidiabetic drugs, ciclosporin, cisapride, midazolam, phenytoin repaglinide, rifabutin, sulphonylureas, tacrolimus, terfenadine, theophylline and zidovudine. Avoid in pregnancy and porphyria. May impair oral contraceptive. May sometimes be hepatotoxic and myelosuppressive. Expensive. Avoid in pregnancy, infants and adrenal disease[c]
Itraconazole	100–200[b] mg/day for at least 14 days capsule or 10 mg/mL liquid[a] 10 mL twice daily for at least 14 days	Expensive. May impair oral contraceptives. May cause cardiac failure. May interact with many drugs, as for fluconazole. Not absorbed in achlorhydria. Avoid in cardiac disease, pregnancy and porphyria[c]
Ketoconazole	200–400 mg/day for at least 14 days (less frequently prescribed)[b]	Hepatotoxic. Expensive. May interact with many drugs as for fluconazole including anticoagulants, antidiabetics, statins, cimetidine, isoniazid, ranitidine, rifampicin. Enhances nephrotoxicity of ciclosporin. May impair oral contraceptive. Avoid in pregnancy and porphyria. Not absorbed in achlorhydria
Posaconazole	400 mg twice daily for at least 14 days available as suspension[a] 200 mg/5 mL	Broad spectrum of activity against numerous yeasts and filamentous fungi. Available as oral suspension and is generally well tolerated. Used routinely for the prophylaxis of invasive fungal infections in immunosuppressed hosts and is an effective treatment of oral candidosis, including azole-resistant disease. May interact with many drugs as for fluconazole. Contraindicated in cardiac disease, liver disease, porphyria and pregnancy. Avoid in breastfeeding
Voriconazole	200–400 mg/day for at least 14 days available as suspension[a] 200 mg/5 mL	Expensive. For fluconazole resistant *Candida albicans*, *Candida dubliniensis* or *Candida krusei* infections. May interact with many drugs as for fluconazole including ciclosporin, midazolam, phenytoin, tacrolimus, theophylline and zidovudine. Contraindicated in cardiac disease, liver disease and pregnancy. May prolong QT interval. Avoid in breastfeeding. Wide range of possible adverse effects. May cause nausea, neuropathy and rash[c]

Intravenous

Drug	Dose	Notes
Amphotericin	0.5 mg/kg for at least 10–14 days	Expensive. May cause nephrotoxicity, arrhythmias, neuropathies and anaphylactoid reactions. Avoid in pregnancy. Liposomal amphotericin may be safer
Caspofungin	Infusion 50 mg i.v. daily	For fluconazole resistant *C. albicans*. Contraindicated in cardiac disease, liver disease and pregnancy. Avoid in breastfeeding. Wide range of possible adverse effects including anaphylaxis[c]
Micafungin	Infusion 100 mg i.v. daily	Prophylaxis of candidosis in haematopoietic stem cell transplantation when fluconazole, itraconazole or posaconazole cannot be used. Significantly hepatotoxic. Contraindicated in liver disease, renal disease and pregnancy. Avoid in breastfeeding

[a]Do not take with food; swish around mouth and swallow; for additional topical effect, do not rinse mouth or eat or drink for 30 minutes.
[b]The higher doses are used in HIV infection.
[c]Check pharmacopoeia for other contraindications, cautions and interactions.

pathways including CYP 3A4. Fluconazole, on the other hand, is more readily cleared from the body. Co-administration of azoles with drugs that induce or accelerate strongly CYP-450 metabolism can result in low or undetectable levels of the azole antifungal. Higher antifungal dosages (particularly of ketoconazole, itraconazole, voriconazole) cannot overcome this interaction.

All azoles are also reversible inhibitors of CYP enzymes. Important drug interactions with azole antifungals arise from inhibition of CYP 3A4, which plays a critical role in the metabolism of a range of drugs used for cardiovascular disease, endocrine disorders including hyperglycaemia, anaesthesia, psychiatric disorders, epilepsy, cancer chemotherapy and treatment of infectious diseases. There can be interactions with many drugs including carbamazepine, ciclosporin, H_2 receptor antagonists, isoniazid, phenobarbitone, phenytoin, rifampicin, statins, sucralfate, terfenadine, tricyclic antidepressants and warfarin. Rifampicin, rifabutin and phenytoin can decrease antifungal levels.

The imidazoles (ketoconazole and miconazole) have more effect on cytochromes than do the triazoles, and the latter thus tend to have less severe adverse effects. However, none of the azoles are entirely benign; hepatotoxicity may be common to all, and the potential for endocrine toxicities exists, particularly at high doses.

Finally, azole resistance is increasingly reported. The development of cross-resistance of *Candida albicans* to different azoles during treatment with a single derivative has been described.

Azoles may thus:
- be hepatotoxic
- displace protein-bound drugs and, thus, enhance the activity of, for example, anticoagulants, producing a bleeding tendency
- interact with a number of drugs. An important interaction is to produce arrhythmias with terfenadine (and in the past with astemizole and cisapride). They may also interfere with the oral contraceptive

- cause antifungal resistance (to ketoconazole, fluconazole, miconazole and itraconazole) and this is now becoming a significant problem in immunocompromised persons, especially those with a severe immune defect, who may show *Candida* species resistant to fluconazole and, sometimes, to other azoles. Voriconazole may then be effective.

If treatment with azoles is ineffective, then culture of candida to determine species, and sensitivities to determine resistance is essential.

Clotrimazole. Clotrimazole is used only topically as a 10 mg troche three times daily, because it can induce gastrointestinal and neurological toxicity. It is less effective than other azoles in patients with HIV infection.

Ketoconazole. Ketoconazole is usually used systemically, 200 to 400 mg/day taken orally with food, since gastric acid is essential for its dissolution. Absorption can be enhanced by taking orange juice, carbonated beverages or glutamic acid. Ketoconazole is poorly absorbed from an empty stomach in HIV/AIDS because of gastric atrophy and reduced acid production, or if there is concurrent use of medications, such as cimetidine, ranitidine and other antacids. It is also poorly absorbed if rifampicin or phenytoin are given. Adverse effects may include nausea, rashes, abdominal pain and pruritus, but especially liver damage. Transient disturbance of liver function (e.g. increased serum aminotransferase concentrations) is so common that regular monitoring with liver function tests is essential in all patients on systemic ketoconazole for more than a few days. Severe liver damage may sometimes occur. Ketoconazole also blocks hormone steroid synthesis and reduces testosterone levels. Adrenocortical suppression may also develop. Drug interactions with ketoconazole are shown in Table 5.11 These adverse effects have restricted its use.

Miconazole. Miconazole is used mainly for topical treatment of various forms of candidosis, such as angular stomatitis. Miconazole buccal tablets or gel exhibit few drug interactions because of low systemic absorption and are generally well tolerated with a good safety profile except if taken concurrently with warfarin. The once-daily dosing schedule may improve patient adherence compared with topical alternatives. Miconazole can be effective for the treatment of chronic atrophic candidosis.

Miconazole is also available for parenteral use against systemic mycoses, but the injection contains polyethoxylated castor oil, which may provoke allergic reactions.

Fluconazole. Fluconazole, unlike some other azoles, has little affinity for cytochromes, which is thought to explain its lower toxicity. Fluconazole is active against most *C. albicans*, though resistance may appear (see below) and active against *Candida dubliniensis, Candida parapsilosis* and *Candida tropicalis*, but less active against *Candida glabrata*, and is inactive against *Candida krusei*. Fluconazole is well absorbed from the gut, even in the absence of gastric acidity, and absorption is rapid and nearly complete within 2 hours. Fluconazole appears to undergo relatively little metabolism in the body, elimination being predominantly renal with a half-life of approximately 30 hours. Fluconazole can therefore be given once daily, in a dose of 50 to 100 mg. It also enters saliva.

Fluconazole has generally been well tolerated, toxicity is mild and infrequent and, with usual doses, fluconazole does not appear to suppress the synthesis of corticosteroid hormones. Drug interactions present less difficulties than those associated with ketoconazole (see Table 5.11 and Chapter 36). An oral suspension of fluconazole is also available. Chronic use of fluconazole in high doses (400 to 800 mg/day) during the first trimester of pregnancy may be associated with certain birth defects in infants. The risk does not appear to be associated with a single, low dose of fluconazole (150 mg). According to the FDA, 'a few published case reports describe a rare pattern of distinct congenital anomalies in infants exposed in utero to high-dose maternal fluconazole (400 to 800 mg/day) during most or all of the first trimester'.

Itraconazole. Itraconazole is an orally active triazole available in 50 and 100 mg capsules and as a 10 mg/mL oral solution. Itraconazole has a long half-life and fewer side effects than ketoconazole, but is expensive, is eliminated hepatically and its use is contraindicated in liver disease. Itraconazole is well absorbed, but absorption is impaired when gastric acid is reduced or when antacids, rifampicin or phenytoin are given. Adverse effects of itraconazole have included altered liver function (but hepatotoxicity is less than that of ketoconazole) and hypokalaemia with hypertension due to accumulation of corticosteroids with an aldosterone-like activity, mild leukopenia, nausea, epigastric pain, headache and oedema. Itraconazole can aggravate or cause cardiac failure, especially in the older patient or one on calcium channel blockers. Drug interactions are shown in Table 5.11.

Voriconazole. Voriconazole is a relatively new triazole antifungal agent, effective against candida species but mainly indicated for the primary treatment of acute invasive aspergillosis. Elevated liver function tests, cardiac QT interval, rash and visual disturbances are the main treatment-related adverse events. Drug interactions are shown in Table 5.11.

Posaconazole. Posaconazole is a relatively new triazole antifungal agent, probably more effective than the others against invasive fungal infections but with more severe adverse effects. Posaconazole acts by disrupting phospholipids, impairing certain enzyme systems such as ATPase and the electron transport system and thus inhibiting synthesis of ergosterol by inhibiting lanosterol 14α-demethylase and accumulation of methylated sterol precursors. Posaconazole can cause QT prolongation, liver dysfunction, rashes and allergies. Drug interactions are shown in Table 5.11.

ANTIVIRAL THERAPY

- Most antivirals (Table 5.13) achieve maximum benefit if given early in the disease.
- Most acute viral infections resolve naturally, though in immunocompromised persons, they may be severe, widespread or persistent.

TABLE 5.13 Antivirals Effective Against Herpesviruses

Virus	Disease	Otherwise Healthy Patient[a]	Immunocompromised Patient[b]
Herpes simplex 1 and 2	Primary herpetic gingivostomatitis	Consider oral 100–200 mg aciclovir tablets 5 times daily, or oral suspension (200 mg/5 mL) 5 times daily for 7 days	Consider aciclovir 250 mg/m^2 i.v. every 8 h. Famciclovir 250 mg three times daily. Caution in renal disease, older patients and pregnancy. Occasionally causes nausea and headache. Valaciclovir 1000 mg can be given orally 2 times daily
	Recurrent herpes labialis	5% aciclovir cream or 1% penciclovir cream every 2 h	Aciclovir tablets 5 times daily, or oral suspension (200 mg/5 mL) 5 times daily. Valaciclovir 2000 mg can be given orally three times daily
	Recurrent herpetic ulcers	Aciclovir tablets 5 times daily, or oral suspension (200 mg/5 mL) 5 times daily	Consider aciclovir 250 mg/m^2 i.v. every 8 h
Herpes varicella zoster	Chickenpox	Consider oral 100–200 mg aciclovir tablets 5 times daily, or oral suspension (200 mg/5 mL) 5 times daily for 7 days	Aciclovir 500 mg/m^2 (5 mg/kg) i.v. every 8 h
	Zoster (shingles)	Consider oral 400–800 mg aciclovir tablets 5 times daily, or oral suspension (800 mg/5 mL) 5 times daily for 7 days. 3% aciclovir ophthalmic ointment for shingles of trigeminal ophthalmic division	Famciclovir 500 mg three times daily. Caution in renal disease, older patients and pregnancy. Occasionally causes nausea and headache. Valaciclovir 2000 mg can be given orally three times daily

[a]In neonate, treat as if immunocompromised.
[b]Aciclovir (systemic preparations): caution in renal disease and pregnancy. Occasional increase in liver enzymes and urea, rashes and CNS effects.

- Immunocompromised patients with viral infections may thus benefit from active antiviral therapy.
- Antiviral resistance is now becoming a significant problem to immunocompromised persons, especially those with a severe immune defect.
- Some antivirals active against herpesviruses and some active against retroviruses, such as HIV, are available, but there are few other antiviral agents of proven efficacy.

Antivirals Active Against Herpesviruses (see Table 5.13)

Antivirals are usually nucleoside analogues, which compete with natural nucleosides to block virus DNA synthesis, or pro-drugs which generally produce greater bioavailability of the active agent. Antivirals against herpes viruses include the following:

- Aciclovir, a guanosine analogue selectively phosphorylated to active form by herpesvirus thymidine kinases has proven efficacy in herpes simplex virus (HSV) infections, including herpes labialis and is fairly safe, though neurotoxic if given intravenously. It is given five times daily. Aciclovir is not effective against cytomegalovirus (which has no such thymidine kinase).
- Valaciclovir is a pro-drug of aciclovir; it has the advantage of a two or three times daily dosing only.
- Penciclovir is a synthetic acyclic guanine derivative which possesses the same antiviral spectrum as, and a similar mechanism of action to that of aciclovir, in that it undergoes phosphorylation in response to HSV viral thymidine kinase and is then further phosphorylated by host cell enzymes into a triphosphate, which selectively inhibits HSV viral DNA replication. It has considerably more bioavailability and a longer intracellular effect than aciclovir, and is generally more effective topically than topical aciclovir, is cheaper than aciclovir but only available as a cream.
- Famciclovir, a pro-drug of penciclovir, is a guanosine analogue that is particularly useful against HSV and varicella-zoster virus (VZV) but produces DNA mutations that may predispose to cancer of the breast or testis.
- Ganciclovir, a guanosine analogue, is active against cytomegalovirus (CMV), but is more toxic than aciclovir, can produce neutropenia, may have carcinogenic activity and, if given with zidovudine, can produce profound myelosuppression.
- Cidofovir is a DNA polymerase chain inhibitor, active against CMV and human papillomaviruses (HPV), but is nephrotoxic and may produce eye damage.

Other Anti-Herpes Agents

- Docosanol is an aliphatic alcohol that inhibits fusion between the plasma membrane and the HSV envelope, thereby preventing viral entry into cells and viral replication. A 10% docosanol cream is available for treating herpes labialis.
- Inosine pranobex (isoprinosine, methisoprinol) is a stimulator of immunity via actions like thymic hormones, active against HSV and HPV. It should be used with caution in gout or renal disease.
- Foscarnet is an organic analogue of inorganic pyrophosphate that selectively inhibits the pyrophosphate-binding site on viral DNA polymerases and can be used for HSV or CMV infections. It is potentially nephrotoxic.

Antiretroviral Agents

Antiretroviral therapy (ART) includes newly developed agents (Tables 5.14 and 5.15) and though effective, all are liable to fairly severe adverse reactions and resistance and many can cause drug interactions. Antiretroviral therapy is fast changing, with newer drug agents offering few side effects, greater durability and a decreased risk of drug resistance. In the past, antiretroviral therapy was described as a three-drug 'cocktail'. More recently, with improved pharmacokinetics and a longer drug half-life, antiretroviral therapy may involve as few as two co-formulated drug agents (see Table 5.15). The current philosophy is to start ART early in HIV infection. They work by blocking a stage of the virus's life cycle and, by doing so, prevent it from replicating. The drugs are organised into six different classes based largely on the stage of the life cycle they inhibit.

Entry or attachment inhibitors

Entry inhibitors prevent HIV attachment by attaching themselves to CD4 cell surface proteins or proteins on the surface of HIV. Some entry inhibitors target the gp120 or gp41 proteins on HIV.

Integrase inhibitors

These inhibit integration of viral nucleic acids into the host cells. Raltegravir (Isentress) can cause abdominal pain, diarrhoea, erythema multiforme and dry mouth. Dolutegravir is a newer integrase inhibitor.

Nucleoside reverse transcriptase inhibitors

Nucleoside reverse transcriptase inhibitors (NRTIs) block HIV reverse transcriptase activity by competing with natural substrates and being incorporated into viral DNA, where they act as chain

TABLE 5.14   Examples of Six Classes of Antiretroviral Agents Targeting Different Parts of the Reproductive Lifecycle of Human Immunodeficiency Virus, and Their Oral Side Effects

	Example	Trade Name	Dose	Possible Oral Side Effects
Entry attachment inhibitors	Fostemsavir	Rukubia	One 600 mg tablet 2×/day	Dry mouth
Integrase inhibitors	Raltegravir	Isentress	One 600 mg tablet 2×/day	Dry mouth, gingivitis, glossitis, dysgeusia
Nucleoside reverse transcriptase inhibitor	Lamivudine	Epivir	One 300 mg tablet 1×/day One 150 mg tablet 2×/day	Dry mouth, oral ulcers
	AZT, zidovudine	Retrovir	One 30 0 mg tablet 2×/day	Erythema multiforme, hyperpigmentation
	Tenofovir	Viread	One 300 mg tablet 1×/day	Dry mouth, erythema multiforme
Non-nuclease reverse transcriptase inhibitors	Etravirine	Intelense	One 200 mg tablet 2×/day	Erythema multiforme, ulcers
	Nevirapine	Viramune	200 mg tablet 2×/day	Erythema multiforme, ulcers
Protease inhibitors	Atazanavir	Reyataz	Two 200 mg capsules 1×/day	Ulcers, dry mouth
	Tipranavir	Aptivus	Two 250 mg capsules + 200 mg Norvir 2×/day	Erythema multiforme
Pharmacokinetic enhancers	Ritonavir	Norvir	Dose varies in combination with other antiretroviral therapy (ART)	Perioral paraesthesia, parotid lipomatosis, dry mouth, taste disturbance, facial oedema
	Cobicistat	Tybost	150 mg 1×/day	Dry mouth

TABLE 5.15   Fixed Dose Combination Antiretroviral Drugs: Examples and Possible Oral Side Effects

Trade Name	Constituents	Dose	Possible Oral Side Effects
Atripla	600 mg efavirenz + 200 mg emtricitabine + 245 mg tenofovir	One tablet 1×/day	Dry mouth, oral ulcers. ? parotid gland enlargement reported
Kivexa	600 mg abacavir + 300 mg lamivudine	One tablet 1×/day	Dry mouth, oral ulcers
Combivir	300 mg zidovudine + 150 mg lamivudine	One tablet 2×/day	Dry mouth, oral ulcers
Eviplera	25 mg rilpivirine + 200 mg emtricitabine + 245 mg tenofovir	One tablet 1×/daily	Dry mouth, erythema multiforme

terminators in the synthesis of pro-viral nucleic acids. The NRTIs often produce adverse effects and, perhaps more significantly, HIV resistance may arise. Among the common effects of many are haematological toxicity, neurological toxicity (including effects on memory, cognition, motor and peripheral nerve function) and enhanced risk of dry mouth ulcers and erythema multiforme (see Table 5.14).

Non-nucleoside reverse transcriptase inhibitors

Non-nucleoside reverse transcriptase inhibitors (NNRTIs) directly bind to HIV reverse transcriptase to inhibit it. NNRTIs suffer from similar disadvantages to NRTIs, especially rashes (see Table 5.14).

Protease inhibitors

Protease inhibitors (PIs) can be anti-HIV (there are also PIs that are anti-HCV (Boceprevir)). Anti-HIV PIs competitively inhibit an HIV aspartyl protease without affecting the human enzyme, and they induce a profound and sustained fall in HIV viral load and restore T-cell counts. Drug-induced lipodystrophy may cause dyslipidaemia and facial lipoatrophy. Taste abnormalities are common and oral and perioral paraesthesia can be disturbing adverse effects. Indinavir, which has activity related to vitamin A analogues, can also produce cheilitis (see Table 5.14).

Pharmacokinetic enhancers

- CCR5 receptor antagonists

These drugs target CD4 protein or the CCR5 or CXCR4 receptors on CD4 (see Table 5.14).

Maturation Inhibitors

These block production of HIV capsid protein p24. Alpha interferon has this effect as do bevirimat and Vivecon.

Combination Therapies (see Table 5.15)

Highly active antiretroviral therapies (HAART) are combinations (CART), involving a protease inhibitor and other antiretroviral drugs, and these have reduced the incidence of opportunistic infections, extended life substantially and decreased the infective load of HIV and other viruses. Such has been the effect of ART and HAART, that orofacial disease caused by HIV/AIDS has now been significantly reduced. Conversely, oral and perioral adverse effects can arise and may sometimes result in patient non-adherence to anti-HIV therapy.

Immune reconstitution syndrome (IRIS) is the term given when ART provokes an inflammatory reaction against residual micro-organisms. Long-term use of ART has been associated with oral warts, erythema multiforme, hyposalivation, toxic epidermal necrolysis, lichenoid reactions, exfoliative cheilitis, oral ulceration and paraesthesia.

TREATMENTS APPROPRIATE FOR PRIMARY OR SECONDARY CARE

Treatments appropriate for primary care are shown in Table 5.16. A specialist opinion may also be called for in the case of other disorders (see Chapter 4).

Contraindications and the most important interactions for drugs used by dental clinicians in primary care and for medical

TABLE 5.16 Primary Care Diagnosis and Management of Main Oral Medicine Conditions (see Table 5.17)

Condition	Typical Main Clinical Features	Investigations That May Aid Diagnosis (In Addition to History and Examination)	Therapeutic Protocols	Evidence Base Available?
Acute necrotising ulcerative gingivitis	Pain, gingival ulceration and bleeding, halitosis	Full blood count Consider HIV	Debridement Metronidazole or amoxicillin	Yes
Aphthous stomatitis	Recurrent oral ulcers only	Full blood count Exclude underlying systemic disease (e.g. iron, folate, vitamin B12)	Chlorhexidine M/W, topical corticosteroids (e.g. hydrocortisone, betamethasone), amlexanox or in adults, topical tetracycline (doxycycline). Specialists may use systemic therapy	Yes (for all)
Allergic reactions	Swelling, erythema or erosions	Allergy testing	Avoid precipitant Consider antihistamines (e.g. loratadine)	Yes
Atypical (idiopathic) facial pain	Persistent dull ache typically in maxilla in an older female	Clinical and imaging to exclude organic disease	Reassurance, CBT GMPs or specialists may use SSRIs or tricyclic antidepressants	Yes (for CBT and tricyclics)
Burning mouth syndrome	Glossodynia	Full blood picture, thyroid function, electrolytes	Reassurance, CBT Topical capsaicin GMPs or specialists may use tricyclic antidepressants or SSRIs	Yes but poor

Continued

TABLE 5.16 Primary Care Diagnosis and Management of Main Oral Medicine Conditions (see Table 5.17)—cont'd

Condition	Typical Main Clinical Features	Investigations That May Aid Diagnosis (In Addition to History and Examination)	Therapeutic Protocols	Evidence Base Available?
Candidosis (including angular stomatitis and denture-related stomatitis)	White or red persistent lesions	Consider smear or biopsy Consider immune defect	Leave out dental appliances and disinfect the appliance Use antifungals intraorally (tablets, creams or gels (e.g. miconazole) or suspensions (e.g. nystatin or fluconazole), regularly for up to 2 weeks Miconazole or fucidin cream applied to commissures	Yes
Chapped lips	Dry, flaking lips	—	Topical petrolatum gel or bland creams	No
Dental infections and pain	Pain usually aggravated by pressure or heat	Oral examination ± radiology	Restorative dentistry; possibly amoxicillin or metronidazole for 5 days	Yes
Erythema migrans	Desquamating patches on tongue	—	Reassurance ± benzydamine	No
Halitosis	Oral malodour	Oral/ENT examination and radiography. Bacterial culture	Treat underlying cause	No
Herpes simplex infection	Oral ulcers, gingivitis, fever	Sometimes PCR or immunostain	Symptomatic ± aciclovir suspension or tablets	Yes
Herpes labialis	Lip blisters	—	Antiviral cream (penciclovir or aciclovir)	Yes
Hyposalivation	Dry mouth May also be dry eyes or a connective tissue disease	Assess salivary flow rate, dry mouth score Exclude drugs, diabetes, Sjögren syndrome (serology — SSA (Ro) antibodies). Consider ultrasound labial gland biopsy or sialography	Preventive dentistry; mouth wetting agents (artificial salivas, of which there are several available) and artificial tears; salivary stimulants (sialogogues) — such as sugar-free chewing gum, or systemic pilocarpine or cevimeline	Yes
Keratosis	Flat, raised or warty white lesion	Biopsy	Stop tobacco, betel or alcohol use Excise if dysplastic	No
Leukoplakia	Flat, raised or warty white or white and red lesion (erythroleukoplakia)	Biopsy	Stop tobacco, betel or alcohol use Excise if dysplastic	No
Lichen planus	Mucosal white or other lesions Polygonal purple pruritic papules on skin May be genital, skin or adnexal involvement	Biopsy ± immunofluorescence	Corticosteroids (e.g. betamethasone or clobetasol propionate) topically. Aloe vera gel may be tried Stop tobacco or any causal drug use	Yes (for corticosteroid and aloe vera)
Pemphigoid	Blisters, mainly in mouth occasionally on conjunctivae, genitals or skin Scarring	Biopsy ± immunostaining	Topical corticosteroids (e.g. betamethasone or clobetasol propionate) Specialists may use tetracycline, dapsone, systemic corticosteroids or other immunosuppressives	Yes
Sinusitis	Pain, nasal discharge	Imaging	Nasal decongestants (e.g. ephedrine) Amoxicillin, doxycycline or clarithromycin for 7 days	Yes

Continued

| TMJ pain-dysfunction | TMJ pain, click, limitation of movement | Rarely imaging or arthroscopy | Reassurance, occlusal splint (overlay appliance), anxiolytics or muscle relaxants (e.g. benzodiazepines such as diazepam or temazepam). Topical NSAIDs | No |

CBT, Cognitive behavioural therapy; *ENT,* ear, nose and throat; *GMP,* general medical practice; *PCR,* polymerase chain reaction; *SSRI,* selective serotonin reuptake inhibitor.

TABLE 5.17   Selected Drugs Prescribed in Primary Care Management: Main Contraindications and Interactions[a]

Drug	Contraindications in Addition to Allergies to the Drug, and Possibly Pregnancy and Breastfeeding	Cautions	Most Important Potential Interactions (Check BNF)
Aciclovir (topical)	—	—	—
Aloe vera	—	Anorexia Inflammatory bowel disease	Digoxin Diuretics Glyburide Hydrocortisone
Amoxicillin	—	Chronic lymphocytic leukaemia Gout Infectious mononucleosis	Anticoagulants Methotrexate
Antihistamines (e.g. promethazine, loratadine)	—	Asthma Cardiac disease Causes drowsiness Diabetes Epilepsy Glaucoma Liver disease Prostatic hypertrophy Renal disease	Alcohol Azoles CNS depressants MAOI Phenothiazines Tricyclic antidepressants
Aspirin	Asthma Children	Bleeding tendency Peptic ulcer	Anticoagulants Corticosteroids Methotrexate NSAIDs Oral hypoglycaemics Phenytoin SSRIs
Benzydamine	—	—	—
Capsaicin	—	—	—
Carbamazepine	Patients with HLA-B1502	Porphyria Blood dyscrasias Cardiac disease Driving or operating machinery Glaucoma Liver disease Renal disease	Alcohol Anticonvulsants Antidepressants CNS depressants Diuretics MAOI Phenytoin Tricyclic antidepressants
Chlorhexidine	—	—	—
Corticosteroids topically	—	Candidosis	—
Diazepam	Children Glaucoma Porphyria	Cerebrovascular disease Depression Driving or operating machinery Liver disease Myasthenia gravis Parkinsonism Respiratory disease	Alcohol Aspirin Clozapine CNS depressants Grapefruit juice

Continued

TABLE 5.17 Selected Drugs Prescribed in Primary Care Management: Main Contraindications and Interactions[a]—cont'd

Drug	Contraindications in Addition to Allergies to the Drug, and Possibly Pregnancy and Breastfeeding	Cautions	Most Important Potential Interactions (Check BNF)
Dihydrocodeine		Asthma Children Hypothyroidism Pancreatitis Renal disease	Alcohol
Fucidin (topical)	—	—	—
Ibuprofen	Arrhythmias Cardiac infarction	Aspirin hypersensitivity Asthma Bleeding problems Cardiac disease Liver disease Older patients Peptic ulcer Renal	Many: check BNF Anticoagulants Baclofen Cardiac glycosides Ciclosporin Corticosteroids Diuretics Nitrates Pentoxifylline SSRIs Tacrolimus Zidovudine
Miconazole			Warfarin
Nystatin	—	Gastrointestinal disturbance	—
Paracetamol	—	Alcoholism Anorexia Liver disease Renal disease	Alcohol Anticoagulants Anticonvulsants Carbamazepine Domperidone Isonicotinic hydrazide Metoclopramide Zidovudine
Penciclovir (topical)	—	—	—
Temazepam	—	CNS depression Driving or operating machinery Glaucoma Myasthenia gravis Respiratory problems	Alcohol CNS depressants Fluvoxamine Itraconazole Ketoconazole Nefazodone
Tetracyclines (e.g. doxycycline)	Children Myasthenia gravis	Lupus erythematosus Neuromuscular diseases Photosensitivity Renal disease	ACE inhibitors Antacids Anticoagulants Barbiturates Iron Lithium Milk Retinoids
Vitamin B$_{12}$	—	—	—

CNS, Central nervous system; MAOI, monoamine oxidase inhibitors; NSAIDs, nonsteroidal antiinflammatory drugs; SNRI, selective noradrenaline reuptake inhibitor; SSRI, selective serotonin reuptake inhibitor.

[a]This list is not complete and there may be other drugs that can interact, including over-the-counter medications, vitamins, minerals or herbal products. Always check BNF or other sources before use. See also http://www.drugs.com/drug-interactions.

clinicians and secondary care management are shown in Table 5.17.

FOLLOW-UP OF PATIENTS

Though it is desirable to offer active treatment for oral lesions, this is not always possible or indicated, and, sometimes, watchful waiting is required, by following up the patient. Sometimes, for example in suspected traumatic ulceration, the diagnosis can only be decided by removing predisposing factors, and then checking progress in 2 weeks to see if the lesion is healing. Patients with chronic conditions can often be followed up in a primary care setting but frequently the care is best shared between the specialist and the primary dental and/ or medical practitioner. Follow-up in secondary care may be indicated when there is:

- a complicated or serious diagnosis (notably Behçet syndrome, cancer, erythroplakia or other potentially malignant disorder with severe dysplasia, HIV infection, pemphigus, etc.)
- a situation where investigations are required, but not possible or appropriate to carry out in a primary care setting
- a situation where therapy may not be straightforward and may require potent agents not available or appropriate to be prescribed in a primary care setting.

ASSESSMENT OF RESPONSE TO TREATMENT

In both primary and secondary care, there is a professional responsibility to assess the effectiveness and outcome of any treatment offered to every patient. Disease severity of most oral conditions can now be estimated using oral disease severity scoring (see Chapter 4) and re-scored after treatment. Since many drugs used in oral medicine have limited evidence for their effectiveness, this assessment is even more important.

Patient-reported outcome measures (PROMS) are equally important in providing evidence of effectiveness of any treatment prescribed (see Chapter 4).

RECOMMENDED READING

BSR and BHPR guideline on prescribing drugs in pregnancy and breastfeeding — Part I: standard and biologic disease modifying anti-rheumatic drugs and corticosteroids. Rheumatology. 55 (9), 2016, 1693—1697.

Carrasco-Labra, A., et al. (Eds.), 2020. How to Use Evidence-based Dental Practices to Improve Your Clinical Decision-making. ADA Publishing, Chicago, IL.

Challacombe, S.J., Alsahaf, S., Tappuni, A., 2015. Recurrent aphthous stomatitis: towards evidence-based treatment? Curr. Oral Health Rep. 2, 158—167.

Cochrane Handbook for Systematic Reviews of Interventions Version 5.1.0, 2011. The Cochrane Collaboration. Available at. www.cochrane-handbook.org (Accessed January 2022).

Khattri, S., Kumbargere Nagraj, S., et al., 2020. Adjunctive systemic antimicrobials for the non-surgical treatment of periodontitis. Cochrane. Database. Syst. Rev. 11, CD012568.

Sadowski, L.A., Upadhyay, R., Greeley, Z.W., Margulies, B.J., 2021. Current drugs to treat infections with herpes simplex viruses-1 and -2. Viruses. 13 (7), 1228.

da Silva, E.L., de Lima, T.B., Rados, P.V., Visioli, F. Efficacy of topical non-steroidal immunomodulators in the treatment of oral lichen planus: a systematic review and meta-analysis. Clin. Oral. Investig. 2021 (9), 5149—5169.

Thakrar, P., Chaudhry, S.I., 2016. Oral ulceration: an overview of diagnosis and management. Prim. Dent. J. 5 (1), 30—33.

Wolff, A., Joshi, R.K., Ekström, J., et al., 2017. A guide to medications inducing salivary gland dysfunction, xerostomia, and subjective sialorrhea: a systematic review sponsored by the world workshop on oral medicine VI. Drugs. R. D. 17 (1), 1—28.

Oral Diseases and Disorders

Oral Ulceration: An Overview

INTRODUCTION

The mouth can be sore for a number of reasons, especially where there are distinct conditions, such as:

- Dry mouth (hyposalivation) — this predisposes to soreness, since the lubricating and protective functions of saliva are reduced and infections, such as candidosis, are more common. It is especially a problem after irradiation to the head and neck.
- Epithelial thinning or breaches can also result in soreness. This occurs in:
  - mucosal inflammation: any inflammatory lesion can cause soreness
  - mucosal atrophy: this is the term often used for thinning of the epithelium, which has a red appearance since the underlying lamina propria shows through. Most commonly seen in geographic tongue (erythema migrans, benign migratory glossitis), atrophy may also be seen in lichen planus or systemic disorders, such as deficiency states (of iron, folic acid or B vitamins)
  - mucosal erosions: this is the term used for localised thinning or superficial breaches of the epithelium, which often initially have a red appearance, since there is little or no damage to the underlying lamina propria. Erosions are common in radiation-induced mucositis and in lichen planus.
  - mucosal ulcers: this is the term used where there is a breach of the epithelium, usually damage to both epithelium and lamina propria, and then a crater forms, sometimes made more obvious clinically by oedema or proliferation causing swelling of the surrounding tissue (Fig. 6.1). When a breach penetrates the full thickness of the epithelium, however, it typically becomes covered by a fibrinous exudate and then has a yellowish appearance. An inflammatory halo, if present, also highlights the ulcer with a red halo, around the yellow or grey ulcer. Ulcers are common in recurrent aphthous stomatitis.

Most other ulcers/erosions are due to local causes, such as trauma or burns, but neoplasms and systemic disorders must always be considered.

- Soreness may also be encountered in an apparently normal mouth with no clinical signs of any of the above. This can be due to:
  - sub-clinical mucosal disease, such as a haematinic deficiency state, particularly of vitamin B_{12}, or anaemia
  - neuropathies, such as in diabetes mellitus
  - burning mouth syndrome/oral dysaesthesia.

ULCERS

Ulcers and erosions can be the final common manifestation of a spectrum of conditions ranging from epithelial damage resulting from an immunological attack (as in pemphigus, pemphigoid or lichen planus) to damage because of an immune defect as in human immunodeficiency virus (HIV) disease and leukaemia, infections as in herpesviruses, tuberculosis and syphilis, or nutritional defects, such as in vitamin deficiencies and some intestinal disease. A useful mnemonic to remember the main causes is 'So many laws and directives' (systemic; malignant; local; aphthae; drugs), and the systemic causes are mainly blood; infections; gastrointestinal and skin diseases ('bigs').

The most important feature of ulceration is to determine whether the ulcer is recurrent (usually local disease) or persistent (Box 6.1), since this may indicate that the ulcer is caused by a chronic condition such as:

- neoplasia, such as carcinoma
- chronic trauma, such as from a rough restoration, appliance or tooth
- systemic disease, such as a blood disorder (e.g. leukaemia); infection, such as syphilis, tuberculosis or a mycosis; gastrointestinal disease, such as Crohn disease or ulcerative colitis; or skin disease, such as lichen planus, pemphigoid or pemphigus.

An important feature is whether one or more than one ulcer is present since malignant tumours usually cause a single

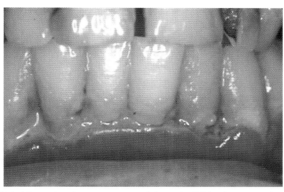

Fig. 6.1 Ulceration in acute necrotising gingivitis destroys the interdental papillae particularly.

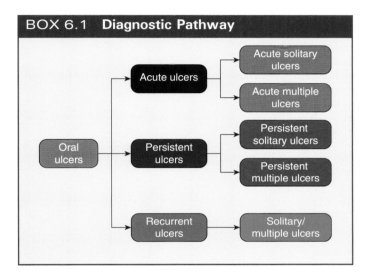

BOX 6.1 **Diagnostic Pathway**

lesion. A single ulcer persisting for greater than 3 weeks without signs of obvious healing must be taken very seriously, as it could be a neoplasm or chronic infection.

Multiple persistent ulcers are mainly caused by:
- **i**nfections
- **b**lood diseases
- **g**astrointestinal diseases
- **s**kin diseases
- **i**mmune defects

Multiple non-persistent ulcers can be caused by aphthae, when the ulcers heal spontaneously, usually within 1 week to 1 month. If this is not the case, an alternative diagnosis should be considered.

Erosions or ulcers on both sides at the commissures of the lips are usually angular stomatitis (cheilitis), but sores are also sometimes caused at the angles by trauma (such as dental treatment) or infection (such as recurrent herpes labialis).

Systemic Disease

A wide range of systemic diseases, especially blood, infectious, gut and skin disorders ('bigs'), may cause oral lesions, which,

because of the moisture, trauma and infection in the mouth, tend to break down to leave ulcers or erosions (Box 6.2).

- Blood (haematological) disease can cause aphthous-like ulceration. Deficiency anaemia may underlie some cases. Mouth ulcers may be seen in leukaemias and myelodysplastic syndromes, associated with cytotoxic therapy, with viral, bacterial or fungal infection, or be non-specific. Other oral features may include purpura, gingival bleeding, lymphadenopathy, recurrent herpes labialis and candidosis. Hypereosinophilic syndrome may also present with ulcers.
- Infective causes of mouth ulcers include mainly viral infections, especially the herpesviruses. Other viruses that may cause mouth ulcers include Coxsackie, enteric cytopathic human orphan (ECHO) and HIV viruses. Bacterial causes of mouth ulcers are less common, apart from acute necrotising (ulcerative) gingivitis. Syphilis, either the primary or secondary stages, and tuberculosis are increasing, especially in HIV/ acquired immunodeficiency syndrome (AIDS). Fungal causes of ulcers are also uncommon in the developed world but are increasingly seen in immunocompromised persons and travellers. Protozoal causes of ulcers, such as leishmaniasis, are rare in the developed world, but are appearing in HIV/AIDS. Other causes are shown in Table 6.1.
- Gastrointestinal disorders may result in soreness or mouth ulcers. Some patients with aphthae-like ulceration may have intestinal disease, such as coeliac disease, causing malabsorption and deficiencies of haematinics, when they may also develop angular stomatitis or glossitis. Crohn disease and pyostomatitis vegetans may cause chronic ulcers. Orofacial granulomatosis (OFG), which has many features reminiscent of Crohn disease, may also cause persistent ulceration.
- Skin (mucocutaneous) disorders that may cause persistent oral erosions or ulceration (or occasionally blisters) include particularly lichen planus, occasionally pemphigoid, and rarely pemphigus, erythema multiforme and epidermolysis bullosa.

Chronic ulcerative stomatitis (CUS) is a mucocutaneous disease characterised by involvement of mucosal surfaces and skin. The disease is seen predominantly among women in the fifth and sixth decades of life. Clinically, CUS patients present with oral erosive or ulcerative lesions that may resemble lichen planus and/or other vesiculobullous lesions. The tongue is the most common location, followed by the buccal mucosa and the gingival tissues. Routine histology may exhibit features of lichenoid mucositis and is often non-diagnostic. Direct immunofluorescence of lesional and perilesional oral mucosa reveals a speckled or finely granular pattern of IgG deposition in the nuclei of keratinocytes, limited to the basal and parabasal layers of the epithelium. Treatment is with topical corticosteroids and/or hydroxychloroquine.

Other causes can include the following:
- lupus erythematosus, Reiter syndrome
- vasculitides: periarteritis nodosa, Wegener granulomatosis and giant cell arteritis

BOX 6.2   Causes of Mouth Ulcers

Systemic Disease

Blood Disorders
- Anaemia
- Haematinic deficiencies
- Leukaemias
- Neutropenia

Infections
- Viruses:
  - herpetic stomatitis
  - HIV
- Chickenpox
  - hand, foot and mouth disease
  - herpangina
  - infectious mononucleosis
- Bacteria:
  - acute necrotising gingivitis
  - syphilis
  - tuberculosis
- Fungi:
  - blastomycosis
  - cryptococcosis
  - histoplasmosis
  - paracoccidioidomycosis
- Parasites:
  - leishmaniasis

Gastrointestinal Disease
- Coeliac disease
- Crohn disease (and orofacial granulomatosis)
- Ulcerative colitis

Skin Disease
- Erythema multiforme
- Lichen planus and lichenoid lesions
- Pemphigoid and variants
- Pemphigus vulgaris
- Chronic ulcerative stomatitis
- Dermatitis herpetiformis
- Epidermolysis bullosa

Others
- Rheumatic diseases:
  - lupus erythematosus

- Sweet syndrome
- Reiter syndrome (reactive arthritis)
- Vasculitides:
  - Wegener granulomatosis
  - periarteritis nodosa
  - giant cell arteritis
- Disorders of uncertain pathogenesis:
  - eosinophilic ulcer
  - necrotising sialometaplasia

Malignant Neoplasms

Oral or Encroaching From Antrum, Salivary Glands, Nose or Skin
- Carcinomas
- Lymphomas
- Sarcomas

Local Causes

Trauma
- Sharp teeth or restorations
- Appliances
- Non-accidental injury
- Self-inflicted
- Iatrogenic

Burns
- Heat
- Cold
- Chemical
- Radiation
- Electric

Aphthae
Recurrent aphthous stomatitis and autoinflammatory disorders (e.g. Behçet syndrome, PFAPA)

Drugs
- Methotrexate
- Bisphosphonates
- Cytotoxics
- NSAIDs
- Nicorandil
- Propylthiouracil

- disorders whose pathogenesis is uncertain: eosinophilic ulcer (traumatic ulcerative granuloma with stromal eosinophilia; TUGSE), necrotising sialometaplasia, sarcoidosis, autoinflammatory syndromes such as periodic fever, aphthae, pharyngitis and adenitis (PFAPA) and Behçet syndrome.

Malignant Ulcers

A range of neoplasms may present with ulcers, most commonly these are carcinomas, but Kaposi sarcoma, lymphomas and other neoplasms may be seen.

Local Causes

- At any age there may be factitious ulceration, especially of the maxillary gingivae, or burns with chemicals of various kinds, heat, cold or ionising radiation.
- In children, they are usually caused by accidental biting, or following dental treatment or other trauma, hard foods or appliance (Fig. 6.2). In child abuse (non-accidental injury), ulceration of the upper labial fraenum may follow a traumatic fraenal tear. Bruised and swollen lips, and even subluxed teeth or fractured mandible, can be other features of child abuse. The lingual fraenum may be traumatised by

TABLE 6.1 Infectious Diseases That May Produce Oral Ulceration

Disease	Causal Agent	Major Manifestations
Herpes simplex[a]	HSV	Fever, oral ulceration, gingivitis, gingivostomatitis, herpes labialis (secondary infection), cervical lymph node enlargement
Herpes zoster[a] (shingles)	VZV	Rash like chickenpox, but limited to dermatome Severe pain Oral ulceration in zoster of maxillary or mandibular division of trigeminal nerve Ulcers on palate and in pinna of ear in Ramsay—Hunt syndrome
AIDS (HIV infection)	HIV	Pneumonia, Kaposi sarcoma, lymphomas, generalised lymphadenopathy, candidosis, herpes simplex virus, hairy leukoplakia, periodontal disease, ulcers
Tuberculosis[a]	Mycobacterium tuberculosis	Ulceration, fever, weight loss, general lymphadenopathy
Syphilis	Treponema pallidum	Chancre, lymphadenopathy, rash, ulceration, mucous patches, gumma
Chickenpox (varicella)[a]	VZV	Rash evolves through macule, papule, vesicle and pustule; rash crops and is most dense on trunk General lymphadenopathy, oral ulcers, cervical lymph node enlargement
Cytomegalovirus[a]	CMV	Glandular-fever-type syndrome (Paul—Bunnell negative), general lymphadenopathy, ulcers in immunocompromised people
Hand, foot and mouth disease	Coxsackie viruses	Rash, minor malaise, oral ulceration (usually mild)
Herpangina	Coxsackie viruses	Fever, sore throat, vesicles and ulcers on soft palate, cervical lymph node enlargement
Infectious mononucleosis	EBV	Fever, pharyngitis, general lymphadenopathy, tonsillar exudate, palatal petechiae, oral ulceration
Mucocutaneous lymph node syndrome (Kawasaki disease)	?	Rash, hands and feet desquamation, general lymphadenopathy, myocarditis, strawberry tongue, labial oedema, pharyngitis
Mycoplasmal pneumonia (atypical pneumonia)	Mycoplasma	Sore throat, fever, pneumonia, erythema multiforme occasionally
Pertussis (whooping cough)	Bordetella pertussis	Cough, fever, occasionally ulceration of lingual fraenum
Toxoplasmosis[a]	Toxoplasma gondii	Glandular-fever-type syndrome (Paul—Bunnell negative), general lymphadenopathy, cough, sore throat
Gonorrhoea	Neisseria gonorrhoea	Urethritis, pharyngitis

[a]Prevalent and often widespread infections in the immunocompromised, high-risk patients such as organ transplant, HIV or leukaemic patients.

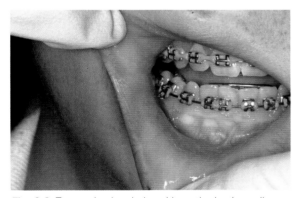

Fig. 6.2 Traumatic ulcer induced by orthodontic appliance.

repeated rubbing over the lower incisor teeth in children with recurrent bouts of coughing as in whooping cough or in self-mutilating conditions. Chronic trauma may produce an ulcer with a keratotic margin.
- Trauma can produce ulceration in adults. Sometimes the lingual fraenum is damaged by trauma in cunnilingus, or the palate in fellatio.

Aphthae (Recurrent Aphthous Stomatitis)

Ulcers (Fig. 6.3), in persons who are otherwise well or at least no systemic disease is evident, are commonly aphthae, though occasionally they are associated with or exacerbated by haematinic deficiencies.

Rarely, similar ulcers are seen in patients with systemic disease such as Behçet syndrome (see Chapter 27), PFAPA and HIV infection (see Chapter 39v).

Drug-Induced Ulceration

Drugs may induce ulcers by producing a local burn or by a variety of mechanisms. Cytotoxic drugs (e.g. methotrexate), NSAIDs, sirolimus, everolimus and nicorandil (a potassium channel activator used in cardiac disorders) or others may be the cause.

DIAGNOSIS

Making a diagnosis of the cause for oral soreness or ulceration is based mainly on the history and clinical features. Key is whether the ulcers are recurrent or persistent, single or

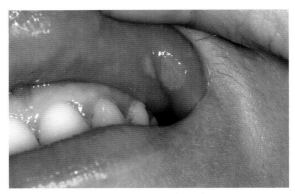

Fig. 6.3 Aphthous ulceration.

	Single Ulcer	Multiple Ulcers
TABLE 6.2 **Differentiation of Mouth Ulcers (Main Causes)**		
Recurrent	Trauma	Recurrent aphthous stomatitis (RAS)
		Behçet syndrome
		Erythema multiforme
		Recurrent herpes
Persistent	Neoplasm	Lichen planus
	Trauma	Pemphigoid
	Chronic infection (syphilis, Tuberculosis, fungal)	Pemphigus
		Drugs
	Drugs	

multiple. The age of onset, number, duration, shape, character of the edge of the ulcer and appearance of the ulcer base should also be noted.

Acute multiple ulcers are often viral in origin; chronic multiple ulcers may be RAS if recurrent, or vesiculobullous diseases if persistent—when biopsy may be indicated.

A chronic single ulcer may be traumatic, drug-induced, a chronic infection (e.g., tuberculosis, syphilis or mycosis) or a neoplasm (Table 6.2).

Ulcers should always be examined for induration (firmness on palpation), which may be indicative of malignancy. Unless the cause is undoubtedly local, general physical examination is also indicated, looking especially for mucocutaneous lesions, lymphadenopathy or fever (Algorithms 6.1–6.6).

Features that might suggest a systemic background to mouth ulcers include:
- Extra-oral features such as:
  - skin lesions
  - ocular lesions
  - anogenital lesions
  - purpura
  - fever
  - lymphadenopathy
  - hepatomegaly
  - splenomegaly
  - chronic cough
  - gastrointestinal complaints (e.g. pain, altered bowel habits, blood in faeces)
  - loss of weight or, in children, a failure to thrive
  - weakness.
- An atypical history or ulcer behaviour such as:
  - onset of ulcers in later adult life
  - exacerbation of ulcers
  - severe aphthae
  - aphthae unresponsive to topical hydrocortisone or triamcinolone.
- Other oral lesions, especially:
  - candidosis
  - herpetic lesions
  - glossitis
  - petechiae
  - gingival bleeding
  - gingival swelling
  - necrotising gingivitis or periodontitis
  - hairy leukoplakia
  - Kaposi sarcoma.

Investigations that may sometimes be indicated include the following (Table 6.3):
- Blood tests: may be useful for excluding possible haematinic deficiencies or other conditions when a systemic cause, such as leukaemia, EBV or HIV infection, is suspected.
- Microbiological and serological investigations: may be needed, especially if microbial causes are suspected.
- HbA1c to exclude diabetes.
- Biopsy: may be needed, especially where there:
  - is a single ulcer persisting for greater than 3 weeks
  - is an ulcer that might have been traumatic in aetiology, but persists for greater than 3 weeks after relief from the trauma
  - is induration
  - are skin lesions
  - are lesions in other mucosae
  - are other related systemic lesions, signs or symptoms.
- Imaging and other special investigations: may be indicated where there are possible lesions, such as tuberculosis, the deep mycoses, carcinoma or sarcoidosis.

TREATMENT

- Treat the underlying cause.
- Remove aetiological factors.
- Ensure any possible traumatic element is removed (e.g. a denture flange).
- Prescribe chlorhexidine 0.2% aqueous mouthwash.
- Maintain good oral hygiene.
- Benzydamine mouthwash or spray, or silver nitrate application to an ulcer may help ease discomfort.

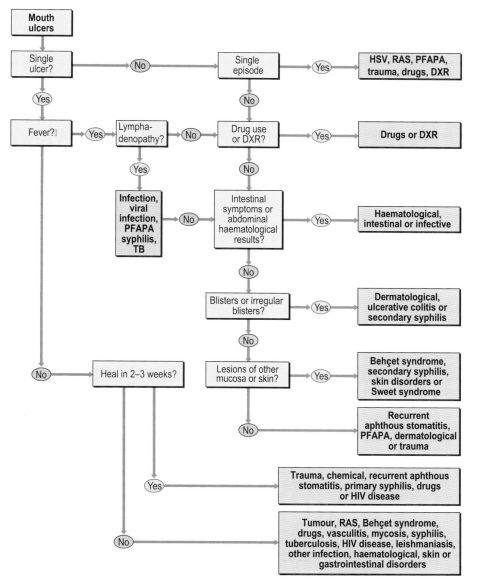

Algorithm 6.1 Oral ulceration. Irradiation; *PFAPA*, autoinflammatory states such as periodic fever, aphthae, pharyngitis, adenitis; *RAS*, recurrent aphthous stomatitis; *TB*, tuberculosis

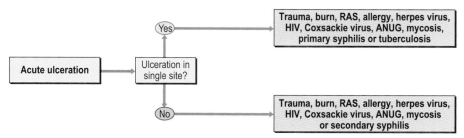

Algorithm 6.2 Acute ulceration. *ANUG*, acute necrotising ulcerative gingivitis.

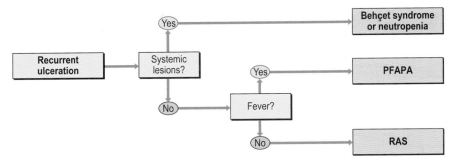

Algorithm 6.3 Recurrent multiple ulcers.

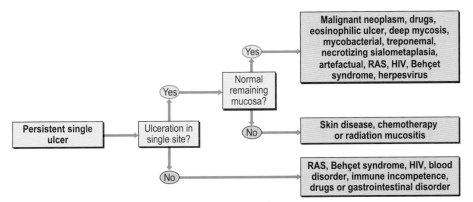

Algorithm 6.4 Persistent single ulcers.

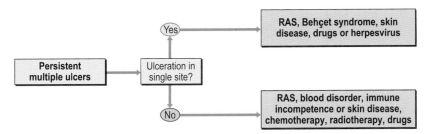

Algorithm 6.5 Persistent multiple ulcers.

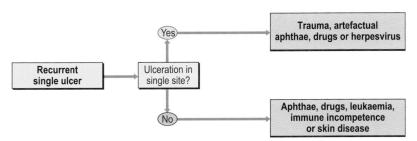

Algorithm 6.6 Recurrent single ulcers.

TABLE 6.3   Aids That Might be Helpful in Diagnosis/Prognosis/Management in Some Patients With Soreness and Ulcers[a]

In Most Cases	In Some Cases
Full blood picture	Blood glucose
Serum ferritin, vitamin B_{12} and corrected whole blood folate levels	Tissue transglutaminase
	ESR
	Serum immunoglobulins
	Serology (HIV, HTLV-1, HSV, VZV, EBV, syphilis, mycoplasma)
	ANA
	ANCA
	Culture and sensitivity
	Biopsy
	ELISA for desmoglein
	Chest radiography

[a]See text for details and glossary for abbreviations.

- Topical corticosteroids are useful in the management of many oral ulcerative conditions where there is no systemic involvement, such as recurrent aphthous stomatitis and oral lichen planus (see Table 6.3). Corticosteroid mouthwash (betamethasone 500 mcg soluble tablets/prednisolone 5 mg tablets/Flixonase 400 mcg nasules), ointment mixed with Orabase dental paste (e.g. clobetasol propionate) and corticosteroid inhalers (e.g. beclomethasone) are often used.

- Patients should not eat or drink for 30 minutes after using the corticosteroid, in order to prolong contact with the lesion.
- Adverse effects are associated with systemic corticosteroid use. With most topical corticosteroids there is little systemic absorption and thus no significant adrenocortical suppression. Candidosis may arise in patients using potent topical corticosteroids.

Recurrent Aphthous Stomatitis

> **KEY POINTS**
> - Ulcers are the most common lesions affecting the oral mucosa.
> - Aphthae are multiple recurrent small, round or ovoid ulcers which have circumscribed margins, erythematous haloes and yellow or grey floors, appearing first in childhood or adolescence.
> - A minor degree of immunological dysregulation underlies aphthae.
> - A family history of aphthae is common.
> - Most patients appear otherwise well and predisposing factors are unclear.
> - Ulcers similar to aphthae (aphthous-like ulcers) may be seen in some immune disorders.
> - Topical corticosteroids control most aphthae.

INTRODUCTION

Recurrent aphthous stomatitis (RAS) is a common condition affecting 10% to 20% of the general population. It is characterised by:

- Multiple recurrent, round or ovoid ulcers known as aphthae, which have circumscribed margins, erythematous haloes and yellow or grey base (Fig. 7.1):
- Typically appear on non-keratinised and mobile mucosae — they are rare on gingivae or palate.
- First onset in childhood or adolescence.
- No systemic disease.
  - It is important to note that individual aphthae last only a limited period of time before they heal spontaneously. Episodes are recurrent which is quite a different history from ulcers that persist without healing, such as malignant ulcers and those associated with vesiculobullous disorders such as pemphigoid and pemphigus. Fortunately, the natural history of RAS is one of eventual remission in most cases, but this may take several years.

EPIDEMIOLOGY

- RAS affects 10% to 15% of the population.
- RAS typically starts in childhood or adolescence.
- There is a slight female predisposition to RAS.
- RAS occurs worldwide though it appears to be more common in the developed world.

PREDISPOSING FACTORS

There is a genetic predisposition shown by a positive family history in about one-third of patients and by an increased frequency of HLA types (HLA-A2, A11, B12 and DR2). There is an association between RAS and inheritance of a single-nucleotide polymorphism of the nitric oxide synthase (NOS2) gene (encoding inducible nitric oxide synthase). RAS has been linked to genes controlling the release of interleukins (IL-1B) and (IL-6). RAS is considered an immune-mediated condition but specific abnormalities of the immune system have not yet been identified.

- Stress underlies RAS in some cases and ulcers appear to exacerbate during school or university examination times.
- Trauma from biting the mucosa or from dental appliances may lead to aphthae in some people.
- Cessation of smoking may precipitate or exacerbate RAS in some cases, but the reason is unclear.
- Haematinic deficiency may be relevant in a minority. In up to 20% of patients, deficiencies of iron, folic acid (folate) or vitamin B are found and sometimes the correction of this may relieve the ulceration. Iron deficiency is usually due to chronic haemorrhage (e.g. from the gastrointestinal or genitourinary tract). Folic acid is found in green leafy vegetables especially, and body stores are small; deficiencies may be dietary, or related to malabsorption or drugs (alcohol,

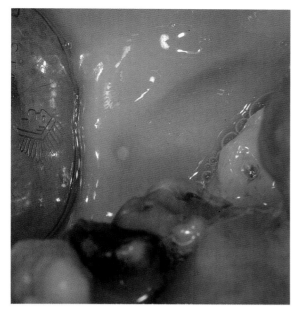

Fig. 7.1 Minor aphthae; typical round shape, yellow base and erythematous halo.

anticonvulsants, carbamazepine and some cytotoxic drugs). Vitamin B_{12} is found especially in meat, is absorbed via intrinsic factor from the gastric parietal cells in the ileum and stored in the liver for about 3 years. Dietary B_{12} deficiency can arise particularly in vegans, in pernicious anaemia and after gastrectomy, and in ileal disease (e.g. Crohn disease). Histamine H2 receptor antagonists (cimetidine, ranitidine, omeprazole) can also impede vitamin B_{12} absorption.

- Endocrine factors are relevant in some women where RAS are related to the fall in progestogen level in the luteal phase of the menstrual cycle, or to the contraceptive pill, and then RAS may regress temporarily in pregnancy.
- Sodium lauryl sulphate (SLS), a detergent in some toothpastes and other oral healthcare products, may be associated with oral ulceration.

Aphthous-Like Ulcers

The diagnosis of RAS is not infrequently misapplied to the similar ulcers (aphthous-like ulcers), which may be seen in a range of systemic conditions (Table 7.3). The history and examination should be directed to eliciting any cutaneous, gastrointestinal, genital, ocular, joint problems or history of fever, which might point to these conditions. They include conditions such as:

- Immune deficiencies such as human immunodeficiency virus (HIV), cyclical neutropenia and other immune defects.
- Behçet disease, where mouth ulcers are seen along with genital ulcers.
- Coeliac disease: in about 3% of patients with recurrent mouth ulcers, coeliac disease (gluten-sensitive enteropathy) — an allergic reaction to gluten in wheat — is seen.

- Crohn disease, where ulcers are seen with an enteropathy.
- Autoinflammatory conditions such as periodic fever, aphthous stomatitis, pharyngitis and cervical adenitis (PFAPA) syndrome — a condition seen in children, appears related to a disorder of innate immunity with complement activation and IL-1β/-18, resolves spontaneously and rarely has long-term sequelae. Corticosteroids are highly effective symptomatically; tonsillectomy and cimetidine treatment have been effective in a few patients.
- Sweet syndrome, in which mouth ulcers are found with conjunctivitis, episcleritis and inflamed tender skin papules or nodules.
- Drug use, especially NSAIDs and nicorandil.

AETIOLOGY AND PATHOGENESIS

The aetiology of RAS is multi-factorial and not entirely clear; therefore aphthae are termed 'idiopathic'. Many studies have explored an infectious aetiology, but there is no evidence of transmissibility and RAS does not at present appear to be infectious, contagious, or sexually shared. It seems likely that a minor degree of immunological dysregulation underlies aphthae, and a genetic tendency to ulceration, and cross-reacting antigens between the oral mucosa and microorganisms may be involved. Reactions to heat shock proteins (HSP) are one possibility. HSP27 is a powerful inductor of interleukin IL-10, a major inhibitor of Th1 response and in RAS, there is a reduced cellular expression of HSP27 and IL-10. Decreased IL-10 suggests a failure of the immune system to suppress inflammation.

Immune mechanisms that appear to play a role in a people with a genetic predisposition to oral ulceration include the following:

- A local cell-mediated immune response to HSP (perhaps induced by infection or agents) involving cytotoxic $CD8^+$ T cells, natural killer (NK) cells, macrophages and mast cells.
- T-helper cells (gamma-delta cells) predominate in the early RAS lesions, along with some NK cells.
- Cytotoxic cells then appear in the lesions and there is evidence for an antibody-dependent cellular cytotoxicity reaction, and neutrophils and NK cells may be involved.
- HSP can block the production of pro-inflammatory cytokines (e.g. tumour necrosis factors (TNFs) and interleukins [IL-1β, IL-6 and IL-8]) through inhibition of NF-κB and mitogen-activated protein kinase (MAPK) pathways or activate anti-inflammatory cytokines (e.g. transforming growth factor-β1), and therefore control the magnitude of the immune response.
- IL-1β and IL-6 gene polymorphisms are associated with an increased risk for RAS. Systemic immunological abnormalities in RAS include increased plasma levels of IL-8 and IL-6. Serum IL-6 (via IL-1β over-production) typically fluctuates in auto-inflammatory syndromes, which also manifest with recurrent ulceration.

- There is increased expression of TNF-α, IL-2, IL-4, IL-5 and interferon-γ in aphthous ulcers.
- There is an overly exuberant inflammation reaction which may be caused by derangement of Toll-like receptor (TLR) gene expression.
- There is decreased constitutive expression of indoleamine 2,3-dioxygenase (IDO) in the oral mucosa in RAS which may lead to the loss of local immune tolerance.
- NOS2 gene polymorphisms implicate a role of inducible nitric oxide synthase.

CLINICAL FEATURES

Patients with RAS have no clinically detectable systemic symptoms or signs. If ulceration affects the genitals or other mucosae, the diagnosis cannot be of RAS alone — rather of aphthous-like ulceration.

There are three main clinical types of RAS (Table 7.1):
- minor aphthous ulcers (~80% of all RAS)
- major aphthous ulcers
- herpetiform ulcers.

Minor Aphthous Ulcers

This type of RAS:
- occurs mainly in the 10- to 40-year age group
- often causes minimal symptoms
- consists of small round or ovoid ulcers 2 to 4 mm in diameter (Fig. 7.2), in groups of only a few ulcers (1—6) at a time, with initially yellowish floors surrounded by an erythematous halo and some oedema, but the floors assume a greyish hue as healing and epithelialisation proceeds
- affects mainly the non-keratinised mobile mucosae of the lips, cheeks, floor of the mouth, sulci or ventrum of the tongue
- heals in 7 to 10 days
- recurs at intervals of 1 to 4 months
- heal without scarring.

Major Aphthous Ulcers

This type of RAS:
- are round or ovoid
- some reach a large size, usually about 1 cm in diameter or even larger
- are found on any area of the oral mucosa, including the keratinised dorsum of the tongue or palate (Fig. 7.3)
- occur in groups of only a few ulcers (1 to 6) at one tihme

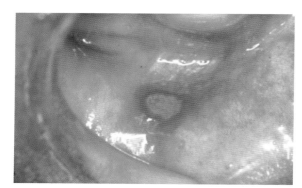

Fig. 7.2 Minor aphthae; small ulcers healing within 7 to 10 days.

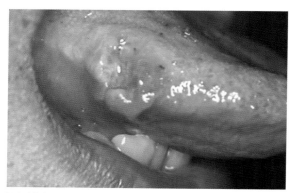

Fig. 7.3 Major aphthae; large ulcer involving the right lateral tongue.

- heal slowly over 10 to 40 days
- are extremely painful
- recur extremely frequently
- may heal with scarring.

Herpetiform Ulceration

This type of RAS:
- is found in a slightly older age group than the other RAS
- is found mainly in females
- begins with vesiculation, which passes rapidly into multiple minute pinhead-sized discrete ulcers (Fig. 7.4)
- increases in size and coalesces to leave large, round, ragged ulcers
- involves any oral site, including the keratinised mucosa but frequently the tongue

TABLE 7.1 Clinical Characteristics of the Different Clinical Types of Aphthae			
	Minor	Major	Herpetiform
Percentage of all aphthae	75—85	10—15	5
Size	Up to 10 mm	>10 mm (some)	<5 mm
Duration (days)	10—14	>14	10—14
Scarring	No	Yes	No

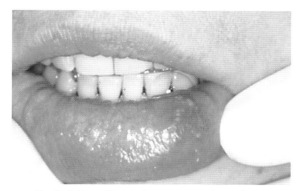

Fig. 7.4 Herpetiform ulcers; many minute ulcers.

- heals in 10 days or longer
- is often extremely painful
- can recur so frequently that ulceration may be virtually continuous.

DIAGNOSIS

A diagnosis of RAS is based on the history and clinical features, as no specific tests are available and is applied to the overall clinical presentation and not a description of individual ulcers. The diagnosis of RAS is not infrequently misapplied to the similar ulcers (aphthous-like ulcers), which may be seen in a range of systemic conditions. The history and examination should be directed to eliciting any cutaneous, gastrointestinal, genital, ocular, joint problems or history of fever, which might point to these conditions. An ulcer severity score may be used to grade the severity of ulceration (Fig. 7.5). Biopsy is rarely indicated and is only usually needed where a different diagnosis is suspected but even vesiculobullous disorders can on occasion present with recurring ulcers. Therefore, to exclude a number of systemic disorders, it is often useful to undertake blood investigations (Table 7.2):

- Full blood picture (haemoglobin, white cell count and differential, red cell indices)
- Red cell folate assay
- Serum ferritin levels (or other iron studies)
- Vitamin B_{12} measurements
- Calcium measurements (low in coeliac disease)
- Tissue transglutaminase and IgA anti-endomysial antibody assays (positive in coeliac disease)
- ESR.

TREATMENT

Disorders where aphthous-like ulcers are also seen (Table 7.3) should be excluded and RAS managed as follows:

1. Correct predisposing factors
2. Relieve pain and heal present ulcers
3. Prevent new ulcers
   Predisposing factors should be corrected (Algorithm 7.1):

- Trauma: patients should avoid hard or sharp foods (e.g. toast, potato crisps) and brush their teeth atraumatically (e.g. by using a small-headed, soft toothbrush).
- If SLS is implicated, this should be avoided; a number of SLS-free toothpastes are available (e.g. Biotene; Kingfisher; Sensodyne Pronamel).
- Any iron or vitamin deficiency should be corrected once the cause of that deficiency has been established.
- If there is an obvious relationship to certain foods, these should be excluded from the diet.
- The occasional patient who relates ulcers to the menstrual cycle or to an oral contraceptive may benefit from suppression of ovulation with a progestogen or a change in the oral contraceptive.
  Relief of pain and reduction of ulcer duration.
- Good oral hygiene should be maintained; chlorhexidine or triclosan mouthwashes may help. An SLS-free toothpaste such as Sensodyne ProNamel may help.
- Anti-inflammatory agents: topical agents, such as benzydamine, amlexanox or diclofenac in hyaluronan may help in the management of discomfort in RAS.
- Active treatment is indicated if the patient has significant discomfort (Tables 7.4–7.6):
  - The ulcer severity can be scored, as well as an oral health index. This may give an indication of whether topical or systemic therapy is needed and allow both the clinical response to therapy to be assessed and a patient-reported outcome.
  - Topical corticosteroids can often control minor or major RAS. Topical corticosteroids are the primary therapeutic agents used to treat ulcerative mucosal lesions, which have an immunologically based aetiology such as aphthae (Fig. 7.6). A mild potency agent such as hydrocortisone may be effective but more typically a medium potency corticosteroid such as betamethasone or a higher potency one such as fluocinonide or beclomethasone is required, moving to a super-potent topical corticosteroid (e.g. clobetasol) if the benefit is inadequate (see Tables 5.5 and 34.5). Patients should be instructed to apply a small quantity of the agent three times daily, refraining from eating and drinking for the subsequent 0.5 hours. In long-term use, candidosis can arise and thus topical antifungal medication such as Nystatin may be prudent. The more major concern — of adrenal suppression with long-term and/or repeated application — has rarely been reported. Topical preparations (apart from super potent halogenated corticosteroids when used several times a day) appear not to cause a significant problem. Larger and recalcitrant ulcers can be treated by intralesional therapy such as triamcinolone injections. Topical tetracycline (a capsule of 100 mg doxycycline dissolved in 10 mL water) as a mouth rinse may provide relief and reduce ulcer duration but must be avoided in children under 12 years old who might ingest the tetracycline and develop tooth staining. It is most effective in herpetiform RAS.

If RAS fails to respond to these measures, systemic immunomodulators may be required, under specialist supervision.

Ulcer severity score

Date:	Consultant:
Name:	M/F:
Hospital no.	Diagnosis:
DoB:	Management:

Characteristic	Descriptor	Score
Average **size** (mm)	Average size of ulcers (mm) **Maximum score 20**	
Average **number**	Average number of ulcers per episode **Maximum score 20**	
Average **duration** (weeks)	1 week = 2 (e.g. 0.5 week = 1, 1.5 weeks = 3) **Maximum score 10**	
Ulcer-free period (weeks)	10 minus the average ulcer-free period in weeks **Maximum score 10**	
Pain	1 (slight discomfort)–10 (interfering with eating) **Maximum score 10**	
Site (circle) **Group 1** Labial mucosa Buccal mucosa Buccal sulcus Soft palate Ventral of tongue Lateral of tongue Floor of mouth	**Group 2** Hard palate Attached gingiva Alveolar ridge Dorsum of tongue Pillars of fauces Tonsils Uvula	1 for each site in group 1 2 for each site in group 2 **Maximum score 10**	
TOTAL		

2 mm	3 mm	4 mm	6 mm	8 mm	10 mm	12 mm
○	○	○	○	○	○	○

Evidence of scarring	Y	N

Fig. 7.5 Ulcer severity score.

TABLE 7.2   Investigations That Might be Helpful in Diagnosis/Prognosis/Management in Some Patients Suspected of Having Recurrent Aphthous Stomatitis or Aphthous-Like Ulcers*

In Most Cases	In Some Cases
Full blood picture	Biopsy rarely
Serum ferritin, vitamin B_{12}, folate and calcium levels	G6PD and TPMT levels*
ESR	Blood glucose*
Serum immunoglobulins	Blood pressure*
IgA antiendomysial antibodies	DEXA (dual-emission X-ray absorptiometry) scan*
Antibodies to tissue transglutaminase (anti-TTG)	Endoscopy/gastroscopy and jejunal biopsy

*If systemic immunomodulation considered.

TABLE 7.3   Some Disorders With Aphthous-Like Oral Ulceration

Disease	Comment
Viral infections (EBV, HIV or HTLV-1)	Chapter 37
Coeliac disease	Chapter 55
Crohn disease	Chapter 32
Behçet disease	Ulcers may be more severe than typical aphthae, and patients also have recurrent genital ulceration, cutaneous and ocular disease and other gastrointestinal, neurological, renal, joint and haematological abnormalities (see Chapter 27). MAGIC syndrome is a variant.
Chronic neutropenia	Can give rise to superficial oral mucosal ulceration without any significant periodicity.
Cyclic neutropenia	Cyclic reduction in circulating levels of neutrophils about every 21 days. Affected patients develop oral ulceration, fever, cutaneous abscesses, upper respiratory tract infections and lymphadenopathy. Other oral complications include severe gingivitis and aggressive periodontitis. Treated with recombinant granulocyte colony stimulating factor.
Sweet syndrome	Acute neutrophilic dermatosis
Autoinflammatory diseases	(e.g. PFAPA syndrome [periodic fever, aphthae like ulceration, pharyngitis and cervical adenitis]). Rare, tends to occur in young children, self-limiting, and non-recurrent. May respond to cimetidine (via suppression of T lymphocyte function), corticosteroids, tonsillectomy.

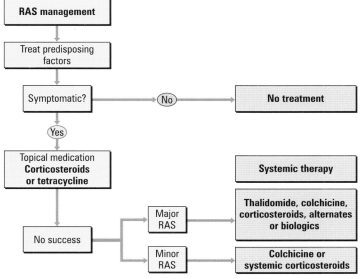

Algorithm 7.1 RAS management.

TABLE 7.4   Regimens That Might be Helpful in Management of Patients Suspected of Having Aphthae (see also Table 7.6)

Regimen	Use in Primary Care	Use in Secondary Care (Severe Oral Involvement and/or Extraoral Involvement)
Beneficial	Chlorhexidine	Corticosteroids (systemically) (e.g. prednisolone) Thalidomide
Likely to be beneficial	Corticosteroids (topical) (e.g. hydrocortisone, betamethasone 500 mcg soluble tablets) Tetracycline 2.5% mouthwash (adults only) Doxycycline mouthwash Vitamin B_{12}	Azathioprine Ciclosporin Colchicine Pentoxifylline
Emergent treatments		Adalimumab Etanercept Infliximab
Supportive	Benzydamine Diet with little acidic, spicy or citrus content Lidocaine gel SLS-free toothpaste	

TABLE 7.5   Treatment Regimens for Recurrent Aphthous Stomatitis

Treatment[a]	Examples of Preparations Available	Particularly Suitable for
Covering agents	Orabase	Reducing pain
Topical analgesics/anaesthetics/anti-inflammatory agents	Benzydamine hydrochloride mouthwash or spray Lidocaine gel	Reducing pain
Topical antiseptics	Doxycycline 100 mg daily as mouthwash Chlorhexidine gluconate 0.2% mouthwash	Hastening healing
Topical mild potency corticosteroids	Hydrocortisone oromucosal tablets 2.5 mg once daily or triamcinolone 0.1% in carboxymethylcellulose paste if available applied to dried areas with moistened finger	Frequently recurring or severe ulcers. Continued use may reduce frequency
Topical moderate or high potency corticosteroids (see Chapter 5)	Beclomethasone dipropionate aerosol 2 puffs (100 µg) spray onto affected area to a maximum of 8 puffs/day Betamethasone sodium phosphate one 500 mcg tablet dissolved in 10 mL of water used as a mouthwash, held in mouth for a minimum of 3 min. qds when ulcers present, bd as maintenance	Inaccessible sites (e.g. soft palate). Use may reduce recurrences
Vitamin B_{12}	Cobalamin 50 µg daily	
Systemic immunomodulatory agents	Oral prednisolone 30 mg for 5 days, reduce by 5 mg every 2 days until stopped Or colchicine 500 mcg three times a day Or pentoxifylline 400 mg three times a day Or azathioprine 50—100 mg daily Or thalidomide 50—200 mg once a day 3—8 weeks	Severe RAS, or aphthous-like ulceration

[a]Children under 6 cannot be expected to rinse and expectorate effectively; avoid preparations that cannot be safely swallowed. Avoid tetracycline preparations, even as a mouthwash, in children under 12. Systemic agents all have potential significant adverse effects.

These include systemic corticosteroids (e.g. prednisolone) and other immunomodulatory agents (e.g. azathioprine, colchicine, pentoxifylline, ciclosporin, dapsone, interferon or anti-TNF agents). Vitamin B_{12} may have beneficial effect even in the absence of unproven deficiency.

FOLLOW-UP OF PATIENTS

Long-term follow-up in primary care is usually adequate for most patients with minor RAS. Patients with severe RAS or aphthous-like ulcers usually need to be managed in secondary care.

TABLE 7.6   Therapies for Aphthae Shown to Have Benefit in at Least One Controlled Trial

Agent	Main Preparations	Route	Daily Dose (Adults)	Possible Main Adverse Effects/ Contraindications
Mild Disease				
Chlorhexidine	0.12% or 0.2% aqueous mouthwash or 1% gel	Topical	4 times daily[a]	Superficial tooth staining (reduce coffee, tea, red wine intake)
Corticosteroids	In adhesive base (carmellose), or as pellet, spray or cream	Topical	Applied to ulcers 4 times daily[a]	Oral candidosis (recommend adding antifungals to more potent corticosteroids because of this possible risk)
Severe Disease				
Corticosteroids	Tablet or capsule	Systemic	Orally 30–60 mg[b]	Hypertension Diabetes Weight gain Osteoporosis Peptic ulceration Adrenal suppression
Thalidomide	Tablet	Systemic	Orally 50 mg[a]	Teratogenic Drowsiness Peripheral neuropathy

[a]For 2 or more weeks, repeated if ulcers recur.
[b]1-week treatment, reducing dose over a further week.

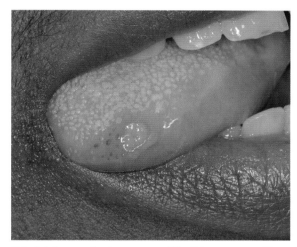

Fig. 7.6 Aphthae on the tongue are difficult to manage with pastes.

EMERGENT TREATMENTS

If RAS fails to respond to topical measures, systemic immunomodulators may be required, under specialist supervision. These include anti-tumour necrosis factor alpha agents such as pentoxifylline, thalidomide, infliximab, etanercept, adalimumab, but often either their efficacy has not been well proven or they have unacceptable adverse effects. For example, thalidomide can be effective against severe RAS but is rarely employed since it is teratogenic and can produce neuropathies.

RECOMMENDED READING

Brocklehurst, P., Tickle, M., Glenny, A.M., Lewis, M.A., Pemberton, M.N., et al., 2012. Systemic interventions for recurrent aphthous stomatitis (mouth ulcers). Cochrane Database Syst. Rev. 12 (9), CD005411.

Burton, M.J., Pollard, A.J., Ramsden, J.D., Chong, L.Y., Venekamp, R.P., 2019. Tonsillectomy for periodic fever, aphthous stomatitis, pharyngitis and cervical adenitis syndrome (PFAPA). Cochrane Database Syst. Rev. 12, CD008669.

Sand, F.L., Thomsen, S.F., 2013. Efficacy and safety of TNF-α inhibitors in refractory primary complex aphthosis: a patient series and overview of the literature. J. Dermatolog. Treat. 24, 444.

Taylor, J., Brocklehurst, P., Glenny, A.M., Walsh, T., Tickle, M., Lewis, M.A., et al., 2013. Topical interventions for recurrent aphthous stomatitis (mouth ulcers). Cochrane Database Syst. Rev. 9, CD010881.

Lichen Planus

- Lichen planus (LP) is a common chronic mucocutaneous condition.
- Lesions of LP are typically bilateral and affect the buccal mucosae, mainly.
- Diagnosis is clinically supported by biopsy.
- Management usually includes topical corticosteroids.
- There is a low but significant malignant potential.
- Lichenoid reaction is a term used when a putative aetiological factor can be identified. Aetiological factors include drugs, dental materials, graft-versus-host disease, hepatitis C and other factors.

INTRODUCTION

Oral lichen planus (OLP) is chronic inflammatory mucocutaneous, immune-mediated condition that can affect stratified squamous epithelia — the skin, oral mucosa and genitalia (Fig. 8.1).

Epidemiology

- LP is not uncommon and has a prevalence of 1% of adults.
- It usually affects persons between the ages of 30 to 65 years.
- OLP is about twice as common in females as in males.
- OLP is seen worldwide.

Predisposing Factors (Fig. 8.2)

OLP is not a classical autoimmune disorder, and the precise aetiology of this condition is unknown (Fig 8.2).

- There is no definitive immunogenetic basis established for OLP, but studies have reported various HLA associations. An increase in HLA-B15, Bw57, B5, B7, BX, DR2 and a decrease in the frequency of HLA-DQ1, DR4 and B18 has been documented for OLP.
- A genetic basis for OLP is supported by the fact that several familial cases have been reported. Genetic polymorphisms of several cytokines have been proposed, however, further studies are required.

- Stress has been widely held to be an important aetiological factor in OLP, but remarkably few studies have objectively examined stress. A statistically significant difference has been found in the psychological profiles of patients affected by OLP (a tendency to be depressed and anxious), but the chronic discomfort that can afflict patients with OLP can itself be a stressing factor.
- Infectious agents have been studied but the evidence is sparse.
- Lesions clinically and histologically similar to OLP, 'lichenoid lesions', are sometimes caused by:
  - dental restorative materials (mainly amalgam and gold)
  - chronic graft-versus-host disease, seen in bone marrow (haemopoietic stem cell) transplant patients
  - infection with hepatitis C virus in some populations, such as those from southern Europe and Japan
  - a variety of other systemic disorders, such as hypertension and diabetes, but this is probably a manifestation of a reaction to the drugs used
  - drug and vaccine use: antidiabetic drugs; antirheumatic drugs (NSAIDs mainly, but also others); antihypertensive agents, such as beta-blockers, thiazides and diuretics; antimalarials, such as quinacrine; many other drugs; occasionally, hepatitis B vaccine, omalizumab or tumour necrosis factor α (TNF-α) antagonists
  - thyroid disease (or medications to treat thyroid disease).

AETIOLOGY AND PATHOGENESIS

LP is a complex disease, resulting through the interplay of genetic, environmental and gene-environment interactions. LP is an immune-mediated condition mediated by cytotoxic CD8$^+$ T cells directed against basilar keratinocytes resulting in vacuolar degeneration and lysis of basal cells. However, it is not a classical autoimmune disorder and no autoantibodies have been identified. The antigen(s) responsible for LP are unknown, but studies have revealed an LP-specific epidermal antigen. The earliest features of LP are changes in, and close to, the basal epithelium. The appearance of antigen-processing cells (Langerhans cells) is one of the first observable changes. A band-like dense mononuclear inflammatory cell infiltrate, mainly of T CD8$^+$ cells, then appears in the upper lamina propria, representing a local cell-mediated immunological response (Fig. 8.3). The NF-κB path is thereby activated with a change of NF-κB-dependent pro-inflammatory cytokines,

including TNF-α, and interleukins IL-8 and IL-6. T-cell cytokines such as TNF-α and interferon-γ (IFN-γ) then cause apoptosis (controlled cell death) in the epithelial basal keratinocytes. The basal keratinocytes degenerate and die, undergoing flattening and hydropic changes causing intercellular spaces to appear, with splitting of epithelium away from the basement membrane — termed basal cell liquefaction. Round or ovoid 'colloid bodies' (also termed cytoid, globular, hyaline, Civatte and Sabouraud bodies) appear mainly in the epithelial spinous layer and in the lamina propria. Immune deposits (typically fibrin and sometimes IgM) are seen in the colloid bodies and at the basement membrane zone, and probably represent non-specific exudation, not autoantibodies. The rest of the epithelium appears to react with thickening of the spinous

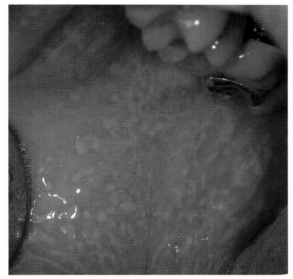

Fig. 8.1 Papuloreticular lichen planus in the most common site.

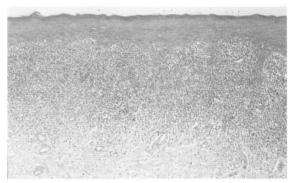

Fig. 8.3 Histopathology of lichen planus showing the subepithelial T cell infiltrate.

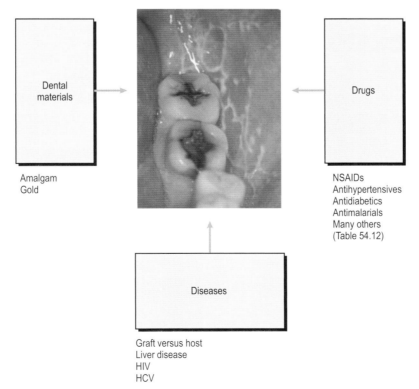

Dental materials

Amalgam
Gold

Drugs

NSAIDs
Antihypertensives
Antidiabetics
Antimalarials
Many others
(Table 54.12)

Diseases

Graft versus host
Liver disease
HIV
HCV

Fig. 8.2 Factors implicated in pathogenesis of lichen planus.

(acanthosis) and granular cell layers (hyperparakeratosis) or hyperorthokeratosis — which accounts for the clinical white lesions. The rete ridges adopt a 'saw tooth' configuration (more commonly than in skin lesions). Epithelial atrophy and even erosions can appear — leading to discomfort and the appearance of red lesions and/or ulceration.

CLINICAL FEATURES

OLP may occur in isolation, or oral lesions may precede, accompany or follow LP affecting other stratified squamous epithelia or appendages but there are no known predictive factors for this involvement.

The clinical picture is mainly of white lesions but is often mixed. Six clinical types of OLP lesions have been described (Table 8.1):

1. reticular, a network of raised white lines termed striae (reticular pattern)
2. papular, white papules (Fig. 8.4)
3. plaque-like, white patches simulating leukoplakia (Fig. 8.5)
4. red atrophic areas — OLP is one of the most common causes of desquamative gingivitis (Fig. 8.6)
5. ulcerative/erosive — persistent, irregular and painful erosions with a yellowish slough (Fig. 8.7)
6. bullous.
   OLP typically presents as lesions which are:
- mostly white
- almost always bilateral and symmetric
- reticular (the most recognised form of OLP), but may be papular or plaque-like and associated with red atrophic areas in the posterior buccal mucosa bilaterally

TABLE 8.1 Oral Lichen Planus Subtypes

Type	Frequency (%)
Reticular	92
Atrophic	44
Plaque-type	36
Papular	11
Ulcerative	9
Bullous	1

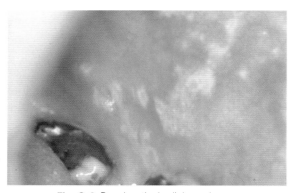

Fig. 8.4 Papuloreticular lichen planus.

- occasionally on the dorsum of the tongue where they may be reticular, papular or plaque-like and associated with red atrophic or erosive areas
- occasionally on the gingiva, as a white lacework of white striae and papules, or as 'desquamative gingivitis' (may also develop in about 25% of patients with ulcerative/erosive OLP and can be the initial or the only sign of oral involvement)
- rarely on the lips — usually a white lacework of white striae and papules

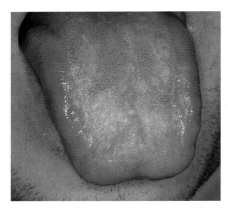

Fig. 8.5 Lichen planus of the plaque type, resembling leukoplakia.

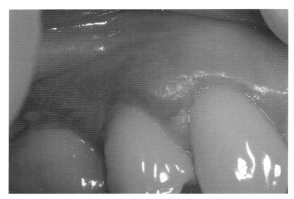

Fig. 8.6 Atrophic lichen planus causing desquamative gingivitis.

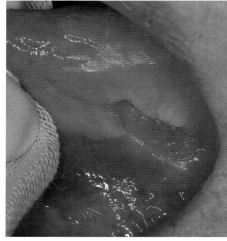

Fig. 8.7 Erosive lichen planus resembling lupus erythematosus.

- rarely on the palate — usually a white lacework of white striae and papules.
  - OLP is often asymptomatic, especially when there are only white lesions but there may be soreness from atrophic areas of thin, red mucosa or erosions, especially when eating or drinking substances which are acidic or spicy. Mild oral discomfort or a burning sensation are the common complaints in most symptomatic cases but in some the discomfort can be severe.
  - OLP has periods of relapses and remissions.
  - The reported incidence of cutaneous lesions in patients presenting with OLP ranges from 4% to 44%.

PROGNOSIS

Often the onset of LP is slow, taking months to reach its peak. It often clears from the skin within 18 months, but in a few people persists for many years. Oral lesions are usually persistent. In people with dark skin there may be pigmentary incontinence with dark areas appearing (post-inflammatory pigmentation) (Fig. 8.8). Extraoral lesions may be present at, or follow the onset of, OLP but a careful history and examination may reveal latent lesions or lesions previously considered due to another disorder. For example, genital LP is not uncommon in patients who complain only of gingival lesions (vulvo-vaginal-gingival syndrome).

OLP has a premalignant potential of less than 1%/year, and predominantly in non-reticular lesions (Fig. 8.9).

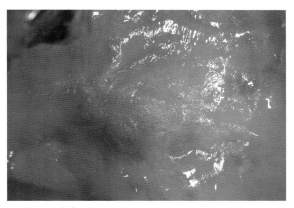

Fig. 8.8 Pigmentary incontinence in lichen planus.

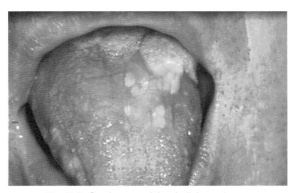

Fig. 8.9 Carcinoma arising in lichen planus.

Extraoral Lesions

LP may also cause lesions elsewhere, including:
- Skin: rash characterised by lesions, which are:
  - **p**urple or pink
  - **p**olygonal
  - **p**ruritic (itchy)
  - **p**apules — often crossed by fine white lines (Wickham striae) (Fig. 8.10).

  It is most often seen on the front (flexor surface) of the wrists, lower back, ankles and shins. Trauma may induce new skin lesions (Koebner phenomenon).
- Skin appendages: in up to 10% of cases, there is nail involvement, usually a minor change (Fig. 8.11), but occasionally resulting in shedding or destruction of the nail. The scalp may also be affected in different patterns, but most frequently as lichen planopilaris with scattered areas of scarring alopecia.
- Anogenital mucosae:
  - up to 20% of females may have concurrent genital LP, usually vulval and often asymptomatic.

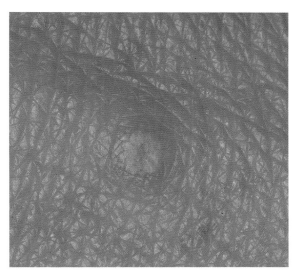

Fig. 8.10 Skin papules in lichen planus with whitish Wickham striae.

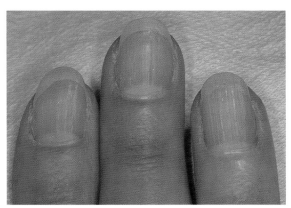

Fig. 8.11 Nail changes in lichen planus.

- the 'vulvo-vaginal-gingival syndrome' is uncommon and involves a variable timing of onset of gingival, vulval and vaginal lesions. The oral lesions may include an isolated desquamative gingivitis, with minimal involvement of other oral mucosal sites, and may lead to complications including loss of sulcal depth and fibrous banding of the buccal mucosa. It is very important for the dentist to enquire about genital involvement as early intervention with ultrapotent topical corticosteroids will prevent the significant vulval scarring and vaginal stenosis that ensues. Lacrimal duct stenosis and oesophageal strictures may also occur.
  - the peno-gingival syndrome and anal LP are less common and less incapacitating if treated early.
- Ocular mucosae: conjunctival involvement with scarring is a recognised complication of LP.

DIAGNOSIS

LP is often fairly obviously diagnosed from the clinical features, but it can sometimes closely simulate other conditions, such as:
- lupus erythematosus
- chronic ulcerative stomatitis
- keratosis
- carcinoma.
  Lichenoid lesions that may need to be excluded include:
- drug-induced lesions
- dental-material-induced lesions (Fig. 8.12)
- graft-versus-host disease
- hepatitis C virus infection.
  Lichenoid lesions clinically resemble OLP, but may:
- be unilateral
- be associated with erosions
- resolve on discontinuation of any offending drug.
  Skin testing for hypersensitivity to drugs or dental materials is only rarely of clinical value.
  Lichenoid lesions histopathologically are more likely to be associated with:
- a mixed cellular infiltrate including plasma cells and eosinophils
- a deeper infiltrate

- a perivascular infiltrate
- parakeratosis
- colloid bodies in the epithelium
- basal cell autoantibodies.

The firm diagnosis of OLP, therefore, relies upon biopsy and histopathological examination of lesional tissue, and can be aided by direct immunostaining which typically shows a ragged fibrin band at the basement membrane. However, often the histological and immunological findings revealed are no more than 'consistent with lichen planus', but this at least serves to exclude other conditions. Other investigations may sometimes be indicated (Table 8.2).

TREATMENT

Patient information is an important aspect in management. The severity of the oral lesions can be measured using an Oral Disease Severity Score (ODSS), and the effect on the patient can be assessed by a quality-of-life score. Unfortunately, although the natural history of cutaneous LP is one often of remission, OLP remits completely only in a few if any patients, and there are no cures currently available. Treatment is indicated for the discomfort of symptomatic OLP (Algorithm 8.1), i.e., mainly for atrophic or ulcerative OLP and significant reductions in the ODSS can be achieved.

Predisposing factors should be corrected:
- Consider removal of dental amalgams or other materials if the lesions are clearly closely related to these, or unilateral. Unfortunately, no tests, such as patch tests, will reliably indicate which patients might benefit.
- Consult with other physicians if there is HCV infection or other systemic background, or if drugs are implicated, and a relevant specialist if skin, genital or ocular involvement is possible.
- Improvement in oral hygiene may result in some subjective benefit, particularly for gingival LP. Chlorhexidine mouthwashes may help.
- Symptoms can often be controlled with topical medication. Benzydamine hydrochloride (0.15%) spray or mouthrinse or lidocaine gel applied to painful areas can be helpful.

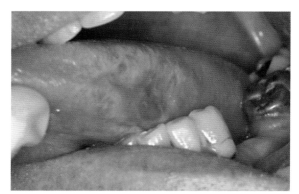

Fig. 8.12 Lichenoid lesions related to an amalgam restoration on the molar tooth.

| TABLE 8.2 **AIDS That Might Be Helpful in Diagnosis/Prognosis/Management in Some Patients Suspected of Having Lichen Planus** ||
In Most Cases	In Some Cases
Biopsy ± direct immunofluorescence	Full blood picture Serum ferritin, vitamin B₁₂ and folate levels Smear or culture candida ssp. Serology (HCV, HIV) Thyroid function and thyroid antibodies Patch testing Blood pressure Blood glucose Dermatological/gynaecological/ophthalmic opinions

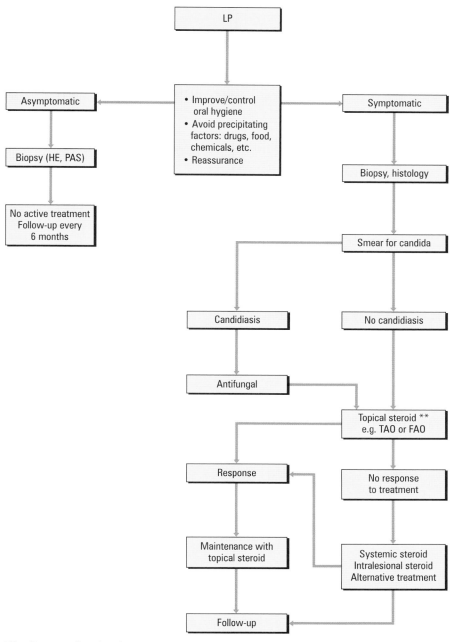

HE = Haematoxylin and eosin
PAS = Periodic acid–Schiff
**TAO = Triamcinolone acetonide 0.1% in Orabase
FAO = Fluocinolone acetonide 0.1% in Orabase/solution

Algorithm 8.1 Management of lichen planus.

- Sodium-lauryl sulphate (SLS) is a foaming agent added to toothpastes that exacerbates symptoms and SLS-free toothpastes should be advised.

There are many therapies suggested (Table 8.3).

Topical corticosteroids can often control OLP. Topical corticosteroids are the primary therapeutic agents used to treat ulcerative mucosal lesions which have an immunologically based aetiology such as LP. A mild potency agent such as hydrocortisone may be effective but more typically a medium potency corticosteroid such as betamethasone (as a mouthwash) or a higher potency one such as beclomethasone are required, moving to a super-potent topical corticosteroid (e.g. clobetasol ointment) if the benefit is inadequate. Patients should be instructed to dissolve one betamethasone tablet in 10 mL of water and use as a mouthwash for 3 minutes up to four times daily and refrain from eating and drinking for the subsequent 30 minutes. In long-term use, candidosis can arise and thus topical antifungal medication such as miconazole or

TABLE 8.3   Regimens That Might Be Helpful in Management of Patient Suspected of Having Lichen Planus

Regimen	Use in primary care	Use in secondary care (severe oral involvement and/or extraoral involvement)
Beneficial	Topical corticosteroids **Prednisolone:** 5 mg dissolved in 10 mL of water as a mouthwash 3–4 times daily **Betamethasone sodium phosphate:** 500 microgram tablet dissolved in 10 mL of water as a mouthwash up to 4 times daily **Flixonase 400 mcg nasules:** 1 flixonase nasule emptied in 10 mL of water as a mouthwash twice daily. 1 mL of Nystatin oral suspension may be added to reduce risk of oral candidiasis. **Clobetasol ointment (0.05%):** to affected areas once daily **Fluticasone propionate spray, 50 microgram/puff:** to affected areas 3 times daily **Beclomethasone spray, 100 microgram/puff:** to affected areas 3–4 times daily	Systemic corticosteroids
Likely to be beneficial	Aloe vera Hyaluronic acid Topical tacrolimus Topical pimecrolimus	Hydroxychloroquine Azathioprine Ciclosporin Hydroxychloroquine Mycophenolate mofetil
Emergent treatments		Biologic agents
Supportive	Benzydamine Diet with little acidic, spicy or citrus content Smoking cessation Sodium-lauryl sulphate (SLS)-free toothpaste	

Nystatin may be prudent. The more major concern of adrenal suppression with long-term and/or repeated application has rarely been addressed, although topical steroid preparations (apart from super potent halogenated corticosteroids, such as clobetasol, when used several times a day) appear not to cause a significant problem. For intractable ulcerative OLP lesions, intralesional injections of triamcinolone acetonide have been used.

In studies, topical tacrolimus or pimecrolimus are also effective. There have been cases reported of carcinoma developing in OLP treated with tacrolimus, though a causal relationship is not established and the FDA have therefore produced an Advisory Note.

Alternative therapies that have been employed include aloe vera and calendula officinalis.

Severity-Dependent Treatment

Mild Oral Lichen Planus (ODSS <20)

Topical aloe vera may help symptomatically but topical corticosteroids are the mainstay of therapy, although erosive and gingival lesions are often recalcitrant. High-potency corticosteroids, such as clobetasol, fluocinonide or fluticasone, may initially be employed and should then be changed to a lower-potency drug (e.g. hydrocortisone hemisuccinate, triamcinolone acetate or fluocinolone). Topical creams or pastes can be applied in a suitable customised tray to be worn at night.

Moderate Oral Lichen Planus (ODSS 20 to 30)

If there is severe or extensive oral involvement, topical tacrolimus may be of significant benefit. Often a high- or super-potent topical corticosteroid is needed in the management of OLP-related desquamative gingivitis recalcitrant to other therapies. Hydroxychloroquine may be tried for 6 months to assess benefit or short courses of oral prednisolone may be helpful.

Severe Oral Lichen Planus (ODSS >30)

In severe OLP in multiple sites, patients may require systemic corticosteroids (prednisolone) or other immunomodulatory agents such as mycophenolate mofetil or azathioprine.

FOLLOW-UP OF PATIENTS

OLP carries a small potential for malignant development, less than 1% per year, necessitating regular monitoring which can be carried out by the general dental practitioner. Clinical photography is helpful in monitoring. If changes are noted in a lesion at follow-up, then an additional biopsy or biopsies should be performed. It is important to offer advice and support in reducing modifiable risk factors.

RECOMMENDED READING

Alrashdan, M.S., Cirillo, N., McCullough, M., 2016. Oral lichen planus: a literature review and update. Arch. Dermatol. Res. 308 (8), 539–551.

Escudier, M., Ahmed, N., Shirlaw, P., et al., 2007. A scoring system for mucosal disease severity with special reference to oral lichen planus. Br. J. Dermatol. 157 (4), 765–770.

Fitzpatrick, S.G., Hirsch, S.A., Gordon, S.C., 2014. The malignant transformation of oral lichen planus and oral lichenoid lesions: a systematic review. J. Am. Dent. Assoc. 145 (1), 45–56.

Giuliani, M., Troiano, G., Cordaro, M., et al., 2019. Rate of malignant transformation of oral lichen planus: a systematic review. Oral Dis. 25 (3), 693–709.

Gupta, S., Ghosh, S., Gupta, S., 2017. Interventions for the management of oral lichen planus: a review of the conventional and novel therapies. Oral Dis. 23 (8), 1029–1042.

Lodi, G., Manfredi, M., Mercadante, V., Murphy, R., Carrozzo, M., 2020. Interventions for treating oral lichen planus: corticosteroid therapies. Cochrane Database Syst. Rev. 2, CD001168.

Ramos-García, P., González-Moles, M.Á., Warnakulasuriya, S., 2021. Oral cancer development in lichen planus and related conditions-3.0 evidence level: a systematic review of systematic reviews. Oral Dis. 27 (8), 1919–1935.

Lumps and Swellings: An Overview

INTRODUCTION

Swelling and lumps in the mouth are common. Patients may notice a lump because it is sore, or it is noticed by the tongue which often detects even very small swellings. Some individuals discover and worry about normal anatomical features, such as the parotid papilla, foliate papillae on the tongue, or the pterygoid hamulus. Some examine their mouths out of idle curiosity, and some through fear (perhaps after hearing of someone with 'mouth cancer'). In contrast, many oral cancers are diagnosed far too late, often after being present several months, because the patient ignores the swelling. Some 'lumps' become ulcers, as in various bullous lesions, infections and in malignant neoplasms.

Many different conditions may present as oral lumps or swellings, causes include the following:

- The mouth's normal anatomy, such as tongue foliate or circumvallate papillae (Figs 9.1 and 9.2).
- Developmental lumps: unerupted teeth and tori are common causes of hard swellings related to the jaws. Cysts and hamartomas (**benign tumour of normal tissues that are found in the region in which they grow**) may present as a swelling. Hamartomas include lymphangiomas and haemangiomas (also known as angiomas). Lymphangiomas are benign neoplasms of lymphatic channels that present as a colourless, sometimes finely nodular soft mass. Bleeding into lymphatic spaces causes sudden purplish discolouration. If bleeding in the tongue is extensive, it is a rare cause of macroglossia. If in the lip, it is a rare cause of macrocheilia. Diagnosis can be confirmed, if necessary, by excision biopsy.

Haemangiomas are vascular malformations that are red, purple or blue, painless, soft and sometimes fluctuant and usually blanch on pressure. Most appear in infancy, but about 15% develop later. They are common on the tongue, lip vermilion or buccal mucosa. Diagnosis may be assisted by aspiration, ultrasonography, radiography, angiography, MRI and MRI-angiography. Differentiation is from lymphangioma, telangiectasia, purpura, Kaposi sarcoma and epithelioid angiomatosis. Management may be active, with removal of the haemangioma, or by simple observation (since some 50% regress spontaneously in childhood). Cryosurgery or laser (Nd-YAG, carbon dioxide, pulsed tuneable dye or copper vapour) are the main treatments. Alternatively, sclerosant injection (propranolol, boiling water, absolute alcohol, sodium tetradecyl sulphate, sodium morrhuate or ethanolamine oleate), compression sutures (Popescu) or (rarely) arterial embolisation can be used.

- Inflammatory lumps: dental abscess is one of the most common causes of oral swellings. Non-infective inflammatory causes include fibrous lumps, Crohn disease, orofacial granulomatosis and sarcoidosis. Salivary gland inflammation can cause swelling in sialadenitis or in Sjögren syndrome.
- Fibrous lump or nodule ('fibroepithelial polyp'): this is a pedunculated or broadly sessile, sometimes ulcerated, firm or soft, lump seen mainly on the buccal mucosa usually with a normal overlying mucosa overlying proliferated connective tissue. It is termed an 'epulis' if on the gingival margin. It is common and is probably caused by chronic irritation causing fibrous hyperplasia. Excision biopsy helps differentiate it from any other soft tissue tumour. The flange of a denture impinging on the vestibular mucosa may stimulate a similar reactive hyperplasia — the so-called denture granuloma or denture-induced hyperplasia (denture granuloma; epulis fissuratum). This is a painless, firm swelling with a smooth pink surface usually in the buccal sulcus related to an ill-fitting lower complete denture, especially anteriorly lying parallel with the alveolar ridge and sometimes grooved or ulcerated by the denture flange. Several ridges with a fairly firm consistency may develop. Denture granulomas are common, found mainly in middle-aged or older patients and the diagnosis is clear-cut if the lesion is in relation to a denture flange. If ulcerated, it may mimic carcinoma (rarely). Diagnosis is clinical, but excision biopsy may be indicated. The denture flange should be relieved, to prevent recurrence.
- Allergic: angioedema can produce diffuse swelling, typically of rapid onset. Oedema of slower onset may be orofacial granulomatosis.
- Traumatic: haematoma may cause a swelling at the site.
- Hormonal: pregnancy may result in generalised gingival swelling (pregnancy gingivitis) or a discrete lump (pregnancy

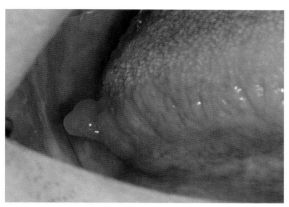

Fig. 9.1 Foliate papillae.

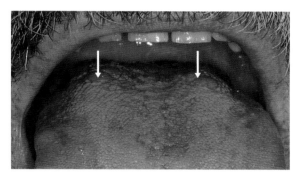

Fig. 9.2 Circumvallate papillae.

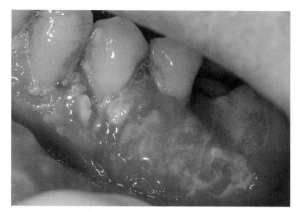

Fig. 9.3 Carcinoma causing gingival swelling.

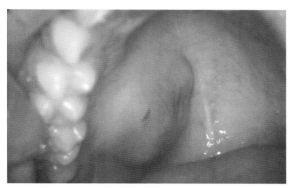

Fig. 9.4 Salivary neoplasm causing palatal swelling.

epulis — really a pyogenic granuloma). Diabetes predisposes to periodontal abscesses and occasionally giant cell lesions are seen in hyperparathyroidism. Sialosis is a painless swelling of major salivary glands that often has a hormonal basis, for example in diabetes.

- Drug induced: a range of drugs can produce gingival swelling — most commonly implicated are phenytoin, ciclosporin and calcium channel blockers. Drugs such as chlorhexidine occasionally cause a reactive salivary gland swelling.
- Benign neoplasms, such as fibromas or salivary gland tumours, may be seen. Malignant neoplasms may include carcinoma (Fig. 9.3), lymphoma, Kaposi sarcoma, malignant salivary gland tumours and others (Fig. 9.4). Occasionally, metastatic malignant disease or leukaemia may present as a lump.
- Viral lesions: mumps virus can cause acute sialadenitis. Papillomas (Fig. 9.5), common warts (verruca vulgaris), genital warts (condyloma acuminatum) and focal epithelial hyperplasia (Heck disease) are all caused by human papilloma viruses (HPV). A higher prevalence is seen in patients with sexually shared infections or in people who are immunocompromised, as in HIV/AIDS. Papillomas are uncommon in the mouth, but typically seen on the fauces, soft palate or tongue, usually less than 5 mm diameter and with whitish filiform projections. Warts are relatively uncommon but not rare in the mouth: verrucae vulgaris are usually transmitted

from skin lesions, and found predominantly on the lips whereas condyloma acuminata, transmitted from genital or anal lesions, are found mainly on the tongue or palate. Diagnosis is confirmed by biopsy and will differentiate from other tumours. They are managed with podophyllum or imiquimod, excision, laser, or electro- or cryosurgery. In contrast to epithelial polyps, warts are composed of normal connective tissue beneath proliferated epithelium.

- Pyogenic granuloma (Fig. 9.6).
- Fibro-osseous lesions: fibrous dysplasia and Paget disease can result in hard jaw swellings.
- Deposits: amyloid disease and other deposits can cause swellings.
- Obstruction to salivary glands can cause swellings (mucoceles or obstructive sialadenitis).

DIAGNOSIS

- Position: the anatomical position of the lump should be defined as accurately as possible. The proximity of the lump to other structures (e.g. teeth, dentures) should be noted. Does the swelling have an orifice, or sinus? If fluid is draining from the opening, is it clear, cloudy or purulent? Other similar or relevant changes elsewhere in the oral cavity should be noted (Box 9.1).

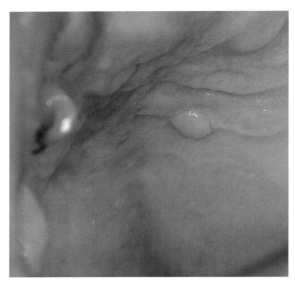

Fig. 9.5 Papilloma causing palatal swelling.

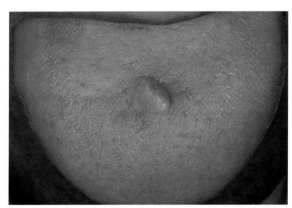

Fig. 9.6 Pyogenic granuloma on the tongue.

- Midline lesions tend to be developmental in origin (e.g. torus palatinus; see Chapter 10).
- Determine whether the lump is bilateral, since most neoplastic lumps are unilateral.
- Number of swellings, particularly with regard to whether the lesion is bilaterally symmetrical and thus possibly anatomical. Multiple or extraoral lesions suggest an infective or occasionally developmental origin.
- Size: the size should always be measured and recorded. A diagram or photograph may be helpful. Thus significant changes that may occur later can be recognised. In contrast, vague comments describing the swelling as 'medium' or 'large' are unhelpful.
- Shape: many swellings have characteristic shapes that point towards the diagnosis. Thus swelling of the parotid gland often fills in the space between the posterior border of the mandible and the mastoid process.
- Colour and temperature: brown or black pigmentation may be due to a variety of causes, such as naevi or rarely

BOX 9.1   **Causes of Oral Lumps and Swellings**

- Normal anatomy
- Lesions:
  - developmental
  - inflammatory
  - allergic
  - traumatic
  - hormonal
  - drug-induced
  - neoplasms
  - fibro-osseous lesions
  - others

melanoma. Purple or red may be due to an angioma, granuloma (see Fig. 9.6) or Kaposi sarcoma. Is the lump pale in colour (suggesting underlying fibrosis, or soft tissues stretched over bony enlargement); red (suggesting inflammation); or deep red (suggesting haemangioma or giant-cell epulis)? Any variations in colour within the lump (e.g. a 'pointing' abscess) should be observed. The skin and mucosa overlying acute inflammatory lesions, such as an abscess, is frequently red and warm.
- Tenderness: inflammatory swellings, such as an abscess, are characteristically tender, although clearly palpation must be gentle to avoid excessive discomfort to the patient.
- Discharge: note any discharge from the lesion (e.g. clear fluid, pus, blood).
- Movement: the mobility of any swelling should be tested to determine if it is fixed to adjacent structures or the overlying skin/mucosa, such as often happens with a malignant neoplasm.
- Consistency: lumps may vary from soft and fluctuant to hard. Fluctuation refers to the presence of fluid within a swelling, such as a cyst, and is a sign elicited by detecting movement of fluid when the swelling is compressed. Palpation may then help assessment of its contents and these can be put into such categories as fluid (fluctuant because of cyst fluid, mucus, pus or blood), soft, firm or hard like a carcinoma (indurated). Palpation may cause the release of fluid (e.g. pus from an abscess) or cause the lesion to blanch (vascular) or occasionally cause a blister to appear or expand (Nikolsky sign). Sometimes palpation causes the patient pain (suggesting an inflammatory lesion). The swelling overlying a bony cyst may crackle (like an eggshell) when palpated. Palpation may disclose an underlying structure (e.g. the crown of a tooth under an eruption cyst) or show that the actual swelling is in deeper structures (e.g. submandibular calculus). Bimanual palpation should be used when investigating lesions in the floor of the mouth, cheek, and occasionally the tongue.
- Surface texture: the surface of a swelling may vary from the uniform smooth texture of many fibrous lumps to the

BOX 9.2   Less Common Conditions That May Present as Oral Lumps or Swellings

Normal
- Pterygoid hamulus
- Parotid papillae
- Foliate papillae
- Unerupted teeth

Developmental
- Haemangioma
- Lymphangioma
- Maxillary and mandibular tori

Genetic
- Hereditary gingival fibromatosis
- Neurofibromatosis

Cystic
- Eruption cysts
- Developmental cysts
- Cysts of infective origin

Inflammatory
- Abscess
- Pyogenic granuloma
- Crohn disease
- Orofacial granulomatosis
- Sarcoidosis
- Wegener granulomatosis
- Infections
- Insect bites
- Others

Traumatic
- Haematoma
- Epulis
- Epithelial polyp
- Denture granulomas

Hormonal
- Pregnancy epulis/gingivitis
- Oral contraceptive (pill gingivitis)
- Brown tumour of hyperparathyroidism

Drugs
- Phenytoin
- Ciclosporin
- Calcium channel blockers

Neoplasms
- Benign (and warts)
- Malignant

Fibro-Osseous Lesions
- Fibrous dysplasia
- Paget disease

Deposits
- Amyloidosis
- Hypoplasminogenaemia (fibrin deposits)
- Other deposits

Others
Angioedema

---

grossly irregular. The surface characteristics should be noted: papillomas have an obvious anemone-like appearance; carcinomas and other malignant lesions tend to have a pebbly surface and may ulcerate. Abnormal blood vessels suggest a neoplasm.

- Ulceration: some swellings such as squamous cell carcinoma may develop superficial ulceration. The character of the edge of the ulcer and the appearance of the ulcer base should also be recorded. Ulcers should be examined for induration, which is indicative of malignancy.
- Margin: the margins of the swelling may be well or poorly defined. This may give some indication of the underlying pathology. Thus, ill-defined margins are frequently associated with malignancy, whereas clearly defined margins are more suggestive of a benign growth.
- Associated swelling: some conditions are associated with multiple swellings of a similar nature inside or outside the mouth (e.g. neurofibromatosis).

- The nature of many lumps cannot be established without further investigation.
- Any teeth adjacent to a lump involving the jaw should be tested for vitality, and any caries or suspect restorations investigated.
- The periodontal status of any involved teeth should also be determined.
- Imaging is required whenever lumps involve the jaws, or may so do, and should show the full extent of the lesion and possibly other areas. Special radiographs (e.g. of the skull, sinuses and salivary gland function), CT scans, MRI or ultrasonography may, on occasions, be indicated. Photographs may be useful for future comparison.
- The medical history should be fully reviewed, as systemic disorders may be associated with intra-oral or facial swellings (Box 9.2). Blood tests may be needed, particularly if there is suspicion that a blood dyscrasia or endocrinopathy may underlie the development of the lump.

10

Lumps and Swellings in the Oral Cavity

INTRODUCTION

Many of the different anatomical sites around the oral cavity share common aetiologies for most of the soft tissue swellings that might occur. However, the salivary glands and bone have very different and specialised tissues and thus very different swellings. These are considered in Chapters 11 (salivary glands) and 13 (bone swellings). The principles of diagnosis of lumps and swellings are:

- history including rate of increase
- size
- colour (especially whether red, blue or brown)
- contour (whether outline and margins of lesion can be defined)
- consistency (e.g. hard or soft)
- degree of Pain
- site.

LUMPS AND SWELLINGS IN THE LIPS

Lip or facial swelling may be diffuse or localised (Boxes 10.1 and 10.2).

- Lip or facial swelling that appears rapidly over a few minutes or up to an hour may be caused by an insect bite or sting, or angioedema.
- Lip or facial swelling that appears over a few hours or days is most commonly inflammatory in origin, often caused by trauma or infection (cutaneous, dental (odontogenic) or rarely systemic.
- Lip or facial swelling that appears over days or weeks may occasionally be caused by granulomatous disorders (e.g. Crohn disease, orofacial granulomatosis or sarcoidosis) (Fig. 10.1).

- Facial swelling that appears over weeks or months is occasionally due to systemic infections (such as tuberculosis, Leishmaniasis or a deep mycosis), a neoplasm (such as lymphoma or salivary gland tumour), deposits such as amyloidosis, or endocrine conditions (e.g. corticosteroid therapy, Cushing disease, hypothyroidism, acromegaly, diabetes mellitus).
- Facial swelling is commonly of very slow onset in masseteric hypertrophy and in obesity.
- Facial swelling that is persistent may be caused by:
  - fluid as in vascular lesions or lymphangiomas
  - solids such as primary neoplasms or metastases, deposits (e.g. amyloidosis) or foreign material (as in lip augmentation with silicone or other fillers).
- Localised swellings in the lip or face may be congenital as in haemangioma (Fig. 10.2) or lymphangioma but more usually are seen after trauma, or in infections, inflammatory conditions such as granulomatous disorders, or pyogenic granuloma, foreign bodies (including fillers) or caused by neoplasms or deposits.
- Pyogenic granuloma is a reactive vascular lesion, often trauma induced and sometimes associated with pregnancy. Typically, a pyogenic granuloma is a small (<3 cm) red painless mass that bleeds easily, ulcerates and grows rapidly, and is frequently seen on the lip, gingival margin or tongue. Treatment is excision to exclude angiomatous proliferations, chancre, carcinoma or Kaposi sarcoma.

LUMPS AND SWELLINGS IN THE GINGIVA

Gingival swelling is often very localised (then sometimes termed an 'epulis' from the Greek, meaning 'upon the gum'; plural 'epulides') (see below), but may be more generalised, or

BOX 10.1   Main Causes of Swelling of Lips/Face

- Haemangioma
- Mucocele
- Allergy
- Inflammation
- Trauma
- Granulomatous condition (e.g. Crohn disease, orofacial granulomatosis, sarcoid) including foreign bodies
- Neoplasm (e.g. carcinoma, salivary gland neoplasm, lymphoma)

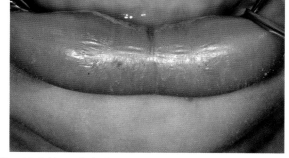

Fig. 10.1 Lip and gingival swelling in orofacial granulomatosis.

BOX 10.2   Less Common Causes of Swelling of Lips/Face

Lip swelling is most commonly inflammatory in origin — caused by cutaneous or dental (odontogenic) infections or trauma.

Congenital (e.g. Haemangioma, Lymphangioma, Ascher Syndrome [see Chapter 54])
- Cysts in soft tissues or bone (especially mucocele or cystic neoplasm)

Infective
- Oral or cutaneous infections, cellulitis, fascial space infections
- Systemic infections
- Insect bites/stings (can be traumatic)
- Papillomas and warts

Traumatic
- Traumatic or post-operative oedema or haematoma
- Surgical emphysema

Immunological/Inflammatory
- Allergic angioedema (see also Drugs: Table 33.15)
- C1 esterase inhibitor deficiency (hereditary angioedema)
- Crohn disease, orofacial granulomatosis or sarcoidosis
- Cheilitis glandularis

Endocrine and Metabolic
- Cushing syndrome and disease
- Myxoedema
- Nephrotic syndrome
- Obesity
- Systemic corticosteroid therapy
- Neoplasms
- Carcinomas
- Lymphoma
- Oral, salivary and antral tumours

Foreign Bodies (Including Cosmetic Fillers)
- Deposits
- Amyloidosis

Others
- Masseteric hypertrophy (facial rather than lip swelling)
- Bone disease
- Fibrous dysplasia
- Paget disease

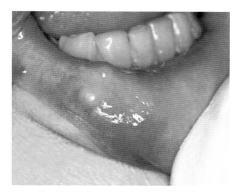

Fig. 10.2 Haemangioma of the lip.

can involve most of the gingivae. Imaging and biopsy may be required for diagnosis. Most gingival lumps originate in the gingival tissues, but some arise from the underlying tissues such as from the bone (Box 10.3).

More generalised gingival swelling is fairly common, often localised to the maxillary anterior gingivae in hyperplastic gingivitis arising as a consequence of mouth-breathing. Generalised gingival swelling is commonly drug-induced, usually aggravated by poor oral hygiene and starting interdentally, especially labially. Affected papillae are firm, pale and enlarge to form false vertical clefts. Granulomatous disorders such as orofacial granulomatosis (see also Chapter 32), Wegener granulomatosis (see Chapter 3) and plasma cell gingivitis may present with localised or more generalised swelling.

Generalised gingival swelling may occasionally be congenital (hereditary gingival fibromatosis [HGF]) which usually presents with firm pink slow-growing swellings; due to deposits such as fibrin in the rare condition hypoplasminogenaemia; or due for example, to leukaemia — when there may be other features such as purpura and/or ulceration (Fig. 10.3).

Epulides (Localised Gingival Swellings)

The main types of epulis include:
- *Fibrous epulides* (irritation fibromas; fibroepithelial polyp) are most common; they typically form narrow, firm, pale swellings of an anterior interdental papilla and may ulcerate (Fig. 10.4). Fibrous epulides may result from local gingival

BOX 10.3   Detailed List of Causes of Lumps on the Gingiva

Gingival Origin
- Inflammation
- Irritation fibroma (fibrous hyperplasia)
- Hyperplastic gingivitis
- Fibrous epulis (fibroepithelial polyp)
- Pyogenic granuloma
- Pregnancy tumour
- Peripheral giant cell granuloma
- Peripheral ossifying fibroma
- Abscesses
- Chronic gingivitis
- Granulomatous conditions
  - Crohn disease
  - Orofacial granulomatosis
  - Sarcoidosis
  - Wegener granulomatosis (see Chapter 54)
  - Tuberculosis
  - Deep mycoses
- Neoplasms
  - Carcinoma
  - Leukaemia
  - Lymphoma
  - Kaposi sarcoma
  - Melanoma
  - Metastasis
  - Papilloma
  - Traumatic neuroma
  - True fibroma
  - Verruciform xanthoma
- Drugs
  - Phenytoin
  - Ciclosporin
  - Calcium channel blockers
- Deposits
  - Amyloidosis
  - Hypoplasminogenaemia
  - Oral focal mucinosis
- Cysts
  - Gingival cysts
  - Lateral periodontal cyst
  - Inflammatory cysts
  - Peripheral odontogenic keratocyst
- Exostoses
- Fibrous epulis
- Giant cell tumour
- Hereditary
- Hereditary gingival fibromatosis
- Torus
- Exostosis
- Naevus

Central Lesions Perforating the Jawbone
- Odontogenic tumours
- Adenomatoid odontogenic tumour
- Ameloblastoma
- Ameloblastic fibroma
- Calcifying epithelial odontogenic tumour
- Odontogenic fibroma
- Squamous odontogenic tumour
- Calcifying odontogenic cyst
- Odontoma
- Malignant neoplasms

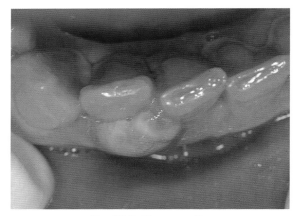

Fig. 10.3 Fibrous epulis.

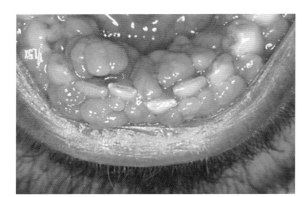

Fig. 10.4 Ciclosporin-induced gingival swelling (extreme example).

irritation, leading to fibrous hyperplasia. They are usually pink and firm but cannot be distinguished clinically with certainty from neoplastic epulides or the usually softer and redder pyogenic granulomas, or giant cell granulomas. Epulides are common, but rarely are they true neoplasms (Box 10.4).

- *Pyogenic granulomas* are common lesions, especially in children and teens, where there are local factors, including inadequate oral hygiene, malocclusion and orthodontic appliances, and in pregnancy (pregnancy epulis; epulis gravidarum) (lesions themselves not histologically distinguishable). Pyogenic granuloma commonly affects the gingiva,

BOX 10.4 Main Causes of Gingival Lumps or Swelling

- Inflammation
- Granulomatous conditions (e.g. Crohn disease, sarcoidosis or orofacial granulomatosis)
- Neoplasms
- Drugs

the lip or the tongue. It may be caused by chronic irritation and appears predisposed in patients who have had organ transplantation.

- *Giant cell epulides* (giant cell granulomas) are reactive lesions seen mainly in children, caused by local irritation or resulting from proliferation of giant cells persisting after resorption of deciduous teeth. Classically, a giant cell epulis is a swelling with a deep-red colour (although older lesions tend to be paler) and it often arises interdentally, but only anterior to the permanent molar teeth.
- *Neoplastic epulides* may be carcinomas, lymphomas, sarcomas or represent metastatic disease.

Treatment

- Radiography and excision biopsy.
- Excision and removal of local irritants (e.g. calculus).

DRUG-INDUCED GINGIVAL OVERGROWTH

Drug-induced gingival overgrowth (DIGO) can be caused by a number of disparate drugs (see Table 33.16), mainly phenytoin, ciclosporin and calcium channel blockers, as an adverse reaction. Swelling typically arises from the interdental papillae and is aggravated by poor oral hygiene.

Aetiology and Pathogenesis

The multidrug resistance 1 (MDR1) gene may modify the inflammatory response to drugs and thereby play a role in the pathogenesis. Causal drugs may include the following:

- Phenytoin: which is used mainly for the control of grand mal epilepsy. Histology shows marked thickening of epithelium with long overgrowths into the connective tissue. Fibroblasts show increased mitotic activity, but are not increased in number, and the collagen fibre component is not increased.
- Ciclosporin (cyclosporin): an immunosuppressive drug particularly used to suppress the cell-mediated response after organ transplants, but only one-third of patients may develop gingival swelling, more commonly children.
- Calcium channel blockers (especially nifedipine): which are mainly used as anti-hypertensive agents. Increased numbers of fibroblasts containing strongly sulphated mucopolysaccharides may be demonstrated histochemically; their cytoplasm contains numerous secretory granules, suggesting an increased production of acid mucopolysaccharides.
- Amphetamines.

Clinical Features

Drug-induced gingival swelling usually starts interdentally, with the palatal and lingual gingiva usually involved less than buccal and labial gingiva. Papillae are firm, pale and enlarge to form false vertical clefts (see Fig. 10.4), which may later involve the marginal and even attached gingiva.

The earlier lesions may be softer and redder, sometimes giving the impression of 'bubbling up' behind the existing papillae. The enlargement is characteristically firm, pale and tough with coarse stippling, but these features may take several years to develop. Older lesions may become red if inflamed. The enlargement rarely affects edentulous sites.

There is no correlation between the extent of overgrowth and the drug dose, its serum level, or the age and gender of the patient. The swelling is aggravated if oral hygiene is poor; there is a positive correlation between the severity of overgrowth and gingival inflammation, plaque score, calculus accumulation and pocket depths.

Excessive body hair growth (hypertrichosis) is commonly associated.

Diagnosis

This is usually a clinical diagnosis.

Treatment (see also Chapters 4 and 5)

Treatment of DIGO often poses problems as the patient often really needs to be on the responsible medication. The patient's level of plaque control often needs improvement and a chlorhexidine mouthwash may be helpful. Excision of enlarged tissue may be indicated, but difficult if the tissue is very firm and fibrous. Healing may be slow, possibly hampered by infection of the large wound. Unfortunately, the gingival enlargement readily recurs, although this is less likely with meticulous oral hygiene, particularly if the drug has been stopped. The physician may be willing to substitute another drug. Therefore:

- treat predisposing factors
- improve oral hygiene
- undertake gingivoplasty where indicated.

Follow-up of Patients

Long-term follow-up as shared care is usually appropriate.

HEREDITARY GINGIVAL FIBROMATOSIS

Hereditary gingival fibromatosis presents with gingival enlargement which begins in puberty, is painless, slowly progressive and dependent to a great extent on oral hygiene. The hyperplastic tissues are usually firm to palpation. It is not unusual for the fibromatosis to completely cover the teeth.

Symmetrical fibromatosis of the tuberosities presents as a generalised, soft, smooth-surfaced, painless enlargement of the tissues — usually over the posterior maxillary alveolus and typically bilaterally.

The most common form of HGF (HGF-1) maps to chromosome 2p21 and is caused by mutation in the *SOS1* (Son of sevenless-1) gene (a guanine nucleotide-exchange factor that mediates the coupling of receptor tyrosine kinases to Ras gene activation) or to chromosome 5q13-q22. An autosomal dominant form of HGF may be associated with hypertrichosis.

Syndromic forms of HGF (e.g. Rutherford, Cross, Laband and Ramon syndromes) have other types of inheritance and associations (see Chapter 54).

LUMPS AND SWELLINGS IN THE PALATE

Lumps in the palate are usually due to unerupted teeth or bone conditions (especially torus palatinus) (Fig. 10.5). Other lumps, which warrant imaging and often biopsy, can be due to fibrous lumps, papillomas, odontogenic infections (Fig. 10.6), odontogenic cysts, nasopalatine cyst, granulomatous disorders (e.g. sarcoidosis), lymphoid hyperplasia and neoplasms (e.g. carcinoma, melanoma, salivary neoplasms, antral neoplasms, disseminated neoplasms, lymphomas, Kaposi sarcoma) (Box 10.5).

Many of these conditions are described elsewhere in the text.

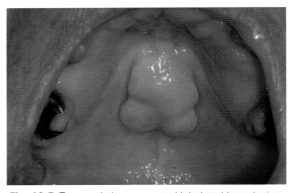

Fig. 10.5 Torus palatinus: a central lobulated bony lesion.

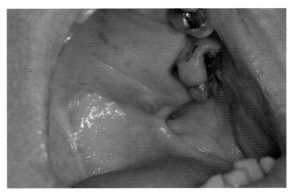

Fig. 10.6 Dental abscess arising from the non-vital third molar.

> ### BOX 10.5   Main Causes of a Lump in the Palate
>
> - Unerupted tooth
> - Torus palatinus
> - Dental abscess
> - Fibrous lump (fibroepithelial polyp)
> - Papilloma
> - Neoplasm (e.g. carcinoma, lymphoma, salivary gland neoplasm, Kaposi sarcoma, antral neoplasm)
> - Others (e.g. allergies, syphilis, sarcoidosis and other granulomas, follicular lymphoid hyperplasia, necrotising sialometaplasia)

Fibrous Lump Or Nodule ('Fibroepithelial Polyp')

Fibrous lump or nodule ('fibroepithelial polyp') is usually a pedunculated or broadly sessile, sometimes ulcerated, hard or soft, lump in the palate. It may resemble a papilloma. Excision biopsy is warranted.

Papilloma

Papilloma is a benign epithelial neoplasm with an anemone-like appearance, caused by human papillomavirus: HPV 6 or 11. Common in HIV-infected people and increased after therapy with HAART (see Chapter 39), papilloma is often a small, white or pink, cauliflower-like, sessile or pedunculated lesion, less than 1 cm in diameter. Most common at the junction of the hard and soft palate, the lip, gingiva or tongue may occasionally be affected. Papillomas in the mouth appear to be and remain benign, unlike papillomas of the larynx or bowel, which may undergo malignant transformation, but they are best removed and examined histologically to establish the diagnosis. Excision must be total, deep and wide enough to include any abnormal cells beyond the zone of the pedicle. Cryosurgery or pulse dye laser or carbon dioxide (CO_2) laser may be used. Some use salicylic acid, imiquimod or topical podophyllum resin paint but the latter is potentially teratogenic and toxic to brain, kidney and myocardium.

Follicular Lymphoid Hyperplasia

Follicular lymphoid hyperplasia of the palate is a rare benign lymphoproliferative lesion that closely resembles lymphomas, clinically and/or histopathologically. It presents as a firm, painless, non-ulcerated, non-fluctuant and slowly growing swelling of the palate. The typical histologic features include multiple germinal centres with a rim of well-differentiated B lymphocytes together with a mixed, mainly mononuclear infiltrate with plasmacytoid lymphocytes.

Lymphomas

(See also Burkitt lymphoma, Hodgkin disease and non-Hodgkin lymphoma (see Chapter 54).)

Lymphomas are malignant tumours that originate in lymph nodes and lymphoid tissue, and can originate from any type of lymphocyte, but mostly from B cells. HIV/AIDS and immunosuppression predispose. Painless enlarged cervical lymph nodes are the initial complaint in 50% of cases, but a lymphoma may occasionally produce primary or secondary oral tumours appearing as swellings, often of the pharynx, palate, tongue, gingivae or lips. Involvement of Waldeyer ring is common in non-Hodgkin lymphomas.

Patients with lymphoma develop a secondary immunodeficiency, when herpes zoster, herpetic stomatitis and oral candidosis may be seen. Diagnosis is from clinical findings (generalised lymph node enlargement and hepatosplenomegaly), imaging (hilar and abdominal lymph node enlargement), lymphangiography and biopsy (lymph node or lesional). Treatment is usually with chemotherapy.

Kaposi Sarcoma

Kaposi sarcoma is a malignant neoplasm of endothelial cells caused by Kaposi sarcoma herpes virus (KSHV — also known as HHV-8 or human herpesvirus 8). Kaposi sarcoma is seen especially in HIV/AIDS when this is contracted sexually or via blood-borne routes, and also in other immunosuppressed patients. Usually, oral lesions are part of more widespread disease. Kaposi sarcoma early oral lesions are red, purple or brown macules (Fig. 10.7), later becoming nodular, extending, ulcerating and disseminating. Kaposi sarcoma typically involves the palate or gingivae. Diagnosis is confirmed by biopsy: epithelioid angiomatosis, haemangiomas, lymphomas and purpura may need to be differentiated. Management is treatment of the underlying predisposing condition if possible, and then radiotherapy or vinca alkaloids systemically or intralesionally.

Antral Carcinoma

Antral carcinoma is rare, usually squamous carcinoma, seen mainly in older males — the only identified predisposing factor being occupational exposure to wood dust. Initially asymptomatic, it may cause swelling or pain in the face or palate when the carcinoma invades. Symptoms depend on the main direction of spread:

- Oral invasion: causes pain and swelling of palate, alveolus or sulcus; teeth may loosen.
- Ocular invasion: causes pain and swelling, ipsilateral epiphora, diplopia or proptosis.
- Nasal invasion: causes nasal pain and swelling, obstruction or a blood-stained discharge.

Diagnose from radiographs, MRI (opaque antrum and later destruction of antral wall or floor) and biopsy. Manage by surgery (sometimes with radiotherapy). Prognosis is 10% to 30% 5-year survival.

LUMPS AND SWELLINGS IN THE TONGUE

Tongue swelling is usually because of an isolated lump typically acquired and caused by trauma, infection or a neoplasm (Box 10.6, Figs 10.8—10.10). Biopsy and other investigations are usually indicated. Ectopic thyroid tissue in the tongue is rare, and usually presents as a persistent single symptomless nodule in the posterior midline dorsum of tongue lingual thyroid. It is important not to remove this without establishing there is adequate thyroid tissue present in the neck.

BOX 10.6   Main Causes of Enlarged Tongue
• Allergy • Trauma • Infection • Angioma • Neoplasm

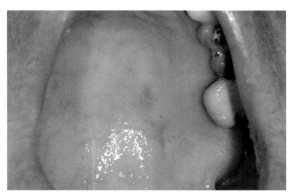

Fig. 10.7 Kaposi sarcoma — early lesions present as bluish macules over the greater palatine vessels. Later, swelling appears.

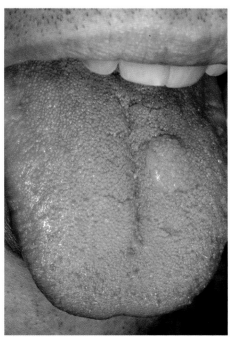

Fig. 10.8 Lingual lump caused by abnormal healing after trauma.

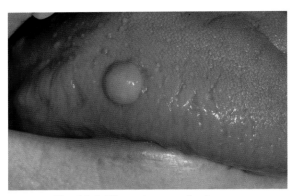

Fig. 10.9 Fibrous lump on the tongue.

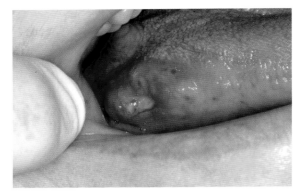

Fig. 10.10 Tongue cancer, presenting as a persistent lump that has ulcerated.

BOX 10.7   Less Common Causes of Tongue Swelling/Lumps

- Acromegaly
- Allergic reaction (see also Drugs: Chapter 33)
- Amyloidosis
- Angioedema
- Beckwith syndrome
- Congenital micrognathia
- Deep mycosis
- Down syndrome
- Fibrous lump
- Foreign body
- Granular cell tumour
- Granulomatous conditions (Crohn disease, OFG, sarcoidosis)
- Median rhomboid glossitis
- Haemangioma
- Hypothyroidism
- Infection
- Leishmaniasis
- Leukaemia
- Lymphangioma
- Lingual thyroid
- Mucopolysaccharidosis
- Multiple endocrine neoplasia syndrome
- Neoplasms (carcinoma, lymphoma, Kaposi sarcoma, salivary gland neoplasms, metastases others)
- Oedema
- Papilloma
- Pellagra
- Pernicious anaemia
- Pyogenic granuloma
- Simpson–Golabi–Behmel syndrome (see Chapter 54)
- Syphilis
- Trauma
- Tuberculosis
- Traumatic ulcerative granuloma with stromal eosinophilia (TUGSE)

Diffuse swelling is usually acquired and caused by trauma, infection or allergy (angioedema). Sudden swelling of the tongue can arise due to an allergic reaction or an adverse drug effect. Rare acquired causes are of slow onset over weeks or months and include amyloidosis (then often with purpura; Chapter 55) and other deposits (Box 10.7), or parasites such as cysticercosis.

Diffuse swelling of the tongue (macroglossia) may occasionally have congenital causes including: lymphangioma (see Chapter 55); haemangioma (see Chapter 55); neurofibromatosis (see Chapter 55); Down syndrome; cretinism; Hurler syndrome (a mucopolysaccharidosis); and multiple endocrine adenomatosis (Chapter 54).

The tongue may get somewhat wider in edentulous persons who do not wear dentures (false macroglossia):
- In true macroglossia, the tongue is indented by teeth, or too large to be contained in the mouth.

- Severe macroglossia can cause cosmetic and functional difficulties including in speaking, eating, swallowing and sleeping. Surgery may be indicated.

RECOMMENDED READING

Ahmed A, Naidu A. Towards better understanding of giant cell granulomas of the oral cavity. J Clin Pathol. 2021 ;74(8):483–490.

Barsoum F, Prete BRJ, Ouanounou A. Drug-Induced Gingival Enlargement: A Review of Diagnosis and Current Treatment Strategies. Compend Contin Educ Dent. 2022;43(5):276–285.

Léauté-Labrèze C. Medical management of vascular anomalies of the head and neck. J Oral Pathol Med. 2022 https://doi.org/10.1111/jop.13324. Epub ahead of print.

Quaranta A, D'Isidoro O, Piattelli A, Hui WL, Perrotti V. Illegal drugs and periodontal conditions. Periodontol 2000. 2022;90(1):62–87.

Lumps and Swellings in the Salivary Glands

INTRODUCTION

Swelling in the region of the salivary glands may arise from the gland or an intra-salivary lymph node, or other tissue (Box 11.1). Ultrasonography, other imaging and biopsy are often indicated.

- The most common salivary lesion causing a swelling is the mucocele, usually caused by extravasation of saliva from a damaged minor salivary gland duct and seen in the lower labial mucosa, sometimes caused by retention within a gland (Fig. 11.1). On the floor of the mouth, a large mucocele may be termed a 'ranula' from its likeness to the belly of a frog (Latin rana = frog).
- Sialadenitis (inflammation of the salivary gland) is another common cause of salivary gland swelling (Box 11.2). Sialadenitis may be caused by infection or may be non-infective (e.g. in Sjögren syndrome or sarcoidosis).
- In children and young people, the most common cause of swelling of one or more of the major glands is viral sialadenitis (mumps).
- In older children, recurrent sialadenitis (juvenile recurrent parotitis), is of uncertain cause but is probably a group of conditions variously caused by genetic factors, ductal obstruction, ductal ectasia (dilatations), or less commonly, diseases such as Sjögren syndrome or sarcoidosis.
- In adults, salivary swelling is most commonly obstructive (e.g. a salivary stone or calculus [sialolith]) or inflammatory in origin (e.g. infective sialadenitis, Sjögren syndrome, sclerosing sialadenitis [IgG4 syndrome] and sarcoidosis) (Fig. 11.2).
  - Salivary swelling may rarely be caused by systemic infections such as tuberculosis.
  - Salivary swelling may be caused by neoplastic disease: when it is typically a unilateral lump (Fig. 11.3), or other disorders (e.g. sialosis) when it is typically diffuse and often bilateral.
- Salivary swelling may be painful or painless and this may help differential diagnosis (Table 11.1). Salivary swelling can also be caused by:
  - fluid: as in trauma (oedema or haematoma), mucocele or vascular lesions
  - solids: such as deposits (e.g. amyloidosis, haemochromatosis) or foreign material
  - swelling of intra-salivary lymph nodes.

The main conditions apart from salivary gland neoplasms (Chapter 12) causing swellings are summarised alphabetically below.

MUCOCELES

Cystic lesions of minor salivary glands, that mostly appear in the lower labial mucosa, buccal mucosa or ventral tongue; mucoceles are fluctuant bluish lesions mostly caused by trauma to the duct, leading to mucous extravasation (extravasation mucoceles). This type of mucocele is not, however, lined by epithelium, and, therefore, is not a true cyst. Occasional mucoceles are caused by saliva retention (retention mucoceles), especially on the floor of the mouth when they may resemble a frog belly and are termed 'ranula'. Mucoceles are diagnosed clinically but it is important to differentiate from a cystic neoplasm, this being most likely in the upper lip (usually a canalicular adenoma).

Most mucoceles either resolve spontaneously or can be excised, ligated or removed with cryosurgery. Ranula may respond to the sclerosant picibanil, commonly used for thyroglossal duct cysts.

Smoking, and its accompanying nicotinic stomatitis, frequently produces transient palatal minor gland outlet obstruction and a mucocele, but damage to the duct or outlet obstructions are most commonly encountered, although also. Superficial mucoceles may be seen in lichen planus.

BOX 11.1 Main Generalised Causes of Salivary Gland Swelling

- Obstruction
- Sialadenitis
- Sjögren syndrome
- Sialosis
- Neoplasm

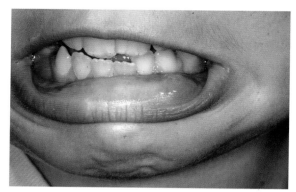

Fig. 11.1 Mucocele in the most common site — the lower labial mucosa.

BOX 11.2 Main Causes of Lumps in the Salivary Glands

Salivary gland swellings may be caused mainly by lymph nodes or other lesions, or salivary:

- Cyst (mucocele or cystic neoplasm)
- Calculus or other obstruction to salivary flow
- Deposits (e.g. amyloidosis, haemochromatosis)
- Hamartoma (branchial cyst, angioma, lymphangioma)
- Hypersensitivity (allergic sialadenitis)
- IgG4 syndrome (Kuttner tumour — chronic sialadenitis)
- Infection (usually bacterial or viral sialadenitis)
- Necrotising sialometaplasia
- Neoplasm (epithelial or mesenchymal)
- Sarcoidosis
- Sialosis
- Sjögren syndrome

MUMPS (ACUTE VIRAL SIALADENITIS; EPIDEMIC PAROTITIS)

Mumps is a common acute viral disease, which principally affects the parotid salivary glands. It is:

- caused by an RNA paramyxovirus (the mumps virus)
- binds to sialic acid receptors on the surface of gland cells
- transmitted by direct contact or by droplet spread from saliva
- characterised by a longish incubation period of 2 to 3 weeks
- followed by immunity to further attacks.

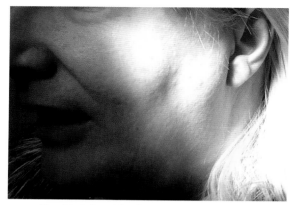

Fig. 11.2 Parotid salivary gland enlargement.

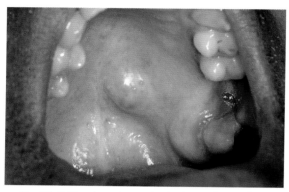

Fig. 11.3 Neoplasm in a palatal minor salivary gland.

Typically, the patient with mumps suffers an acute onset of:

- painful salivary swelling (parotitis), usually bilaterally, although in the early stages, only one parotid gland may appear to be involved. There is no significant hyposalivation. In approximately 10% of cases, the submandibular glands are also affected; rarely, these may be the only glands involved. Generally, the salivary swelling persists for about 7 days and then gradually subsides. An episode is associated with:
  - trismus
  - fever
  - malaise.

Mumps less commonly (and mainly in adults) has extra-salivary manifestations involving organs other than the salivary glands, including:

- orchitis; rarely, oophoritis and thyroiditis; ensuing infertility is rare
- pancreatitis
- meningoencephalitis.

The diagnosis is on clinical grounds, but confirmation, if needed, is by demonstrating a fourfold rise in serum antibody titres to mumps S and V antigens between acute serum and convalescent serum collected 3 weeks later. Other viruses can rarely produce parotitis. No specific antiviral agents are available, so treatment is symptomatic involving:

- analgesics
- adequate hydration
- reducing the fever.

TABLE 11.1 Differentiation of Salivary Lumps

Type of Swelling Symptoms	DIFFUSE		DISCRETE	
	Painful	Painless	Painful	Painless
Main causes	Sialadenitis Lymphadenitis Neoplasm	Sialadenitis Sialosis Neoplasm Sarcoidosis Sjögren syndrome Hamartoma (e.g. angioma) Deposits (e.g. amyloidosis, haemochromatosis)	Abscess Neoplasm Sialometaplasia	Cyst Neoplasm Hamartoma (e.g. angioma)
Investigations	US FNAC MRI or CT Biopsy Sialoendoscopy if obstructive	US FNAC Biopsy Chest radiography Serology SACE Adenosine deaminase	US FNAC MRI or CT	US FNAC

CT, Computerised tomography; *FNAC*, fine needle aspiration cytology; *MRI*, magnetic resonance imaging; *US*, ultrasound imaging.

Patient isolation for 6 to 10 days may be advisable since the virus is in saliva and infectious during this time. Mumps can be prevented with MMR vaccine. This protects against three diseases: measles, mumps and rubella. It is recommended that children get two doses of MMR vaccine, starting with the first dose at 12 through 15 months of age, and the second dose at 4 through 6 years of age.

OBSTRUCTION (OBSTRUCTIVE SIALADENITIS, 'MEALTIME SYNDROME')

Obstruction of a minor salivary gland duct or a ductal tear may produce a mucocele (see above). Obstruction is fairly common in the submandibular duct or gland and is usually caused by calculi and small stones. It is rare in parotid and more likely to be a mucus plug, fibrous stricture, or neoplasm than stones (see also Chapter 12). Uncommon causes of duct obstruction include:
- oedema from irritation of the duct by, for example, a denture clasp
- 'physiological' duct obstruction due either to duct spasm or an abnormal passage of the parotid duct through the buccinator or in relation to the masseter muscles
- neoplasm
- stricture.

Obstruction may be asymptomatic but typically there is pain and swelling of the gland at meals ('mealtime syndrome') and there can be a consequent bacterial sialadenitis. Prolonged duct obstruction produces atrophy, particularly of serous acini, such as in the parotid gland:

It is important to differentiate from other causes of salivary swelling:
- inflammatory: mumps, bacterial sialadenitis
- Sjögren syndrome, sarcoidosis: duct obstruction; neoplasms (see Chapter 12); others including sialosis, drugs
- Mikulicz disease (sclerosing sialadenitis, IgG4 syndrome).

It is sometimes possible to clinically determine the cause of major duct obstruction if calculus is palpable or visible. Ultrasound may help but sialoendoscopy or radiography (but 40% of stones are radiolucent) can be diagnostic, and MRI/CT or sialography if necessary. Management is the surgical removal of the obstruction (lithotripsy, interventional sialoendoscopy, Storz balloon or Dormia basket removal, or incisional removal).

SARCOIDOSIS

An uncommon chronic granulomatous reaction of unknown aetiology, prevalent particularly in black females, sarcoidosis may present with cervical lymphadenopathy, enlarged salivary glands and hyposalivation. Other oral lesions may occasionally precede systemic involvement but Heerfordt syndrome (salivary and lacrimal swelling, facial palsy and uveitis), mucosal nodules, gingival hyperplasia or labial swelling are rare.

Diagnosis is by lesional biopsy, chest radiography, gallium scan, raised serum angiotensin-converting enzyme and adenosine deaminase, to differentiate from Crohn disease, tuberculosis and foreign body reactions. Biopsy of minor salivary glands reveals granulomas in up to 20% of patients with sarcoidosis, particularly in those with hilar lymphadenopathy. Clinical trials guiding evidence for treatment are lacking due to the rarity of disease, heterogeneous clinical course but management is with intralesional corticosteroids or systemic corticosteroids, especially if the lungs or eyes are involved.

SIALADENITIS (BACTERIAL)

Sialadenitis most commonly manifests in the parotid gland (parotitis). The organisms most commonly isolated from bacterial ascending sialadenitis are α-haemolytic streptococci, such as *Streptococcus viridans* and *Staphylococcus aureus*, the latter frequently being penicillin-resistant. Reduced salivary flow allows retrograde access of bacteria from the oral cavity, associated with:

- dehydration: such as following gastrointestinal surgery
- radiotherapy for oral or salivary tumours
- salivary gland or duct abnormalities or obstruction
- Sjögren syndrome.

Acute parotitis presents with:
- painful, swollen salivary glands
- redness of the overlying skin
- pus may exude from the parotid duct (if the infection localises as a parotid abscess it may point externally through the overlying skin or, rarely, into the external acoustic meatus)
- trismus
- pyrexia
- cervical lymphadenopathy
- leukocytosis.

Diagnosis is on clinical grounds, but ultrasound may help. Investigations may be needed to exclude hyposalivation (see Chapter 20). Management is as follows:

- Collect pus for a stained smear, culture and antibiotic sensitivity testing.
- Body temperature should be noted.
- Cervical lymphadenopathy should be excluded.
- Antibiotic therapy should be commenced orally. The antibiotic of choice is flucloxacillin, with erythromycin as an alternative if the patient is penicillin-allergic.
- Any fluctuant swelling should be surgically drained.
- Supportive therapy, such as ensuring an adequate fluid intake, analgesics and attention to good oral hygiene, is important.

Once the acute condition has resolved, correctable factors, such as mucus plugs, strictures or calculi should be treated. If treatment is inadequate, or predisposing factors are not eliminated, chronic bacterial sialadenitis may develop. Unfortunately, serous acini may atrophy when salivary outflow is chronically obstructed, and this further reduces salivary function.

SIALADENOSIS (SIALOSIS)

Sialadenosis is an uncommon, benign, non-inflammatory, non-neoplastic bilaterally symmetrical and painless enlargement of salivary glands. A variety of causes are recognised, most associated with autonomic neuropathy, including:

- drugs (sympathomimetic agents such as isoprenaline, phenylbutazone, isoprenaline, antithyroid drugs and phenothiazines)
- alcohol abuse with or without accompanying liver cirrhosis
- endocrine conditions:
  - diabetes mellitus
  - pregnancy
  - acromegaly
  - following oophorectomy.

Nutritional disorders:
- malnutrition
- anorexia nervosa
- bulimia
- cystic fibrosis and pancreatitis.

Sialadenosis usually affects both parotids with soft, painless general enlargement of the glands. A useful guide to whether the patient is simply obese or has parotid enlargement is to observe the outward deflection of the ear lobe, which is seen in true parotid swelling. The diagnosis of sialadenosis is one of exclusion, based mainly on history and clinical examination. Investigations indicated may include:

- Blood tests: for raised glucose levels or abnormal liver function.
- Ultrasound: rarely, a bilateral space-occupying lesion such as a salivary neoplasm, cyst or lymphoid neoplasm may present difficulties in differentiation from sialadenosis, and then ultrasound may help.
- Sialography: reveals enlarged but otherwise normal glands, although salivary secretion is not impaired. However, if a bilateral space-occupying lesion, such as a salivary neoplasm, cyst, or lymphoid neoplasm presents difficulties in differentiation, sialography or MRI may help.
- A biopsy is rarely needed. The affected glands show acinar hypertrophy, which appears related to autonomic neuropathy.
- Sialochemistry shows raised potassium and calcium levels, which are not found in other causes of parotid enlargement.

No treatment is available. If investigations have revealed a likely cause such as alcoholism or diabetes, then sialadenosis may be resolved when alcohol intake is reduced, or glucose control is instituted.

Eosinophilic Sialodochitis

Eosinophilic sialodochitis is a rare cause of recurrent salivary gland swelling associated with eosinophil-rich mucus plugs or evidence of eosinophilic infiltration around the larger salivary gland ducts on biopsy. It is characterised by the swelling of the salivary glands, which may be painful, with an itch of the skin overlying the affected gland. Stringy secretions from the parotid or submandibular duct are often noted. The aetiology is unknown, although the most accepted hypothesis is that it is an allergic process.

RECOMMENDED READING

Atkinson, C., Fuller, J., Huang, B., 2018. Cross-sectional imaging techniques and normal anatomy of the salivary glands. Neuroimaging Clin. N. Am. 28 (2), 137–158. doi: S1052-5149(18)30001-7 [pii].

Dawes, C., Wong, D.T.W., 2019. Role of saliva and salivary diagnostics in the advancement of oral health. J. Dent. Res. 98 (2), 133–141. https://doi.org/10.1177/0022034518816961.

Isa, A.Y., Hilmi, O.J., 2009. An evidence based approach to the management of salivary masses. Clin. Otolaryngol. 34 (5), 470–473. https://doi.org/10.1111/j.1749-4486.2009.02018.x.

Rzymska-Grala, I., Stopa, Z., Grala, B., et al., 2010. Salivary gland calculi - contemporary methods of imaging. Pol. J. Radiol. 75 (3), 25–37.

Salivary Neoplasms

KEY POINTS
- A wide range of uncommon neoplasms can affect the salivary glands. Most are epithelial neoplasms, present as unilateral swelling of the parotid and are benign. The 'rule of nines' is an approximation that states that 9 out of 10 salivary gland tumours:
  - affect the parotid
  - are benign
  - are pleomorphic salivary adenomas (PSAs).
- Intra-oral salivary gland neoplasms are more likely to be malignant compared with those in major glands.
- Treatment of all neoplasms is largely surgical.

INTRODUCTION

The wide range of different neoplasms that can affect the salivary glands has been classified by the World Health Organization (Box 12.1). The epithelial neoplasms, which are the most important, can be memorised by the mnemonic 'A Most Acceptable Classification' — most are benign, but some are malignant (Tables 12.1 and 12.2):
- **A**denomas: benign
- **M**ucoepidermoid tumour: intermediate level of malignancy (see below)
- **A**cinic cell tumour: intermediate malignancy (see below)
- **C**arcinomas such as adenoid cystic carcinoma, polymorphous low-grade adenocarcinoma and others.

Most salivary gland neoplasms are epithelial, presenting as a unilateral swelling of the parotid and most are benign (Fig. 12.1). This can be remembered by the 'rule of nines' (an approximation) that states that 9 out of 10 salivary gland neoplasms:
- affect the parotid

- are benign
- are pleomorphic salivary adenomas (PSAs).

The next most common neoplasm is carcinoma. Other neoplasms of major salivary glands are usually monomorphic adenomas (such as adenolymphomas), mucoepidermoid tumours or acinic cell tumours. Minor gland neoplasms are more often malignant (see Fig. 12.1).

EPIDEMIOLOGY

- Salivary gland neoplasms are uncommon.
- Most salivary gland neoplasms are seen in older people. In adults, 10% to 25% are malignant but in children, 50% are malignant.
- There is overall a female predisposition to salivary gland neoplasms.
- Salivary gland neoplasms are more common in certain geographical locations. Inuits, for example, have an increased prevalence.
- There is a correlation between the salivary gland and breast cancer.

AETIOLOGY AND PATHOGENESIS

The aetiology is largely unknown, but associations have included:
- Tobacco smoking: at least in Warthin tumour.
- Infections such as:
  - Kaposi syndrome herpesvirus (KSHV) infection or Epstein—Barr virus (EBV) infection in Warthin tumour

---

BOX 12.1   WHO Classification of Salivary Gland Tumours

Non-neoplastic epithelial lesions
- Nodular oncocytic hyperplasia
- Lymphoepithelial sialadenitis

Benign epithelial tumours
- Pleomorphic adenoma
- Basal cell adenoma
- Warthin tumour
- Oncocytoma
- Salivary gland myoepithelioma
- Canalicular adenoma
- Cystadenoma of salivary gland
- Ductal papillomas
- Sialadenoma papilliferum
- Lymphadenoma
- Sebaceous adenoma
- Intercalated duct adenoma and hyperplasia
- Striated duct adenoma
- Sclerosing polycystic adenoma
- Keratocystoma

Malignant epithelial tumours
- Mucoepidermoid carcinoma
- Adenoid cystic carcinoma
- Acinic cell carcinoma
- Secretory carcinoma
- Microsecretory adenocarcinoma
- Polymorphous adenocarcinoma
- Hyalinizing clear cell carcinoma
- Basal cell adenocarcinoma

- Intraductal carcinoma
- Salivary duct carcinoma
- Myoepithelial carcinoma
- Epithelial-myoepithelial carcinoma
- Mucinous adenocarcinoma
- Sclerosing microcystic adenocarcinoma
- Carcinoma ex pleomorphic adenoma
- Carcinosarcoma of the salivary glands
- Sebaceous adenocarcinoma
- Lymphoepithelial carcinoma
- Squamous cell carcinoma
- Sialoblastoma
- Salivary carcinoma NOS and emerging entities

Mesenchymal tumours specific to the salivary glands
- Sialolipoma

Soft Tissue Tumours
- Haemangioma

Haematolymphoid Tumours
- Hodgkin lymphoma
- Diffuse large B-cell lymphoma
  - Extranodal marginal zone B-cell lymphoma

Secondary Tumours
Morphology code of the International Classification of Diseases for Oncology and the Systematized Nomenclature of Medicine (http://snomed.org). Behaviour is coded /0 for benign tumours, /3 for malignant tumours and /1 for borderline or uncertain behaviour.

TABLE 12.1   The More Common Benign Salivary Gland Epithelial Neoplasms

Neoplasm	Comment
Pleomorphic salivary adenoma (PSA)	Most common
Warthin tumour	Second most common benign neoplasm; associated with tobacco smoking; often multiple, sometimes bilateral; frequency increasing
Oncocytoma	Older patients affected May follow irradiation May be bilateral
Canalicular adenoma	Most common in the upper lip, and older patients

TABLE 12.2   The More Common Malignant Salivary Gland Epithelial Neoplasms

Neoplasm	Comment
Carcinoma ex-pleomorphic salivary adenoma	Variable prognosis
Acinic cell carcinoma	Mainly in parotid Poor prognosis
Mucoepidermoid carcinoma	Most common malignancy
Adenoid cystic carcinoma	Poor prognosis

- EBV infection, at least in salivary lymphoepithelial carcinomas in Asian patients and Inuits
- Simian virus 40 (SV40) infection, at least in PSA.
- Occupation: rubber manufacturing, plumbing industry, woodworking, hairdressing, mineral exposure (nickel, chromium, cement, asbestos, silica).
- Ionising radiation exposure, as in:

- survivors of the atomic explosions in Japan in 1945 (mucoepidermoid carcinomas, pleomorphic adenomas and Warthin tumours)
- the use of iodine-131 in the treatment of thyroid disease
- radiotherapy to the head and neck, including cranial irradiation
- radiographs to the head and neck
- exposure to ultraviolet radiation.
- Other radiation: concern about mobile telephones predisposing to epithelial parotid gland malignancy and mucoepidermoid carcinoma has not been resolved, though they may almost double the risk of head tumours according to some studies.

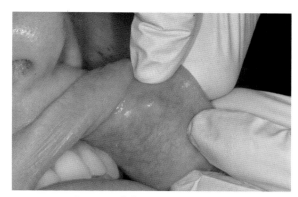

Fig. 12.1 Salivary neoplasm in lip.

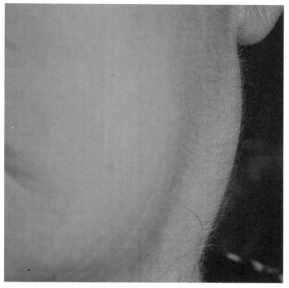

Fig. 12.2 Salivary gland (parotid) neoplasm.

- Genetics:
  - genes expressed or altered in salivary neoplasms include particularly the pleomorphic adenoma gene 1 (PLAG1) on chromosome 8 and changes in 19p, particularly at 19p13 in PSAs
  - p53 and Mcm-2 in areas of malignant transformation in PSAs and recurrences
  - C-kit expression is common in salivary gland cancers
  - MECT1-MAML2 gene rearrangement is seen in most mucoepidermoid carcinomas with cyclic AMP response element-binding protein (CREB)-regulated transcription coactivator (CRTC1-MAML2) rearrangement in high-grade neoplasms
  - MYB-NFIB translocations have been identified in adenoid cystic carcinomas
  - ETV6-NTRK3 translocation is seen in mammary analogue secretory carcinoma, a newly described salivary gland neoplasm.

CLINICAL FEATURES

The main clinical feature of a neoplasm is salivary gland swelling (Fig. 12.2; see also Fig. 9.4). A swelling, especially if persistent, may be a neoplasm in the gland or an intrasalivary lymph node. A history of gradual painless gland enlargement suggests a benign process. A malignant neoplasm may also be symptomless but is suggested by:
- facial palsy
- sensory loss
- pain
- difficulty swallowing
- trismus
- rapid growth.

A clinical examination may reveal an obvious swelling in the case of the parotid outlining the gland anteriorly to the ear and causing eversion of the ear lobe. However, some neoplasms are small, and the presentation may be of pain only.

The gland affected may be relevant:
- parotid neoplasms are largely PSAs

- submandibular gland neoplasms are also usually PSAs, but malignant neoplasms contribute up to one-third of all submandibular neoplasms
- sublingual gland neoplasms are exceedingly rare, but virtually all are malignant
- minor salivary glands neoplasms are PSAs in around 50%, and most of the remainder are malignant, such as carcinomas and adenoid cystic carcinomas. Minor salivary gland neoplasms most commonly arise in the palate but may be seen in the buccal mucosa or upper lip, rarely in the tongue or lower lip.

DIAGNOSIS

- A detailed history and examination are essential (Table 12.3).
- Ultrasonography (US) is diagnostically useful and readily available. Due to their relatively superficial anatomic location, distinct borders and homogeneous echotexture, the major salivary glands are ideally positioned for ultrasonographic assessment, the advantages which include high diagnostic accuracy, non-invasiveness, lack of radiation exposure, as well as high reproducibility and low costs. Benign neoplasms are typically hypoechoic but with defined margins. Irregular shape, irregular borders, blurred margins and a hypoechoic inhomogeneous structure are suggestive of malignancy.
- Ultrasound-guided fine-needle aspiration (US-FNA) cytology is almost invariably indicated since the US alone cannot give equivocal results. However, negative or non-diagnostic cytologic results cannot always guarantee the lesion is benign; careful consideration of US features and cytological results is necessary to avoid false reassurance.

TABLE 12.3   Aids That Might Be Helpful in Diagnosis/Prognosis/Management in Some Patients Suspected of Having Salivary Neoplasm[a]

In Most Cases	In Some Cases
Ultrasound	Sialography
Biopsy	Full blood picture
MRI	Serum ferritin, vitamin B_{12} and corrected whole blood folate levels
	ESR

[a]See text for details and glossary for abbreviations.

TABLE 12.4   Regimens That Might Be Helpful in Management of Patient Suspected of Having Salivary Neoplasm

Regimen	Use in Secondary Care
Likely to be beneficial	Excision
Unproven effectiveness	Radiotherapy
	Chemotherapy
Emergent treatments	Bortezomib
	Cetuximab
	Dasatinib
	Gefitinib
	Lapatinib
	Trastuzumab

Preoperative needle biopsy has a high neoplasm detection rate in experienced hands, more if ultrasound- or CT-guided, although some advocate leaving this until perioperatively if malignancy is likely because neoplasm cells can be seeded in the needle track.

- MRI particularly (or CT) is a sensitive means of neoplasm detection when the US suggests a neoplasm or the result is equivocal. Reports are now emerging of the successful use of PET or PET/CT.
- Sialography may reveal a filling defect or gland displacement but is relatively imprecise and non-specific.

TREATMENT

- Early detection carries the best prognosis.
- Surgical excision is the treatment of choice both for benign and malignant neoplasms; the main hazard is facial nerve damage and palsy. Even PSAs require early removal since, in a minority of cases, carcinoma arises (carcinoma ex-PSA).
- Some malignant salivary neoplasms, such as adenoid cystic carcinoma, invade bone and neural tissues preferentially and therefore wide excision is required.
- Radiotherapy is sometimes used as an adjunct post-operatively in the treatment of malignant neoplasms where the prognosis is poor, or for palliation. Adverse effects may cause hyposalivation, hearing loss, optic nerve damage and mastoiditis (Chapter 53).
- Chemotherapy has had some beneficial but transient effects, has not significantly increased survival, is usually palliative alone and has adverse effects (Chapter 53). Agents trialled have included cisplatin, carboplatin, cyclophosphamide, epirubicin, gemcitabine, vinorelbine, mitoxantrone, doxorubicin, paclitaxel and 5-fluorouracil as single agents or in various combinations.

EMERGENT THERAPIES

- Targeted therapies are emerging but thus far have failed to improve local control or survival. Since C-kit is overexpressed in many salivary gland carcinomas, clinical trials with single-agent imatinib have been tried but proved negative. Bortezomib has been trialled but has not been reliably beneficial. Expression of epidermal growth factor receptor EGFR (ErbB1 and ErbB2) has provided a rationale for trials with trastuzumab, cetuximab, gefitinib and lapatinib. Vascular endothelial growth factor (VEGF) might also be a sensible target (Table 12.4).

FOLLOW-UP OF PATIENTS

Long-term follow-up in secondary care is usually appropriate.

SPECIFIC SALIVARY GLAND NEOPLASMS

The more important neoplasms only are discussed here.

BENIGN NEOPLASMS

Pleomorphic Salivary Adenoma (Mixed Salivary Gland Tumour)

PSA appears to originate from ductal epithelium, which proliferates to contribute to duct-like spaces, sheets of epithelial cells and sometimes areas of squamous metaplasia (Fig. 12.3). There are also areas reminiscent of connective tissue, such as cartilage. The admixture of epithelial elements with what resembles fibrous, myxoid or cartilage tissue, leads to the name 'mixed tumour'. These lesions usually have a thin fibrous capsule, but this is not complete and neoplastic cells may be seen in or outside the capsule. Various genetic abnormalities can be seen — especially involving chromosomes 8 and/or 12, and PLAG-1 and HMG1-C genes.

PSA is the most common salivary gland neoplasm, and:
- usually a slow-growing, lobulated, rubbery swelling with the normal overlying skin, but a bluish appearance if intraoral
- usually benign. However, it recurs if excision is inadequate (around 3% recur in 5 years). The neoplasm is poorly encapsulated and parotid adenomas are in an intimate relationship with the facial nerve, both of which make complete excision difficult to guarantee.

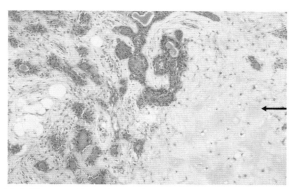

Fig. 12.3 Pleomorphic salivary adenoma with characteristic epithelial islets and chondroid matrix (*arrowed*).

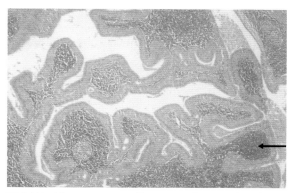

Fig. 12.4 Warthin tumour; papillary cystadenoma lymphomatosum (lymphocytes arrowed).

Malignant change in PSA (carcinoma ex-pleomorphic adenoma) is uncommon and is actually a category of tumours rather than a single type — and there are both aggressive and indolent versions. These neoplasms should be:

- Further qualified as to type/grade of carcinoma and extent, since both intracapsular and minimally invasive neoplasms have a fair prognosis. Malignant change though uncommon is suggested clinically by:
  - rapid growth
  - pain
  - fixation to deep tissues
  - facial palsy.
- Malignant change is confirmed histopathologically by obvious malignant features within the benign cellular picture.

Warthin Tumour (Papillary Cystadenoma Lymphomatosum or Adenolymphoma)

Warthin tumour is found virtually only in the parotid, and:
- is found mainly in smokers, in people with autoimmune disease, or those exposed to radiation
- accounts for about 1:10 parotid neoplasms
- is benign
- is multiple in about 20% and bilateral in 5%
- may rarely be associated with other salivary neoplasms such as PSA, or another malignant disease.

Columnar cells surround lymphocytes in a folded (papillary) lining to cystic spaces (Fig. 12.4). Chromosome 11q and 19p translocations may be present.

Oncocytoma (Oncocytic or Oxyphil Adenoma)

Oncocytoma is exceedingly rare, and:
- is found virtually only in the parotid
- in 20% of cases is in people exposed to radiation
- is extremely rare
- affects mainly the older patient
- is benign.

The characteristic of this neoplasm is that it consists of cords of large eosinophilic cells with small nuclei (oncocytes).

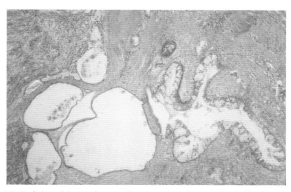

Fig. 12.5 Adenoid cystic carcinoma showing typical 'Swiss-cheese' appearance.

MALIGNANT NEOPLASMS

Adenoid Cystic Carcinoma

Adenoid cystic carcinoma is rare, and:
- slow-growing
- malignant, with a tendency to infiltrate, spread perineurally and metastasise.

Rounded islands of small darkly staining cells surrounding multiple clear areas of varying size (Swiss-cheese appearance) are characteristic (Fig. 12.5). Adenoid cystic carcinomas are graded based on pattern, with solid areas correlating with a worse prognosis. They occasionally transform to highly aggressive pleomorphic high-grade carcinomas with frequent nodal metastases. Chromosome 6q, 8q and 12q abnormalities may be present and several chromosome regions (e.g. 1p32-p36, 6q23-q27) are of prognostic interest.

Acinic Cell Tumour

Acinic cell tumour is very rare, and:
- is found virtually only in the parotid
- is usually malignant, although all grades of malignancy have been reported and, although generally considered of low-grade malignancy, they can recur, metastasise, or even prove lethal. Acinic cell tumours comprise large cells with a granular basophilic cytoplasm with spaces between some cells.

The cells resemble serous cells of normal salivary glands. Aggressive histopathological parameters (anaplasia, necrosis and mitoses) are predictive of poor outcomes.

Mucoepidermoid Carcinoma

Mucoepidermoid carcinoma accounts for up to 10% of salivary gland neoplasms:

- is slow growing
- most frequent salivary gland tumour of the young
- may resemble a mucocele.

The mucoepidermoid tumour consists of large pale mucus-secreting cells (hence 'muco') surrounded by squamous epithelial cells (hence 'epidermoid') (Fig. 12.6). Chromosome 11q and 19p translocations may be present, with HER-2 gene overexpression. This neoplasm is graded using standard schemes in a 3-tier manner with the intermediate-grade category showing the most variability between grading systems and thus the most controversy in management. The MECT1-MAML2 translocation t(11;19)(q21;p13) may prove to be an objective marker that can help to further stratify difficult cases.

Non-Epithelial Salivary Neoplasms

- Malignant lymphomas are the next most common neoplasms found in salivary glands. Sjögren syndrome is recognised as predisposing to lymphomas. An intermediate stage between the salivary gland swelling in Sjögren syndrome and lymphomas is termed the 'benign lymphoepithelial lesion', a histological rather than a clinical condition. It has recently been suggested that the lymphoepithelial lesion represents a localised lymphomatous process.

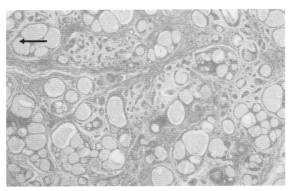

Fig. 12.6 Mucoepidermoid tumour; mucus-secreting cells arrowed.

HIV disease also predisposes to lymphomas, mainly non-Hodgkin lymphomas, which are EBV-related (Chapter 53).

- Others (e.g. juvenile haemangioma).
- Secondary neoplasms.
- Unclassified neoplasms.
- Tumour-like lesions (benign lymphoepithelial lesion, sialosis, oncocytosis).

RECOMMENDED READING

Jensen, S.B., Vissink, A., Firth, N., 2019. Salivary Gland Disorders and Diseases. In: Farah, C., Balasubramaniam, R., McCullough, M. (Eds.), Contemporary Oral Medicine. Springer, Cham.

Odell, E., 2017. Cawson's Essentials of Oral Pathology and Oral Medicine, 9th Ed. Elsevier.

Lumps and Swellings in the Jaws

INTRODUCTION

The most common cause of jaw swelling is developmental enlargements (e.g. tori or exostoses), which are benign, painless, broad-based and self-limiting, usually with normal overlying mucosa and typically require no intervention.

Jaw swelling is less commonly due to odontogenic causes (unerupted teeth, infections, cysts or neoplasms) (Box 13.1).

Jaw swelling may occasionally be caused by non-odontogenic inflammatory or neoplastic disorders, metabolic or fibro-osseous diseases (Box 13.2).

Tumour metastases to the mouth are rare but are typical to the jaws, especially the posterior mandible.

Imaging and other investigations (often biopsy) are almost invariably required to assist the diagnosis of jaw swelling.

Many of these conditions are discussed elsewhere in the text. Here we discuss, alphabetically, other relevant but uncommon or rare, conditions.

ANEURYSMAL BONE CYST

An aneurysmal bone cyst is a rare lesion, which is actually not a cyst since it is unlined. It is a benign, locally destructive multiloculated blood-filled cystic lesion of bone which has recently been re-classified as an osteoclastic giant cell-rich tumour (WHO 2020).

The aetiology remains obscure: approximately one-third appears to be associated with other bone disorders, such as a giant cell lesion, fibrous dysplasia (FD) and ossifying fibromas. This rare lesion presents as an asymptomatic hard swelling of the jaw, sometimes following a history of trauma. It may occur in any part of the skeleton. Radiographs show a unilocular or multilocular translucency with a honeycomb or soap-bubble appearance. Preoperative aspiration shows bloody fluid with a low haematocrit, differentiating it from undiluted blood in a vascular anomaly, such as haemangioma. Diagnosis is confirmed by histology, which shows numerous capillaries and blood-filled spaces, areas of haemorrhage associated with multinucleated giant cells and irregular areas of osteoid. Treat by thorough curettage or excision.

CHERUBISM

Cherubism is a disorder characterised by abnormal bone tissue in the jaw. Beginning in early childhood, both the lower jaw (the mandible) and the upper jaw (the maxilla) become enlarged as bone is replaced with painless, cyst-like growths. Cherubism is a rare genetically determined jaw disease, which closely resembles FD except for the autosomal dominant inheritance. The cause of cherubism is believed to be traced to a genetic defect resulting from a mutation of the *SH3BP2* gene from chromosome 4p16.3 with variable expression. This gene plays a major role in bone homeostasis. Due to its rare occurrence, there is as yet no comprehensive understanding of the natural history and clinical course of the disease.

Clinical features: painless symmetrical enlargement at the angles of the mandible and in the maxilla leads to the typical 'cherubic' facial appearance. Cherubism presents at 2 to 4 years of age, lesions growing progressively until puberty when they arrest or regress. Expansion of the alveolar bone results in irregular spacing and premature loss of teeth and possible disturbances to a developing dentition (Fig 13.1) Imaging shows well-defined multilocular radiolucencies in the mandible, but maxillary lesions are less clearly defined. Blood chemistry is normal, although there may be a raised alkaline phosphatase during active growth periods.

Histologically, the lesions consist of loose vascular connective tissue with numerous multinucleated giant cells and, as in FD, there is fibrous replacement of bone. Other fibro-osseous lesions and giant cell lesions of bone (giant cell granuloma, hyperparathyroidism, giant cell tumours) should be excluded. Treatment of cherubism is as for FD (see also Noonan syndrome, Chapter 54).

BOX 13.1   Most Frequent Causes of Jaw Swelling

- Congenital (torus palatinus, torus mandibularis, exostosis)
- Odontogenic (teeth, infections, cysts or neoplasms)

BOX 13.2   Detailed List of Causes of Jaw Swellings

- Congenital (e.g. torus, exostosis)
  - Odontogenic
  - Cysts
  - Infections
  - Neoplasms
  - Post-operative or post-traumatic oedema or haematoma
  - Unerupted teeth
- Non-odontogenic
  - Infections
  - Cysts
  - Neoplasms (e.g. myeloma, histiocytoses)
  - Pseudotumours (e.g. haemophilic pseudotumour)
  - Foreign bodies
  - Bone disease
  - Fibrous dysplasia
  - Cherubism
  - Neoplasms (e.g. sarcomas)
  - Osteomas (and Gardner syndrome)
  - Paget disease

EXOSTOSES

Bone prominences are not uncommon in the jaws and are given different names which are site-specific. Torus palatinus is found only in the midline of the hard palate (see below). Torus mandibularis is found only on the lingual surface of the mandible, near the premolar teeth. Buccal exostosis is found only on the facial surface of the alveolar bone, usually in the maxilla. Exostoses typically appear in early adulthood, are painless and may slowly enlarge over time. Bone prominences usually require no treatment and have no malignant potential.

Bony proliferations in other sites are considered to be usually either trauma-induced inflammatory periosteal reactions (exostoses) or true neoplasms (osteomas). Unless such a bony prominence is specifically located, is pedunculated or is associated with an osteoma-producing syndrome such as Gardner syndrome (Chapter 54), there is no way to differentiate exostosis from osteoma, even histopathologically.

FIBROUS DYSPLASIA

FD is an uncommon disorder characterised by the replacement of an area of bone with fibrous tissue. Mutations in the signalling protein gene GNAS 1 may be involved. FD usually presents as a painless bony hard swelling, most often in a child and in the maxilla or adjacent bones. The maxillary sinus is often involved, when there may be encroachment on the orbit (causing proptosis) and nasal cavity (causing obstruction). Expansion of the alveolar bone leads to a disruption of occlusion, displacement of teeth and possibly failure of eruption of teeth. Lesions appear to stabilise with skeletal maturation.

Three types of FD are recognised:

- Monostotic (MFD), in which there is a single lesion in only one bone.
- Polyostotic (PFD), in which several lesions are present in one or more bones.
- Albright syndrome, PFD plus cutaneous pigmentation (cafe-au-lait type) on the same side as the bony lesion, and precocious puberty (see Chapter 54).

Radiographically, there is either a translucent cystic appearance in the affected bone, or mottled opaque areas likened to ground glass. The lesions are often ill-defined and may extend to, but not cross, suture lines. Serum calcium and phosphate levels are normal but, in many, the serum alkaline phosphatase level is high and urinary hydroxyproline is increased (findings similar to those in Paget disease). Microscopically, the lesion consists of fibrous tissue that replaces the normal bone and gives rise to osseous trabeculae by metaplasia (Fig. 13.2). The osseous tissue is composed of irregular ('Chinese characters') trabeculae of woven bone lined by osteoblasts. Focal degeneration of fibrous tissue accounts for the cystic spaces seen macroscopically. The treatment of choice to correct any cosmetic defect is conservative surgery, preferably after the cessation of normal skeletal growth. The lesion is not radio-sensitive; irradiation may cause sarcomatous change.

GIANT CELL GRANULOMA

The central giant cell granuloma is an uncommon lesion only seen in the tooth-bearing regions of the jaws, most commonly in the mandible and typically in the second and third decades. The true nature of these lesions is unknown but, as they are invariably destructive, the term 'reparative' giant cell granuloma would appear to be inappropriate. Lesions may be symptomless or simulate a malignant neoplasm clinically and radiographically. Occasionally, the lesion erodes through the cortical bone where it presents as a domed, purplish submucosal swelling. Radiography shows an ill-defined area of radiolucency and there may be resorption of the roots of related teeth. Microscopy shows multinucleated giant cells irregularly distributed in a cellular stroma of plump, spindle-shaped cells which is often highly vascular. There may be areas of new and old haemorrhage with haemosiderin pigment deposition. These histopathological features are indistinguishable from the focal lesions of hyperparathyroidism, which can only be excluded by the appropriate serological tests (calcium and phosphate levels and alkaline phosphatase). Although central giant cell granulomas may recur following curettage, they virtually never metastasise.

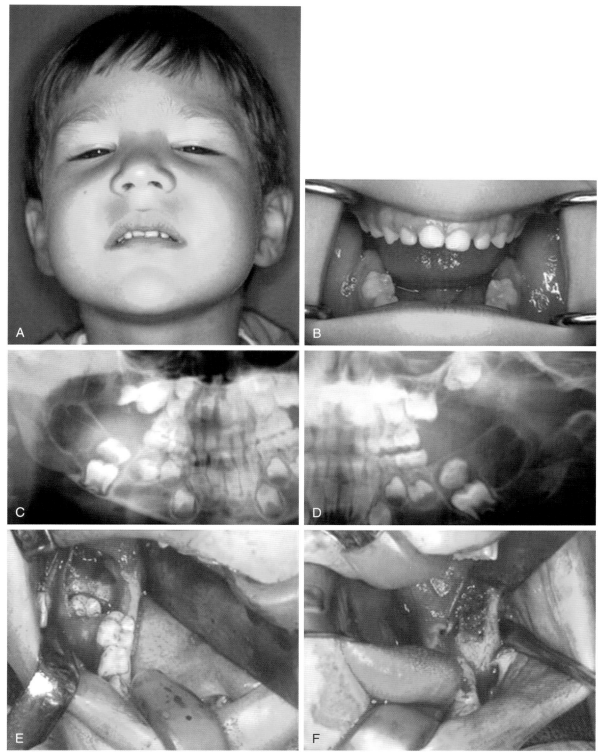

Fig. 13.1 The radiographic appearance of cherubism in a 5-year-old boy. Panoramic radiograph showing bilateral radiolucent lesions in the mandible and maxilla. (A) Clinical appearance showing bilateral extra-oral swellings. (B) Intraoral bilateral swelling of retro-molar areas. (C, D) Radiographic appearances showing displacement of second molar tooth buds superior to the first molar buds. (E, F) Removal of superficial bone to allow development of molar buds.

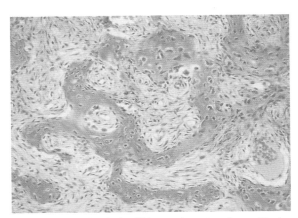

Fig. 13.2 Fibrous dysplasia: Chinese characters formed by bone.

METASTATIC TUMOURS IN THE JAWS

The jaws are not a common site for clinically obvious metastases ('secondaries') but sub-clinical secondary deposits can also occur. The mandible is involved four times as frequently as the maxilla, especially in the premolar and molar regions. In up to one-third of patients, the jaw lesions are the first manifestation of a tumour.

Most metastases originate from primary cancers of the breast, lung, kidney, thyroid, stomach, liver, colon, bone or prostate via lymphatic or haematogenous spread, and present as a lumps, ulceration, pain, swelling, tooth loosening, sensory change or pathological fracture. Metastases from the bronchus, breast, kidney or thyroid gland are usually destructive and osteolytic. Prostatic metastases tend to be osteoblastic and may be confused radiographically with chronic osteomyelitis, Paget disease or cemental lesions.

OSTEOID OSTEOMA AND OSTEOBLASTOMA

These are benign bone tumours that are uncommon in the skeleton generally and rare in the jaws, and their microscopic features are similar, with a vascular stroma in which there are trabeculae of osteoid surrounded by numerous, and darkly staining osteoblasts, but they have distinctive clinical and radiological features.

Osteoid osteoma is usually seen in adolescents and young adults, most frequently in the femur and fibia, is often painful (particularly at night) and has a characteristic central radiolucent area or nidus surrounded by a rim of densely sclerotic bone of variable thickness.

Osteoblastoma, on the other hand, shows progressive growth without the osteosclerotic rim and is rarely painful.

OSTEOMA

Osteoma is a benign bone neoplasm that grows by the continuous formation of lamellar bone. Osteomas are usually unilateral, painless, hard smooth swellings covered by normal oral mucosa. Multiple osteomas, cutaneous cysts or fibromas and polyposis coli are features of Gardner syndrome (Chapter 54); an autosomal dominant syndrome in which the polyps in the large bowel may become malignant. Should a patient have multiple bony growths or lesions, not in the classic torus or buccal exostosis locations, Gardner syndrome should be excluded.

PAGET DISEASE OF BONE

Paget disease is a monostotic or polyostotic progressive skeletal disease with a genetic predisposition and affecting more males than females. The affected bone areas show osseous swelling and often deformation, chronic pain and fractures. Many cases are asymptomatic for a long time resulting in a late diagnosis.

The aetiology is unclear and the incidence appears to be decreasing. Viruses, particularly paramyxoviruses such as canine distemper or measles virus, have been implicated — but with little evidence. There is a strong genetic component; 15% to 20% have a first-degree relative with Paget disease. Mutations in sequestosome 1/p62 gene (SQSTM1/p62) are seen in about one-third of patients with a genetic background, and in 5% to 15% of patients with no family history. SQSTM1/p62 protein is a selective activator of the transcription factor NFB, which plays an important role in osteoclast differentiation and activation in response to the cytokines RANK-ligand and interleukin-1.

Paget disease is characterised by the total disorganiaation of the normally orderly remodelling of bone and an anarchic alternation of bone resorption and apposition ('reversal lines') (Fig. 13.3), often with severe bone pain. In early lesions, bone destruction predominates (osteolytic stage) and there may be bowing of long bones, especially the tibia with occasional pathological fractures, some broadening/flattening of the chest and spinal deformity. As disease activity declines, bone apposition increases (osteosclerotic stage) and bones enlarge. If the skull is affected, a headache may be present. Constriction of skull foraminae may cause cranial neuropathies, e.g. hearing loss. The maxilla often enlarges, particularly in the molar region, with the widening of the alveolar ridge and any dentures may appear to become too tight. The dense bone, hypercementosis and loss of lamina dura make extractions difficult, and there is a liability to haemorrhage and infection.

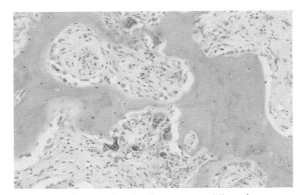

Fig. 13.3 Paget disease showing bone reversal lines from resorption/deposition with a 'mosaic pattern'.

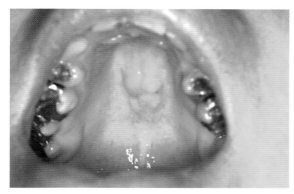

Fig. 13.4 Torus palatinus: central palatal symptomless bony mass.

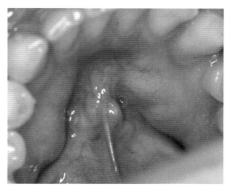

Fig. 13.5 Torus mandibularis: symptomless, bilateral bony masses.

Diagnosis is supported by imaging, biochemistry and histopathology. In early lesions, large irregular areas of relative radiolucency (osteoporosis circumscripta) are seen, but later there is increased radio-opacity, with the appearance of an irregular 'cotton wool' pattern. There is a progressive thickening of the diploe and base of the skull as well as the sphenoid, orbital and frontal bones. Isotope bone scanning shows localised areas of very high uptake. Increase in plasma alkaline phosphatase and urine hydroxyproline levels, but little or no changes in serum calcium or phosphate levels. Differential diagnosis includes other fibro-osseous lesions, such as FD, and conditions with a raised alkaline phosphatase, such as osteomalacia, hyperparathyroidism and osteoblastic metastatic deposits (e.g. prostate carcinoma).

Treatment: Bisphosphonates have become the favoured treatment and are recommended for most patients with active Paget disease who are at risk for further skeletal complications. Bisphosphonate treatment inhibits osteoclastic bone resorption and should be initiated early to prevent secondary complications. A single dose of 5 mg i.v. zoledronate as the treatment of choice in patients without contraindications appears effective.

TORUS PALATINUS AND TORUS MANDIBULARIS

Torus palatinus and mandibularis are common developmental benign exostoses more common in Asians, especially Koreans.

They appear in late teens or adulthood and may become more apparent as they enlarge with increasing age. They have a smooth or nodular surface and are of no consequence apart from occasionally interfering with denture construction. The two types are not necessarily associated one with another:

- Torus palatinus occurs in the centre of the hard palate, is of variable size and configuration (Fig. 13.4).
- Torus mandibularis is lingual to the lower premolars and usually bilateral (Fig. 13.5).

RECOMMENDED READING

Auskalnis, A., Bernhardt, O., Putniene, E., et al., 2015. Oral bony outgrowths: prevalence and genetic factor influence. Study of twins. Medicina (Kaunas). 51 (4), 228–232.

Corral-Gudino, L., Tan, A.J., Del Pino-Montes, J., Ralston, S.H., 2017. Bisphosphonates for Paget's disease of bone in adults. Cochrane Database Syst. Rev. 12, CD004956. https://doi.org/10.1002/14651858.CD004956.pub3.

Matthies, L., Rolvien, T., Pakusa, T.J., et al., 2019. Osteoid osteoma of the mandible – clinical and histological findings. Anticancer Res. 39 (1), 291–296.

Papadaki, M.E., Lietman, S.A., Levine, M.A., Olsen, B.R., Kaban, L.B., Reichenberger, E.J., 2012. Cherubism: best clinical practice. Orphanet. J. Rare. Dis. 7 Suppl 1(Suppl 1), S6.

Odontogenic Cysts and Tumours

KEY POINTS Odontogenic cysts are common, may be asymptomatic and often are first detected on routine imaging:
- Radicular cysts are the most common 45%
- Dentigerous cysts are the second most common 16%
- Odontogenic keratocysts are the third most common cysts and are sometimes associated with Gorlin syndrome (naevoid basal cell carcinoma syndrome or basal cell naevus syndrome) 10%
- Odontogenic tumours are rare, may be asymptomatic and detected on routine imaging
- Most odontogenic tumours are odontomas (75%)
- Ameloblastoma is the next most common and may recur after removal
- Malignant odontogenic tumours are very rare in comparison with benign lesions

INTRODUCTION

Odontogenic cysts and tumours are defined as lesions of the jaws and gingiva derived from odontogenic epithelium.

ODONTOGENIC CYSTS

A cyst is a pathological cavity having liquid, semi-liquid or gaseous contents. It is frequently, but not always, lined with epithelium.

Most cysts of the jaws arise from odontogenic epithelium. These are relatively common lesions — most are inflammatory cysts (about 50% of all jaw cysts), dentigerous cysts (20%) or odontogenic keratocysts (keratocystic odontogenic tumours; 10%).

There is an overall male predominance.

Most odontogenic cysts are benign.

Aetiology and Pathogenesis

The main pathogenic factors include the following:
- Epithelial proliferation — either stimulated by inflammation in the case of radicular cysts, or occurring from a mutated oncogene in the case of keratocystic odontogenic tumours and probably also the glandular odontogenic cyst (GOC).
  - Hydrostatic or osmotic factors: may play a part in cyst growth since the cyst wall acts as a semipermeable membrane.
  - Bone resorbing factors: such as prostaglandins and collagenase.

Clinical Features

Odontogenic cysts are often discovered as an incidental finding on imaging (Fig. 14.1). They are generally symptomless, slow-growing and may reach a large size before they give rise to symptoms, such as:
- swelling: cysts in bone initially produce a smooth bony hard lump with normal overlying mucosa, but as the bone thins, it may crackle on palpation rather like an egg shell (termed 'egg shell cracking'). When the overlying bone is resorbed, the cyst may show through as a bluish fluctuant swelling (Fig. 14.2)
- discharge: usually into the mouth
- pain: due to secondary infection.

Diagnosis

The diagnosis of an odontogenic cyst is based on an adequate history, clinical examination and appropriate investigations, such as pulp vitality testing and radiographs (both intraoral and extraoral) of associated teeth, together with aspiration and analysis of cyst fluids, and histopathology (Table 14.1).

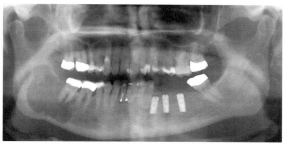

Fig. 14.1 Mandibular odontogenic tumour revealed on dental pantomograph.

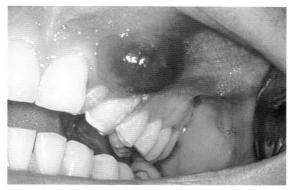

Fig. 14.2 Odontogenic cyst arising from the non-vital lateral incisor.

Treatment

Odontogenic cysts are managed either by enucleation or by marsupialisation:

- Enucleation is the complete removal of the cyst: the benefit is that all the cyst tissue is available for histological examination, and the cyst cavity will usually heal uneventfully with minimal aftercare. Enucleation is potentially problematic; however, since if the cyst involves the apices of adjacent vital teeth, surgery may deprive the teeth of their blood supply and render them non-vital.
- Marsupialisation is the partial removal of the cyst: the benefit is that it is somewhat less invasive than enucleation and tooth vitality is retained, but it requires considerable aftercare and good patient cooperation in keeping the cavity clean whilst it resolves. In order to keep the cavity open, a 'bung' or acrylic plug is usually inserted in the opening, often attached to a denture or acrylic splint. The bung stops most food collecting in the cavity, but the cavity must still be

syringed by the patient after each meal. Healing is slower than after enucleation: marsupialised cyst cavities may take up to 6 months to close down to the extent of becoming 'self-cleansing'. The other disadvantage of marsupialisation is that not all the cyst lining is available to histopathological examination, and this could lead to misdiagnosis.

Inflammatory Cysts

Inflammatory cysts are by far the most common of all jaw cysts and arise in association with a non-vital tooth.

Aetiology and Pathogenesis

The epithelial lining of inflammatory cysts is derived from the rests of Malassez, which proliferate to produce thick, irregular, often incomplete squamous epithelium, with granulation tissue forming the cyst wall in the denuded areas (Fig. 14.3). Depending on the nature of the inflammatory response, there may be areas of chronic inflammation, or acute inflammation with abscess formation. Cholesterol crystal clefts are often present, and mucous cells may be found. The cyst fluid is usually watery but may be thick and viscid with cholesterol crystal clefts giving it a shimmering appearance. The cysts have capsules of collagenous fibrous connective tissue and cause bone resorption and may become quite large.

Radicular Cyst

- This is associated with the apex of a non-vital tooth. Occasionally, a radicular cyst may develop on the lateral aspect of a root, where the stimulus has been an inflammatory reaction arising from necrotic pulp in a lateral root canal. Radicular cysts are rare in the primary dentition but are seen especially where:
- a non-vital pulp is infected
- endodontic treatment has failed
- a root has fractured and there is a perforation
- a root is retained.

Residual radicular cysts. These arise where an inflammatory cyst (usually a radicular cyst) remains after the removal of the non-vital tooth or root from which it arose.

TABLE 14.1 Aids That Might Be Helpful in Diagnosis/Prognosis/Management in Some Patients Suspected of Having Odontogenic Cyst or Tumour[a]	
In Most Cases	**In Some Cases**
Radiography	MRI
Biopsy	Aspiration

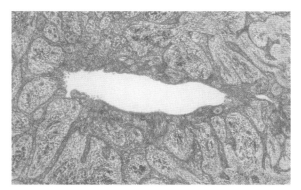

Fig. 14.3 Developing radicular cyst.

Diagnosis

The diagnosis is based on history, clinical examination and appropriate investigations, such as pulp vitality testing and radiographs (both intraoral and extraoral) of associated teeth, aspiration and analysis of cyst fluids, and histopathology. These cysts are usually 1 to 2 cm in diameter with a well-defined, unilocular radiolucency with a sclerotic margin.

Treatment

The treatment of inflammatory cysts depends on whether or not the involved non-vital tooth is to be retained. Conventional intra-canal endodontic treatment may lead to the resolution of very small radicular cysts, but regular radiographic review is necessary until there has been complete resolution of the cyst. If, when the tooth has been root-filled, the cyst does not resolve, or if the cyst is of such a size that it is unlikely to resolve with endodontic treatment alone, surgery is indicated — either enucleation or marsupialisation combined with extraction of the non-vital tooth.

Follow-Up

This is mainly in primary care.

Developmental Cysts

Dentigerous Cyst

Dentigerous cyst is the second most common odontogenic cyst. It surrounds the crown of a tooth and arises as an expansion of the follicle caused by separation of the reduced enamel epithelium from the enamel.

Clinical features. The dentigerous cyst is most frequently found in areas where unerupted teeth are found — mandibular third molars, maxillary third molars and maxillary canines, in decreasing order of frequency. These cysts may grow to a large size, displace the tooth with which they are associated, or rarely cause resorption of adjacent tooth roots.

Diagnosis. Diagnosis is usually made by clinical and radiographic assessment — when the follicular space exceeds 5 mm from the crown, it is likely that a cyst is present. However, odontogenic keratocysts and ameloblastomas may occasionally mimic the radiological appearances of follicular cysts.

Treatment. Treatment may be either marsupialisation, allowing the tooth to erupt, or enucleation, with removal of the associated tooth.

Eruption Cysts

Eruption cysts are considered as minor soft tissue forms of dentigerous cysts. In these cases, the involved teeth are usually prevented from eruption by dense fibrous tissue overlying them. They often burst spontaneously before eruption of the associated tooth and only require excision if impeding normal eruption. Then, a narrow window can be excised over the erupting tooth.

Follow-up. This is mainly in secondary care.

Odontogenic keratocyst (OKC)

This is the third most common odontogenic cyst, occurring in 10% to 20% of cases. It can be associated with the naevoid basal cell carcinoma syndrome or basal cell naevus syndrome (Gorlin syndrome). Most arise from rests of odontogenic epithelium that remain in the alveolus after tooth development. A third may be associated with mutations or deletions of the PTCH gene on chromosome 9q, a tumour suppressor gene. Loss of gene activity leads to the release of a brake on the cell cycle mediated through the *Hedgehog* (Hh) signalling pathway. The remainder may be associated with other alterations of the signalling pathway. The effect is for cyst linings to enlarge with a tendency to recurrence after removal.

Clinical features. The OKC may have many clinical appearances and may be seen over a wide age range. Most involve the mandibular angle and may expand to occupy the major part of the ramus as a radiolucent lesion. They may sometimes be multilocular. They may resorb the cortical plates and expand into the soft tissues, envelop unerupted teeth giving a dentigerous appearance or displace teeth but not resorb them. OKCs are generally painless and often grow to a large size before giving rise to symptoms, unless they become secondarily infected.

Diagnosis. Diagnosis may be suggested by clinical features supported by imaging. The radiological appearance is characteristic with a sharply demarcated and corticated margin. They are typically multilocular. The cyst lining usually has a characteristic appearance of a regular keratinised stratified squamous epithelium, commonly five to eight cell layers thick and without rete pegs (Figs. 14.4 and 14.5). There is a well-defined basal layer predominantly of columnar, but occasionally cuboidal, cells that show palisading of nuclei. Desquamated keratin is always present within the cyst lumen, and the fibrous wall is usually thin. Cysts may be multilocular and have microscopic daughter cysts.

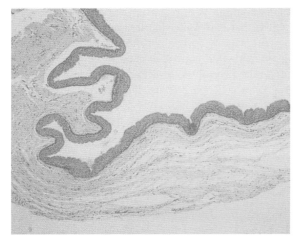

Fig. 14.4 Keratocystic odontogenic tumour (low power view).

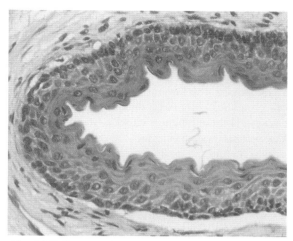

Fig. 14.5 Keratocystic odontogenic tumour (high power).

Treatment. Gorlin syndrome is highly likely if the lesions are bilateral and/or in young people. Cysts must be completely excised to minimise the risk of recurrence.

Follow-Up. This is mainly in secondary care. Long-term clinical and radiographic follow-up is mandatory as recurrences may occur many years after initial treatment.

Other developmental odontogenic cysts are uncommon and their pathogenesis is far from clear. They include:

Gingival cysts of adults

These arise from epithelial rests in the gingivae and are found only in soft tissue in the lower premolar areas.

Gingival cysts of infants

These arise from remnants of the dental lamina and are located in the corium below the surface epithelium. They are generally asymptomatic. Bohn nodules and Epstein pearls are similar lesions with which gingival cysts sometimes are confused (see Chapter 53).

Lateral periodontal cysts

These are most commonly associated with the mandibular premolar area and occasionally with the maxillary anterior region and arise from the post-functional dental lamina. As described earlier, cysts of inflammatory origin are found to lie on the lateral aspect of a non-vital tooth and are diagnosed on histology.

Glandular odontogenic cysts (GOC)

These are very rare developmental cysts accounting for less than 0.5% of all odontogenic cysts. They usually present in the anterior mandible as a painless, slow-growing swelling and a large, mul-tiloculated, well-defined radiolucency. GOC contain mucous cells and duct-like structures that may mimic central mucoepidermoid

carcinoma. Characteristic histopathological features include epithelial spherules/'knobs'/whorls, cuboidal eosinophilic cells, goblet cells, intraepithelial glandular/microcystic ducts, variations in lining width, ciliated cells and mucous pools/mucous-lined crypts, which, with the expression of p53 and Ki67, may aid the diagnosis. GOC may recur following curettage.

Calcifying epithelial odontogenic cysts

Calcifying epithelial odontogenic cyst is extremely rare, with a wide age range. Either jaw of either sex may be affected, but most are anterior to the first molar. Clinically, there is a slowly enlarging, painless swelling of the jaws, which, on radiographic examination, appears as a well-defined unilocular radiolucency containing flecks of opacity associated with calcifications within cyst lining. It is diagnosed by finding ghost and ameloblast-like cells histologically. Treatment is usually enucleation.

Follow-Up

Follow-up is mainly in secondary care.

ODONTOGENIC TUMOURS

Odontogenic tumours may classified simply into:
- Benign epithelial tumours e.g. ameloblastomas, adenoma-toid odontogenic tumour, and calcifying epithelial odonto-genic tumour
- Benign mixed epithelial and mesenchymal tumours, e.g. ameloblastic fibroma and odontomes
- Benign mesenchymal tumours e.g. odontogenic fibroma and odontogenic myxoma
- Fibro-osseous lesions
- Malignant neoplasms e.g. ameloblastic carcinoma

or

A. **Odontogenic tumours consisting predominantly of epithelium arise from odontogenic epithelium** (remnants of the dental lamina, reduced enamel epithelium, rests of Serres, rests of Malassez),
B. **Odontogenic tumours of mixed origin** consist both of odontogenic epithelium and odontogenic mesenchyme.
C. **Odontogenic tumours originating from the odontogenic mesenchyme** (dental follicle, dental papilla, pulp, peri-odontal ligament)

Most odontogenic tumours are odontomas and benign.

Treatment and Follow-Up of Patients With Odontogenic Tumours

Secondary care is usually appropriate.

A. Odontogenic Tumours of Epithelial Origin
Ameloblastoma

The ameloblastoma is the most common odontogenic neoplasm. There are several subtypes that include the solid/

multicystic (most frequent), unicystic, desmoplastic and metastasising ameloblastoma. All are benign. Most have been shown to harbour the V600E mutation in the BRAF gene or mutations of the SMO gene.

Clinical features and diagnosis. Ameloblastomas are more frequent in males and usually appear after the age of 40 years. The tumour is not uncommon in people of African heritage compared to the lower incidence in white people.

The initial detection of an ameloblastoma is likely to be a 'chance finding', but when the tumour is evident clinically, there is a slow-growing, painless, expansile swelling of bone. 75% are found in the mandible, most in the posterior mandible and often involve the ramus. The lesion expands to produce progressive facial deformity, and intraorally, there may be evidence of malocclusion and mobile teeth.

Diagnosis. A monocystic (unicystic) or polycystic ('soap bubble') radiolucency is evident. Diagnosis is confirmed by histological examination of a biopsy specimen. Ameloblastomas are composed of epithelial cells arranged as a peripheral layer of ameloblast-like cells around a central area of cells resembling stellate reticulum (Fig. 14.6). Two main histological types are seen: follicular and plexiform types. In the follicular type, discrete islands (follicles) of epithelial cells are evident, whereas in the plexiform type, the epithelium forms continuous anastomosing strands. Enamel formation is not evident, presumably because no odontogenic mesenchyme is present to give the critical inductive forces. Histological variations may be seen. There appears to be little correlation between these histological patterns and the clinical course of the tumour.

Treatment. Ameloblastomas expand rather than destroy bone. The treatment of choice, therefore, is surgical excision of the tumour together with removal of a margin of normal bone but retention of the lower border of the mandible.

Metastatic dissemination is very rare and usually occurs by aspiration to the lungs following longstanding local disease or previous surgical intervention.

Adenomatoid Odontogenic Tumour

This is an uncommon and benign odontogenic tumour.

Clinical features and diagnosis.
- most commonly occurs in the second and third decades of life
- most cases are seen in females
- most occur in the anterior maxilla
- resembles a dentigerous or radicular cyst

Clinically, the lesion presents as a gradually increasing intrabony swelling, which is occasionally painful.

On radiographs, the tumour appears as a unilocular radiolucency sometimes with radio-opaque foci. A clinical provisional diagnosis should include either a lateral periodontal cyst or a dentigerous cyst, particularly as, in the latter case, the tumour is sometimes associated with an unerupted tooth.

Histologically the tumour is encapsulated and consists of sheets and strands of epithelial cells (Fig 14.7).

Treatment. Enucleation

Calcifying Epithelial Odontogenic Tumour (Pindborg Tumour)

Clinical features and diagnosis. This is rare, benign, but aggressive tumour that has been reported in all age groups but usually over the age of 40 years. It presents as a progressive painless swelling of the jaws, most frequent in the mandibular premolar-molar region or as a chance radiological finding. Radiographically, the tumour usually appears as a radiolucency that may mineralise, leading to mixed radiolucency.

Histological examination:
- Sheets of epithelial cells in fibrous tissue
- Amyloid deposition in the connective tissue that may become mineralised.

Treatment. The tumour may be locally infiltrative and therefore excision is required with a small margin.

Enamel Pearls

Rarely, disturbances in odontogenesis cause small deposits of enamel, termed enamel pearls (enamelomas), usually between the roots of the first permanent molars. No treatment is required.

B. Odontogenic Tumours of Mixed Origin
Ameloblastic Fibroma

Clinical features and diagnosis. Ameloblastic fibroma is a tumour that occurs in young adults (15 to 25 years) presenting as a slow, painless jaw expansion and appears as a unilocular radiolucency. It may be very destructive in the growing facial bones.

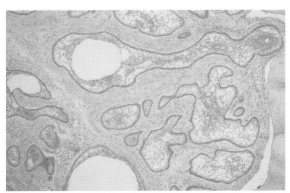

Fig. 14.6 Ameloblastoma.

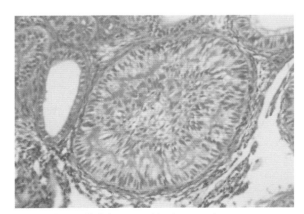

Fig. 14.7 Adenomatoid odontogenic tumour.

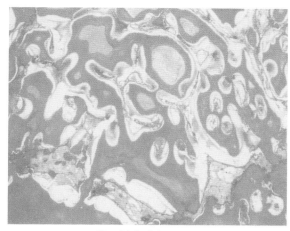

Fig. 14.8 Odontome.

They appear as multi or unilocular swellings that can displace teeth or prevent their eruption.

Histologically, odontogenic epithelium is present as small islands or elongated strands. The odontogenic mesenchyme resembles the dental papilla. Malignant change is a rare finding.

Treatment (see also Chapters 4 and 5). Excision with a small margin.

Odontomes

These are the commonest odontogenic tumour comprising calcified hamartomatous malformations of dental hard tissues and consist of dental tissues in normal relationship one to another (Fig. 14.8). **Odontomes have been classified according to the type and spatial arrangement of the dental tissues as follows:**

- compound type (compound composite odontomes): consist of multiple small simple denticles embedded in fibrous connective tissue within a fibrous capsule. Multiple lesions may be seen in Gardner syndrome (Chapter 54)
- complex type (complex composite odontomes): consist of an irregular mass of all the dental tissues.

Clinical features. Odontomes typically present in children and adolescents, more commonly in females than males, and show a distinct predilection for the premolar-molar region of the mandible. They are formed from the dental lamina. They may rarely erupt, but more usually, they may go unnoticed or, if located over the crown of an unerupted tooth, may prevent its eruption. They may displace adjacent teeth or impede eruption.

Diagnosis. Radiographically, the lesions appear as small well-defined radio-opacities.

Treatment (see also Chapters 4 and 5). The lesions should be excised, but considerable mechanical difficulty may be encountered.

C. Odontogenic Tumours of Mesenchymal Origin

Odontogenic Myxoma (Myxoma of the Jaws)

Clinical features and diagnosis. Odontogenic myxoma is the third most common odontogenic tumour. It usually occurs in adolescents and young adults (10 to 40 years), more frequently in females than males, and usually in the posterior region of the mandible. Maxillary lesions are characterised by extensive involvement of the alveolar bone, antrum, and zygomatic process. Clinically, the myxoma is an intrabony lesion that slowly expands the bony cortex and only perforates later. The lesion is rarely painful, but there may be loosening and displacement of the teeth.

Radiographic examination shows a well-defined unilocular or multilocular ('soap bubble') radiolucency, which may extend between the roots of the teeth and, thus, a scalloped margin is seen.

On microscopic examination of biopsy specimens, spindle/stellate shaped cells are present in an intercellular mucoid stroma, sometimes containing nests of epithelial cells. Fibrous tissue and collagen are frequently evident throughout the lesion ('fibromyxoma'). The ground substance permeates between medullary bone trabeculae.

Treatment. Myxomas permeate and, therefore, should be treated with surgical excision of the tumour and removal of a margin of normal bone.

Odontogenic Fibroma

Clinical features and diagnosis. Odontogenic fibroma is a rare benign tumour that may be peripheral or central. The tumour generally presents in close relation to the root of a tooth, the crown of an unerupted tooth, or in the site of a tooth that is congenitally missing. Histologically, the lesion consists of fibrous tissue that has a similar appearance to the dental pulp.

Treatment. Conservative enucleation is the treatment of choice.

RECOMMENDED READING

WHO classification of tumors of odontogenic and maxillofacial bone tumors (El-Naggar et al. 2017)

Cawson's essentials of oral pathology and oral medicine. Edward Odell. 9th editon, 2017. Chapter 10 and 11.

Cervical Lymphadenopathy

INTRODUCTION

Discrete swellings in the neck are often due to lymph node enlargement (cervical lymphadenopathy) but may occasionally be caused by disorders in:

- the salivary glands
- the thyroid gland
- other structures.

More diffuse swelling of the neck may be caused by obesity or:

- oedema (inflammatory or allergic)
- haematoma
- malignant infiltration
- surgical emphysema.

The location of a lump or swelling in the neck will often give a good indication of the tissue of origin, and the age of the patient may also help suggest the most likely diagnoses (Box 15.1). The history of the duration of the lesion is also relevant: one that has been present since an early age is likely to be of congenital origin, while a lump appearing in later life and persisting may be malignant.

The most common complaint in the neck is of swelling and/or pain in the cervical lymph nodes (Box 15.2) (cervical lymphadenopathy), although a wide range of diseases may present with lesions in the neck (Fig. 15.1). Over a quarter of the lymph nodes in the body are connected with lymph nodes situated in the head and the neck. The tonsil is lymphoid tissue located between the pillars of the fauces, and there is similar material in the posterior third of the tongue (lingual tonsil) and the posterior wall of the pharynx (adenoids). These three areas form a ring of lymphoid tissue around the oropharynx (Waldeyer ring). It is not surprising then that many diseases of the lymphoid tissue present primarily in the head and neck.

The dental surgeon can often detect serious disease through neck node examination. Tenderness, consistency and mobility as well as history should be documented. Both anterior and posterior cervical nodes should be examined as well as other nodes. Liver and spleen should be included if systemic disease is a possibility. Generalised lymphadenopathy with or without enlargement of other lymphoid tissue such as liver and spleen (hepatosplenomegaly) suggests a systemic cause.

CLINICAL FEATURES

The patient may be aware that they have lymphadenopathy, usually termed 'glands in the neck'. The main complaint with respect to cervical lymph nodes is usually of swelling. Tenderness may have drawn the patient's attention to their presence.

The history should include:

- date of onset of symptoms;
- details of any swelling, e.g. duration and character
- unilateral or bilateral; cervical or generalised
- pain experienced, such as duration, character, radiation
- aggravating and relieving factors
- associated phenomena.

The duration of the lymphadenopathy is vital.

Acute less than 6 weeks — Lymph nodes that are tender and mobile may be inflammatory (lymphadenitis). Lymph nodes swollen from acute infections are usually tender, soft and discrete, Chronic greater than 6 weeks — chronic infections give firm lymph nodes. In systemic infective disorders, the nodes are usually firm, discrete, tender and mobile.

Nodes that are increasing in size and are hard or fixed to adjacent tissues may be malignant. Nodes that are enlarged and firm and matted or rubbery may be due to leukaemia. In the lymphomas, particularly, the nodes may be rubbery, matted together and fixed to deeper structures.

AETIOLOGY AND PATHOGENESIS

Lymph nodes can enlarge in a number of disorders (see Box 15.2), often because of disease in the local area of drainage, sometimes because of disease affecting the wider lymphoreticular system (lymph nodes, liver and spleen).

BOX 15.1 Most Common Causes of Swellings in the Neck at Different Ages

Child (First Decade)
- Lymphadenitis due to viral respiratory tract infection
- Kawasaki disease

Adolescent and Teenager (Second Decade)
- Lymphadenitis due to viral respiratory tract infection
- Bacterial infection
- Glandular fever syndromes, including HIV infection
- Toxoplasmosis

Adult (Third and Fourth Decades)
- Lymphadenitis
- Glandular fever syndromes, including HIV infection
- Malignancy

After Fourth Decade
- Lymphadenitis
- Malignancy

BOX 15.2 Main Causes of Cervical Lymph Node Enlargement

Infections
- Viral upper respiratory tract: an enlarged jugulodigastric (tonsillar) lymph node is common
- Oral or local bacterial in the drainage area (dental, scalp, ear, nose or throat): e.g. streptococcal, staphylococcal, uncommonly mycobacterial lymphadenitis
- Systemic:
  - viral (e.g. infectious mononucleosis, cytomegalovirus, HIV infection)
  - bacterial, including syphilis, tuberculosis, brucellosis
  - fungal, including histoplasmosis
  - parasitic: toxoplasmosis, leishmaniasis, tularaemia

Malignant Disease
- In the drainage area (usually oral, scalp, ear, nose or throat; rarely thyroid or gastric)
- Lymphoreticular (leukaemia, lymphoma)
- Langerhans histiocytosis

Inflammatory Disorders
- Connective tissue disorders, e.g. lupus
- Orofacial granulomatosis
- Crohn disease
- Sarcoidosis

Others
- Drug-induced hypersensitivity syndrome (e.g. phenytoin)
- Mucocutaneous lymph node syndrome (Kawasaki disease)
- Rosai–Dorfman disease (rare non-neoplastic histiocytosis)

Enlargement of the cervical lymph nodes alone usually arises because they are involved in an immune response to an infectious agent in the area of drainage that could be anywhere on the face, scalp and nasal cavity, sinuses, ears, pharynx and oral cavity. Such lymphadenitis only rarely leads to suppuration. The local cause may not always be found, however, despite a careful search; for example, young children (especially those of African heritage) occasionally develop a *Staphylococcus aureus* lymphadenitis (see below) or a similar problem due to atypical *Mycobacteria* (non-tuberculous mycobacteria [NTM]) (usually in a submandibular node) in the absence of any obvious portal of infection or any clear explanation for their susceptibility. *Mycobacterium avium-intracellulare* complex (MAC) is the main organism involved but sometimes *M. kansasii* or *M. scrofulaceum* are implicated. These bacteria are common in soil and infection may be via the oral cavity; chemotherapy with antituberculous agents may be used, but most lesions clear spontaneously over several months.

Enlargement of cervical lymph nodes alone may also occur when there is reactive hyperplasia to a malignant tumour in the drainage area or metastatic infiltration. The latter may cause the node to feel distinctly hard, and it may become bound down to adjacent tissues ('fixed'), may not be discrete, and may even, in advanced cases, ulcerate through the skin. Most disease is detected in nodes in the anterior triangle of the neck, which is bounded superiorly by the mandibular lower border, posteriorly and inferiorly by the sternomastoid muscle, and anteriorly by the midline of the neck. Nodes in this site drain most of the head and neck except the occiput and back of the neck. Lymphadenopathy in the anterior triangle of the neck alone is often due to local disease, especially if the nodes are enlarged on only one side.

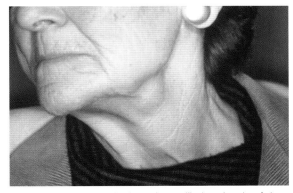

Fig. 15.1 Visible swelling in the submandibular triangle of the neck.

Generalised lymph node enlargement, including cervical nodes, sometimes with liver and/or spleen involvement, may occur in:
- Systemic infections, such as the glandular fever syndromes. Lymphadenitis in tuberculosis may also lead to neck swelling (scrofula) and suppuration (cold abscess).
- Inflammatory lesions, such as connective tissue diseases and granulomatous conditions (Crohn disease, orofacial granulomatosis and sarcoidosis); and mucocutaneous lymph node syndrome (MLNS) (Kawasaki disease).
- Drug reactions (see Chapters 5 and 33).

- Neoplasms of the lymphoreticular system, such as lymphomas, leukaemias and histiocytoses (see Box 15.2). In some, there is clinical involvement of the whole reticuloendothelial system, with generalised lymph node enlargement (detectable clinically in the neck, groin and axilla) and enlargement of both liver and spleen (hepatosplenomegaly).

Infective Inflammatory Conditions

Viral infections with predominantly upper respiratory and oral manifestations:

- Usually cause fever and malaise.
- Usually several anterior triangle nodes — especially the jugulodigastric nodes — are enlarged, often bilaterally. Posterior triangle nodes are not enlarged and there is, of course, no generalised lymph node enlargement nor hepatosplenomegaly unless there are systemic complications or lesions elsewhere.
- Any viral upper respiratory infection from the common cold to viral tonsillitis can be responsible for enlarged cervical nodes (see Box 15.2).
- Oral viral infections that may cause cervical lymph node swelling are mainly those that also produce mouth ulcers such as:
  - herpes simplex stomatitis
  - Herpangina (Coxsackie A6)
  - occasionally, herpes zoster of the trigeminal nerve (see Chapter 38).

Viral Infections With Multiple Systemic Manifestations

In these disorders, there are typically fever and malaise and perhaps a rash, and there are usually several anterior and often posterior triangle nodes enlarged, with generalised enlargement and, in some instances, hepatosplenomegaly. Infections implicated are mainly:

- hand, foot and mouth disease (Coxsackie A16) (see Chapter 37)
- viral exanthemata (chickenpox, measles, rubella)
- glandular fever syndromes (Epstein–Barr virus, human herpesvirus 6, cytomegalovirus infections and HIV/AIDS).

Acute Non-Specific Bacterial Infections

Probably the most common presentation of cervical lymphadenopathy. Any bacterial infection in the area of drainage, such as an odontogenic infection (e.g. dental abscess, pericoronitis), sinusitis or a boil in the nose, can cause enlargement of anterior cervical lymph nodes. Usually only one or two nodes are enlarged, often unilaterally and only in the anterior triangle in most instances. However, lesions on the back of the scalp or neck may cause enlargement of posterior cervical nodes.

Acute Specific Bacterial Infections

Occasionally, specific acute bacterial infections involve lymph nodes, particularly in young children who can develop acute lymphadenitis caused by *S. aureus* in the absence of any detectable entry point for the organism. These infections, usually of a submandibular lymph node, should be treated with antibiotics — usually flucloxacillin because the *S. aureus* is often penicillinase-producing. If the lesion is fluctuant and pointing, surgical drainage is needed.

Chronic Specific Bacterial Infections

- Tuberculosis and atypical mycobacterial (non-tuberculous) infections (see Chapter 40)
- Actinomycosis
- Secondary syphilis (see Chapter 40)
- Brucellosis
- Cat-scratch disease (Bartonella)
- Lyme Disease

Chronic Granulomatous Disease

A rare genetic immune defect of leukocyte function in which neutrophils and macrophages fail to kill catalase-positive bacteria, such as staphylococci. Patients suffer from recurrent pyogenic infections and may develop suppurating cervical lymph nodes showing granulomas on biopsy. Need referral for investigation.

Parasitic: Toxoplasmosis, Leishmaniasis, Filariasis

For these conditions, see Chapter 40.

Non-Infective Inflammatory Conditions

- Connective tissue diseases: cervical lymph nodes may be enlarged in rheumatoid arthritis or lupus erythematosus.
- MLNS: Kawasaki disease (see Chapter 54).
- Granulomatous diseases: sarcoidosis (see Chapter 32), Crohn disease (see Chapter 32), orofacial granulomatosis (see Chapter 32).
- Drug-induced hypersensitivity syndrome (DIHS): also therefore called drug rash with eosinophilia and systemic symptoms (DRESS), is a severe immune-mediated reaction involving macrophage and T-lymphocyte activation and cytokine release, usually characterised by fever, rash and multiorgan failure, occurring 1 to 8 weeks after exposure to various drugs (see Table 33.15). Diagnosis is supported by a finding of eosinophilia and abnormal liver function tests. There may be reactivation of herpesviruses including HHV-6, HHV-7, CMV and/or EBV. The mortality from drug hypersensitivity syndrome is estimated at around 8%. Specialist medical care is indicated with immediate withdrawal of all suspect medicines, followed by supportive care, typically with systemic corticosteroids.

Neoplastic Conditions

Metastases

The neoplasms that usually metastasise to cervical lymph nodes are mainly head and neck cancers including:

- Oral squamous carcinoma (Fig. 15.2; see Chapter 53): usually one or more anterior cervical nodes are involved, often unilaterally in oral neoplasms anteriorly in the mouth, but otherwise not infrequently bilaterally.
- Tonsillar: clinically unsuspected tonsillar cancer is the most common cause of metastasis in a cervical node of

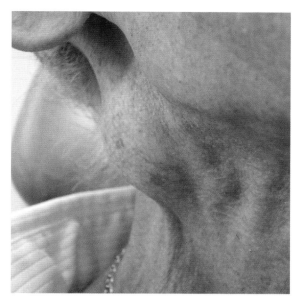

Fig. 15.2 Enlarged jugulodigastric lymph node from metastatic oral squamous cell carcinoma.

unidentified origin. Blind biopsy of the tonsil may reveal a hitherto unsuspected malignancy.

- Nasopharyngeal: clinically unsuspected nasopharyngeal cancer is a common cause of metastasis in a cervical node of unidentified origin. Blind biopsy of the nasopharynx, particularly the fossa of Rosenmuller or tonsil, may reveal a hitherto unsuspected malignancy.
- Laryngeal.
- Thyroid.
- Skin.

Other Metastatic Neoplasms (Other Than Lymphoid)

Rarely, cervical metastases from the stomach or even testicular tumours migrate to the lower cervical nodes, especially the supraclavicular nodes. Occasionally in patients with a malignant cervical lymph node, the primary tumour is never located.

Lymphoid Malignancies

In lymphoid malignancies, there is usually swelling both of anterior and posterior cervical lymph nodes together with generalised lymph node enlargement and often hepatosplenomegaly.

Histiocytoses

Management should be of the underlying Langerhans histiocytosis or Rosai–Dorfman disease (see Chapter 54).

MANAGEMENT OF A PATIENT WITH CERVICAL LYMPHADENOPATHY

Most enlarged lymph nodes have an infectious aetiology. A full blood count, ESR, CRP, serology and SACE (serum angiotensin converting enzyme) levels may help the diagnosis (Table 15.1). If aspects of the clinical picture suggest chronic infection or malignancy, such as persistent fevers or weight loss, chest

TABLE 15.1 Investigations That Might Be Helpful in Diagnosis/Prognosis/Management in Patients With Cervical Lymphadenopathy Thought Related to Infection/Inflammation[a]

In Most Cases	In Some Cases
Full blood picture	ANA
ESR	RF
CRP	SACE
	Serology and DNA studies for viral or bacterial diseases, or toxoplasmosis (throat swabs)
	Tuberculin test
	Interferon Gamma Release Assay e.g. QuantiFERON®—TB Gold In-Tube test (QFT—GIT) orT—SPOT®.TB test (T—Spot)
	US-FNA
	Chest imaging
	MRI neck
	Biopsy

[a]See text for details and glossary for abbreviations.

TABLE 15.2 Investigations That Might Be Helpful in Diagnosis/Prognosis/Management in Patients With Cervical Lymphadenopathy Thought Related to Malignant Disease[a]

In Most Cases	In Some Cases
Full blood picture	ESR
Ultrasound	Thyroid scan
FNA	Examination under anaesthetic
MRI/CT/PET CT	Blind biopsy of nasopharynx/tonsil
Biopsy	

[a]See text for details and glossary for abbreviations.

imaging, MRI scan and lesional biopsy should be pursued sooner (Table 15.2). Fine-needle aspiration (FNA) of the cervical lymph nodes is the most reliable diagnostic method for many disorders, including tuberculosis (see Chapter 40). If TB is suspected, chest radiographs, a tuberculin skin test and culture for mycobacterial organisms are indicated, even if the results of at least two are often negative.

RECOMMENDED READING

Chorath, K., Prasad, A., Luu, N., Go, B., Moreira, A., Rajasekaran, K., 2021. Critical review of clinical practice guidelines for evaluation of neck mass in adults. Braz. J. Otorhinolaryngol. 88 (4), 625–632. https://doi.org/10.1016/j.bjorl.2021.03.005.

Costagliola, G., Consolini, R., 2021. Lymphadenopathy at the crossroad between immunodeficiency and autoinflammation: an intriguing challenge. Clin. Exp. Immunol. 205 (3), 288–305. https://doi.org/10.1016/j.crad.2020.12.021.

Meadows, O., Sarkodieh, J., 2021. Ultrasound evaluation of persistent cervical lymph nodes in young children. Clin. Radiol. 76 (4), 315.e9–315.e12. https://doi.org/10.1016/j.crad.2020.12.021.

Angioedema

KEY POINTS
- Angioedema is life-threatening oedema of the subcutaneous or submucosal tissues.
- Angioedema can be hereditary or acquired.
- Neck oedema may compromise the airway.
- Most cases are allergic in nature.
- Emergency treatment is with intramuscular adrenaline (epinephrine).

INTRODUCTION

This is a potentially lethal condition. Angioedema manifests with the rapid development of oedematous swelling of the lip(s), tongue and oral or facial swelling (Fig. 16.1). This can be life-threatening as oedema may also involve the neck and compromise the airway. The swelling in angioedema is usually relatively transient and the skin does not scale.

The disorder may be acquired or hereditary. Acquired forms may be of allergic origin (histaminergic angioedema) or non-allergic.

Allergic angioedema is a type 1 hypersensitivity response seen mainly in those with an atopic tendency. The hereditary form (hereditary angioedema or HAE) is caused by a deficiency of the complement component C1 esterase inhibitor — C1-INH. Acquired angioedema may be drug-induced (mainly by angiotensin-converting enzyme [ACE] inhibitors and non-steroidal antiinflammatory drugs [NSAIDs]) or complement-mediated (due to an acquired deficiency of C1-inhibitor). Occasionally, the precipitating agent is not clearly identified.

All types of angioedema may be aggravated by the oral contraceptive pill (OCP) or hormone replacement therapy.

ALLERGIC ANGIOEDEMA

Epidemiology
- Allergic angioedema is common — far more common than HAE.
- It occurs mainly in adults.
- It is most prevalent in females.
- No known geographic incidence.

Aetiology and Pathogenesis

Allergic angioedema is a type 1 hypersensitivity reaction that may be induced by:
- foods: nuts are a well-known cause but many other foods (e.g. shellfish, eggs, milk) may be implicated
- latex
- drugs, especially:
  - antibiotics
  - aspirin
- other allergens — such as radiocontrast media, hepatitis B immunisation and insect bites/stings.

Allergic angioedema is secondary to mast-cell and basophil activation, with the release of histamine and bradykinin, causing vasodilatation, and increased vascular permeability. The C4 complement component is consumed and thus plasma levels fall, but the levels of C1 and C3 are usually normal. It can be acute or chronic and with or without urticaria ('hives').

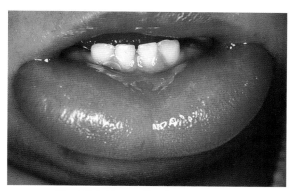

Fig. 16.1 Lip swelling in angioedema.

Other symptoms such as flushing, pruritus, bronchospasm, abdominal pain and vomiting may also be present. Symptoms typically develop within 60 minutes after allergen exposure and last about 24 to 48 hours.

Clinical Features

- The acute oedema, which appears within 60 minutes of antigen exposure, can cause pronounced itchy labial and periorbital swelling and can involve any oral site, but when oedema involves the tongue and neck and extends to the larynx, it can cause rapidly fatal respiratory obstruction.
- Acute allergic oedema usually develops along with urticaria and may be associated with anaphylactic reactions.

Diagnosis

Angioedema is diagnosed clinically and from a history of atopic disease and/or exposure to allergen. Once the initial treatment has been started, laboratory tests for a correct diagnosis of can be performed. Skin prick testing should only be performed where there are appropriate resuscitation facilities and an emergency kit containing injectable adrenaline at hand. Mast cell tryptase levels may be raised. HAE may need to be excluded — HAE has low C4, but normal C3 levels, and absence of C1-INH activity (Table 16.1).

Treatment

Although the swelling is of acute onset and often only mild and transient, there is always the potential of obstruction of the airway and thus urgent treatment is indicated (Table 16.2). If the airway is threatened, urgent hospital care is required and intubation may be needed.

TABLE 16.1 Investigations That Might Be Helpful in Diagnosis/Prognosis/Management in Some Patients Suspected of Having Angioedema[a]	
In Most Cases	**In Some Cases**
Serum complement C3 and C4 levels	Full blood picture
C1 esterase inhibitor activity	ESR

[a]See text for details and glossary for abbreviations.

TABLE 16.2 Regimens That Might Be Helpful in Management of Patient Suspected of Having Allergic Angioedema	
Regimen	**Use in Primary and Secondary Care**
Beneficial	Epinephrine (adrenaline)
Likely to be beneficial	Corticosteroids Antihistamines
Supportive	Avoid allergens

- In severe cases, especially if there is any potential or real threat to the airway, the emergency should be managed with intramuscular adrenaline (epinephrine) and with systemic corticosteroids and/or antihistamines, such as chlorphenamine or loratidine.
- The rare intractable chronic cases may respond to systemic corticosteroids.

DRUG-INDUCED (NON-ALLERGIC) ANGIOEDEMA

Non-allergic orofacial swelling can arise in response to drug exposure — especially to ACE inhibitors — due to a rise in levels of bradykinins and/or altered levels or function of C1 esterase inhibitor. The reaction may manifest after many weeks of drug treatment. Other drugs that may also be responsible can include antidepressants and NSAIDs. People of African heritage may be at particular risk of this adverse drug reaction. Sometimes the precipitating drug is not identified.

The swelling usually affects the lips, although it can be localised to the tongue or soft palate, and is occasionally fatal. The offending drug must be immediately discontinued.

Management is to ensure a patent airway. Adrenaline, antihistamines and corticosteroids may be indicated. Endotracheal intubation or tracheostomy is required in severe cases.

HEREDITARY ANGIOEDEMA (C1 ESTERASE INHIBITOR DEFICIENCY)

HAE mimics the other types of angioedema but is usually a more severe reaction. Despite its hereditary nature, usually as an autosomal dominant trait, the disease may not present until later childhood or adolescence, and nearly 20% of cases are caused by spontaneous genetic mutation.

Epidemiology

- It is uncommon.
- It can occur at any age.
- It occurs equally in both sexes.
- No known geographic incidence.

Predisposing Factors

A genetically determined mutation in the SERPING1 gene results in deficiency of an inhibitor of the enzyme C1 esterase (C1-INH) (type I), or C1-INH is dysfunctional (type II).

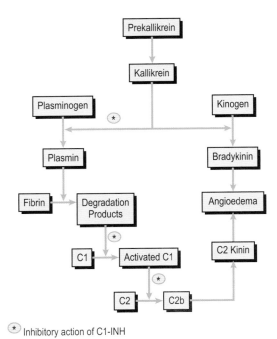

* Inhibitory action of C1-INH

Fig. 16.2 Hereditary angioedema; actions of C1-INH.

TABLE 16.3 Regimens That Might Be Helpful in Management of Patient Suspected of Having Hereditary Angioedema

Regimen	Use in Secondary Care (Severe Oral Involvement and/or Extraoral Involvement)
Beneficial	C1-INH concentrates
	Ecallantide
	Icatibant
	Danazol
	Stanazolol
	Fresh frozen plasma
Supportive	Avoid trauma, stress, alcohol and NSAIDs

NSAIDs, Nonsteroidal antiinflammatory drugs.

Type III is X-linked and seen in women in relation to pregnancy or OCP use linked with F12 gene mutations that encode blood coagulation factor XII. Autoimmune C1-INH deficiency most commonly arises in B-cell lymphoproliferative disorders. In all these types of angioedema, there is continued complement activation after trauma and activation of kinin-like substances that cause a sudden increase in capillary permeability (Fig. 16.2). Alcohol or cinnamon, which are vasodilators, may increase the likelihood of an attack in susceptible patients, as may NSAIDs. Some attacks follow emotional stress.

Clinical Features of C1-INH Deficiency

* Blunt injury is the most consistent precipitating event: the trauma of dental treatment is a potent trigger.
* Abdominal pain, nausea or vomiting, diarrhoea, rashes and peripheral oedema sometimes herald an attack.
* There is an acute onset of non-itchy or painful oedema affecting the lips, tongue, mouth, face and neck region, the extremities and the gastrointestinal tract — with abdominal pain and sometimes diarrhoea. There may be a leucocytosis.
* Angioedema may persist for many hours and even up to 4 days, and throughout, involvement of the airway is a constant threat.
* The mortality may be as high as 30% in some families, but the disease is compatible with prolonged survival if emergencies are avoided or effectively treated.

Diagnosis

Diagnosis of HAE is made from (see Table 16.1):
* family history
* clinical features with a history of oedema after trauma
* blood tests: low C4, but normal C3 levels, and absence of C1-INH activity. In 85% of cases, C1-INH levels are reduced (type I HAE), but in 15% of cases, C1-INH is present though dysfunctional (type II HAE).

Treatment

Precipitants, once identified, should be avoided where possible.

There is no beneficial response to corticosteroids or antihistamines. Management is by avoiding precipitants, and with C1-INH replacement. Other treatments include the bradykinin-receptor antagonist icatibant, the plasma kallikrein inhibitor ecallantide, fresh frozen plasma; plasminogen inhibitors such as tranexamic acid; or androgenic steroids, such as danazol (Table 16.3).

Follow-Up of Patients

Patients with HAE should be under specialist care.

RECOMMENDED READING

Maurer, M., Magerl, M., Ansotegui, I., et al., 2018. The international WAO/EAACI guideline for the management of hereditary angioedema—The 2017 revision and update. Allergy. 73 (8), 1575–1596.

Powell, R.J., Leech, S.C., Till, S., Huber, P.A., Nasser, S.M., Clark, A.T., British Society for Allergy and Clinical Immunology, 2015. BSACI guideline for the management of chronic urticaria and angioedema. Clin. Exp. Allergy. 45 (3), 547–565.

Halitosis (Oral Malodour)

INTRODUCTION

Halitosis, from the Latin for breath *halitus*, is oral malodour. Halitosis is a problem analogous to body odour and is the cause for serious concern by many sufferers since it has negative connotations, affecting not only the patient's self-image but also others' attitudes towards the patient. It is a fairly common complaint, found mainly in adults. Up to one-third of adults over 60 years old report either being conscious of their oral malodour or having been told by others they have it. In some cases, patients may present with pseudo-halitosis, whereby there is a belief that they have bad breath despite their malodour not being perceived or detected, either by those around them or by objective analysis. Halitosis can be divided into extra-oral halitosis, intra-oral halitosis and pseudo-halitosis.

Intra-oral halitosis is formed by volatile compounds, which are produced mainly by many of the same anaerobic bacteria involved in periodontal diseases. These odorous compounds include volatile sulphur compounds (VSCs), aromatic compounds, amines, short-chain fatty or organic acids, alcohols, aliphatic compounds, aldehydes and ketones. The most important VSCs are hydrogen sulphide, dimethyl sulphide, dimethyl disulphide and methyl mercaptan. VSCs can be toxic for human cells even at low concentrations.

Oral malodour is common on awakening (morning breath) and is then usually a consequence of low salivary flow and oral cleansing during sleep. This is termed 'physiological halitosis', rarely has any special significance, and can be readily rectified by eating, oral cleansing and rinsing the mouth with fresh water. Malodour at other times is often the consequence of habits such as smoking or drinking alcohol or of eating various foods such as especially durian, garlic, onion or spices and to some extent cabbage, cauliflower or radish. The avoidance of these habits and foods is the best prevention.

Halitosis is also more common:
- in starvation, probably partly due to oral stagnation
- in those who snore and/or mouth breathe
- in the ovulation phase of the menstrual cycle
- in use of certain drugs:
  - amphetamines
  - chloral hydrate
  - cytotoxic agents
  - dimethyl sulphoxide (DMSO)
  - disulfiram
  - nitrates and nitrites
  - phenothiazines
  - solvent abuse.

AETIOLOGY AND PATHOGENESIS

Halitosis that is not due to the above causes is termed 'pathological halitosis' and is most often a consequence of oral bacterial activity (Fig. 17.1). More than 85% of cases are due to oral causes (oral malodour), but some are due to lung or systemic causes (Table 17.1). In most cases, the aetiology is from anaerobes in the tongue coating or periodontal pockets, or arising from:
- poor oral hygiene (Figs 17.2 and 17.3)
- gingivitis (especially necrotising gingivitis)
- periodontitis
- pericoronitis and other types of oral sepsis
- infected extraction sockets
- debris under bridges or appliances
- ulcers
- dry mouth.

There is no single micro-organism incriminated. Bacteria (especially anaerobes) appear to be the main culprits, the main organisms implicated including:
- *Porphyromonas species*, e.g. *gingivalis*
- *Prevotella species*, e.g. *intermedia, veroralis*
- *Fusobacterium species*, e.g. *nucleatum*
- *Bacteroides species*, e.g. *forsythus*
- *Treponema denticola.*

Other genera that have been implicated in true halitosis include *Actinomyces, Eubacterium, Peptostreptococcus, Selenomonas* and *Leptotrichia*.

There is no obvious consensus on the microbiology, potentially indicating that dysbiosis of normal flora and an

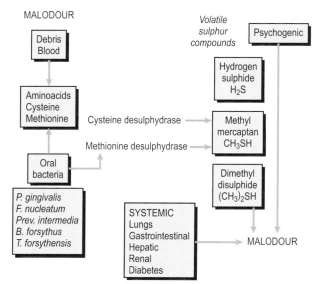

Fig. 17.1 Causes of malodour.

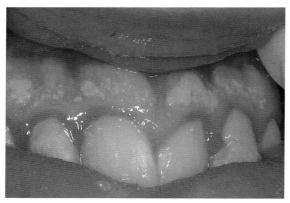

Fig. 17.2 Materia alba and marginal gingivitis.

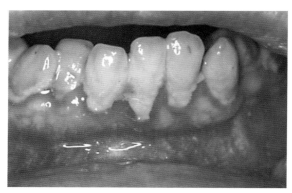

Fig. 17.3 Plaque accumulation and gingivitis.

TABLE 17.1 Factors That Might Be Helpful in Diagnosis/Prognosis/Management in Some Patients With Halitosis (Oral Malodour)[a]	
In Most Cases	**In Some Cases**
Halimetry or organoleptic assessment	Full blood picture
Oral microbiology screen	Blood glucose
	Serum ferritin, vitamin B_{12} and corrected whole blood folate levels
	ESR
	BANA (benzoyl-arginine-naphthyl-amide) test
	Dark field microscopy
	Oral imaging
	Sinus imaging
	Nasendoscopy
	Chest radiography
	Helicobacter pylori serum antibody or endoscopy and rapid urease test or biopsy
	Liver function tests
	Renal function tests
	Urinalysis for the ratio of trimethylamine to trimethylamine oxide
	Psychological assessment

[a]See text for details and glossary for abbreviations.

overgrowth of proteolytic anaerobic bacteria may result from a number of elements with a number of species involved. These include temporary or sustained residence in the oral flora of gut organisms including *Escherichia coli* and Proteus species. It is, however, clearer that although there is much still to learn, the responsible anaerobes produce chemicals that cause the malodour in many instances, and these include:
- VSCs (mainly methyl mercaptan, hydrogen sulphide and dimethyl sulphide)
- volatile aromatic compounds (indole, skatole)
- polyamines (putrescine and cadaverine)
- short-chain fatty acids (butyric, valeric, acetic and propionic acids).

Extra-Oral Halitosis

Halitosis in a very few cases originates distal to the tonsils (extra-oral halitosis) (Box 17.1). Such causes that may be responsible for malodour include the following:
- Respiratory disease: nasal sepsis or foreign bodies, or infection of the paranasal sinuses or respiratory tract may be a cause. In children, the insertion of foreign bodies, such as small toys into the nose, and subsequent sepsis is a common cause of halitosis. At any age, infections in the respiratory tract, such as tonsillitis, bronchitis, bronchiectasis or other lung infections, or tumours in the respiratory tract may be responsible.
- Gastrointestinal disease: gastro-oesophageal reflux may be responsible. Although *Helicobacter pylori* has been suspected as a cause, it is an uncommon aetiology.
- Metabolic disorders:
  - diabetic ketosis: the breath may smell of ketones, especially acetone.
  - hepatic failure: caused by dimethyl sulphide and to a lower extent by ketones in alveolar air.
  - renal failure: dialysis helps reduce halitosis.
- Trimethylaminuria: fish and eggs may produce malodour in this rare metabolic syndrome.

BOX 17.1 Main Causes of Halitosis

- Dry mouth
- Starvation
- Smoking
- Some foods
- Drugs (see Chapter 33 and Algorithm 17.1)
- Oral sepsis
- Systemic disease:
  - respiratory and nasal disease
  - gastrointestinal disease
  - diabetic ketosis
  - hepatic failure
  - renal failure
  - trimethylaminuria
- Psychogenic factors (pseudo-halitosis)

TABLE 17.2 Drugs Which May Cause Halitosis

- Amphetamines
- Arsenic salts
- Bisphosphonates
- Chloral hydrate
- Cytotoxic agents (some)
- Dimethyl sulphoxide
- Disulfiram
- Ethyl alcohol
- Griseofulvin
- Lithium salts
- Metronidazole
- Nitrites and nitrates
- Phenothiazines
- Paraldehyde
- Penicillamine
- Triamterene

Drugs Causing Halitosis

Pharmaceutical therapy is a potential source of extra-oral halitosis, and the nature of the halitosis can vary according to the drug group. The medications that can cause extra-oral halitosis can be categorised into 10 groups: acid reducers, aminothiols, anticholinergics, antidepressants, antifungals, antihistamines and steroids, antispasmodics, chemotherapeutic agents, dietary supplements and organosulphur substances (see Table 17.2).

Pseudo-Halitosis

Psychogenic or psychosomatic factors: Not all persons who believe they have halitosis actually have any objectively confirmed malodour, and the halitosis may then be attributed to a form of delusion, obsessive-compulsive disorder or monosymptomatic hypochondriasis (halitophobia). Halitophobia refers to individuals who refuse to accept objective evidence that excludes an underlying cause and cannot be convinced their breath is not malodorous. Such patients rarely wish to engage with psychological therapy because they fail to recognise their own psychological condition and never doubt they have oral malodour. Attempting to persuade them otherwise is usually futile, although evidence of normality via a halimeter may help. Other people's behaviour, or perceived behaviour, such as apparently covering the nose or averting the face, is typically misinterpreted by these patients as an indication that their breath is indeed offensive. Anxiety may also increase malodour.

DIAGNOSIS

Diagnosis (Algorithm 17.1; Table 17.1) is mainly clinical, made from:
- Full history: many patients will adopt behaviour to minimise their problem, such as covering the mouth when talking, avoiding or keeping a distance from other people, using chewing gum, mints, mouthwashes or sprays designed to reduce malodour, or excessively cleaning their tongue or mouth.
- Assessment of halitosis: usually by simply smelling the exhaled air (organoleptic method) first from the mouth (with nose closed by pinching nostrils) then from the nose (with patient's mouth closed). Some centres are also able to undertake objective measurements of the agents responsible, such as:
  - volatile sulphur compounds, using a halimeter (Interscan Corp., Chatsworth, CA, USA) (Figs 17.4 and 17.5) or using OralChroma, a portable gas chromatograph (Fig. 17.6). Compounds other than VSCs, however, are not usually detected.
  - oral flora, such as by the benzoyl-arginine-naphthylamide (BANA) test or dark field microscopy, which can be helpful, at least for patient education. Culture of oral flora can be helpful to exclude E. coli and other non-oral flora.

Systemic causes if suspected need the opinion of the relevant specialist and possibly, investigations, such as nasendoscopy, chest imaging, H. pylori serum antibody or endoscopy and rapid urease test or biopsy, liver and renal function tests and urinalysis for the ratio of trimethylamine to trimethylamine oxide.

TREATMENT

The management of halitosis currently includes the following:
- Treating the dental or oral cause.
- Patient education.
- Treating the cause: medical input may be required to manage patients with a systemic background to their complaint.
- Avoiding smoking, and foods such as onions, garlic, durian, cabbage, cauliflower and radish.

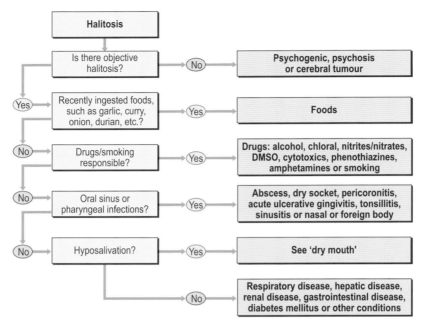

Algorithm 17.1 Halitosis management (DMSO, dimethyl sulphoxide).

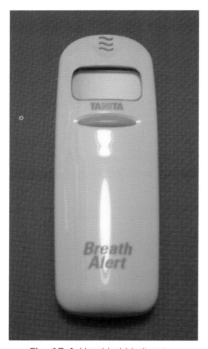

Fig. 17.4 Hand held halimeter.

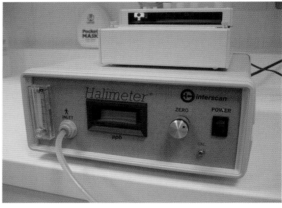

Fig. 17.5 Halimeter.

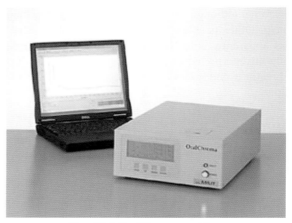

Fig. 17.6 OralChroma machine.

- Eating regular meals and finishing meals with fibrous fruits/vegetables (e.g. carrots, pineapple).
- Ensuring good oral hygiene: dental prophylaxis, tooth brushing, flossing and tongue cleaning (with a brush or scraper; this is best done before going to bed since scraping early during the day may induce retching).
- Using oral healthcare products: there is evidence of benefit mainly from the use of toothpastes and mouthwashes containing:

- chlorhexidine digluconate, or
- triclosan, or
- amine fluoride/stannous fluoride, or
- metal ions.
- Oral antiseptics such as chlorhexidine (which is effective but may cause tooth-staining and occasional other adverse effects), triclosan, cetylpyridinium, essential oils or products with zinc or stannous ions can be helpful. All are reportedly effective at reducing malodour for at least 3 hours. Generally, it is recommended that mouthwashes should be used two or three times daily for at least 30 seconds.

Some products appear effective for longer, such as a toothpaste containing triclosan and a copolymer; and a two-phase mouthwash consisting of natural essential oils, triclosan and cetylpyridinium chloride, plus sodium fluoride.

Using oral deodorants (oral malodour counteractives [OMC]). Chewing gum, parsley, mint, cloves or fennel seeds and the use of proprietary 'fresh breath' preparations may help mask malodour.

- In recalcitrant cases, the specialist empirically may use a 1-week course of metronidazole 200 mg three times daily in an effort to eliminate unidentified anaerobic infections (although metronidazole may itself give rise to mild halitosis).
- Emergent therapies include the use of chemicals or natural products to inhibit the bacterial enzymes responsible for the production of odiferous substances, and even vaccines prepared against the responsible bacteria.

- The use of probiotics including those containing lactobacillus to change the balance of the flora.
- A multitude of anti-malodour products is also available over the counter, testimony to the extent of the perceived or, indeed real, problem of halitosis and also to the fact that few of the preparations are reliably effective.

Patients with halitophobia may benefit referral to a psychiatrist for mental health assessment and appropriate management.

RECOMMENDED READING

Fedorowicz, Z., Aljufairi, H., Nasser, M., Outhouse, T.L., Pedrazzi, V., 2008. Mouthrinses for the treatment of halitosis. Cochrane Database Syst. Rev. 4, CD006701.

Mortazavi, H., Rahbani Nobar, B., Shafiei, S., 2020. Drug-related halitosis: a systematic review. Oral Health Prev. Dent. 18 (1), 399–407.

Porter, S.R., 2011. Diet and halitosis. Curr. Opin. Clin. Nutr. Metab. Care. 14 (5), 463–468.

Torsten, M., Gómez-Moreno, G., Aguilar-Salvatierra, A., 2017. Drug-related oral malodour (halitosis): a literature review. Eur. Rev. Med. Pharmacol. Sci. 21 (21), 4930–4934.

Wu, J., Cannon, R.D., Ji, P., Farella, M., Mei, L., 2020. Halitosis: prevalence, risk factors, sources, measurement and treatment—a review of the literature. Aust. Dent. J. 65 (1), 4–11.

Taste Abnormalities

INTRODUCTION

Taste is the perception accompanying oral intake, attributed to sensory information received from the oral cavity and oropharynx. 'flavour', on the other hand, is a combination of several chemosensory afferents (including taste, texture, temperature and olfaction) perceived while eating. Taste is primarily classified into five types: salty, sweet, bitter, sour and umami.

Previously, it was thought that specific areas on the tongue were responsible for interpreting only one taste quality. However, the current understanding is that the entire tongue is able to perceive each of the taste qualities. The sense of taste is mediated by specialised taste buds — oval bodies made up of groups of neuroepithelial and supporting cells (Fig. 18.1). The neuroepithelial cells are rod-shaped with a peripheral hair-like process projecting into the taste pores at the surface of the overlying mucous membrane (Fig. 18.2). There are five basic tastes, and they do not appear to be detected by structurally different taste buds:

- Salt taste: mediated via sodium chloride (NaCl) ions. Na^+ ions enter the receptor cells via Na^+ channels, causing a depolarisation; calcium ions enter through voltage-sensitive Ca^{2+} channels, and transmitter release occurs and results in increased firing in the primary afferent nerve.
- Sour taste: mediated by protons (H^+), which block potassium channels causing depolarisation, Ca^{2+} entry, transmitter release and increased firing in the primary afferent nerve.
- Sweet taste: receptors bind glucose, which activates adenyl cyclase, thereby increasing cyclic adenosine monophosphate (cAMP), causing phosphorylation of K^+ channels, inhibiting them. Depolarisation occurs, Ca^{2+} enters and transmitter is released, increasing firing in the primary afferent nerve.

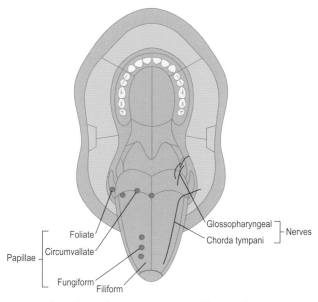

Fig. 18.1 Locations of taste receptors and innervations on tongue.

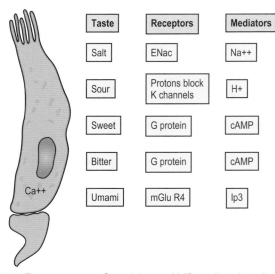

Fig. 18.2 Taste receptor. *Ca*, calcium; *cAMP*, cyclic adenosine monophosphate; *ENac*, epithelial sodium channels; *H*, hydrogen; *Ip3*, inositol triphosphate; *K*, potassium; *mGluR4*, G-protein coupled receptor; *Na*, sodium.

- Bitter taste: bitter substances cause a second messenger (inositol trisphosphate [IP3]) mediated release of Ca^{2+}, resulting in transmitter release and firing of the primary afferent nerve.
- Umami taste: certain amino acids (e.g. glutamate, aspartate) bind to a glutamate receptor (mGluR4) activating a G-protein, raising intracellular Ca^{2+}. Glutamate may also stimulate the NMDA (N-methyl-D-aspartate)-receptor when non-selective cation channels open and Ca^{2+} enters, causing transmitter release and increased firing in the primary afferent nerve.

The terminal branches of the nerve fibres subserving taste end in close relationship to these special neuroepithelial cells. Taste buds are found in the mucous membrane of the tongue, soft palate, fauces and pharynx, and, in the newborn, on the lips and cheeks. Papillae at the front of the tongue have more taste buds compared to the mid-region. Taste buds are also located throughout the oral cavity, in the pharynx, the laryngeal epiglottis and at the entrance of the oesophagus. Sensitivity to all tastes is distributed across the whole tongue and to other regions where there are taste buds (epiglottis, soft palate), but some areas are more responsive to certain tastes than others:

- Fungiform papillae are innervated by the chorda tympani branch of the facial (7th cranial) nerve.
- Foliate papillae are predominantly sensitive to sour tastes. Innervated by the glossopharyngeal (9th cranial) nerve.
- Circumvallate papillae confer a sour/bitter sensitivity to the posterior two-thirds of the tongue. Innervated by the glossopharyngeal (9th cranial) nerve.

Electrical signals generated in the taste cells transmit information via sensory nerves, which arise from the ganglion cells of branches of cranial nerves:

- chorda tympani nerve: via the lingual nerve (cranial nerve V) from the tongue (anterior two-thirds and lateral)
- glossopharyngeal nerve: from the tongue (posterior third)
- vagus nerve: from pharynx and larynx.

All three nerves connect in the brainstem in the nucleus solitarius before proceeding to the thalamus and then to the brain frontal lobe (the insula and the frontal operculum cortex) for the conscious perception of taste and the hypothalamus, amygdala and insula for the 'affective' component of taste — responsible for the behavioural response (e.g. feeding behaviour).

TASTE CHANGES

Taste and olfaction are susceptible to the general sensory phenomenon known as adaptation, i.e. the progressive reduction in the appreciation of a stimulus during the course of continual exposure to that stimulus. Taste exhibits almost complete adaptation to a stimulus — perception of a substance fades to almost nothing in seconds. Both taste and olfaction are also susceptible to genetic, hormonal, age and other factors. The cells of the taste buds undergo continual renewal, with a life span of about 10 days, renewal being modulated by nutrition, hormones and age, and other factors such as drugs and radiation.

- Genetics are important to taste. For example, sensitivity to the bitter taste of phenylthiourea is genetically determined. In contrast, people who have more than the normal number of taste papillae (and taste buds and increased density of fungiform papillae) have extreme sensitivity to n-propylthiouracil (PROP), are called supertasters, and account for 25% of the population (more women than men) — they tend not to like green vegetables and fatty foods.
- Hormones may also influence taste: the sense of taste may vary through the menstrual cycle and may be distorted during pregnancy, often with the appearance of cravings for unusual foods.
- Age affects taste sense; the number of taste buds declines, and there are changes in taste cell membranes involving the altered function of ion channels and receptors with age.
- Drugs can influence taste (Chapter 33). For example, taste can be suppressed by local anaesthetics applied to the tongue. Amiloride blocks Na^+ channels and reduces the ability to taste salt. Adenosine monophosphate (AMP) may block bitterness. Gymnemic acid (from the Indian tree/shrub *Gymnema sylvestre*) decreases sweet perception. The active compounds of artichokes, chlorogenic acid and cynarin, by suppressing sour and bitter taste receptors, enhance sweet taste. Miracle fruit via an active ingredient, 'miraculin', makes sour substances taste sweet.

TASTE ABNORMALITIES

Frequently, when individuals say they cannot taste, the problem is that they cannot appreciate the flavour of food. As the aroma of food contributes to about 75% of its flavour, these individuals have often suffered a loss of smell ability only.

True taste disorders are uncommon but may present as a loss of taste or as an abnormal taste in the mouth or an unpleasant taste. Taste is key in informing whether we find food rewarding, which in turn drives appetite and eating behaviours.

Types of Taste Loss

- Dysgeusia: persistent abnormal taste.
- Hypogeusia: reduced taste function.
- Ageusia: absence of taste. Some have termed the phantom sensation of bitterness as 'phantogeusia' (Table 18.1). Disorders of taste sense can be distressing and sometimes incapacitating, and can even cause anorexia and depression.

TABLE 18.1 Terminology of Taste Disorders

Dysfunction	Sense of Taste
Absence	Ageusia
Diminished	Hypogeusia
Distorted	Dysgeusia
Heightened	Hypergeusia

CAUSES OF TASTE DYSFUNCTION

Taste abnormalities can be caused by anything that interrupts the taste pathways from the mucosa, taste buds, non-myelinated nerves or cranial nerves to the brainstem and brain, or conditions that affect the way the brain interprets taste stimuli (Table 18.2).

- The most common causes of loss of sense of taste are viral upper respiratory tract infections. The loss is often transient and reversible. Among patients with symptomatic COVID-19, smell or taste abnormalities are well described. These features are more common with COVID-19 than with other viral upper respiratory tract infections. Most subjective smell and taste disorders associated with COVID-19 resolve or improve by 4 weeks.
  - Head injury — affects olfaction but also, thereby, decreases the appreciation of food and may be perceived as taste loss.
  - Chronic middle ear infections or otitis media may affect afferent taste fibres of the chorda tympani.
  - Normal ageing produces taste loss.
  - Severe hyposalivation.
  - Burning mouth syndrome.
  - Chronic candida infection.

- Oral mucosal pathology: patients with oral lichen planus (OLP) and tongue involvement have impaired taste function.
- Surgical procedures affecting cranial nerves V, VII, IX or X may alter taste (e.g. dental surgery, tonsillectomy, middle ear surgery, skull base surgery). These include:
  - lingual nerve damage as a result of surgery or even dental injections
  - lingual resections
  - otological surgery that damages the chorda tympani nerve.
- Radiation and chemotherapy: damage taste receptors and decrease salivary flow altering taste perception. Taste loss occurs in up to 75% of patients with head and neck cancer. Alteration of sweet and salty perception in patients receiving systemic chemotherapy may persist up to 3 years after completion of therapy.
- Drugs: such as ACE inhibitors, antibiotics (e.g., metronidazole), and terbinafine, and antithyroid drugs, captopril, cytotoxic agents.
- Metabolic/systemic: renal insufficiency, hepatic insufficiency, thyroid dysfunction, diabetes.
- Hormonal fluctuations: in menstruation and pregnancy or diabetes, hypogonadism, pseudohypoparathyroidism, hypothyroidism and adrenal cortical insufficiency.

TABLE 18.2 Causes of Dysgeusia

Mechanism	Main Causes	Examples	
		Common	**Less Common**
Infection	Upper respiratory tract infections Chronic middle ear infections Chronic candida infection	COVID-19 Influenza Common cold	
Drugs (various effects)	Those causing hyposalivation	See Table 33.17	
Olfaction impaired	Nasopharyngeal pathology	Common cold Influenza Nasal infection Nasal polyps Sinusitis Viral pharyngitis	Head injuries, due to tearing of olfactory fibres and ageing
Oral pathology	Oral lichen planus	Oral lichen planus involving the tongue	
Sensory receptor disorders or environment changes	Oral Hyposalivation Sepsis Smoking Aging (taste bud numbers diminish)	Gastric regurgitation Vitamin (B$_{12}$) or mineral (zinc) deficiency	Chemotherapy Radiation Salivary gland infections
Cranial nerve disorders	Trauma Neuropathies	Trauma to mouth, nose or head, or to lingual, chorda tympani or facial nerves, e.g. oral or middle ear surgery	Bell palsy Disseminated sclerosis
Cerebral disorders	Demyelinating disease Cancer Psychogenic disorders Trauma	Hypochondriasis Lung cancer	Frontal lobe tumours Leukaemia or other brain metastases Parkinson disease

- Neurological: stroke, Parkinson disease, Alzheimer dementia, multiple sclerosis. Rarely, distorted taste can be an early sign of ALS or myasthenia gravis. Gustatory auras (dysgeusia) may manifest as a result of seizure activity in epilepsy.
- Nutritional deficiencies: Decreased zinc, copper and nickel levels; iron deficiency; vitamin B_{12} deficiency.
- Familial dysautonomia (i.e. Riley—Day syndrome): causes absence of taste buds.

DIAGNOSIS

A thorough patient history and a detailed clinical examination are important in evaluating patients presenting with taste disturbance. It is important to establish if the taste disturbance was of acute or gradual onset. Acute may be associated with iatrogenic causes or toxins. A more gradual history may suggest a neurological or neoplastic process.

A full medical history is essential including any precipitating events, medical procedures, medication or cancer therapy.

A complete examination of the oral cavity is advised to pay particular attention to mucosal lesions and salivary flow. Enlargement of the major salivary glands may suggest Sjögren syndrome. Assessment of cranial nerve function may be necessary depending on the clinical history.

Chemical gustometry or electrogustometry testing of the tongue can be performed.

Chemical gustometry may be applied in drops to the tongue, by oral rinsing, or by rapidly dissolving taste strips. Four standardised sizes of filter paper are soaked with strong concentrations of the four basic tastes. The papers are randomly placed on the tongue. Patients then identify the quality of the taste and rate its intensity using the same scale as in whole mouth assessment. Tastes used are:

- sucrose for sweet taste
- vinegar or citric acid to produce sour taste
- sodium chloride for the taste of salt
- quinine for bitter.

Electrogustometric testing is also available. Olfactory function should be evaluated. Further tests may be necessary including full blood count (FBC), serum ferritin, vitamin B_{12} and folate to exclude anaemia, zinc, HbA1c, thyroid stimulating hormone (TSH) and T4 assay, renal function, liver function and if Sjögren syndrome is suspected, testing for anti-Ro antibodies.

Neurological imaging is indicated if the history and clinical examination suggest any unidentified intracranial pathology,

---

TABLE 18.3 Investigations That Might Be Helpful in Diagnosis/Prognosis/Management in Some Patients With Taste Abnormalities[a]

Full blood picture
Serum ferritin, vitamin B_{12} and corrected whole blood folate levels
Serum zinc levels
Blood glucose
Anti-nuclear antibody (ANA)/extractable nuclear antibody (ENA)
Nasendoscopy
Audiometry
Radiography/magnetic resonance imaging (MRI)
Salivary flow rate, culture

[a]See text for details and glossary for abbreviations.

TREATMENT

- Treat the cause, if possible (Table 18.3): supplements of zinc have been successful in some patients.
- Treat any nasal pathology causing impaired olfaction.
- Treat any dry mouth, oral mucosal disorders or haematinic deficiency.
- Consider eliminating any suspect drugs.
- Advise patients to chew food well to increase the release of tastants and saliva production, and drink well. Dietary advice on food preparation and seasoning is helpful. Switching different foods during the meal can decrease the phenomenon of adaptation and can improve taste appreciation.
- Refer for a medical opinion if there are any endocrine or neurological disorders.

RECOMMENDED READING

Barasch, A., Epstein, J.B., 2020. Assessment of taste disorders. BMJ Best Practice. https://bestpractice.bmj.com/topics/en-gb/971. Last accessed 30 January 2022.

Cowart, B.J., 2011. Taste dysfunction: a practical guide for oral medicine. Oral Dis. 17 (1), 2—6.

Doty, R.L., 2019. Treatments for smell and taste disorders: a critical review. Handb. Clin. Neurol. 164, 455—479.

Epstein, J.B., Barasch, A., 2010. Taste disorders in cancer patients: pathogenesis, and approach to assessment and management. Oral Oncol. 46 (2), 77—81.

Hypersalivation

INTRODUCTION

Increased salivary flow (hypersalivation) is also termed sialorrhoea or ptyalism. Drooling is defined as the presence of saliva beyond the margins of the lips but may not be due to hypersalivation.

EPIDEMIOLOGY

True hypersalivation is rare. Drooling is more common. People at the extremes of age, the chronically debilitated or those in chronic care facilities, especially when associated with cerebrovascular events and oesophageal cancer, are especially affected by drooling.

Drooling

Drooling is perfectly normal in healthy infants but usually stops by approximately 18 months of age and is considered abnormal if it persists beyond the age of 4 years.
- Drooling can occur in either gender.
- Drooling has no known geographic incidence.
- Drooling is a problem for many children with cerebral palsy, intellectual disability and other neurological conditions and in adults who have Parkinson disease, cerebral palsy or intellectual disability or have had a stroke (cerebrovascular accident (CVA)), pseudobulbar palsy or bulbar palsy. Drooling in older age may frequently be linked to posture (head forwards and downwards) and difficulty in normal swallowing.

AETIOLOGY AND PATHOGENESIS

Drooling is caused either by increased saliva flow (hypersalivation) that cannot be compensated for by swallowing; by poor oral and facial muscle control in patients with swallowing dysfunction; or by anatomic or neuromuscular anomalies (Table 19.1).

CLINICAL FEATURES

Drooling (Fig. 19.1) impacts on patients, families and/or caregivers:
- Functionally: saliva soils clothing (of patient, peers, siblings, parents and caregivers), furniture, carpets, teaching materials, communicative devices and toys.
- Socially: embarrassment may make it difficult for patients to interact with their peers and can lead to isolation.
- Psychologically: stigmatism is common.
- Clinically: drooling persons are at increased risk of skin maceration, infection periorally and on the neck, chest and hands and aspiration-related respiratory infections. Pulmonary complications are greatest in those with a diminished sensation of salivary flow and hypopharyngeal retention.

DIAGNOSIS

History helps assess the severity and frequency of drooling and the effect on the quality of life of patients and family. Quantitative measurements can be helpful for guiding treatment decisions (Table 19.2): counting the number of bibs or items of clothing soiled each day provides a subjective estimate.

Hypersalivation: Sialorrhoea

Examination

This should include:
- head position and control
- perioral skin condition
- dentition and occlusion: malocclusion, particularly an open bite deformity, is common in patients with cerebral palsy and can make proper oral hygiene difficult to maintain
- tongue size and control and the presence of thrusting behaviours
- tonsil and adenoid size
- gag reflex and intraoral tactile sensitivity

TABLE 19.1 Causes of Drooling

Excessive Saliva Production (Hypersalivation)	Decreased Swallowing	Anatomic Abnormalities	Neuromuscular Diseases
Oral lesions or foreign bodies Neurologic disorders (especially Riley—Day syndrome) Otolaryngologic diseases Pregnancy Gastrointestinal causes Liver disease Drugs and poisons parathion, strychnine (Table 33.3)	Oropharyngeal infections and obstruction Forward and lowered posture of head Dysphagia	Macroglossia or tongue thrusting Surgical defects following major head and neck surgery	Parkinson disease, cerebral palsy, intellectual impairment Stroke, pseudobulbar palsy, bulbar palsy Rabies Anterior opercular syndrome (Foix—Chavany—Marie syndrome)

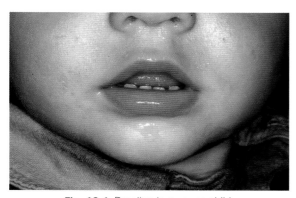

Fig. 19.1 Drooling in a young child.

TABLE 19.2 Clinical Semiquantification of Drooling

Clinical Severity	Clinical Description
Dry	Never drools
Mild	Only lips are wet. Occasional drooling — not every day
Moderate	Frequent drooling. Lips and chin are wet every day
Severe	Constant drooling. Lips, chin and face wet. Clothing soiled, hands moist or wet

TABLE 19.3 Some Drug and Substances Associated With Hypersalivation

Medication	• Adrenergic antagonists (e.g. ephedrine) • Antibiotics (e.g. doxycycline) • Direct cholinergics (e.g. pilocarpine) • Poisons and toxins (e.g. mercury, insecticides)
Medication (psychiatric)	• Acetylcholinesterase inhibitors (e.g. rivastigmine) • Anticonvulsants (e.g. lamotrigine) • Antipsychotics (e.g. clozapine) • Stimulants (e.g. modafinil)
Recreational drugs	• Phencyclidine (PCP) • Ketamine

TABLE 19.4 Investigations That Might Be Helpful in Diagnosis/Prognosis/Management in Patients With Drooling and Hypersalivation[a]

In Most Cases	In Some Cases
Sialometry (an unstimulated whole saliva rate >0.8 mL/min is indicative of hypersalivation)	Psychological assessment Flexible nasopharyngoscopy Lateral neck radiography Magnetic resonance imaging Modified barium swallow Audiography

[a]See text for details and glossary for abbreviations.

- mouth breathing, nasal obstruction and appearance of tissues upon anterior rhinoscopy
- swallowing efficiency: determined by observation, barium swallow or fibreoptic endoscopic evaluation of swallowing
- neurologic examination: cranial nerve examination.

A number of drugs and toxins may be associated with hypersalivation. These may include medicines prescribed in psychiatry, recreational drugs as well as some heavy metals and poisons (Table 19.3).

Investigations (Table 19.4) may include:
- Assessment of salivary flow by spitting into a universal container. If within normal range, then hypersalivation is excluded. An unstimulated whole saliva (UWS) rate higher than 0.8 mL/min is indicative of hypersalivation.

- Flexible nasopharyngoscopy, lateral neck radiography or magnetic resonance imaging (MRI) to detect adenoid hypertrophy.
- Modified barium swallow to help rule out the contraindications to surgical therapy, including oesophageal motility disorders, oesophageal spasm or aspiration.
- Radiosialography, a dynamic study of the salivary glands by 99m Tc-pertechnetate for evaluating salivary secretory function (now rarely used).

- Audiography to detect unilateral hearing impairment in patients considered for tympanic neurectomy or chorda tympani nerve section (because of the risk of hearing loss associated with these procedures).

TREATMENT

Determine whether hypersalivation or drooling without hypersalivation. Treatment is best by a team approach, including at least a(n) otolaryngologist, neurologist, surgeon, dentist, orthodontist, speech and occupational therapists and physiotherapist. The impact of drooling on the quality of life is the most important factor in determining the treatment needs. The goal is to reduce drooling whilst maintaining a moist, healthy oral cavity. Treatment options include medical therapy, radiotherapy and surgery:

- Medical therapy
  - Drooling without hypersalivation:
    - Oral motor training: exercises to improve muscle tone, increase lip closure and promote swallowing.
    - Behaviour therapy: biofeedback and correction of posture.

- Training of nurses in recognition of posture
- Hypersalivation:

Medication to reduce saliva to amounts that can be swallowed (to prevent 'pool and drool') without producing hyposalivation (Table 19.5), by:

- reducing cholinergic activity, either systemically (e.g. atropine-related anticholinergics orally), hyoscine transdermal patch or more locally (e.g. sublingual ipratropium spray). These drugs are contraindicated in patients with asthma, or ocular problems such as glaucoma.
- increasing adrenergic activity (e.g. clonidine patch)
- botulinum toxin type A injected under ultrasound guidance into the parotid and submandibular glands.

- Radiotherapy

Irradiation of the major salivary glands has been used to reduce salivation but has variable success and potential risks of late malignancy.

- Surgery

Surgery (Table 19.6) may be indicated where drooling:

- is caused by hypersalivation
- persists after at least 6 months of conservative therapy; or

TABLE 19.5   Medications Used to Reduce Drooling/Hypersalivation

Agent	Adult Dosage	Potential Adverse Effects Apart From Hyposalivation
Botulinum toxin A	Single injections of 10–40 units, under ultrasound guidance, into major glands	Pain at injection site
Clonidine	50–250 µg twice daily. Titrate for effectiveness	May cause drowsiness and interfere with driving
Ipratropium[a]	Spray 250 µg/mL sublingually as needed	Nausea, urinary retention, blurred vision, glaucoma
Hyoscine[a]	One 1.5 mg patch every day or 300 µg up to three times daily	Pruritus at patch site, urinary retention, irritability, blurred vision, dizziness, glaucoma
Trihexyphenidyl (benzhexol)[a]	1 mg daily	Drowsiness, vertigo, headache, glaucoma, urinary retention

[a]Atropinics — care in older patients and in patients with cardiovascular disease, glaucoma or urinary obstruction; caution with driving; avoid in gastrointestinal obstruction and myasthenia gravis.

TABLE 19.6   Surgical Treatment of sialorrhoea. Useful in patients with neuro-developmental disorders

Surgical Therapy	Effects	Comments
Submandibular gland excision	Can be effective in flow reduction	External scar. General anaesthetic needed
Submandibular duct re-routing to avoid oral cavity	Can be effective in reducing oral salivary flow	General anaesthetic needed. Submandibular gland still functional, ranulae possible
Parotid Gland excision	Not advisable	Facial nerve at risk of damage
Parotid duct re-routing to avoid oral cavity	Can be effective in reducing oral salivary flow	General anaesthetic needed. Gland still functional. Risk of sialocele. Little extra benefit if submandibular gland excised
Parotid duct ligation	Simple procedure	Gland still functional for a while. Risk of sialocele. Little extra benefit if submandibular gland excised

- is moderate to profuse and in a patient whose cognitive function precludes use of conservative therapy.

Surgical procedures to control drooling are aimed at decreasing salivary flow or redirecting it to a location more advantageous to promote swallowing. Procedures include salivary:

- gland excision
- duct rerouting
- duct ligation or
- nerve sectioning (neurectomy) or combinations of the aforementioned.

RECOMMENDED READING

Einhorn, O.M., Georgiou, K., Tompa, A., 2020. Salivary dysfunction caused by medication usage. Physiol. Int. 107 (2), 195—208.

Hockstein, N.G., Samadi, D.S., Gendron, K., Handler, S.D., 2004. Sialorrhea: a management challenge. Am. Fam. Physician. 69 (11), 2628—2634.

Proctor, G.B., 2016. The physiology of salivary secretion. Periodontol 2000. 70 (1), 11—25.

Riva, A., Federici, C., Piccolo, G., Amadori, E., Verrotti, A., Striano, P., 2021. Exploring treatments for drooling in children with neurological disorders. Expert Rev. Neurother. 21 (2), 179—187.

Dry Mouth (Xerostomia and Hyposalivation)

INTRODUCTION

Saliva is essential to oral health, and patients who have decreased salivary flow (hyposalivation) suffer from a lack of oral lubrication, affecting many functions and may develop infections as a consequence of the reduced defences. It is now accepted that xerostomia reflects the sensation of dryness, even in the presence of normal salivary flow, whereas hyposalivation is the term applied when there is a demonstrable reduction in salivary flow.

Dry mouth (xerostomia) is a complaint that is the most common salivary problem and is the subjective sense of dryness that may be due to:
- reduced salivary flow (hyposalivation)
- changed salivary composition.
- mouth breathing
- an increase in the thickness of saliva
- increased oral mucosal keratinisation.

Advancing age is increasingly associated with dry mouth, but this is usually due to medication or disease, rather than age *per se*. Age does, however, result in an increase in adipose tissue and a reduction of salivary acini, salivary secretory reserve and proteins such as MG1 and MG2 mucins but stimulated salivary flow is normal in the unmedicated elderly.

AETIOLOGY AND PATHOGENESIS

- Dry mouth is common in mouth-breathers and during periods of anxiety. Salivation is significantly reduced during sleep. Other than these, the causes can be remembered from the mnemonic 'Money can solve difficult problems' (Medications, Cancer treatments, Salivary disease, Dehydration, Psychogenic)

The main causes of dry mouth are iatrogenic (Chapter 33) and salivary gland diseases:

- Drugs with anticholinergic or sympathomimetic or diuretic activity are the most common cause (Box 20.1, Table 20.1 and Fig. 20.1). There is usually a fairly close temporal relationship between starting the drug treatment or increasing the dose and experiencing the dry mouth. Most reduce flow by 25% to 30% but are reversible. However, the cause for which the drug is being taken may also be important; for example, patients with anxiety or depressive conditions may complain of dry mouth even in the absence of drug therapy (or evidence of reduced salivary flow).
- Irradiation involving the salivary glands can produce profound hyposalivation, such as in treatment for neoplastic conditions in the head and neck, or mantle irradiation in lymphomas, or total body irradiation (TBI) before a haematopoietic stem cell transplant (bone marrow transplant). Chemotherapy and graft-versus-host disease (GVHD) can also induce hyposalivation (Chapter 33).
- Dehydration, as in diabetes mellitus, diabetes insipidus, hyperparathyroidism or any fever, is an occasional cause of hyposalivation. Dehydration is common in the elderly due to reduced fluid intake.
- Disorders affecting salivary glands such as Sjögren syndrome, sarcoidosis and some viral infections (e.g. EBV, CMV, HIV, HCV) may cause hyposalivation.
- Psychogenic causes may underlie the complaint of dry mouth; objective evidence for hyposalivation may be lacking.
- Rarely there is salivary gland aplasia, or cholinergic dysfunction (congenital or autoimmune).

CLINICAL FEATURES

The patient with hyposalivation may complain of dry mouth alone or combined with other features, such as dryness of the eyes and other mucosae (nasal, laryngeal, genital), with other eye complaints (inability to cry, blurring, light intolerance,

BOX 20.1 **Main Causes of Dry Mouth**

Iatrogenic Causes: Drugs (see Table 20.1)
Other Iatrogenic Causes
- Irradiation
- External beam
- Radioiodine
- Graft-versus-host disease

Dehydration (e.g. Diabetes, Hypercalcaemia, Renal Disease, Diarrhoea and Vomiting)
Salivary Gland Disease
- Aplasia (agenesis)
- Cystic fibrosis
- Deposits (haemochromatosis, hyperlipidaemia, amyloidosis)
- Ectodermal dysplasia
- IgG4 syndrome
- Infections (HIV, hepatitis C, EBV, CMV)
- Parotidectomy
- Primary biliary cirrhosis
- Sarcoidosis
- Sjögren syndrome
- Non-specific sialadenitis with primary generalised nodal osteoarthritis (SNOX syndrome)

Neural
- Alzheimer disease
- Anxiety states
- Autonomic cholinergic dysfunction
- Bulimia
- Dysautonomia (Allgrove syndrome [Chapter 56], diabetes, dysautonomia, hypothyroidism)

Psychogenic

TABLE 20.1 **Prescription Drugs Causing Dry Mouths**

- Analgesics
- Anti-cholinergics and anti-spasmodics
- Anti-hypertensives (may cause a compositional change in saliva. α_1-Antagonists and α_2-agonists reduce salivary flow. Beta-blockers [e.g. atenolol and propranolol] reduce protein levels)
- Diuretics
- Anti-psychotics
- Psychotropics (e.g. amitriptyline, nortriptyline, clomipramine) Anti-depressants
- Anti-Parkinson's
- Anti-histamines
- Appetite suppressants
- Anti-diarrhoeals, emetics
- Anti-acne (isotretinoin), arthritic (piroxicam)
- Most recreational drugs

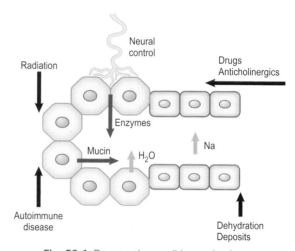

Fig. 20.1 Dry mouth; possible mechanisms.

burning, itching or grittiness), and sometimes voice or other changes (see Sjögren syndrome, Chapter 26).

In hyposalivation, there may be:
- difficulty in swallowing — especially in eating dry foods, such as biscuits (the cracker sign) (note the oesophagus is mainly lubricated by saliva)
- difficulty in controlling dentures
- difficulty in speaking, as the tongue tends to stick to the palate; this can lead to 'clicking' speech
- mouth soreness
- unpleasant taste or change in or loss of sense of taste
- a dry mucosa (Fig. 20.2) — the lips adhere one to another and an examining dental mirror may stick to the mucosa
- lipstick or food debris sticking to the teeth (Fig. 20.3)
- lack of the usual pooling of saliva on the floor of the mouth
- thin lines of frothy saliva may form along the lines of contact of the oral soft tissues or in the vestibule
- saliva not expressible from the salivary ducts
- a characteristic lobulated tongue, usually red, with partial or complete depapillation.

ORAL COMPLICATIONS

Oral complications of hyposalivation may also include:
- halitosis (oral malodour) (Chapter 17)
- dental caries, which tends to involve smooth surfaces and areas otherwise not very prone to caries — such as the lower incisor region. Caries can also involve roots and be severe and difficult to control
- candidosis (Chapter 36), which may cause:
  - burning sensation
  - taste changes
  - intolerance of acids and spices
  - mucosal erythema
  - lingual filiform papillae atrophy
  - angular stomatitis (angular cheilitis)
- ascending (suppurative) sialadenitis (Chapter 11), which presents with pain and swelling of a major salivary gland, and sometimes purulent discharge from the duct.

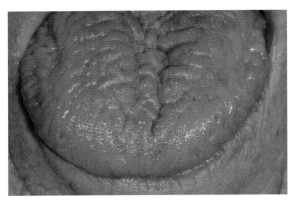

Fig. 20.2 Dryness evident on the tongue.

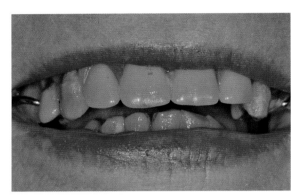

Fig. 20.3 Dryness causing lipstick and food retention.

DIAGNOSIS

Hyposalivation is a clinical diagnosis, made predominantly on the basis of the history and examination and measurement of salivary flow (sialometry). By far the most common cause of hyposalivation is medication and over 1000 drugs on the market have reduced salivary flow as a side effect (see Table 20.1)

There is now a validated **Clinical Oral Dryness Score** (CODS) designed for general use (Fig 20.4). Ten common oral signs of dryness are assessed, and the dryness is categorised as mild, moderate or severe. The aims are to document the degree of salivary dysfunction and to determine the cause (Algorithm 20.1). An additive score of 1 to 3 indicates **mild dryness** which may not need treatment. (Table 20.2). Sugar-free chewing gum chewed for 15 to 20 minutes twice a day may be adequate to maintain oral health and diminution of symptoms. Patients should also be advised of the importance of maintaining hydration, especially the elderly.

An additive score of 4 to 6 indicates **moderate dryness**. Sugar-free chewing gum or mild sialogogues may be required. Saliva substitutes and topical fluorides or fluoride toothpaste may be appropriate. If the reason for the dryness is not apparent, then these patients should be further investigated. Monitor at regular intervals to ensure that the symptoms remain unchanged and that caries development is controlled.

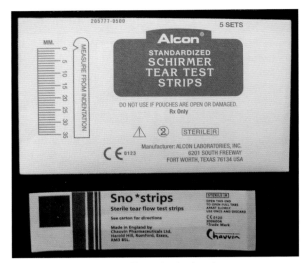

Fig. 20.4 Tests for lacrimation.

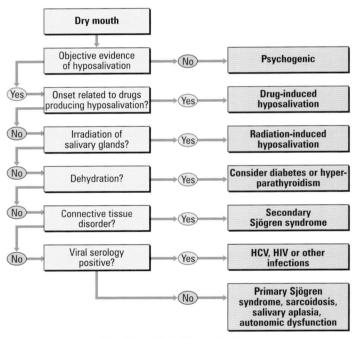

Algorithm 20.1 Diagnosis of dry mouth (see also Chapters 2, 3, 20).

An additive score of 7 to 10 indicates **severe dryness** (see Table 20.2). Saliva substitutes and topical fluorides are usually needed. The cause of the hyposalivation must be determined and Sjogren's syndrome excluded. This usually requires referral and investigation by a specialist in oral medicine or rheumatology department. Patients then need to be monitored regularly to ensure maintenance of oral health, for changing symptoms and signs and further specialist advice if appropriate.

CODS seems to be closely related to both the unstimulated salivary flow and the thickness of the mucin layer over the

TABLE 20.2 Investigations That Might Be Helpful in Diagnosis/Prognosis/Management in Some Patients With Dry Mouth (Xerostomia and Hyposalivation)[a]

In Most Cases	In Some Cases
Sialometry	Sialography
Antinuclear antibodies (ANA)	Ultrasonography
	Salivary gland biopsy
Extractable nuclear antigens (ENA) SS-A	Eye tests, e.g. Schirmer
	Urinalysis
HbA1c	Serum ferritin, vitamin B_{12} and corrected whole blood folate levels
ESR	
Full blood picture	Blood CD4 cell counts
Rheumatoid factor (RF)	Complement levels
	Serum immunoglobulin levels
	Serum immunoglobulin IgG4 levels
	Serum liver function tests and antimitochondrial autoantibodies
	Serum angiotensin-converting enzyme (SACE)
	Serum calcium and phosphate
	Serology — viral (HCV, HIV)
	Thyroid function tests
	Chest radiography
	MRI
	Salivary scinitiscanning
	Psychological assessment

[a]See text for details and glossary for abbreviations.

epithelium (mucosal wetness) suggesting a physiological basis for the feeling of xerostomia

Salivary Studies

It can be helpful to document salivary function through salivary function studies, especially studies of the salivary flow rates (sialometry). Ultrasonography is also useful. Other studies such as sialography, salivary scintiscanning and salivary biopsy, are less commonly used. Sialoendoscopy has no role in the assessment of hyposalivation.

Salivary Flow Rates (Sialometry)

Salivary flow rate estimation is simple, non-invasive, inexpensive but not especially sensitive and a non-specific indicator of salivary gland dysfunction usually carried out by one of two possible methods:

• Unstimulated whole saliva flow rate (this more closely correlates with symptoms of hyposalivation than do stimulated flow rates). The test should be standardised by being carried out first thing in the morning after overnight fasting; no food or drink for at least 1 hour before the test; no smoking for at least 1 hour before the test. Allow the patient to dribble into a measuring container for over 15 minutes. A resting secretion rate of less than 1.5 mL in 15 minutes indicates hyposalivation: in a normal person, the unstimulated whole saliva flow rate exceeds 1.5 mL/15 minutes (0.1 mL/min).

• Stimulated saliva flow rate. Use various means of stimulation, such as 10% citric acid dropped onto the tongue, and

collect parotid saliva using a Carlsson–Crittenden cup placed over one Stensen papilla. A flow of less than 0.5 mL per gland in 5 minutes or less than 1 mL per gland in 10 minutes is decreased. In normal persons, the flow should well exceed 0.5 mL/min/parotid gland.

Ultrasonography

Ultrasonography provides information about the changes to major salivary glands during inflammation. It reveals, for example, decreased echogenicity and volume of submandibular glands in patients with Sjögren syndrome, with high specificity and moderate sensitivity. Recent improvements in ultrasonography techniques have allowed the degree of gland damage to be scored and high scores may indicate Sjogren syndrome (see Chapter 26). It has now become a standard investigation in suspected Sjogren's syndrome.

Sialography

Sialography, in which radio-opaque dye, often iodine-based, is introduced into the salivary duct, is non-specific. It may be of value if there is dilatation or duct obstruction (e.g. by a calculus, though this rarely causes dryness), but carries risks of discomfort and infection. It has largely been superseded by ultrasonography.

Salivary Scintiscanning

Salivary scintiscanning non-invasively examines all major salivary glands simultaneously but is associated with a small radiation hazard since technetium-99 m, a γ-emitting radionuclide is used. It can detect individual non-functioning glands but is not always available and is expensive.

Salivary Gland Biopsy

Although it is perfectly possible to biopsy the parotid or other major glands, there is a small risk of nerve damage or salivary fistula, and an extraoral approach will leave a small scar. Therefore, a biopsy of minor salivary glands is usually done. Minor glands in the palate and lower lip are accessible, but the latter site is preferred both from the aspects of patient comfort and access for the operator and also because the extent and pattern of histopathological changes on labial salivary gland (LSG) biopsy correlate with those in major glands.

Glands in the lower labial mucosa are selected since they are readily biopsied through a simple incision in the labial mucosa under local analgesia. The incision is paramedian, placed in the lower labial mucosa (avoiding any clinically obvious mucosal lesions, which could confuse the diagnosis) and is thus not visible externally. Four to six lobules of salivary glands should be removed. The wound is closed with one or two sutures and, apart from mild discomfort in many and anaesthesia or hypoaesthesia in some cases, complications are rare.

Determination of the Cause of Xerostomia

The history and examination may help to determine the cause of a complaint of xerostomia and determine whether or not there is objective evidence of hyposalivation. It is important to recognise that some patients complaining of dry mouth have no evidence of reduced salivary flow or a salivary disorder; there may then be a psychogenic reason for the complaint.

If there is hyposalivation, investigations may be indicated to exclude systemic causes noted above. Commonly indicated investigations may thus include the following (Table 20.3):

- Eye tests, using Schirmer test of lacrimal flow (see Fig. 20.4), and slit-lamp examination, mainly to exclude Sjögren syndrome (see Chapter 26).
- Urinalysis, mainly to exclude diabetes.
- Blood tests:
  - ESR, CRP or PV — non-specific tests mainly to exclude Sjögren syndrome or sarcoidosis
  - antinuclear antibodies (ANA, ENA) — including SS-A antibodies, mainly to exclude Sjögren syndrome and lupus erythematosus (see Chapters 26 and 34)
  - rheumatoid factor (RF), mainly to exclude Sjögren or SNOX syndrome
  - serum liver function tests, and antimitochondrial autoantibodies to exclude primary biliary cirrhosis
  - serum immunoglobulin levels, a non-specific test mainly to exclude connective tissue diseases
  - serum immunoglobulin IgG4 levels, to exclude IgG4 syndrome (see Chapters 11 and 26)
  - serum angiotensin-converting enzyme (SACE), mainly to exclude sarcoidosis
  - serum calcium and phosphate, mainly to exclude hyperparathyroidism
  - serology, to exclude viral causes
  - blood glucose, to exclude diabetes.

- Imaging:
  - chest radiography, mainly to exclude sarcoidosis
  - ultrasonography, mainly to exclude Sjögren syndrome or neoplasia
  - MRI, mainly to exclude Sjögren syndrome.
- Salivary biopsy may be indicated if there is suspicion of organic disease of the salivary glands.

TREATMENT

- If there is objective evidence of hyposalivation, any underlying cause should, if possible, be rectified; for example, hyposalivation-producing drugs may be changed for an alternative and causes such as diabetes should be treated.
- Efforts should be made to avoid factors that may increase dryness, such as:
  - dry hot environments
  - dry foods such as biscuits
  - drugs (e.g. tricyclic antidepressants or diuretics)
  - alcohol (including alcohol-based mouthwashes)
  - smoking
  - beverages that produce diuresis (coffee and tea).
- The mouth should be hydrated as regularly as possible. The lips may become dry, atrophic and susceptible to cracking and thus should be kept moist using a water-based lubricant or a lanolin-based product rather than one containing petroleum-derived lubricants (e.g. Vaseline). Olive oil, vitamin E or lip balm may help.

TABLE 20.3   Some Salivary Stimulants (Sialogogues) and Salivary Replacements (Mouth Wetting Agents or Saliva Substitutes)

Agent	Use	Comments
Sialogogues		
Pilocarpine (Salagen) or cevimeline	5 mg up to 3 times daily with food. Titrate from once daily	The patient may be unable to see well enough to drive or operate machinery Contraindicated in asthma, chronic obstructive airways disease, glaucoma and pregnancy Care with cardiac disease
Chewing gum (sugar-free)	Regularly	Inexpensive, no adverse effects
Salivix	Malic acid	Pastille
Salivary Replacements		
Glandosane	Sodium carboxymethylcellulose base	Spray
Luborant	Sodium carboxymethylcellulose base	Spray
Oral Balance	Lactoperoxidase, glucose oxidase and xylitol	Gel
Saliva Orthana	Mucin	A spray containing fluoride, or lozenge May be unsuitable if there are religious objections to porcine mucin
Salivace	Sodium carboxymethylcellulose base	Spray
Saliveze	Sodium carboxymethylcellulose base	Spray

TABLE 20.4 Clinical Oral Dryness Score (1 point for each feature)

1. Mirror sticks to both buccal mucosae
2. Mirror sticks to tongue
3. Saliva frothy
4. No saliva pooling on the floor of mouth
5. Tongue shows loss of papillae
6. Altered/smooth gingival architecture (especially anterior)
7. Glassy appearance to oral mucosa (especially palate)
8. Tongue lobulated/fissured
9. Cervical caries (more than two teeth)
10. Debris on palate (excluded under dentures)

Score of 1–3 = mild dryness. May not need treatment or management. Sugar-free chewing gum for 15 minutes twice daily and attention to hydration.

Score 4–6 = moderate dryness. Sugar-free chewing gum or simple sialogogues are needed. Investigate if the reasons for dryness are not clear. Saliva substitutes are helpful. Monitor.

Score 7–10 = severe dryness. Saliva substitutes and topical fluoride are needed. Cause of hyposalivation to be ascertained and Sjogren's excluded. Refer for investigation and diagnosis.

In general, a low COD score (1–3) indicates mild dryness manageable normally in practice, whereas a high COD score (7–10) is an indication for referral for further investigation.

- Mouth wetting agents (salivary substitutes) may help symptomatically. Various means are available, including:
  - water or ice chips: frequent sips of water are generally more effective than synthetic salivary substitutes
  - synthetic salivary substitutes, which vary in properties and patient acceptability, fluoride content and pH (Table 20.4). Synthetic salivary substitutes usually contain carboxymethylcellulose (UK: Glandosane, Luborant (contains fluoride), Salivace, Saliveze. USA: Moi-Stir, Orex, Salivart, Xero-Lube, Mouth-Kote), mucin (Saliva Orthana; also contains xylitol and fluoride) or glycerate polymer (Oral Balance; also contains xylitol, glucose oxidase and lactoperoxidase). A home preparation can be made using ¼ teaspoon of glycerine in 8 ounces of water (approximately 250 mL).
- Salivation may be promoted by using a stimulant: (sialogogue) such as:
  - chewing gums (containing sorbitol or xylitol, not sucrose)
  - diabetic sweets
  - cholinergic drugs such as pilocarpine, bethanechol, cevimeline or anetholetrithione.
- Oral complications, such as dental caries, should be prevented and treated with:
  - dietary control of sucrose intake
  - regular dental checks and monitoring of *Streptococcus mutans* counts
  - topical fluorides (reduce caries risk by reducing demineralisation and by increasing remineralisation)
- full-strength fluoride toothpaste containing 1000 to 1500 ppm fluoride should be used at least twice daily. Higher content pastes may be indicated
  - fluoride rinses of 0.05% sodium fluoride (used before retiring to bed at night)
  - fluoride gel products provided in tightly adapted vacuform mouth guard carriers are also useful. Fluorides may be usefully applied in the dental office, or daily at home (sodium fluoride gels or 0.4% stannous fluoride gels)
  - amorphous calcium phosphate (ACP)
  - glass ionomer restorations can be useful since they release fluoride
  - it is best to wait until a year of no new caries has elapsed before constructing new crowns.
- Oral complications such as candidosis should be treated:
  - a rinse or swab from the oral mucosa should be taken to confirm candidosis if there is soreness and signs of inflammation. A commercial kit such as Ori-cult may be helpful
  - dentures should be left out of the mouth at night, cleaned and stored in sodium hypochlorite solution, benzalkonium chloride or chlorhexidine. Alternatively, after cleaning, leaving to dry is said to disrupt the biofilm
  - chlorhexidine, used in aqueous solution as a mouth rinse, has both antibacterial and antifungal effects, and there may be advantages to its use in dentate patients, due to some effects of chlorhexidine against cariogenic bacteria as well as *Candida*
  - antifungals should be used, until there is no evidence of mucosal erythema and symptoms, and should be continued for at least 2 weeks more, to reduce the risk of recurrence. Topical antifungals tend to be most effective since salivation is low and thus salivary antifungal delivery is not good. Topical antifungals are available as gels or tablets which can be allowed to dissolve intraorally, resulting in contact with mucosa while dissolving in the mouth. However, if the mouth is extremely dry, tablets may not dissolve, and in these cases, liquid products such as suspensions or gels are best. The polyene, nystatin, is effective topically and available as a suspension. Azoles can be given as a suspension or liquid, used as a mouthwash and then swallowed (Chapter 5). Fluconazole, itraconazole and posaconazole are available as suspensions effective against oropharyngeal candidosis, and voriconazole as a liquid – preparation that may find favour for use in patients with dry mouths. An antifungal, such as miconazole gel, should be spread on dentures or appliances before re-insertion.
- Oral complications such as bacterial sialadenitis should be treated:
  - a swab should be collected of any pus expressed from the salivary duct, for bacterial culture and antibiotic sensitivities
  - acute sialadenitis needs treating, usually with a penicillinase-resistant antibiotic, such as flucloxacillin.

RECOMMENDED READING

Al Hamad, A., Lodi, G., Porter, S., Fedele, S., Mercadante, V., 2019. Interventions for dry mouth and hyposalivation in Sjögren's syndrome: a systematic review and meta-analysis. Oral. Dis. 25 (4), 1027–1047.

Baer, A.N., Walitt, B., 2018. Update on Sjögren syndrome and other causes of sicca in older adults. Rheum. Dis. Clin. North. Am. 44 (3), 419–436.

Furness, S., Worthington, H.V., Bryan, G., Birchenough, S., McMillan, R., 2011. Interventions for the management of dry mouth: topical therapies. Cochrane. Database. Syst. Rev. 12, CD008934.

Tan, E.C.K., Lexomboon, D., Sandborgh-Englund, G., Haasum, Y., Johnell, K., 2018. Medications that cause dry mouth as an adverse effect in older people: a systematic review and metaanalysis. J. Am. Geriatr. Soc. 66 (1), 76–84.

Trismus

INTRODUCTION

Trismus (lockjaw) (from the Greek *Trimos* = 'grating', 'grinding') is a restriction in the inability to open the mouth normally. Normal mouth opening in an adult ranges from 35 to 55 mm inter-incisally. The lower limit of the normal maximum opening is 35 mm for females and 40 mm for males. Trismus can have consequences including impaired mastication, difficulty in speaking, achieving adequate oral hygiene and access to oral care. If left untreated, degenerative processes in the masticatory muscles, with disuse atrophy, may ensue.

Many patients with trismus are likely to have a temporo-mandibular disorder (TMD). In some people, such as persons who have received radiation to the head and neck, trismus is often seen in conjunction with difficulty in swallowing. In trismus caused by radiotherapy, hyposalivation and mucositis are also commonly associated challenges. Occasionally, in TMD joint trauma or infection, and rarely in pain-dysfunction syndrome, the joint may become fibrotic or even ankylosed.

AETIOLOGY AND PATHOGENESIS

Limited opening of the jaw is most commonly due to TMD. Myofascial pain and disc displacement without reduction may result in restricted mouth opening. Extra-articular disease with masticatory muscle spasm secondary to trauma or local infection (e.g. pericoronitis around a partially erupted mandibular third molar) may cause limited mouth opening. Occasionally trismus is caused by joint (intra-articular and intra-capsular) disease, or conditions affecting the adjacent soft (peri-capsular) tissues such as scarring, infiltrating neoplasms or oral submucous fibrosis. Up to 38% of patients develop trismus after treatment for head and neck cancer. It is rare for trismus to be the presenting feature of malignancy.

Trismus is usually caused by inflammation and masticatory muscle spasm, or inflexible scarring or other tissues (Box 21.1).

Life-threatening causes include tetanus, malignant neoplasms and fascial space infections. In stroke patients, trismus may appear as a result of CNS dysfunction. Some drugs (e.g. amphetamines and ecstasy (methylenedioxymeth-amphetamine; MDMA)) can cause masticatory muscle spasm which forcibly causes bruxism and difficulty in mouth opening.

DIAGNOSIS

Except for those cases caused by acute trauma and tetanus, trismus tends to develop slowly, and some patients may not be aware until the interincisal distance is less than 20 mm (Fig. 21.1). A simple diagnostic test is the so-called 'three finger test', in which the patient is asked to insert three of their fingers into the mouth. If all three fingers can fit between the incisors, mouth opening is considered normal but if less than three can be inserted, trismus is likely.

The cause should be sought (Algorithm 21.1; Table 21.1) and a thorough history and clinical examination should be undertaken. Lymphadenopathy, severe trismus of less than 15 mm, the pain of non-myofascial origin, progressive worsening symptoms and a suspicious intraoral soft tissue lesion may alert the clinician of an underlying malignancy. An imaging examination must be performed to exclude malignancy in the pharynx and infratemporal regions as well as the TMJ, jaws and parotid salivary glands. Panoramic radiography has limited ability to demonstrate the extent of lesions or soft tissue involvement or to detect bony destruction in malignancy when compared to computed tomography (CT). Where malignancy is suspected, more advanced imaging is warranted, including CT and magnetic resonance imaging (MRI).

TREATMENT

The underlying condition should be treated where possible. Trismus treatment should begin early in the progression of the trismus since it then is likely to be more effective, and easier on

BOX 21.1 Causes of Trismus

Acute Trismus
- Infection:
  - pericoronitis
  - odontogenic infection with spread involving masticatory muscles, TMJ, bone or fascial spaces
  - TMJ or bone infections
  - tonsillar or pharyngeal infections
  - parotitis
  - otitis
  - tetanus
- Trauma:
  - jaws
  - facial soft tissues
- Postoperative:
  - third molar teeth removal
  - other jaw and oral surgery
  - associated with haematoma
  - local anaesthetic injection trauma to pterygoid muscles
- Drug-related:
  - psychotomimetics such as ecstasy
  - extra-pyramidal reaction to anti-emetics (e.g. metoclopramide)
  - malignant hyperthermia
  - temporomandibular joint disorders

Sub-acute Trismus
- Tumour infiltration of muscles or joints
- Chronic infection
- Temporomandibular joint disorders

Chronic Trismus
- Soft tissue scar formation or TMJ damage after surgery, trauma, radiation or burns
- Submucous fibrosis
- Scleroderma
- Rheumatoid arthritis
- Temporomandibular joint disorders
- TMJ ankylosis
- Masticatory muscle disorders (e.g. myotonia, myositis ossificans)
- CNS disease: Suprabulbar palsy, multiple sclerosis

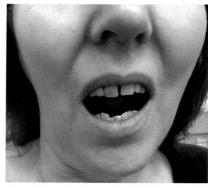

Fig. 21.1 Trismus in severe temporomandibular pain-dysfunction syndrome.

Management of trismus includes passive and active physiotherapy with a range of simple and inexpensive devices. 'Range of motion' devices provide passive motion which, applied several times per day, provides significant improvement in opening and reduction in inflammation and pain. It is important to record the initial opening (inter-incisal distance) before starting therapy and keep a patient logbook. Then the patient should open and close the mouth with assisted opening five times, holding the open position to the maximum opening that can be sustained *without pain* for 5 seconds. They should do this five times per day. The most common way to achieve such passive motion is by using tongue spatulas (depressors) which can be stacked, forced and held between the teeth in an attempt to lever the mouth open slowly over time. The use of stacked tongue depressors and/or corkscrew-like devices has fallen out of favour due to the oral and dental trauma associated with their use. The most commonly used devices to treat trismus are the TheraBite System and The Dynasplint Trismus System. The Therabite (Platon Medical Ltd., Eastbourne, UK) functions similarly to the spatula systems. Patients using spatulas or the Therabite may gain up to 1.5 mm of sustainable opening gains per week, and thus may need to exercise for up to 10 weeks to achieve useful oral opening. Many patients will need to continue to mobilise and stretch daily at least once each day, for life.

Continuous passive motion devices are also commercially available (e.g. Dynasplint; Stevensville, Maryland, USA). More sophisticated and expensive devices can be custom made for each patient.

Pentoxifylline, a methylxanthine derivative used to treat vascular diseases such as intermittent claudication, has been reported to have anti-tumour necrosis factor, vasodilator and anti-inflammatory effects. Endogenous tocopherol can scavenge reactive oxygen species generated during oxidative stress. The use of a combination of pentoxifylline with tocopherol has

the patient. If treatment is delayed, the difficulty in reversing trismus increases. If the local infection is the cause, the source should be removed, drainage instituted and antibiotics prescribed. In most cases, a soft diet is advisable. Symptomatic relief may include anti-inflammatory analgesics such as nonsteroidal antiinflammatory drugs (NSAIDs), muscle relaxants such as benzodiazepines, warmth, physical therapy and 'range of motion' devices. Warmth is best applied with moist hot towels placed on the affected area for 15 minutes every hour. Soft lasers, splints and botulinum toxoid have also been employed.

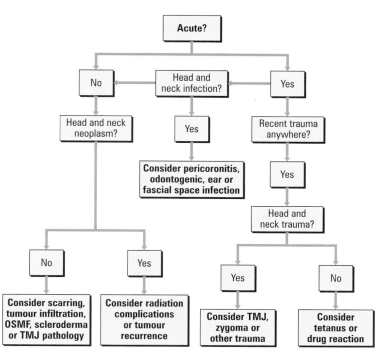

Algorithm 21.1 Diagnosis of trismus.

TABLE 21.1 Investigations That Might Be Helpful in Diagnosis/Prognosis/Management in Some Patients With Trismus	
In Most Cases	**In Some Cases**
Panoramic radiography of TMJs	CT/MRI
	Nasendoscopy
	Ultrasound
	Biopsy
	Anti-topoisomerase 1 antibodies (or anti-Scl-70)
	Anti-CCP antibodies
	Psychological assessment

proven effective in the treatment of post-radiotherapy fibrosis in head and neck cancer patients.

In rare cases, persons with severe limitations to opening may need cricothyrotomy or intubation.

Tetanus is a medical emergency and should be treated with antimicrobials (penicillin or metronidazole), tetanus immunoglobulin and muscle relaxants (e.g. diazepam).

In all cases, maintenance of oral hygiene is of particular importance.

RECOMMENDED READING

Beddis, H.P., Davies, S.J., Budenberg, A., Horner, K., Pemberton, M.N., 2014. Temporomandibular disorders, trismus and malignancy: development of a checklist to improve patient safety. Br. Dent. J. 217 (7), 351–355.

Johnson, J., Carlsson, S., Johansson, M., Pauli, N., Rydén, A., Fagerberg-Mohlin, B., 2012. Development and validation of the gothenburg trismus questionnaire (GTQ). Oral. Oncol. 48 (8), 730–736.

Johnson, J., Johansson, M., Rydén, A., Houltz, E., Finizia, C., 2015. Impact of trismus on health-related quality of life and mental health. Head. Neck. 37 (11), 1672–1679.

Watters, A.L., Cope, S., Keller, M.N., Padilla, M., Enciso, R., 2019. Prevalence of trismus in patients with head and neck cancer: a systematic review with meta-analysis. Head. Neck. 41 (9), 3408–3421.

Erythema Migrans

KEY POINTS
- Erythema migrans or 'geographic' tongue or benign migratory glossitis is a common genetic condition, where the tongue dorsum has red patches with a white margin that vary in appearance over time. It may cause a sore tongue
- Treatment is symptomatic only and patients need mainly reassurance
- Fissured tongue often has related erythema migrans

INTRODUCTION

Erythema migrans (geographic tongue, benign migratory glossitis) is a common cause of a sore tongue, where the tongue has red patches that resemble a map ('geographic' tongue) (Fig. 22.1). It is unrelated to erythema migrans of the skin (Lyme disease).

Epidemiology

- Occurs in 1% to 2% of adults.
- May be seen at any age.
- Can occur in either gender.
- No known geographic incidence.

AETIOLOGY AND PATHOGENESIS

- There is a genetic background; there is:
  - often a family history
  - sometimes an HLA association (an increased incidence of HLA-Cw6, DR5 and DRW6 antigens and a decrease in B51 antigen), and an increased incidence of HLA-B15 in atopic patients with erythema migrans
  - an association with IL-1B polymorphism +3954
  - increased Il-6 positivity in the epithelium.
- Patients with fissured tongues often have erythema migrans.
- Patients with erythema migrans are typically non-smokers.
- Some patients with erythema migrans have:
  - psoriasis, probably about 4% of cases. Some have a family history of psoriasis. Histologically there is epithelial thinning at the centre of the lesion with an inflammatory infiltrate mainly of polymorphonuclear leukocytes (PMNLs), reminiscent of psoriasis — even in patients without psoriasis (Fig. 22.2)
  - atopic allergies, such as hay fever, and a few relate the discomfort or oral lesions to various foods (e.g. cheese)
  - diabetes mellitus.
- People with Down syndrome have a higher prevalence of erythema migrans.

CLINICAL FEATURES

- Erythema migrans typically involves the dorsum of the tongue, sometimes the ventrum, and rarely other areas on the oral mucosa.
- There are irregular, pink or red depapillated map-like areas, which change in shape, increase in size and spread or move to other areas, sometimes within hours (Figs 22.3–22.7).
- The red areas are often surrounded by distinct yellowish, slightly raised margins.
- There is increased thickness of the intervening filiform papillae.
- It is often asymptomatic.
- A small minority complain of soreness and these patients are virtually invariably middle-aged. If sore, this may be noted especially with acidic foods (e.g. tomatoes, strawberries, pineapple, eggplants or others), walnuts or some cheese. Why the condition should give rise to symptoms after it has presumably been present for decades is unclear.
- Many patients with a fissured tongue (scrotal tongue) also have erythema migrans.

DIAGNOSIS

- The diagnosis is clinical mainly from the history of a migrating pattern and the clinical appearance.
- Very similar lesions may be seen in psoriasis and Reiter syndrome (transiently).
- There also may be confusion with glossitis, lichen planus and lupus erythematosus.

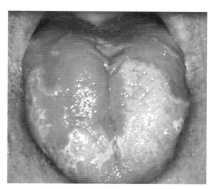

Fig. 22.1 Erythema migrans (geographic tongue), showing typical red lesions with irregular creamy borders.

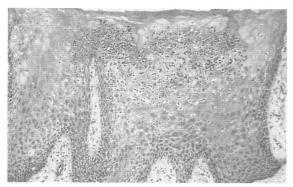

Fig. 22.2 Erythema migrans (geographic tongue), showing typical histopathological features of intra-epithelial foci of leukocytes, resembling psoriasis.

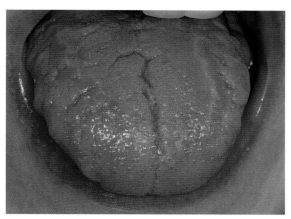

Fig. 22.3 Erythema migrans (geographic tongue), showing typical lesions in a fissured tongue — a common association.

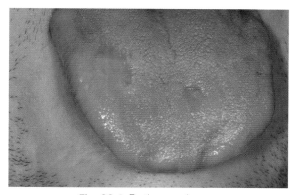

Fig. 22.4 Erythema migrans.

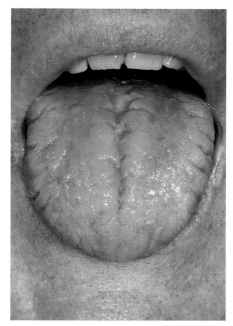

Fig. 22.5 Erythema migrans.

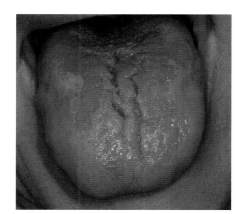

Fig. 22.6 Erythema migrans.

- Blood examination may rarely be necessary to exclude anaemia if there is confusion with a depapillated tongue of glossitis (Table 22.1).

TREATMENT (SEE ALSO CHAPTERS 4 AND 5)

- Patient information is an important aspect of management. Over 20 layers of epithelium per day are shed from the tongue dorsum which is why the pattern can change so quickly. The term 'benign migratory glossitis' is reassuring to patients

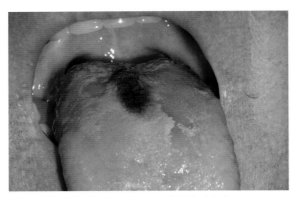

Fig. 22.7 Erythema migrans with black hairy tongue.

TABLE 22.1 Aids That Might Be Helpful in Diagnosis/Prognosis/Management in Some Patients Suspected of Having Erythema Migrans[a]
In Some Cases
Full blood picture
Serum ferritin, vitamin B_{12} and corrected whole blood folate levels
ESR
Blood glucose

[a]See text for details and glossary for abbreviations.

- There are isolated reports of management with vitamin B, zinc, tetracyclines, corticosteroids or ciclosporin but immunosuppressive agents are not indicated and should be avoided. Reassurance remains the best advice that can be given (Table 22.2). Chewing gum or using benzydamine topically can afford symptomatic relief if essential, without adverse effects.

TABLE 22.2 Regimens Used for Management of Patients Suspected of Having Oral Erythema Migrans	
Regimen	
Supportive	Benzydamine rinse
	Chewing gum
	Diet with little acidic, spicy or citrus content
	Lidocaine
	Reassurance

FOLLOW-UP OF PATIENTS

Long-term follow-up is rarely appropriate.

RECOMMENDED READING

Assimakopoulos, D., Patrikakos, G., Fotika, C., Elisaf, M., 2002. Benign migratory glossitis or geographic tongue: an enigmatic oral lesion. Am. J. Med. 113 (9), 751—755.

González-Álvarez, L., García-Pola, M.J., Garcia-Martin, J.M., 2018. Geographic tongue: predisposing factors, diagnosis and treatment. A systematic review. Rev. Clin. Esp. 218 (9), 481—488.

González-Álvarez, L., García-Martín, J.M., García-Pola, M.J., 2019. Association between geographic tongue and psoriasis: a systematic review and meta-analyses. J. Oral. Pathol. Med. 48 (5), 365—372.

Picciani, B.L., Domingos, T.A., Teixeira-Souza, T., et al., 2016. Geographic tongue and psoriasis: clinical, histopathological, immunohistochemical and genetic correlation—a literature review. An. Bras. Dermatol. 91 (4), 410—421.

Picciani, B.L.S., Santos, L.R., Teixeira-Souza, T., et al., 2020. Geographic tongue severity index: a new and clinical scoring system. Oral. Surg. Oral. Med. Oral. Pathol. Oral. Radiol. 129 (4), 330—338.

Red and White Lesions

RED LESIONS

Introduction

Red oral lesions are commonplace in the mouth and are usually caused by inflammation in, for example, mucosal infections such as candidiasis (Fig. 23.1). However, they can also be sinister and signify severe epithelial dysplasia or malignant neoplasms. Red lesions, especially if persistent, can be:

- Focal: the lesion of most concern is erythroplakia, since it is usually dysplastic. Carcinoma or telangiectasia can also cause red lesions.
- Multifocal: these lesions are often caused by candidiasis or lichen planus.
- Discoid: these are prominent on the dorsum of the tongue in erythema migrans (geographic tongue).
- Diffuse: candidiasis is the most common cause, but these lesions may be caused by mucositis, haematinic deficiency states and infections.
- Linear: these may be seen on the tongue in deficiency states.
  The causes of red lesions can be remembered from the acronym BLING (Blood disorders, Lichen planus, Infection or inflammation, Neoplastic and pre-neoplastic and Geographic tongue).

Aetiology and Pathogenesis

Mucosal Inflammation

Most red lesions are inflammatory (Box 23.1), the most common being caused by:

- Viral stomatitis (e.g. herpes simplex stomatitis) (Chapter 37).
- Candidiasis (Chapter 36):
  - denture-related stomatitis is a form of chronic atrophic candidiasis consisting of inflammation of the mucosa beneath a dental appliance (usually a complete upper denture), such that the hard palate is red (see Fig. 23.1)

- acute oral atrophic candidiasis may complicate corticosteroid or antibiotic therapy, particularly with long-term, broad-spectrum antimicrobials, and causes widespread erythema and soreness of the oral mucosa, especially of the tongue sometimes with thrush (pseudomembranous candidiasis)
  - erythematous oral candidiasis may complicate HIV disease and causes focal or widespread erythema and soreness of the oral mucosa, often in the palate, and sometimes with thrush
  - median rhomboid glossitis is usually detected by the patient or dental professional as a persistent red, rhomboidal depapillated area in the midline of the dorsum of the tongue, just anterior to the circumvallate papillae.
- Deep mycoses (Chapter 36), which are rare in the developed world, except in HIV disease and other immunocompromised persons:
  - histoplasmosis
  - cryptococcosis
  - blastomycosis
  - paracoccidioidomycosis.
- Iatrogenic
  - radiation-induced mucositis (mucosal barrier injury or MBI) is common after irradiation of tumours of the head and neck if the radiation field involves the oral mucosa. Arising within 3 weeks of the irradiation, there is generalised erythema, and sometimes ulceration
  - chemotherapy-induced mucositis is common after chemotherapy. Fluorouracil and cisplatin almost always cause mucositis. Etoposide, melphalan, doxorubicin, vinblastine, taxanes and methotrexate are also particularly stomatotoxic. Arising within 1 to 2 weeks of the therapy, there is generalised erythema, and sometimes ulceration
  - Check point inhibitors, particularly PD-1, e.g. pembrolizumab and CTLA-4 inhibitor Ipilimumab

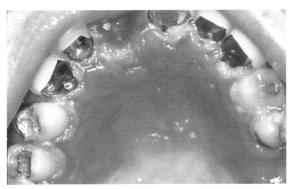

Fig. 23.1 Denture-related stomatitis; red lesions are usually inflammatory in origin.

BOX 23.1 Causes of Red Lesions

Localised
- Inflammatory
- Herpes or other viral infections
- Candidiasis
- Other mycoses
- Granulomatous conditions (Crohn disease, orofacial granulomatosis, sarcoidosis)
- Plasma cell gingivitis
- Reiter syndrome (reactive arthritis)
- Graft-versus-host disease
- Drugs (e.g. causing candidiasis, mucositis or lichenoid lesions)
- Epithelioid angiomatosis
- Reactive lesions:
  - pyogenic granulomas
  - peripheral giant cell granulomas
- Atrophic lesions:
  - geographic tongue
  - lichen planus
  - lupus erythematosus
  - erythroplasia
  - avitaminosis B_{12}
- Burns
- Vascular anomalies (e.g. angiomas)
- Purpura
- Telangiectases (hereditary haemorrhagic telangiectasia or scleroderma)
- Angiokeratomas (Fabry disease)
  - neoplasms
  - giant cell tumour
  - squamous carcinoma
  - Kaposi sarcoma
  - Wegener granulomatosis

Generalised
- Candidiasis
- Avitaminosis B complex
- Mucositis irradiation or chemotherapy induced
- Polycythaemia

used as immunotherapy for cancer patients are also frequently associated with mucositis particularly lichenoid reactions.

- Immunological reactions, such as lichen planus, plasma cell gingivostomatitis, granulomatous disorders (sarcoidosis, Crohn disease, orofacial granulomatosis), amyloidosis and graft-versus-host disease.

Reactive Lesions

These include. for example. pyogenic granulomas and peripheral giant cell granulomas.

Erosions

These are caused by burns, and vesiculobullous disorders, such as lichen planus, erythema multiforme, mucous membrane pemphigoid and pemphigus.

Atrophy

These are caused by:
- erythroplakia: one of the more important causes of a localised red lesion, since it is pre-neoplastic (see Chapter 51)
- erythema migrans (geographic tongue): manifests with irregular depapillated red areas, which change in size and shape, usually in the dorsum of the tongue
- lichen planus and lupus erythematosus: may present with atrophic red areas in some forms. These may be visible in any part of the oral mucosa including the lips
- desquamative gingivitis: a fairly common problem in which the gingivae show chronic desquamation and is a term that denotes a particular clinical picture and not a diagnosis in itself. Many of the patients are middle-aged women. Desquamative gingivitis is mainly a manifestation of:
  - mucocutaneous disorders, usually. Most gingival atrophy is related to lichen planus, but pemphigus, chronic ulcerative stomatitis and other conditions may need to be excluded. Most of these conditions are acquired, but a few are congenital with a strong hereditary predisposition, such as epidermolysis bullosa.
- chemical damage, such as reactions to sodium lauryl sulphate in toothpaste
- allergic responses
- drugs.

Some patients make no complaint, but others complain of persistent gingival soreness, worse when eating spices, or acidic foods, such as tomatoes or citrus fruits. Most patients are seen only when vesicles and bullae have broken down to leave desquamation, and the clinical appearance is thus of erythematous gingivae, mainly labially, the erythema and loss of stippling extending apically from the gingival margins to the alveolar mucosae. The desquamation may vary from mild almost insignificant small patches to widespread erythema with a glazed appearance. In addition to a full history and examination, biopsy examination and histopathological and immunological investigations are frequently indicated. Conditions that should be excluded include:

- reactions to mouthwashes, chewing gum, medications and dental materials
- candidiasis
- lupus erythematosus
- plasma cell gingivitis
- Crohn disease, sarcoidosis and orofacial granulomatosis
- leukaemias
- factitial (self-induced) lesions.
  The treatment of desquamative gingivitis consists of:
- Making a diagnosis
- improving the oral hygiene
- minimising irritation of the lesions
- specific therapies for the underlying disease where available
- local or systemic immunosuppressive, notably corticosteroids or immunomodulatory drugs.
  Corticosteroid creams used overnight in a soft polythene splint may help.
- Iron or vitamin deficiency states: may cause glossitis or other red lesions.

Purpura

Bleeding into the skin and mucosa is usually caused by trauma (Box 23.2), occasional small traumatic petechiae at the occlusal line (or elsewhere) are seen in otherwise healthy patients (Fig. 23.2). Less common causes include (Box 23.3):

- angina bullosa haemorrhagica: an idiopathic, fairly common, cause of purpura or blood blisters, seen only in the mouth, pharynx or oesophagus, mainly in the soft palate, in older persons and induced by trauma
- a blood platelet disorder such as thrombocytopenia: red or brown pinpoint lesions (petechiae) or diffuse bruising

(ecchymoses) are seen, mainly at sites of trauma, such as at the junction of the hard and soft palate (and often extraorally).

Vascular Anomalies (Angiomas and Telangiectasia)

These can be caused by:

- dilated lingual veins (varices): these may be conspicuous in the older in the ventrum of the tongue and may cause unnecessary alarm. Similar lesions may be seen in the lip
- haemangiomas: these are usually small isolated developmental anomalies or hamartomas. Rarely, orofacial angiomas may be more extensive and part of the Sturge—Weber syndrome (haemangioma with epilepsy and hemiplegia; see Chapter 54

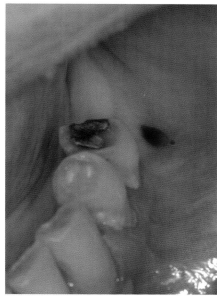

Fig. 23.2 Petechiae from trauma.

BOX 23.2 Causes of Oral Purpura

- Trauma
- Suction or trauma from:
  - appliances
  - habits
  - coughing
  - vomiting
- Localised oral purpura (angina bullosa haemorrhagica)
- Platelet disorders
- Autoimmune thrombocytopenia (idiopathic thrombocytopenic purpura)
- Drugs
- Aplastic anaemia
- Leukaemia
- Amyloidosis
- Infections:
  - infectious mononucleosis
  - rubella
  - HIV infection
- Gammopathies
- Vascular disorders
- Scurvy
- Ehlers—Danlos syndrome

BOX 23.3 Causes of White Oral Lesions

Congenital (e.g. leukoedema, Fordyce spots, white sponge naevus)
Lichen planus, lichenoid reactions, lupus erythematosus
Infections:
    Candidiasis (candidal leukoplakia)
        Hairy leukoplakia
        Syphilitic mucous patches and keratosis
        Koplik spots (measles)
        Some papillomas
        Neoplasms and potentially premalignant oral epithelial lesions:
Carcinoma
Leukoplakia
Keratoses:
    Frictional keratosis (and cheek/lip biting)
    Smoker's keratosis
    Snuff-dipper's keratosis

- telangiectasias (dilated capillaries): these may be seen after irradiation of the mouth and in various systemic disorders, such as hereditary haemorrhagic telangiectasia, systemic sclerosis and primary biliary cirrhosis.

Neoplasms

Red neoplasms include the following:
- peripheral giant cell tumour
- angiosarcomas, such as Kaposi sarcoma: a common neoplasm in HIV/AIDS, appears in the mouth as red or purplish areas or nodules, especially seen on the palate
- squamous cell carcinoma

- Wegener granulomatosis
- lymphoma.

Diagnosis

Diagnosis of red lesions is mainly clinical; lesions should also be sought on the skin or other mucosae. It may be necessary to take a blood picture (including blood and platelet count) and assess haemostatic function or exclude vitamin deficiencies, and/or aspiration, biopsy or imaging may be indicated (Algorithm 23.1 and Table 23.1).

Treatment

Treatment is of the underlying cause.

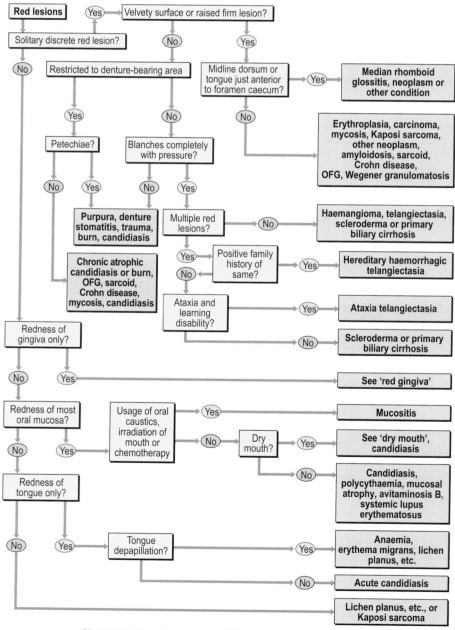

Algorithm 23.1 Red lesions. *OFG*, Orofacial granulomatosis.

TABLE 23.1 **Investigations That Might Be Helpful in Diagnosis/Prognosis/Management in Some Patients With Persistent Red Lesions**[a]	
In Most Cases	**In Some Cases**
Biopsy	Aspiration
	Diascopy (blanching on pressure)
	Full blood picture
	Serum ferritin, vitamin B_{12} and corrected whole blood folate levels
	Erythrocyte sedimentation rate
	Microbiological swabs

[a]See text for details and glossary for abbreviations.

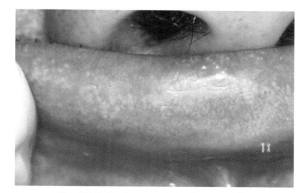

Fig. 23.3 Fordyce spots in the upper lip.

WHITE LESIONS

Introduction

Lesions in the mouth may be white because there is material (e.g. candidiasis or material alba (debris from poor oral hygiene)) on the epithelial surface, or the epithelium is thickened (e.g. in keratosis, lichen planus or leukoplakia).

An acronym by which to remember the causes is CLINK:

- congenital (e.g. leukoedema and white sponge naevus)
- Lichen planus (see Chapter 8)
- infections (e.g. candidiasis or hairy leukoplakia) (see Chapters 36 and 39)
- neoplastic and potentially premalignant oral epithelial lesions (see Chapter 49)
- keratosis.

Some other common conditions are yellowish rather than white in colour, such as Fordyce spots/granules and geographic tongue but they may cause diagnostic confusion. Burn, scars, grafts and furred or hairy tongue may also be white.

Fordyce Spots

Fordyce spots, also known as Fordyce granules, are creamy yellowish soft granules beneath the oral mucosa, usually seen along the border between the vermilion and the oral mucosa of the upper lip (Fig. 23.3) and in the buccal mucosa, particularly, inside the commissures, and also in the retromolar regions and lips. They are sebaceous glands containing neutral lipids similar to those found in skin sebaceous glands, but they are not associated with hair follicles.

Probably 80% of the population have Fordyce spots but they are not usually evident in infants (though they are present histologically), appearing clinically in children after the age of 3 years, increasing during puberty and then again in later adult life. They are noticeable mainly in adults, more prominent in men and seem to be more obvious:

- with advancing age
- patients with greasy skin
- in hyperlipidaemia
- Muir-Torre syndrome.

Fordyce spots are totally benign, though the occasional patient or physician becomes concerned about them or misdiagnoses them as, for example, candidiasis or lichen planus. No treatment is reliable or indicated, other than reassurance.

Keratosis

(A) Frictional keratosis

Frictional keratosis is a benign, trauma-induced lesion of the oral mucosa, usually caused by a parafunctional habit. The most common sites are the buccal mucosa, the lateral/ventral tongue, and the lower labial mucosa. It presents as asymptomatic, poorly demarcated, thickened, shaggy, white plaques. Linea alba (occlusal line) is a simple line of frictional keratosis seen in the buccal mucosae, horizontally aligned with the occlusal surfaces of the teeth, sometimes with small vertical lines coincident with the interdental areas. It is a benign lesion. Patients should be reassured.

(B) Smoker's keratosis

Leukoedema

Leukoedema is not a mucosal disease — simply the description of very faint whitish lines in some normal buccal mucosae, seen very often in people of African heritage. It is the result of fluid accumulation within keratinocytes. The whitish lines are bilateral and disappear if the mucosa is stretched (a diagnostic test). A biopsy is rarely necessary. The condition is benign.

White Sponge Naevus

White sponge nevus is a rare autosomal dominant disorder caused by a mutation in genes associated with keratin-4 or keratin-13. The lesions appear at birth, early childhood or adolescence and usually present bilaterally as asymptomatic, thick, white plaques, usually on the buccal mucosa, ventral tongue, lip mucosa and soft palate. It is a benign inherited condition. There is no effective treatment.

Other White Lesions

White lesions can be due to materia alba (debris from poor oral hygiene) but are mainly traumatic or inflammatory in cases such as candidiasis or hairy leukoplakia.

Diagnosis

Collections of debris (materia alba) or fungi (candidiasis) may look white, but these can usually easily be wiped off with a dry sterile gauze swab. Other lesions appear white usually because they are composed of thickened keratin, which looks white when wet, and these lesions, being inherent in the mucosa, will not wipe away with a gauze swab.

White lesions are usually painless but can be focal, multi-focal, striated or diffuse, and these features may give a guide to the diagnosis. For example:

- Focal lesions are often caused by cheek-biting (Fig. 23.4), at the occlusal line (Fig. 23.5), where there are collapsed bullae (Fig. 23.6) or leukoplakia (Fig. 23.7).
- Multifocal lesions are common in thrush (pseudomembranous candidiasis) and lichen planus.
- Striated lesions are typical of lichen planus.
- Diffuse white areas are seen in the buccal mucosa in leukoedema, and in the palate in stomatitis nicotina.

Diagnosis of white lesions is mainly clinical; lesions should also be sought on the skin or other mucosae. Haematological tests and/or biopsy may be indicated (Algorithm 23.2; Table 23.2).

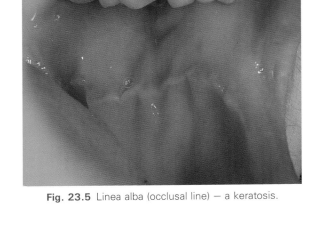
Fig. 23.5 Linea alba (occlusal line) — a keratosis.

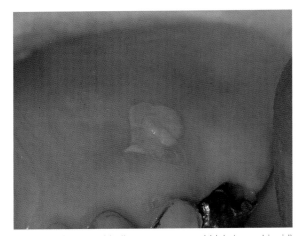
Fig. 23.6 Collapsed bullae can appear whitish (pemphigoid).

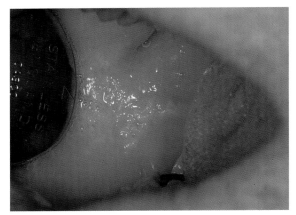
Fig. 23.4 Cheek biting is seen mainly around the occlusal area.

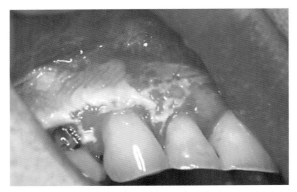
Fig. 23.7 Leukoplakia on the gingivae.

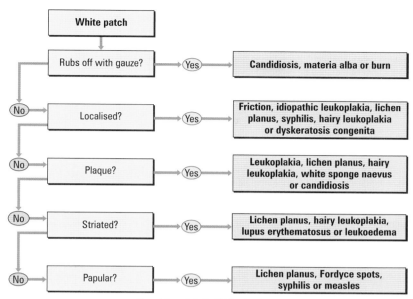

Algorithm 23.2 White lesions.

TABLE 23.2 Investigations in the Diagnosis/Prognosis/Management in Some Patients With Persistent White Lesions (Where the Lesion Does Not Wipe Off With a Gauze Swab)	
In Most Cases	**In Some Cases**
Biopsy	Full blood picture
	Serum ferritin, vitamin B_{12} and folate levels
	ESR
	Microbiological swabs
	Viral serology (hepatitis C virus, human immunodeficiency virus)
	Syphilis serology

Treatment

Treatment is usually of the underlying cause.

RECOMMENDED READING

Epstein, J.B., Gordon, S., 2013. Managing patients with red or red-white oral lesions. J. Can. Dent. Assoc. 79, d95.

Warnakulasuriya, S., 2019. White, red, and mixed lesions of oral mucosa: a clinicopathologic approach to diagnosis. Periodontol. 2000. 80 (1), 89—104.

Pigmented Brown or Black Lesions

INTRODUCTION

Oral mucosal discolouration, which ranges from brown to black may be due to extrinsic (exogenous) or intrinsic (endogenous) causes, the latter usually being more important. Extrinsic causes are usually superficial and intrinsic are usually deep in or beneath mucosa.

AETIOLOGY AND PATHOGENESIS

The most common causes of intrinsic pigmentation are racial (physiological), vascular, freckles, naevi, macules and melanomas. Main extrinsic causes include drugs, smoking and tattoos. Causes are shown in Boxes 24.1 and 24.2.

Extrinsic Discolouration

Extrinsic discolouration is rarely of serious consequence, usually being caused by coloured foods, drinks or drugs, when both mucosae and teeth may be discoloured. Causes include:
- Foods and beverages, such as beetroot, red wine, fruit juices, coffee and tea.
- Confectionery, such as liquorice and coloured candies.
- Drugs, such as chlorhexidine, iron salts, griseofulvin, crack cocaine, minocycline, bismuth subsalicylate, lansoprazole and HRT, and stains such as gentian violet and toluidine blue.
- Tobacco: may cause extrinsic brown staining and may also cause intrinsic pigmentary incontinence, with pigment cells increasing and appearing in the lamina propria — especially in persons who smoke with the lighted end of the cigarette within the mouth (reverse smoking), as practised in some Asian communities. Tobacco is a risk factor for potentially malignant disorders and cancer.
- Betel: this may cause a brownish-red extrinsic discolouration, mainly on the teeth and in the buccal mucosa, with an irregular epithelial surface that has a tendency to desquamate. Betel chewing is seen mainly in women from South and Southeast Asia; the mucosa epithelium is often hyperplastic, and histologically brownish amorphous material from the betel quid may be seen on the epithelial surface and intra- and intercellularly, with the ballooning of epithelial cells. This betel chewer's mucosa is not known to be precancerous, but betel use predisposes to submucous fibrosis and potentially malignant disorders and cancer.
- Black or brown hairy tongue (Fig. 24.1). Black hairy tongue affects mainly the posterior tongue; the filiform papillae are excessively long. The discolouration may vary from yellow to brown to black and usually involves the anterior and middle thirds of the dorsal tongue. It appears to be caused by the accumulation of epithelial squames and proliferation of chromogenic micro-organisms. It is more common:
  - in smokers
  - in people with hyposalivation
  - where the diet is soft
  - where various agents are used antimicrobials (penicillin, cephalosporin, chloramphenicol, streptomycin and tetracycline), corticosteroids, oxygenating mouth rinses, NSAIDs and psychotropics
  - where oral hygiene is wanting and also seen with much greater frequency in drug addicts, alcoholics and patients infected with HIV.

The discontinuation of smoking, oxygenating mouth rinses, and antibiotics may help the condition resolve. Patients with black hairy tongue may also find the condition improved by:
- increasing their oral hygiene
- using a tongue scraper
- brushing the tongue before retiring at night, with a hard toothbrush and cold water
- using sodium bicarbonate mouthwashes
- eating pineapple or sucking a peach stone
- chewing gum.

Superficial transient brown discolouration of the dorsum of the tongue and sometimes other soft tissues may be caused by

BOX 24.1 Common Causes of Brown Pigmented Mucosal Lesions

Intrinsic: Increased Melanin
- Racial
- Ephelis (freckle)
- Pigmentary incontinence
- Melanotic macule
- Naevus
- Hypoadrenalism (Addison disease)
- Malignant melanoma
- Drugs
- Vascular

Extrinsic: Exogenous Pigments
- Amalgam tattoo
- Smoking
- Ornamental tattoo
- Graphite tattoo
- Drugs and heavy metals

BOX 24.2 Further Causes of Hyperpigmentation

Localised
- Ephelis (freckle)
- Melanotic macule
- Naevus
- Amalgam, graphite, carbon, dyes, inks or other tattoos
- Black hairy tongue
- Extravasated haemorrhage:
  - haematoma
  - ecchymosis
  - purpura
  - petechiae
- Kaposi sarcoma
- Malignant melanoma
- Vascular: hamartomas, haemangiomas
- Melanoacanthoma
- Pigmented neuroectodermal tumour
- Verruciform xanthoma
- Epithelioid angiomatosis

Multiple or Generalised
- Genetic:
  - racial (physiological)
  - Peutz–Jeghers syndrome
  - Carney syndrome (Chapter 54)
  - isolated mucocutaneous melanotic pigmentation (IMMP)
  - Laugier–Hunziker syndrome (Chapter 54)
  - Lentiginosis profusa
  - Leopard syndrome (Chapter 54)
- Drugs (Table 33.12)
- Metals (bismuth, mercury, silver, gold, arsenic, copper, chromium, cobalt, manganese)
- Smoking
- Endocrine:
- Pregnancy
- Post-inflammatory
- Addison disease
- Albright syndrome
- Nelson syndrome
- Others:
  - haemochromatosis
  - HIV/AIDS
  - Wilson disease
  - Gaucher disease
  - generalised neurofibromatosis
  - incontinentia pigmenti
  - thalassaemia
  - Whipple disease

cigarette smoking, tobacco or betel chewing, some drugs (such as iron salts), some foods and beverages (such as coffee and tea), liquorice and chlorhexidine. Such discolouration is easily brushed off. Topical podophyllin and tretinoin have been advocated by some.

Intrinsic Discolouration

Intrinsic discolouration may have more significance than the extrinsic type. Normal intrinsic pigmentation is due to melanin, produced by melanocytes — dendritic cells prominent in the basal epithelium. This originates from the amino acid tyrosine, which is converted to dihydroxyphenylalanine (DOPA) and thence to melanin. The colour can vary from brown to blue or black, depending on the amount and location of the melanin. Increased melanin or the number of melanocytes, or other materials can cause intrinsic (endogenous) hyperpigmentation.

Vascular abnormalities are a common cause of oral and perioral discolouration. These may be developmental, e.g. hamartomas, traumatic leading to extravasated haemosiderin, e.g. haematomas, or melanin, e.g. melanotic macules (see Box 24.2).

There are a number of miscellaneous lesions that can be associated with blue-brown discolouration and these include pyogenic granuloma, peripheral ossifying fibroma, mucoceles, lymphomas and metastatic cancers.

Generalised Hyperpigmentation

Generalised pigmentation, often affecting the gingivae mainly, is common in persons of Asian or African origin, and is racial (Figs 24.2 and 24.3).
- Racial pigmentation: this is the most usual cause of patchy or generalised brown oral mucosal pigmentation, caused by melanin. Seen mainly in people of African or Asian heritage, it can also be noted in patients of Mediterranean

descent, sometimes even in some fairly light-skinned people. It is most obvious in the anterior labial gingivae and palatal mucosa, and the pigmentation is usually symmetrically distributed. Patches may be seen elsewhere. Pigmentation may be first noted by the patient in adult life and then incorrectly assumed to be acquired rather than congenital in origin.

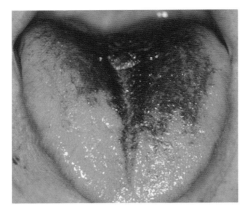

Fig. 24.1 Black hairy tongue.

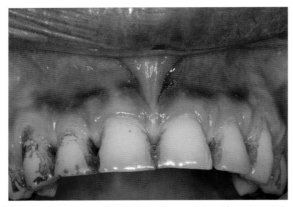

Fig. 24.2 Racial pigmentation (the teeth are stained from betel chewing and poor oral hygiene).

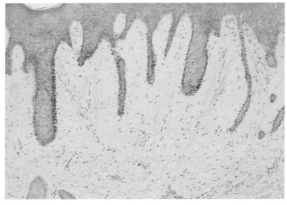

Fig. 24.3 Racial pigmentation showing melanin-containing cells in the basal epithelium.

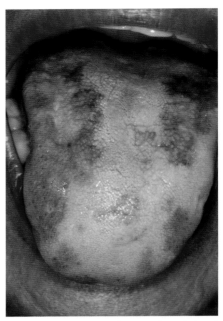

Fig. 24.4 Post-inflammatory hyperpigmentation of the dorsum of the tongue, in oral lichen planus

- Drugs: generalised hyperpigmentation or pigmentation may be induced sometimes with the pigmentation of the skin or other areas:
  - Smoking tobacco is a fairly common cause (smoker's melanosis).
  - Antimalarials produce a variety of colours in the mucosa, ranging from yellow with mepacrine to blue-black with amodiaquine.
  - Zidovudine and adrenocorticotrophic hormone (ACTH) therapy may both produce brown pigmentation
  - Busulphan, some other cytotoxic drugs, oral contraceptives, phenothiazines and anticonvulsants may also occasionally produce, or increase, brown pigmentation.
  - Minocycline may cause blackish discolouration of the teeth, gingivae and bone, palate, skin and sclera.
  - Gold may produce purplish gingival discolouration.
  - Many of the other heavy metals formerly implicated in producing oral pigmentation (such as mercury, lead and bismuth) are not used therapeutically now, although industrial or accidental exposures still occur, fortunately rarely. Metallic sulphides deposited in the tissues are seen especially where oral hygiene is poor, and bacteria produce sulphides, resulting in pigmentation at the gingival margin (e.g. lead line).
- Hypoadrenalism (Addison disease): uncommon but may cause generalised or patchy hyperpigmentation due to excessive production of ACTH, which has activities similar to melanocyte-stimulating hormone (MSH). Addison disease is usually autoimmune (idiopathic), but hypoadrenalism may be seen in HIV disease. Hyperpigmentation is generalised but is most obvious in areas normally pigmented (e.g. the areolae of nipples, genitalia), skin flexures and sites

- Chronic inflammation, such as in lichen planus, can result in melanin drop-out, especially in persons with pigmented skin. This oral pigmentation (pigmentary incontinence or post-inflammatory hyperpigmentation) is often gingival or buccal but sometimes lingual (Fig. 24.4). It may be termed post-inflammatory hyperpigmentation.

of trauma. The oral mucosa may show patchy hyperpigmentation. Patients with Addison's disease also typically have weakness and weight loss, and hypotension.

- Nelson syndrome: this is a rare condition caused by ACTH overproduction in response to adrenalectomy, usually for breast cancer.
- Melanin pigmentation increases under hormonal stimulation, either by MSH, or in pregnancy, or rarely due to the action of ACTH, the molecule of which is similar to MSH, or under the influence of other factors (e.g. smoking).
- Peutz–Jeghers syndrome: a rare autosomal-dominant condition, in which oral and circumoral patchy brown pigmentation is seen with small-intestinal polyps (circumoral melanosis with intestinal polyposis). A similar condition without intestinal polyps has been termed isolated mucocutaneous melanotic pigmentation (IMMP); both conditions may be associated with various malignant neoplasms (see Chapter 49 and 53).

Localised Areas of Pigmentation

Localised areas of pigmentation may be caused by the above but are usually caused by:

- Embedded amalgam (Fig. 24.5). An amalgam tattoo is the most common cause of a single patch of macular blue-black pigmentation, does not change significantly in size or colour, is painless and is usually seen in the mandibular gingiva or at least close to the teeth or an apicectomy where there has been a retrograde amalgam root-end filling. The diagnosis is clinical, but the lesion may be radio-opaque. Tattoos are best excised to confirm the diagnosis and exclude naevi or melanoma.
- Embedded graphite (graphite tattoo) may be seen, for example, where a pencil lead has broken off in the mucosa. Tattoos are best excised to exclude naevi or melanoma.
- Other foreign bodies.

Local Irritation/Inflammation

- Melanotic macules (Fig. 24.6): these are usually single, brown, collections of melanin-containing cells. Melanotic macules are flat and mostly smaller than 1 cm and contain increased melanin, do not change rapidly in size or colour, are painless and are seen particularly on the vermilion border of the lip and on the palate. They are seen mainly in white people and are innocuous. Most arise slowly, but occasionally they rapidly appear. They are best removed to exclude melanoma.
- Naevi: these are blue-black lesions formed from increased melanin-containing cells (naevus cells) usually smaller than 1 cm. Some 60% are papular, they do not change rapidly in size or colour, are painless and are seen particularly on the palate. Approximately half of naevi are histologically of the intradermal (intramucosal) type when the melanin is in the lamina propria, one-third are blue naevi, others are compound naevi, and some are junctional. There is no evidence that naevi, except rare junctional naevi, progress to melanoma. However, naevi may clinically resemble

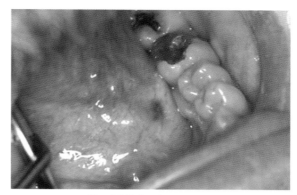

Fig. 24.5 Amalgam tattoo

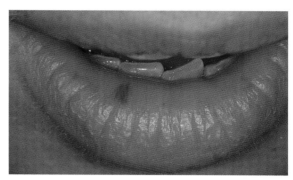

Fig. 24.6 Labial melanotic macule

melanomas and are therefore usually best removed to exclude melanoma. The melanocyte-specific gene (MSG-1) is expressed in some cases of malignant melanoma but is absent in all benign naevi.

- Malignant melanoma: this is rare but may arise in apparently normal mucosa or a pre-existent pigmented naevus, usually in the palate or maxillary gingivae. About one-third of melanomas arise in areas of hyperpigmentation. Mucosal melanoma of the oral cavity may present as a painless bleeding mass, ulceration, area of discolouration or with ill-fitting dentures. Features suggestive of malignancy include a rapid increase in size, change in colour, ulceration, pain, the occurrence of satellite pigmented spots or regional lymph node enlargement. However, up to 15% of melanomas are amelanotic. Superficial melanomas have a better prognosis than nodular ones. Radical excision is indicated.
- Other neoplasms, such as Kaposi sarcoma, pigmented neuroectodermal tumour or palatal pigmentation from ACTH-producing bronchogenic carcinoma.
- Melanoacanthoma: in some adults of African descent, larger lesions, from 5 to 20 mm in diameter, termed 'melanoacanthomas', may be seen. These are seen mainly in the buccal mucosa or palate in females, may appear rapidly and are probably reactive rather than neoplastic lesions. They are best removed.

DIAGNOSIS AND MANAGEMENT

The nature of hyperpigmentation can sometimes only be established after further investigation (Table 24.1).

Management of Generalised or Multiple Hyperpigmentation

Systemic causes should be excluded, and therefore, the following may be indicated:

- Blood pressure: to exclude Addison disease (hypotension is characteristic).
- Plasma cortisol levels: to exclude Addison disease (low levels found).
- An ACTH stimulation (Synacthen) test: to exclude Addison's disease (an impaired response is typical).
- Endocrinological or gastroenterological opinions.
- HIV serology or opinion.
- Bone imaging to exclude Albright syndrome (Chapter 54).

Management of Localised Hyperpigmentation

- Radiographs may be helpful, as they can sometimes reveal amalgam, graphite or a foreign body, or (in pigmented neuroectodermal tumour of infancy) bone rarefaction. In the latter, the urinary catecholamines are raised.
- Biopsy. If early detection of oral melanomas is to be achieved, all pigmented oral cavity lesions should be viewed with suspicion. The consensus of opinion is that a lesion with the following clinical features is seriously suggestive of being a malignant melanoma, and is best biopsied at the time of definitive operation:
  - a solitary raised lesion
  - a rapid increase in size
  - change in colour
  - ulceration
  - pain
  - evidence of satellite pigmented spots
  - regional lymph node enlargement.
- Photographs may be useful for future comparison of size and colour.

TABLE 24.1 Investigations That Might Be Helpful in Diagnosis/Prognosis/Management in Some Patients with Pigmented Lesions[a]

In Many Cases	In Some Cases
Biopsy	Full blood picture
	Serum ferritin, vitamin B_{12} and corrected whole blood folate levels
	HIV test
	Blood pressure
	Plasma cortisol
	ACTH stimulation test
	Oral radiography
	Chest radiography
	Urinary catecholamines
	Endocrine opinion
	Gastroenterological opinion

[a]See text for details and glossary for abbreviations.

Management is of the underlying condition. Excision biopsy of isolated hyperpigmented lesions is often recommended to exclude malignancy, and because of the malignant potential of some others (particularly the junctional naevus) and for cosmetic reasons. This is particularly important if the lesions are raised or nodular or have clinical features as above seriously suggestive of being malignant melanoma.

RECOMMENDED READING

Alawi, F., 2013. Pigmented lesions of the oral cavity: an update. Dent. Clin. North. Am. 57 (4), 699–710.

Lambertini, M., Patrizi, A., Ravaioli, G.M., et al., 2018. Oral pigmentation in physiologic conditions, post-inflammatory affections and systemic diseases. G. Ital. Dermatol. Venereol. 153 (5), 666–671.

Meleti, M., Vescovi, P., Mooi, W.J., et al., P2008. Pigmented lesions of the oral mucosa and perioral tissues: a flow-chart for the diagnosis and some recommendations for the management. Oral. Surg. Oral. Med. Oral. Pathol. Oral. Radiol. Endod. 5 (105), 606–616

Rosebush, M.S., Briody, A.N., Cordell, K.G., 2019. Black and brown: non-neoplastic pigmentation of the oral mucosa. Head. Neck Pathol. 13 (1), 47–55.

Cheilitis

Inflammation of the lips (cheilitis) has a broad differential and includes, inflammatory causes such as eczema (also termed exfoliative cheilitis), granulomatous as seen in oral Crohn's or orofacial granulomatosis (Chapter 32), trauma from repeated picking or habits such as lip licking, the infection which may be primary or secondary, drug-induced, e.g. isotretinoin, auto-immune conditions such as lichen planus (Chapter 8), lupus erythematosus or the immunobullous diseases (Chapters 30 and 31), actinic cheilitis or graft versus host disease (Table 25.1). The diagnosis is often made from the history and clinical findings, but in certain conditions where there is a risk of malignant change, a biopsy may be required, e.g. actinic cheilitis.

This chapter will focus on actinic cheilitis and exfoliative cheilitis.

ACTINIC CHEILITIS

Actinic cheilitis (actinic keratosis, solar keratosis, solar cheilosis; solar cheilitis) from the Greek *aktino* = rays and *cheili* = lips) is common in sun-overexposed individuals and is essentially a burn. Chronic actinic cheilitis is a potentially malignant disorder caused by chronic exposure to solar radiation. Although numerous studies have assessed the association between actinic cheilitis and squamous cell carcinoma (SCC), no accurate data is available on the rates of malignant transformation.

Epidemiology

- A number of studies have placed the rate at approximately 10% to 30%. Up to 95% of cases of SCC of the lips are preceded by actinic cheilitis. Thus, early diagnosis and treatment are essential.

- Although it can occur at any age, the disease is more common in older adults in their fifth to eighth decade.
- Most prevalent in men.
- The frequency is higher in geographical areas with high ultraviolet (UV) radiation, in open-air workers and people with fair skin.

Predisposing Factors

Ultraviolet light from the sun can damage the lips and skin. The vermilion of the lower lip is almost at the right angles to rays of the sun and is poorly protected by keratin and melanocytes. Commonly seen in Caucasians in the tropics, less in people with darker skin types. Particularly at risk are people whose lifestyles include much time spent outdoors, especially farmers, sailors, fishermen, windsurfers, skiers, mountaineers, golfers, etc.

Other forms of radiation including arc-welding can occasionally cause similar damage. Actinic cheilitis rarely may be an early manifestation of genetic susceptibility to light damage, as in xeroderma pigmentosum. Immune defects (including immunosuppression in organ transplant recipients) also predispose to malignant transformation.

Clinical Features

Actinic cheilitis is most common on the lower lip, with sparing of the oral commissures. In the early acute stages, the lip may be red and oedematous with cracks or ulcers. Repeated exposure to UV radiation over long periods produces chronic tissue changes and the lip may become dry, scaly and atrophic. Lesions may appear as a smooth or scaly, friable patch or can involve the entire lip, later, becoming palpably thickened with small greyish-white plaques (Fig. 25.1). The border between the vermilion and the skin or

TABLE 25.1   Differential Diagnosis of Cheilitis

- Trauma/habit — lip licking
- Inflammatory, e.g. eczema/ exfoliative cheilitis
- Granulomatous — e.g. oral Crohn disease, orofacial granulomatosis
- Drugs, e.g. isotretinoin
- Lichen planus
- Lupus erythematosus
- Immunobullous disorders, e.g. pemphigus vulgaris, mucous membrane pemphigoid
- Actinic cheilitis
- Graft versus host disease

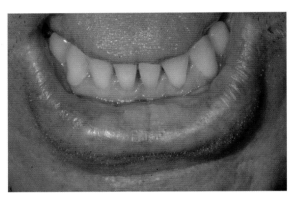

Fig. 25.1 Chronic actinic cheilitis.

mucosa becomes indistinct. Eventually, warty nodules may form, which may evolve into SCC. Suspicious features include pain, chronic ulceration, a speckled area, generalised atrophy with focal areas of whitish thickening, persistent flaking and crusting.

Diagnosis

A careful history and a biopsy are indicated. A biopsy should be taken from an area representative of the lesion's severity, as well as from areas with atrophy, ulceration or induration. Histologically, the epithelium in actinic cheilitis can present with hyperkeratosis, hyperparakeratosis, atrophy, acanthosis or loss of polarity of the basal keratinocytes. Various degrees of dysplasia and/or carcinoma may occur. The differential diagnosis includes lupus erythematosus, lichen planus, leukoplakia, SCC and a variety of forms of cheilitis such as exfoliative cheilitis and contact cheilitis.

Treatment

Prevention is advised, especially in high-risk individuals (patients with photosensitivity disorders, xeroderma pigmentosum, transplant recipients and those taking immunosuppressive drugs), and those whose exposure to UVB is high. Wearing broad-brimmed hats, using a broad-spectrum sunscreen

TABLE 25.2   Regimens That Might Be Helpful in Management of Patient Suspected of Having Solar Cheilosis

Regimen	Use in Secondary Care
PDT	Photodynamic therapy (PDT)
Surgery	Cryotherapy, electrodessication, CO_2 laser ablation, YAG laser therapy, surgical excision with the advancement of a mucosal flap (vermilionectomy; lip shave)
Topical	5- Fluorouracil 5% Imiquimod 5% 3% Diclofenac in 2.5% hyaluronic acid
Supportive	Sunscreens and sun protection

(protection against both UVA and UVB rays) applied generously and reapplied, and avoiding mid-day sun exposure is advised.

Management of established actinic cheilitis is required both to relieve symptoms and to endeavour to prevent the development of OSCC. In a recent systematic review of 49 studies, the highest success rates were seen with surgical approaches, laser therapy (mainly ablative CO_2 laser) or photodynamic therapy with aminolaevulinic acid. However, these approaches require specialist expertise and are expensive.

Topical chemotherapeutic approaches, e.g. topical applications of fluorouracil (5-FU) or 5% imiquimod have a good success rate of approximately 75% and are straightforward to prescribe and administer. Repeated courses over 2 to 3 weeks provide incremental success.

Less successful approaches (30% to 50%) include 3% diclofenac with 2.5% hyaluronic acid, and 0.015% ingenol mebutate or trichloroacetic acid (Table 25.2).

Following treatment, regular use of protective sunscreen is advised.

Follow-Up

Actinic cheilitis carries a potential for malignant development, necessitating periodic clinical check-ups. If there is any change causing concern, during the follow-up visits, a biopsy or additional biopsies should be performed.

EXFOLIATIVE CHEILITIS

Exfoliative cheilitis is an uncommon inflammatory condition affecting the vermilion border of one of both lips that result in peeling, cracking, pain or burning and is a significant cause of morbidity (Fig. 25.2). It is often ongoing with fluctuations in severity. Patients frequently search tirelessly for a solution and try numerous ointments and balms to ease symptoms. Making the diagnosis is essential as early as possible to break the habits that patients develop, explain the underlying cause and introduce optimal multidisciplinary approaches to management. The precise cause is unknown, but it is frequently associated with atopy or seborrheic dermatitis and is therefore often considered to be a localised form of eczema. There is very little literature on this condition.

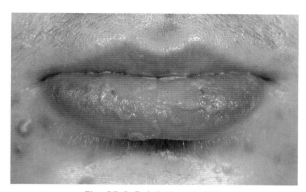

Fig. 25.2 Exfoliative cheilitis

Epidemiology

- Patients may present in adolescence or early adulthood although later presentation is also seen.
- Males and females may be affected.
- Age of onset varies.

Predisposing Factors

An underlying tendency to eczema is present in about 40% of patients. Additionally, underlying mental health problems are also frequently present ranging from stress and anxiety to combined anxiety and depression, obsessive-compulsive disorders and eating disorders. Contact dermatitis may be relevant in a significant proportion of patients. Secondary infection is also very frequent.

Clinical Features

Patients slowly develop a tendency to dry, peeling lips at the onset. They find themselves picking and peeling the dry skin away and start to apply copious amounts of emollient. This harbours bacteria and yeasts and needs to be minimised. Patients complain of pain, burning and discomfort. There is a large psychological morbidity which further exacerbates a tendency to anxiety or depression. Patients start to avoid wetting their lips in the shower and guard their lips trying as little as possible to have any contact with liquid or food. Some drink through a straw and allow large amounts of keratin to sit on the lip surface.

Diagnosis

This is a clinical diagnosis. A careful history is required to exclude another cause such as a drug. A biopsy is not indicated.

Swabs of the nose and mouth for microscopy, culture and sensitivity are vital and need to be repeated frequently. Patch testing is valuable.

Treatment

Modification of unhelpful habits such as lip licking is important. Limiting Vaseline or lip balms to occasional use. Wiping away the loose keratin each morning after a shower is important followed by twice daily application of topical tacrolimus 0.1% for 6 weeks to start with. This can be continued as needed to control the inflammation but to be avoided if direct sunlight is likely during the day. Maintenance with twice-weekly use ongoing is essential. Treating infection in the nose and mouth with antibiotics and anti-fungals is important. Antiseptic mouthwashes are also used daily (twice weekly chlorhexidine and five-times weekly hydrogen peroxide). Good oral hygiene is paramount. Avoid any identified allergic contact substances. Finally, and most importantly, a psychological assessment is recommended for those with mental health problems. Without this combined approach treatment will be unlikely to be successful.

Follow-Up

Initially quarterly and then as needed. Regular bacterial swabs needed. Ongoing psychological support is very helpful.

RECOMMENDED READING

Almazrooa, S.A., Woo, S.B., Mawardi, H., Treister, N., 2013. Characterization and management of exfoliative cheilitis: a single-center experience. Oral Surg. Oral Med. Oral Pathol. Oral Radiol. 116 (6), e485–e489.

Jadotte, Y.T., Schwartz, R.A., 2012. Solar cheilosis: an ominous precursor. J. Am. Acad. Dermatol. 66 (2), 187–198.

Lai, M., Pampena, R., Cornacchia, L., Pellacani, G., Peris, K., Longo, C., 2019. Treatments of actinic cheilitis: a systematic review of the literature. J. Am. Acad. Dermatol. 83 (3), 876–887.

Salgueiro, A.P., de Jesus, L.H., de Souza, I.F., Rados, P.V., Visioli, F., 2019. Treatment of actinic cheilitis: a systematic review. Clin. Oral. Investig. 23 (5), 2041–2053.

Vieira, R.A.M.A.R., Minicucci, E.M., Marques, M.E.A., Marques, S.A., 2012. Actinic cheilitis and squamous cell carcinoma of the lip: clinical, histopathological and immunogenetic aspects. An. Bras. Dermatol. 87, 105–114.

Zhang, Q.Q., Xu, P., Sun, C., Liu, L.J., Jiang, W.W., 2020. Topical tacrolimus with different frequency for exfoliative cheilitis: a pilot study. J. Dermatolog. Treat. 23, 1–5.

Systemic Oral Diseases and Disorders

Sjögren Syndrome

KEY POINTS
- Sjögren syndrome (SS) is a chronic inflammatory autoimmune disorder characterised by diminished salivary and lacrimal gland secretion (sicca complex) and other exocrine glands.
- It is an autoimmune exocrinopathy.
- 95% of SS patients are women.
- SS can occur alone (primary SS) or alongside another autoimmune disease (secondary SS) such as lupus, rheumatoid arthritis and systemic sclerosis.
- Dry mouth predisposes to difficulty in speaking and swallowing.
- Complications may include oral infections, caries, candidiasis, sialadenitis and lymphoma.
- Diagnosis is confirmed by confirmation of hyposalivation, detection of serum ENA autoantibodies anti-Ro (SS-A) and other investigations including ultrasound and a labial salivary gland biopsy.

Treatment mainly symptomatic with sialogogues and salivary substitutes (mouth-wetting agents), maintenance of oral health and preventive dentistry.

INTRODUCTION

Sjögren syndrome (SS) is a chronic inflammatory autoimmune disorder in which immunocytes damage the salivary, lacrimal and other exocrine glands and is thus termed an autoimmune exocrinopathy. Dry mouth (xerostomia due to hyposalivation) and dry eyes (keratoconjunctivitis sicca) are seen with lymphoid infiltrates in salivary, lacrimal and other exocrine glands, and serum autoantibodies as discussed later (Fig. 26.1). Additional symptoms can include dryness of the skin, nose, throat and vagina; arthralgia and myalgia; peripheral neuropathies; pulmonary, thyroid and renal disorders; and lymphoma. SS has two major forms (Table 26.1):

- Primary Sjögren syndrome (pSS): in which dry eyes and dry mouth are seen in the absence of a connective tissue disease.
- Secondary Sjögren syndrome (sSS) is more common: dry eyes and dry mouth are seen together with other autoimmune diseases:
  - rheumatoid arthritis (RA)
  - systemic lupus erythematosus (SLE)
  - polymyositis
  - scleroderma
  - mixed connective tissue disease
  - primary biliary cholangitis (previously termed primary biliary cirrhosis).

EPIDEMIOLOGY

- Population prevalence of between 0.5% and 1.6% adults.
- SS can affect any age, but the onset is most common in middleage or older.
- The great majority of patients affected by SS are women, with a female-to-male ratio greater than 9:1.
- Two age peaks; the first after menarche (20s to 30s) and the second following menopause (mid-50s).
- There is no known geographic incidence to SS.

PREDISPOSING FACTORS

- Female gender. The high prevalence in females suggests a possible role for oestrogen and/or androgen deficiency. Females have higher baseline immunoglobulin levels and higher incidence of autoimmune diseases compared with males.

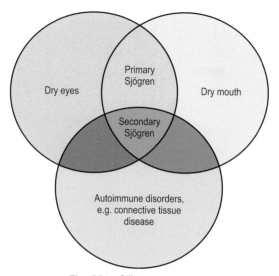

Fig. 26.1 Sjögren syndrome.

- Age peaks in 20s to 30s and after menopause
- SLE, RA, systemic sclerosis (scleroderma) — overlap with SS
- Genetic risk factors such as:
  - human leukocyte antigen (HLA) class II markers A1, B8 and DR3/DQ2, especially with HLADRB1*15-DRB1*0301, are linked with susceptibility to SS
  - signal transducer and activator of transcription 4 (STAT-4), interferon (IFN) responsive factor (IRF), immunoglobulin (Ig)-like transcript 6 (ILT6)
  - people with SS also more commonly have family members with other autoimmune disorders.
- Environmental risk factors, including possibly viral infections. A Sjögren-like syndrome can be produced by:
- viruses (Epstein—Barr virus (EBV), hepatitis C virus, retroviruses (human immunodeficiency virus [HIV], human T lymphotropic virus 1 [HTLV-1])
- IgG4 syndrome
- graft-versus-host-disease (see Chapter 34)
- SNOX syndrome (nonspecific sialadenitis, primary generalised nodal osteoarthritis, xerostomia).

AETIOLOGY AND PATHOGENESIS

SS is an autoimmune exocrinopathy. The pathogenesis of salivary gland damage is multifactorial, involving immunological, genetic, hormonal and viral components. In animal models of SS, environmental triggers such as infection by viruses and/or oestrogen deficiency can lead to the activation of mucosal epithelial cells. This leads to the activation of the innate and adaptive immune systems with the secretion of autoantibodies. This results in a cycle of immune-system activation that leads to tissue damage.

Multiple viruses have been implicated to have a role, although none have been shown to be causal. Lymphocytic infiltrates and salivary gland epithelial cells on biopsy have been found to have EBV DNA and antigens. Adenovirus infection has been showed to redistribute SS-B/La localisation, possibly inducing autoimmunity. Viruses can induce expression of B cell—activating factor (BAFF) by salivary gland epithelial cells via Toll-like receptor (TLR)- and IFN-dependent and -independent pathways. In mice at least, IRF5 and STAT4 gene polymorphisms are involved in the activation of type I IFN pathways, the isolated stimulation of innate immunity resulting in dryness, which precedes lymphocytic infiltrates in salivary glands. Immunologically activated or apoptotic glandular epithelial cells might drive autoimmune-mediated tissue injury with upregulation of type I IFN-regulated genes, abnormal expression of BAFF (a member of the tumour necrosis factor (TNF) family that promotes B-cell maturation, proliferation and survival) and activation of the interleukin (IL)-23 type-17 helper T cell pathway.

In SS, IFN-γ is upregulated, and CD40 can be further induced by IFN-γ and IL-1β cytokines. The antigen CD40 is constitutively expressed by salivary ductal epithelial cells and endothelial cells and on infiltrating lymphocytes but not by acinar cells, myoepithelial cells or fibroblasts. CD40 enhances expression of adhesion molecule intercellular adhesion molecule-1 (ICAM-1)/CD54.

In SS, salivary glands express functional TLRs including TLR2, -3 and -4. TLR-induced signalling typically culminates in activation of nuclear factor (NF)-κB, mitogen-activated protein kinase (MAPK) pathways and IRF, as well as production of inflammatory and immune cytokines.

TABLE 26.1 Sjögren Syndrome: Comparison of Subtypes		
Feature	**SS-1**	**SS-2**
Connective tissue disease	–	+
Oral involvement	More severe	Less severe
Ocular involvement	More common	Less common
Recurrent sialadenitis	More common	Less common
Lymphoma	More common	Less common
Main serum autoantibody	Ro/(La)	Ro, anti-CCP, rheumatoid factor, lupus autoantibodies

anti-CCP, cyclic citrullinated peptide; *SS*, Sjögren syndrome.

In SS, there may be intrinsic activation of epithelial cells through the MAPK pathway.

SS progresses through a number of stages:

- SS pathogenesis is related mainly to B-cell dysregulation, in part, from the survival and activation of self-reactive B cells, which produce tissue-damaging pathogenic autoantibodies. The presence of ectopic germinal centres in salivary glands highlights the B-cell activation. In pSS, the level of BAFF is increased in both the serum and salivary glands and provides a link between innate immunity and autoimmunity in disease pathogenesis.
- Early hypergammaglobulinaemia and autoantibody production: serum autoantibodies (especially antinuclear antibodies SS-A [Ro] and SS-B [La]) are common in pSS (~75%). ANAs (~90%), rheumatoid factor (~50%), antithyroglobulin antibodies (~25%) and antibodies to lacrimal and salivary gland extracts can also be seen.
- Decreased salivary gland function with early periductal lymphocytic infiltration and antibody deposition in the submandibular and parotid glands. Lymphocytic infiltration of the submandibular, parotid and lacrimal glands with B and T (mainly CD4) lymphocytes and plasma cells causes progressive exocrine glandular acinar destruction along with interstitial lung disease and mild renal disease.
- Large B-cell lymphoma.

The autoimmune response in SS usually mainly affects exocrine glands, particularly the salivary, lacrimal and vaginal. The epithelial cells in salivary glands of patients with SS are activated, bearing characteristics of antigen-presenting cells — inappropriate expression of class II HLA and costimulatory molecules. Salivary gland epithelial cells may participate in the development of the glandular inflammatory reactions via the expression and function of several TLR molecules. TLR signalling and antigen presentation may drive the autoimmune response and local autoantibody production in SS.

The autoantibodies found in SS are commonly against ribonucleoproteins, especially Ro (SS-A or SS-A) and La (SS-B) autoantibodies. There may also be other autoantibodies (e.g. alpha-fodrin, alpha-amylase, muscarinic M3 receptor, carbonic anhydrase, actin, salivary duct). There is periductal infiltration initially mainly by B but later mainly by T lymphocytes (Fig. 26.2).

Activated $CD4^+$ T helper type 1 (Th1) lymphocytes, B cells, macrophages and dendritic cells, as well as a network of cytokines including IFN-γ, TNF-α and IL-1β, cause tissue destruction and dysfunction, and IL-6 often acts as the end-stage effector cytokine in this cascade. IL-6 is upregulated in serum, peripheral circulating lymphocytes and saliva of SS patients and significantly correlates with the degree of infiltration in the gland and the number of extraglandular features.

The distribution of the membrane pore channel (water channel) protein aquaporin-5 is abnormal in SS, and the neurogenic regulation of the salivary gland also becomes impaired. Antimuscarinic 3 receptor antibody plays an important role in cholinergic hyperresponsiveness in SS.

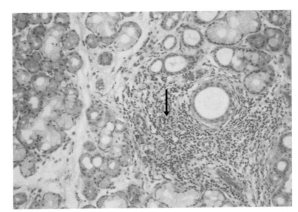

Fig. 26.2 Sjögren syndrome: histopathology showing dense lymphocytic periductal infiltrate (focal sialadenitis) (*arrowed*).

Salivary gland biopsies show foci of lymphocytic infiltrates, with anti-Ro— and anti-La—producing B cells present in the infiltrates. There is lymphocyte-mediated destruction of exocrine glandular acini, but, although the gland acini atrophy, the duct epithelium tends to persist and proliferates. The fully developed lesion of SS in major glands thus appears as a dense mass of lymphocytes interspersed by islands of epithelium, a pattern termed the 'benign lymphoepithelial lesion' (BLL). Occasionally, BLL exists in the absence of serological and other features of SS.

B-cell lymphoproliferation may eventually lead to pseudolymphoma or even true lymphoma.

CLINICAL FEATURES

The early manifestations may be nonspecific, such as fatigue, arthralgia and Raynaud phenomenon, and it can be 8 to 10 years from the initial symptoms to full-blown disease. SS ultimately presents with a clinical spectrum that ranges from an organ-specific autoimmune process to a systemic disorder (Box 26.1). It manifests as dryness of the mouth and eyes, fatigue and joint pain in more than 80% of patients. Other autoimmune disorders associated with SS may include SLE, scleroderma, mixed connective tissue disease, primary biliary cholangitis, hyperthyroidism (Graves disease) or hypothyroidism (Hashimoto thyroiditis). Mothers with SS can pass autoantibodies across the placenta into the foetal circulation — leading to foetal heart block.

Features of SS may include:

Glandular Presentation

- Eye symptoms — dry, itchy, burning or gritty eyes, redness, light intolerance, sensitivity to wind. The lacrimal glands may swell.
- Mouth symptoms (often the presenting feature) — dry mouth (xerostomia) (Fig. 26.3), soreness, burning, difficulty eating dry foods such as biscuits (the cracker sign), difficulty in swallowing dry foods, altered or decreased taste sensation, difficulty speaking for long periods (a clicking quality of the

BOX 26.1 Sjögren Syndrome Main Features

Oral Signs and Symptoms
- Dry mouth
- Cracker sign
- Burning
- Salivary swelling and sialadenitis
- Caries
- Candidiasis
- Abnormal taste
- Halitosis

Ocular Signs and Symptoms
- Foreign body sensation
- Inability to tear
- Light intolerance

Others
- Fatigue
- Constitutional symptoms
- Raynaud phenomenon
- Purpura
- Musculoskeletal
- Vasculitis
- Interstitial nephritis
- Peripheral neuropathy
- Cerebral vasculitis, transverse myelitis or demyelinating lesions
- Lymphadenopathy or lymphoma
- Interstitial pneumonitis
- Facial pain
- Venous thromboembolism
- B-cell lymphoma

speech as the tongue tends to stick to the palate), dental decay, difficulties in controlling dentures, halitosis, ascending (suppurative) sialadenitis, increased fungal and bacterial infections. Dentists are often first to detect these symptoms.

- Episodic swelling and tenderness of major salivary glands may be caused by bacterial ascending infection (acute sialadenitis; Fig. 26.4). Salivary gland enlargement is usually caused by the SS inflammatory process. Occasionally it is massive and associated with enlargement of the regional lymph nodes, a condition called 'pseudolymphoma'. Rarely is due to true lymphoma.

Oral and salivary gland examinations are important. The mouth may appear dry, and on examination there may be objective:
- hyposalivation
- tendency of the mucosa to stick to a dental mirror
- food residues (Fig. 26.5)
- lack of salivary pooling
- frothiness of saliva and absence of frank salivation from major gland duct orifices
- a characteristic tongue appearance; lobulated, usually red, surface with partial or complete depapillation
- in advanced cases — obviously dry and glazed oral mucosae.

Extraglandular Presentation (Fig. 26.6)

- Fatigue — often severe, may be the main complaint.
- Constitutional symptoms — fever, involuntary weight loss or night sweats.
- Raynaud phenomenon.
- Skin — palpable purpura, vasculitis or subacute cutaneous lupus.
- Musculoskeletal — arthritis, arthralgia and myalgia. SS patient often have a nondeforming inflammatory arthritis that involves the small joints of the hands and feet.
- Vasculitis — vasculitic skin disease (manifesting as a skin rash). Rarer — vasculitis of medium-sized vessels. Vasculitis

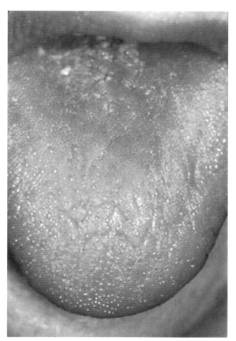

Fig. 26.3 Sjögren syndrome showing dry mouth.

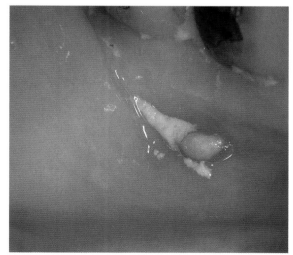

Fig. 26.4 Sjögren syndrome showing food residues in vestibule.

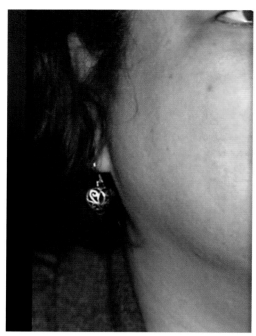

Fig. 26.5 Sjögren syndrome showing salivary swelling.

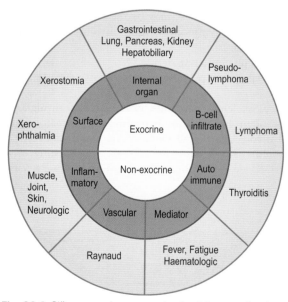

Fig. 26.6 Sjögren syndrome — extraglandular complications.

is associated with the presence of anti-Ro and anti-La antibodies and serum cryoglobulins.

- Renal — interstitial nephritis or cryoglobulinaemia-associated glomerulonephritis.
- Peripheral neuropathy — a small fibre neuropathy is the most common form of neuropathy in SS. Patients with neuropathy commonly have neuropathic pain. On examination, light touch, vibratory sensation and proprioception are affected.

TABLE 26.2   Risk Factors for the Development of Lymphoma
Recurrent swelling of parotid glands
Splenomegaly, lymphadenopathy or both
Purpura
Score of >5 on the EULAR Sjögren's Syndrome Disease Activity Index
Rheumatoid factor
Cryoglobulinaemia
Low C4 level
CD4 T-cell lymphocytopenia
Presence of ectopic germinal centres
Focus score of >3

- Central nervous system — cerebral vasculitis, transverse myelitis or demyelinating lesions.
- Lymph nodes — benign lymphadenopathy or lymphoma.
- Pulmonary chronic bronchitis or bronchiolitis or interstitial pneumonitis.
- Facial pain — burning mouth syndrome, trigeminal neuralgia, sensory neuropathies, motor dysfunction (facial nerve most commonly involved).
- Venous thromboembolism — deep vein thrombosis (DVT) and pulmonary embolism (PE).
- The risk of B-cell lymphoma is markedly 15- to 40-fold among patients with pSS, as compared with the general population. *Lymphoproliferative diseases* are mostly seen as mucosa-associated lymphoid tissue (MALT) or can develop into monoclonal gammopathies (e.g. Waldenström macroglobulinaemia); non-Hodgkin diffuse large B-cell lymphoma or extranodal marginal zone B-cell lymphomas. Most lymphomas complicating SS arise in mucosal extranodal sites, especially the salivary glands. Most are low-grade marginal zone B-cell lymphoma (MZL) with long-term survival. MZL is diagnosed from broad strands of monocytoid B cells surrounding and invading epimyoepithelial islets, and monotypic immunoglobulin expression. The treatment and prognosis of SS lymphoma depend on the lymphoma type and stage. Lymphomas may be most likely where there is severe clinical disease and if there has been cytotoxic chemotherapy or salivary irradiation. Pseudolymphoma or frank lymphoma should be suspected when there is:
  - persistent salivary gland enlargement
  - lymphadenopathy
  - hepatosplenomegaly (Table 26.2).

Risk factors for the development of lymphoma include (see Table 26.2):
- recurrent swelling of parotid glands
- splenomegaly, lymphadenopathy or both
- purpura
- score of >5 on the EULAR Sjögren's Syndrome Disease Activity Index (ESSDAI)
- rheumatoid factor
- cryoglobulinaemia

- low C4 level
- CD4 T-cell lymphocytopenia
- presence of ectopic germinal centres
- focus score (FS) of >3.

BLLs of the salivary glands do not necessarily require surgical treatment. For lymphomas, an oncological opinion is indicated; chemotherapy or rituximab may be required. Lymphomas have also been treated with radioimmunotherapy.

DIAGNOSIS OF SJÖGREN SYNDROME

A subjective feeling of dry mouth (xerostomia) is common in the general population, although reduced salivary flow (hyposalivation) is not always confirmed by objective studies. Indeed, of older people, some 16% to 25% complain of xerostomia — usually caused by drugs. SS is one cause of hyposalivation. The diagnosis of SS is confirmed mainly from the history, clinical examination and investigation findings including:

- ocular symptoms
- oral symptoms
- ocular signs
- autoantibodies and other blood tests
- salivary gland studies (Table 26.3).

The ACR–EULAR Classification Criteria for Primary SS is illustrated in Box 26.2. A diagnosis of pSS is defined as a score of 4 or more on the basis of this criteria:

- FS of $\geq 1 = 3$
- presence of anti-SSA antibodies = 3
- SICCA ocular staining score of $\geq 5 = 1$
- Schirmer test of ≤ 5 mm/5 minutes = 1
- unstimulated whole salivary flow of ≤ 0.1 mL/min = 1.

If SS is suspected and there is objective hyposalivation, specialist referral is warranted because a range of investigations may be needed, as the differential diagnosis may include:

- Viral infections:
  - hepatitis C virus
  - HIV
  - HTLV-1
  - EBV.
- Sarcoidosis
- IgG4 syndrome
- SNOX syndrome
- Glandular deposits in:
  - haemochromatosis
  - lipoproteinaemias
  - amyloidosis
  - lymphomas.

AUTOANTIBODIES AND OTHER BLOOD TESTS

Blood tests may be indicated to:

- Ro (SS-A) autoantibodies are the hallmark antibodies in pSS. They are present in approximately 70% and associated with earlier disease onset, glandular dysfunction and extraglandular manifestations as well as with other B-cell activation markers. Recent studies suggest that La (SS-B) antibodies on their own are not associated with SS but with Ro autoantibodies reflect more severe SS. Autoantibody assays (ANA and ENA) can be extremely helpful in diagnosis and are readily available, inexpensive and fairly noninvasive.
- ESR or CRP (raised in SS).
- Exclude anaemia (common in RA and SS).

TABLE 26.3 Investigations That Might Be Helpful in Diagnosis/Prognosis/Management in Patients Suspected of Having Sjögren Syndrome

Investigation	Typical Findings	Comments
Sialometry	Reduced salivary flow rate	Nonspecific, but noninvasive, useful, readily available and often used
Lacrimal flow	Reduced on Schirmer test	Nonspecific, but noninvasive, readily available and often used
Autoantibodies	ANA ENA: Ro (La) Rheumatoid factor (RF) Serum immunoglobulin levels Serum immunoglobulin IgG4 levels Serum complement CD4 counts Cryoglobulins Full blood picture Serum ferritin, vitamin B_{12} and corrected whole blood folate levels ESR	Noninvasive, readily available and often used. La on its own is not linked with SS but with Ro indicates more severe SS
Ultrasonography	Hypoechogenicity	Noninvasive, readily available and often used Severity score related to SS
Salivary gland biopsy	Focal lymphocytic infiltrate Acinar atrophy Fibrosis	More specific, invasive, readily available and routinely used
Sialography	Sialectasis	Nonspecific, uncommonly used

- Examine for CD4 levels, serum complement and immuno-globulin levels, cryoglobulins and monoclonal immunoglobulins (may help lymphoma prediction).
- Exclude similar syndromes seen in IgG4 syndrome (raised IgG4 levels), sarcoidosis (raised serum ACE levels) and infections (e.g. hepatitis C virus, EBV, HTLV-1 or HIV) (serologically tested).

SALIVARY GLAND STUDIES

Salivary gland functional studies such as sialometry, and ultrasound may be indicated (Box 26.2, Table 26.3, Algorithms 26.1 and 26.2). Labial gland biopsy is a gold standard investigation, and major salivary gland biopsy is occasionally used. Sialography and scintigraphy are rarely used.

Salivary Flow Measurements (Sialometry)

Objective evidence of diminished salivary flow includes a:
- decreased resting secretion rate of whole saliva less than 1.0 mL in 10 minutes: this is more closely associated with symptoms of xerostomia than are stimulated flow rates
- decreased stimulated flow rate.

Ultrasonography

Useful for evaluating salivary gland disease and has replaced other diagnostic techniques, such as sialography and salivary scintigraphy because it is inexpensive and noninvasive. The diagnosis is considered positive for SS if the major glands show hypoechoic areas, echogenic streaks and/or irregular gland margins on ultrasound. It is also helpful in excluding lymphoma. Ultrasonography of the major salivary glands may reveal multiple hypoechoic or anechoic areas in the four main salivary glands (parotid and submandibular glands) and may be helpful in diagnosis or longitudinal assessment. Ultrasound assessment is not yet formally included among the classification criteria.

Salivary Gland Biopsy

Biopsy of salivary glands in the diagnosis of SS can show focal sialadenitis — the characteristic histopathological feature. LSG histology, if used with an FS, provides a reproducible and objective evaluation of severity of inflammation. A focus is defined as an aggregate containing 50 or more mononuclear cells; the FS is the number of such aggregates in each 4-mm^2 area. The mononuclear cells are predominantly T helper inducer cells. The FS is reliable only where gland lobes with acinar atrophy and interstitial fibrosis are excluded and where an adequately large specimen is examined. The threshold FS generally used for diagnosis of SS is one focus per 4 mm^2. However, other features such as fibrosis or fatty atrophy, duct dilatation and hyperplasia are nonspecific. Focal sialadenitis in an adequate LSG biopsy (at least four to five lobules) appears to be sensitive and disease-specific but invasive. It remains an important investigation for SS.

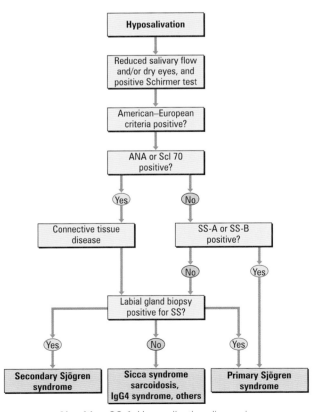

Algorithm 26.1 Hyposalivation diagnosis.

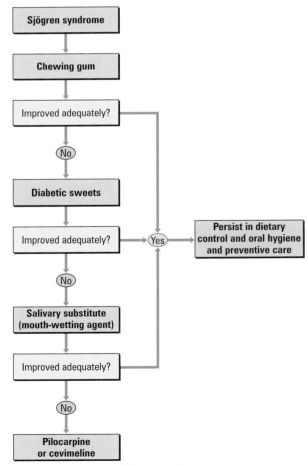

Algorithm 26.2 Sjögren syndrome management.

Sialography

Sialography in SS may show peripheral sialectasis; this is the most typical finding, it is most sensitive using oil-based contrast media and is seen particularly in parotid glands. It may correlate with histologic scores and scintigraphy but is not universally used.

Salivary Scintiscanning

Salivary scanning (scintigraphy) may show diminished radionuclide uptake and spontaneous secretion, or reduced secretion following citric acid or pilocarpine stimulation. Changes correlate with sialographic, flow rate and LSG histological changes but are nonspecific, and so it is not routinely used.

Magnetic Resonance Imaging

Magnetic resonance imaging (MRI) can be helpful in quantifying glandular parenchyma according to the size of nodules and ducts, cavities' structure and functional glandular changes.

Disease Activity Assessments

Two indexes for the assessment of disease activity in pSS have been validated. The EULAR Sjögren's Syndrome Patient Reported Index (ESSPRI) is a patient-administered questionnaire that assesses mouth and eye dryness, fatigue and pain. The EULAR Sjöögren's Syndrome Disease Activity Index (ESSDAI is used in clinical trials to assess systemic complications of the disease in 12 domains. The clinical oral dryness score (CODS) is a useful clinical adjunct to indicate the clinical impact of hyposalivation.

TREATMENT

- SS remains an incurable condition because no therapeutic modality has been identified that reliably modifies the course of the disease.
- Patient information and understanding are an important aspect in management.

- A patient who has dry eye symptoms should be referred to a specialist ophthalmologist. Ocular involvement is assessed by:
  - Schirmer test for lacrimal flow
  - tear break-up time (stain with fluorescein and lissamine)
  - ocular staining score (OSS) (stain with fluorescein and lissamine)
  - corneal abrasions (stain as aforementioned or Rose Bengal)
  - methylcellulose eye drops or ligation or cautery of the nasolacrimal duct may be appropriate care
  - anticholinergics, antihistamines and diuretics may exacerbate eye dryness and should be avoided if possible.
- Other aspects of care include the following, for which the dental professional is the expert (Table 26.4):
  - Dry mouth: sip water or other fluids throughout the day; protect the lips with lip salve; take small bites of food; eat slowly; eat soft, creamy foods (casseroles, soups) or cool foods with a high liquid content (melon, ice cream); and moisten foods with water, gravies, sauces, extra oil, dressings, sour cream, mayonnaise or yoghurt.
  - Advise the patient to avoid: mouth-breathing; any drugs that may produce hyposalivation (e.g. tricyclic antidepressants); alcohol (including in mouthwashes); smoking; caffeine (coffee, some soft drinks); dry foods, such as biscuits (or moisten in liquid first); spicy foods; and oral healthcare products containing sodium lauryl sulphate, which may irritate the mucosa. A humidifier may also help.
  - Salivary substitutes may help symptomatically. Those that are available include: methylcellulose; Saliva Orthana and Oralbalance are particularly useful because they contain fluoride (e.g. Glandosane or Luborant), or mucin. However, there may be religious or cultural objections to use of mucin.
  - Saliva stimulating agents (sialogogues): chewing gums (containing xylitol or sorbitol, not sucrose); diabetic sweets; cholinergic drugs, such as pilocarpine or cevimeline that stimulate salivation.
- Oral complications should be avoided or managed by:
  - avoiding sugary foods

TABLE 26.4 Regimens That Might Be Helpful in Management of Patient Suspected of Having Sjögren Syndrome		
Regimen	**Use in Primary Care**	**Use in Secondary Care (Severe Oral Involvement and/or Extraoral Involvement)**
Beneficial	Sialogogues Avoid systemic pilocarpine for patients with respiratory disease (e.g. chronic bronchitis, asthma and chronic obstructive pulmonary disease)	Corticosteroids Hydroxychloroquine Anti-CD20 (rituximab)
Emergent treatments	Electrostimulation	Anti—B cell—activating factor (belimumab)
Supportive	Antifungals Humidifier Moist diet Mouth-wetting agents	

- good oral hygiene
- using topical fluorides
- using chlorhexidine mouthwash.
- Dental caries is best controlled by dietary control of sucrose intake, and the daily use of fluorides as toothpastes, mouthwashes and gels (1% sodium fluoride gels or 0.4% stannous fluoride gels).
- Candidiasis may cause soreness or burning and should be treated with antifungals until there is neither erythema nor symptoms. Topical antifungals in liquid form, such as nystatin suspension, are the most effective and acceptable. Other preparations such as miconazole are also effective. Fluconazole and itraconazole are available as suspensions (effective against oropharyngeal candidiasis), and voriconazole as a liquid. Dentures should be left out of the mouth at night and stored in sodium hypochlorite solution or chlorhexidine to disinfect. An antifungal, such as miconazole gel, or nystatin ointment should be spread on the denture before reinsertion.
- Bacterial sialadenitis needs treating with a penicillinase-resistant antibiotic, such as flucloxacillin.
- A specialist physician or rheumatologist should be referred to when the patient suffers any connective tissue or other systemic disorders. Patients with severe extraglandular manifestations are usually treated with systemic corticosteroids, hydroxychloroquine and other immunosuppressive drugs (methotrexate, mycophenolate sodium, azathioprine and cyclosporine). To date, no immunomodulatory drug has proven to be efficacious in pSS. The monoclonal anti-CD20 antibody rituximab tends to be the biologic of choice. There appears to be little benefit from use of infliximab and etanercept in studies. Belimumab, an inhibitor of BAFF, is an emerging treatment option. Salivary stimulation by intraoral electrical devices may emerge as a viable treatment.

FOLLOW-UP OF PATIENTS

SS, particularly the primary type, and especially when clinically severe, carries a small potential for lymphoma development, necessitating regular monitoring. If there is any change causing concern, particularly the development of a salivary swelling or lump, lymphadenopathy or hepatosplenomegaly, a specialist opinion should best be obtained. Clinical and investigative risk factors have been discussed earlier. Routine assessment of oral microbiology is useful to exclude secondary infection and candidiasis.

IgG4-Related Disease

IgG4-related disease is a multisystem immune-mediated fibroinflammatory condition. It is characterised by mass formation with abundant infiltration of IgG4-bearing plasma cells.

Many cases were previously classified as Mikulicz disease, Küttner tumour and orbital pseudotumour (idiopathic orbital inflammation).

IgG4-related disease presents with enlargement of one of more salivary gland(s) and/or lacrimal gland(s). Histologically it is characterised by a dense polyclonal lymphoplasmacytic infiltrate, storiform fibrosis and obliterative phlebitis. IgG4-bearing plasma cells are nearly always present, as is an increased ratio of IgG4- to IgG-containing plasma cells. Serum immunoglobulin IgG4 is increased. Complications include multifocal fibrosclerosing disease with autoimmune pancreatitis, retroperitoneal fibrosis, tubulointerstitial nephritis, autoimmune hypophysitis and Riedel thyroiditis.

In IgG4-related disease compared with SS, the incidence of dry eyes, dry mouth and arthralgias is lower, whereas allergic rhinitis, bronchial asthma, sclerosing pancreatitis, interstitial nephritis and interstitial pneumonitis are more common; IgG4-related disease is *not* associated with anti-Ro/SS-A and anti-La/SS-B autoantibodies. The condition may mimic many neoplastic, inflammatory and infectious diseases. There is good responsiveness to systemic corticosteroids or anti-CD20 (rituximab). Early recognition is important to minimise organ damage.

Snox Syndrome

Up to 25% of patients with primary generalised nodal osteoarthritis may present with xerostomia and hyposalivation. Patients are Ro autoantibody and rheumatoid factor negative. There is associated nonspecific sialadenitis on labial gland biopsy without focal lymphocytic infiltrates, and no evidence of increased risk of lymphoma development.

RECOMMENDED READING

Price, E.J., Rauz, S., Tappuni, A.R., et al., 2017. The British Society for Rheumatology guideline for the management of adults with primary Sjögren's syndrome. Rheumatology (Oxford). 56 (10), 1643—1647. Erratum in: Rheumatology (Oxford). 2017 Oct 1;56(10),1828.

Ramos-Casals, M., Brito-Zerón, P., Bombardieri, S., et al., 2020. EULAR recommendations for the management of Sjögren's syndrome with topical and systemic therapies. Ann. Rheum. Dis. 79 (1), 3—18.

Shiboski, C.H., Shiboski, S.C., Seror, R., et al., 2017. 2016 American College of Rheumatology/European League Against Rheumatism classification criteria for primary Sjögren's syndrome: a consensus and data-driven methodology involving three international patient cohorts. Ann. Rheum. Dis. 76, 9—16.

Vivino, F.B., Carsons, S.E., Foulks, G., et al., 2016. New treatment guidelines for Sjögren's disease. Rheum. Dis. Clin. North Am. 42, 531—551. https://www.sjogrens.org/.

Behçet Syndrome

KEY POINTS
- Behçet syndrome (BS) (also known as Behçet disease) is a systemic variable vessel vasculitis that involves the mucosa, skin, joints, eyes, arteries, veins, nervous system and the gastrointestinal system.
- There is an association with human leukocyte antigen (HLA)-B51.
- BS is characterised by unpredictable relapses and remissions and presents with a wide spectrum of clinical manifestations.
- Patients with BS need specialist advice, multidisciplinary team care and systemic immunomodulation.

INTRODUCTION

Behçet syndrome (BS)/Behçet disease is a systemic variable vessel vasculitis that involves the mucosa, skin, joints, eyes, arteries, veins, nervous system and the gastrointestinal system.

EPIDEMIOLOGY

- Turkey has the highest prevalence, present in 420/100,000. The prevalence of BS is approximately 0.64/100,000 in the United Kingdom and up to 0.33/100,000 in the United States.
- Onset of the disease usually occurs in the third or fourth decade of life.
- BS affects men and women equally, although some regional variability exists. Men have more severe sequelae.
- The disease is found worldwide but is most common in people from the Mediterranean area and Asia, China, Korea and Japan (along the 'silk road' which extended from Japan to the Middle East and Mediterranean countries). In those countries, it is a leading cause of blindness.
- There are no proven predisposing factors for BS. Dental and periodontal therapies may be associated with a flare-up of oral ulcers in the short term but may decrease their number in longer follow-up. Periodontal status tends to be worse and may be associated with disease severity.

AETIOLOGY AND PATHOGENESIS

The aetiology of BS is unknown (Fig. 27.1):
- There is a genetic predisposition to BS — which is strongly associated with human leukocyte antigen (HLA)-B*51 (HLA-B*5101). The frequency of HLA-B51 along the Silk Route ranges between 50% and 80% among patients with BS (<25% in the population). In contrast, the frequency of HLA-B51 in Northern Europe and the United States is approximately 15% among patients with BS against 5% in the general population.
- The most widely accepted theory behind its pathogenesis is that an environmental stimulus elicits an abnormal immune response in a genetically susceptible host. A possible pathogenic role of certain bacterial antigens that have cross-reactivity with human peptides has been proposed. Heat shock proteins, streptococcal antigens, *Helicobacter pylori*, herpes simplex virus and parvovirus B19 have been implicated.
- Many immunologic findings in BS are similar to those seen in RAS, with various T lymphocyte abnormalities and increased polymorphonuclear leukocyte motility. There is increased T cell (T helper type 1 [Th1]) activity, cells infiltrating into lesions expressing interferon (IFN)-γ and reacting against heat shock proteins. Proinflammatory cytokines interleukin (IL)-12, IL-18 and tumour necrosis factor alpha (TNF-α) are increased, and some, such as IL-12, are potent inducers of Th1 immune reactions. IL-2 and IL-6 cytokines and T regulatory cells (Treg cells) also play a major role. Th17 cells can contribute to the development of the disease with their proinflammatory cytokine IL-17. IL-21 may promote Th17 effectors and suppress Treg cells. Th2 may also play a role.
- Circulating autoantibodies against a number of components, including intermediate filaments found in mucous

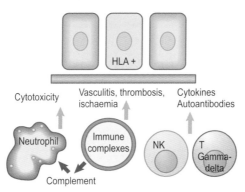

Fig. 27.1 Pathogenesis of Behçet syndrome.

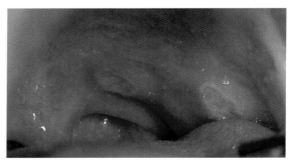

Fig. 27.2 Aphthous-like ulcers in Behçet syndrome: the most common feature.

membranes, cardiolipin and neutrophil cytoplasm, are present, but it is not clear whether they play a role in pathogenesis or are induced by cell damage. There are raised levels of acute phase proteins and circulating immune complexes and changed levels of complement.

- Vasculitis: usually leukocytoclastic vasculitis underlies many of the clinical features (erythema nodosum, arthralgia, uveitis) as in established immune complex diseases/vasculitis. Immunocytes (mostly CD4 cells), B cells and neutrophils infiltrate perivascularly.
- Hypercoagulability is also a feature. Von Willebrand factor, endothelin-1,2, thromboxane and thrombomodulin are increased and factor V Leiden and prothrombin mutations are associated with thromboses in BS.

CLINICAL FEATURES

BS is a chronic multisystem and sometimes life-threatening vasculitis, characterised mainly by:

- Oral aphthous-like ulceration: in 90% to 100% of cases (Fig. 27.2) is the most common and usually the initial manifestation of BS. Oral ulcers precede the diagnosis by 7.5 ± 10 years. However, only a few patients with aphthous-like ulceration progress to BS. The minor form is by far the most common in BS, followed by the major and herpetiform variants.
- Recurrent painful genital ulcers that tend to heal with scarring: in 64% to 88% of cases. Genital ulcers are especially common in females with BS, resemble RAS and precede the diagnosis by 1 to 2 years. In women, ulcers most commonly affect the labia, and in men, the scrotum is regularly involved.
- Ocular lesions: precede the diagnosis by 1 to 2 years. Ocular disease is seen in 30% to 70% of patients and is more frequent and severe in men. Uveitis with conjunctivitis (early) and hypopyon (late), retinal vasculitis (posterior uveitis), iridocyclitis and optic atrophy can arise.
- Central nervous system (CNS) lesions are predominantly subtentorial (affecting cerebellum, brainstem and spinal cord), with meningoencephalitis, cerebral infarction, psychosis, cranial nerve palsies, hemiparesis and quadriparesis.
- Skin lesions are described in approximately 80% of patients and include erythema nodosum-like lesions, papulopustular lesions and acneiform nodules. Venepuncture is, in some patients, followed by pustulation, but this phenomenon (pathergy) is not seen often in UK or US patients.
- Cardiac or large vein thrombosis (of the inferior vena cava and cranial venous sinuses), can be life-threatening.
- Involvement of the joints, epididymis, heart, intestinal tract and vascular system.
- It is associated with increased mortality due to involvement of the CNS, lungs and large vessels, bowel perforation and gastrointestinal haemorrhage.
- A range of nonspecific signs and symptoms may precede the onset of the mucosal membrane ulcerations. This includes a history of malaise, myalgias and migratory arthralgias without overt arthritis. The mucocutaneous variant (oral and genital ulceration with cutaneous manifestations) is the most common clinical phenotype seen in the United Kingdom and the United States.

DIAGNOSIS

Because BS is rare and the established features overlap those of many other diseases, the condition can be difficult to diagnose. The International Study Group (ISG) for BS criteria 1990 (Table 27.1) suggests the diagnosis should be made on clinical grounds alone—on the basis of oral aphthous-like ulcers plus two or more of:

- recurrent genital ulceration
- eye lesions

TABLE 27.1 Features of Behçet Syndrome (The International Study Group for Behçet Disease Criteria 1990)

Major Criteria	Minor Criteria
• Aphthous-like oral ulcers • Genital ulcers • Ocular lesions • Central nervous system (CNS) lesions • Skin lesions	• Arthralgia: large joint arthropathies that are subacute, nonmigratory, self-limiting and nondeforming • Superficial or deep migratory thrombophlebitis, especially of lower limbs • Thromboses of large veins, such as the dural sinuses or venae cavae • Intestinal lesions: inflammatory bowel disease with discrete ulcerations • Lung disease: pneumonitis • Renal disease: haematuria and proteinuria

TABLE 27.2 Investigations That Might Be Helpful in Diagnosis/Prognosis/Management in Some Patients Suspected of Having Behçet Syndrome

In Most Cases	In Some Cases
Full blood picture Serum ferritin, vitamin B_{12} and folate levels Erythrocyte sedimentation rate Human leukocyte antigen analysis (HLA-B51) Ophthalmological opinion Rheumatological opinion Neurological opinion Dermatology opinion Thiopurine methyltransferase levels	Serum immunoglobulins Serum complement Cardiolipin antibodies Pathergy test

- skin lesions
- pathergy reaction: a greater than 2-mm diameter erythematous nodule or pustule forming 24 to 48 hours after sterile subcutaneous puncture of the forearm skin.

The International Criteria for Behçet's Disease (ICBD) (2013) include oral aphthous ulcers, genital ulceration and ocular lesions, each given 2 points, whereas 1 point was assigned to each of skin lesions, vascular manifestations and neurologic manifestations. A patient scoring 4 points or greater is classified as having BS. In clinical practice, the ISG 1990 criteria are generally used to distinguish BS from complex aphthosis (continual oral/oral + genital), the majority of whom do not progress to BS.

The differential diagnosis is from other oculomucocutaneous syndromes such as:
- sweet syndrome: oral ulcers, conjunctivitis, episcleritis, inflamed tender skin papules or nodules
- erythema multiforme: erosions, target (iris) lesions
- pemphigoid: bullae, erosions
- pemphigus: erosions, flaccid skin bullae
- Reiter syndrome: ulcers, conjunctivitis, keratoderma blenorrhagica
- ulcerative colitis
- syphilis
- lupus erythematosus
- mixed connective tissue disease.

There are no specific tests for the diagnosis of BS (Table 27.2). Findings of HLA-B51, raised serum immunoglobulin D (IgD) and antibodies to cardiolipin are supportive of a diagnosis of BS. Disease activity may be assessed by serum levels of acute phase proteins (erythrocyte sedimentation rate, C reactive protein).

TREATMENT

The effects of BS may be cumulative, especially with neurological, vascular and ocular involvement; one main problem is ophthalmic involvement, which can result in blindness. Mortality, although low, can result from neurological involvement, vascular thromboses, bowel perforation or cardiopulmonary disease or as a complication of immunosuppressive therapy.

In the face of such serious potential complications, patients with suspected BS should be referred early for specialist advice and typically require systemic immunomodulation (Table 27.3). A multidisciplinary approach is necessary for optimal care. The goals of treatment are to prevent irreversible organ damage and to alleviate symptoms. Patient information is an important aspect in management:
- Treatment for aphthous-like ulcers in BS includes tetracycline mouthwash and topical corticosteroids. Benzydamine hydrochloride and lidocaine are helpful for symptomatic relief.
- If the ulcers in BS fail to respond to topical measures as used in recurrent aphthae, systemic immunomodulators may be required, under specialist supervision. Systemic therapy with colchicine, and dapsone is often useful for mucocutaneous lesions. In refractory cases, thalidomide, azathioprine or biological agents, such as TNF-α antagonists (infliximab, etanercept), may be necessary.

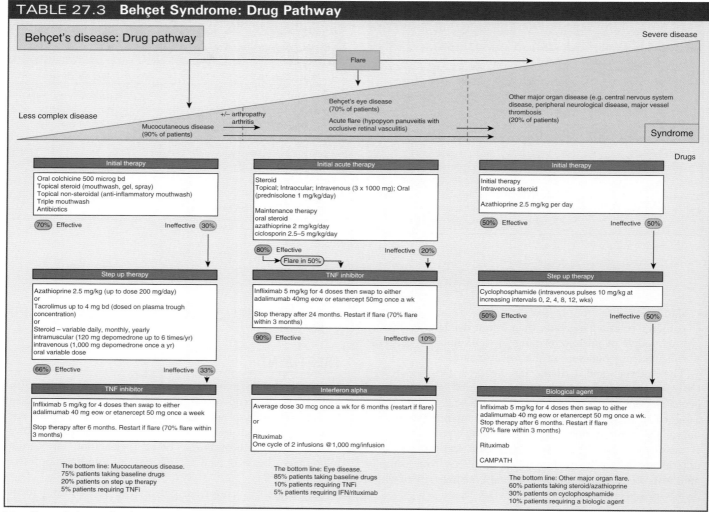

TABLE 27.3   Behçet Syndrome: Drug Pathway

https://www.behcets.nhs.uk

FOLLOW-UP OF PATIENTS

Long-term follow-up as shared care is usually appropriate.

RECOMMENDED READING

Davatchi, F., Chams-Davatchi, C., Shams, H., et al., 2017. Behçet's disease: epidemiology, clinical manifestations, and diagnosis. Expert Rev. Clin. Immunol. 13 (1), 57–65.

Hatemi, G., Christensen, R., Bang, D., et al., 2018. 2018 update of the EULAR recommendations for the management of Behçet's syndrome. Ann. Rheum. Dis. 77 (6), 808–818.

Taylor, J., Glenny, A.M., Walsh, T., et al., 2014. Interventions for the management of oral ulcers in Behçet's disease. Cochrane Database Syst. Rev. (9), CD011018.

Erythema Multiforme

KEY POINTS

- Erythema multiforme (EM) is an acute, often recurrent, hypersensitivity reaction.
- The cause of EM may remain elusive, but herpes simplex virus, other infections and occasionally drugs are implicated.
- EM affects the mouth with serosanguinous exudates on the lips and widespread ulceration.
- Some patients develop lesions on other mucosae or skin.
- Treatment usually involves corticosteroids.

INTRODUCTION

Erythema multiforme (EM) is an acute, often recurrent, hypersensitivity reaction affecting mucocutaneous tissues, seen especially in males, and characterised by serosanguinous exudates on the lips, mouth ulceration and sometimes lesions on other mucosae. Target-like lesions may occur on the skin with or without mucosal lesions. It is now considered a distinct entity from Stevens-Johnson syndrome (SJS) (see Chapter 29).

Most cases are thought to be triggered by an infection most frequently Herpes simplex virus but *Mycoplasma pneumoniae*, Epstein Barr virus and other infections are associated.

SJS and toxic epidermal necrolysis (TEN), on the other hand, form a distinct spectrum and are usually drug-induced; Chapter 33). They form a spectrum and lie within the group of severe cutaneous adverse reactions (SCARs). These hypersensitivities, predominantly drug, reactions though rare (affecting approximately 1 or 2:1,000,000 annually) are medical emergencies as they are potentially fatal.

EPIDEMIOLOGY

- EM is uncommon.
- Young adults 20 to 40 years of age are affected; 20% of cases occur in children.
- It is slightly more common in males.
- It is seen worldwide.
- There may be a genetic predisposition to EM, with several possible human leukocyte antigen (HLA) associations HLA-B15 (B62), HLA-B35, HLA-A33, HLA-DR53 and HLA-DQB1*0301: in patients with recurrent EM.

AETIOLOGY

The trigger for EM is unclear in most patients but, where a trigger can be identified, it is mainly due to an infection. Box 28.1 includes many potential associations.

- Infective agents: herpes simplex virus is implicated in 15% to 20% of cases of EM and 70% of recurrent EM (herpes-associated EM; HAEM). It is not usually isolated from lesions but follows 7 to 10 days after infection. Numerous other organisms, particularly mycoplasmas, have also been implicated.
- Drugs have been implicated, though these are more typically associated with the distinct SJS-TEN spectrum. However, where suspected these include NSAIDs, anticonvulsants, allopurinol and antimicrobials
- Immune conditions: such as systemic lupus erythematosus or following immunisation such as Bacille Calmette-Guerin (BCG) or hepatitis B immunisation
- Food additives or chemicals: such as benzoates, nitrobenzene, perfumes and terpenes.

PATHOGENESIS

EM is associated with the appearance of cytotoxic T lymphocytes in the epithelium that induce apoptosis in keratinocytes and results in necrosis. The infiltrate is mainly T lymphocytes, macrophages and neutrophils. Herpes-associated EM appears to be the result of a cell-mediated immune reaction to the precipitating agent. It is proposed that the HSV-DNA fragments in the skin or mucosa initiate a specific

BOX 28.1   Possible Causes of Erythema Multiforme

Infections — These Are the Most Likely Cause for Erythema Multiforme

- Viruses:
  - herpes simplex virus 1 and 2
  - Coxsackie viruses
  - human immunodeficiency virus
  - Parapoxvirus orf
  - varicella zoster virus
- Cytomegalovirus
  - Epstein-Barr virus
  - hepatitis C
- Bacterial:
  - *Mycoplasma pneumoniae*
- Streptococci
- Fungal:
  - histoplasmosis

Drugs (see Table 33.7) More likely to Be Linked to Stevens-Johnson Syndrome—Toxic Epidermal Necrolysis

- Allopurinol
- Anticonvulsants, e.g. carbamazepine, phenytoin, lamotrigine
- Sulphamethoxazole and other sulpha drugs
- Antimicrobials, e.g. aminopenicillins, cephalosporins

Vaccines

- Bacille Calmette-Guerin
- Diphtheria-tetanus
- Hepatitis B
- Smallpox

Immune Disorders

- Graft-versus-host disease
- Inflammatory bowel disease
- Polyarteritis nodosa
- Sarcoidosis
- Systemic lupus erythematosus

Food Additives or Chemicals

- Benzoates
- Nitrobenzene
- Perfumes
- Terpenes

Radiation Therapy

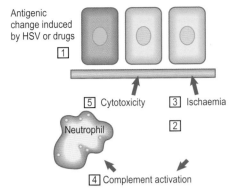

Fig. 28.1 Aetiopathogenesis of erythema multiforme (see text).

CLINICAL FEATURES

EM may present a wide spectrum of severity, from the much more common mild limited disease (minor EM) often involving only the mouth or skin, to a more severe form referred to as EM major (Table 28.1).

Oral Lesions

Most patients with EM (70%), of either minor or major forms, have oral lesions, which typically are self-limiting and:
- Precede lesions on other stratified squamous epithelia or may arise in isolation.
- Present with:
  - lips that become swollen and cracked, bleeding and crusted (Fig. 28.2)
  - lesions on the non-keratinised mucosae and most pronounced in the anterior mouth (Fig. 28.3)
  - +/− macules on skin that progress through to blisters and ulceration
  - recur in about 25%; the periodicity can vary from weeks to years, attacks usually lasting 10 to 20 days occurring once or twice a year.
- Resolve after about six episodes though may be ongoing.

Skin Lesions

Skin lesions seen more frequently in major EM:
- commonly affect the distal extremities, especially the extensor surfaces of the arms, legs, elbows, knees, dorsum of hands and feet
- vary in type (hence the term erythema *multiforme*) but are usually macules that are symmetric, round, erythematous and slightly pruritic or non-itchy and may evolve into papules or plaques that frequently display a circumferential pallor and evolve into the typical target or iris lesions. The well-demarcated centre of the papule may form a blister and then a necrotic ulcer, which results in a depressed white, yellow or grey area surrounded by a red edge and then a pale oedematous ring; a bright red margin may surround this pale ring. Patients may also present with raised atypical

T-cell-mediated type IV hypersensitivity response resulting in the presence of HSV-specific T cells, which generate interferon-γ (IFN-γ). This cytokine then amplifies the immune response and stimulates the production of additional cytokines and chemokines, which aids the recruitment of further reactive T cells to the area. These cytotoxic T cells, natural killer (NK) cells or chemokines can all induce epithelial damage. See Figure 28.1.

TABLE 28.1 Differentiation of Erythema Multiforme From Stevens-Johnson Syndrome—Toxic Epidermal Necrolysis

	Oral Erosions	Erosions of Other Mucosae	Skin Target Lesions	Other Skin Lesions	Body Surface Area Epidermal Detachment (%)
Erythema multiforme minor	+	−	± Typical targets		<10
Erythema multiforme major	+	+	± Typical targets		<10
SJS and TEN overlap	+	+	−	Flat atypical targets	10–30
TEN	+	+	−	Dark red macular lesions and bullae	>30

ªSee text for details and glossary for abbreviations.

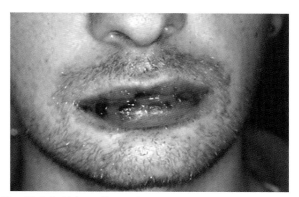

Fig. 28.2 Labial swelling and crusting in erythema multiforme.

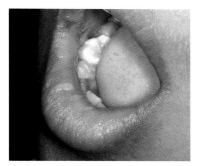

Fig. 28.3 Erythema multiforme.

targets lesions (without the double erythematous ring). Skin involvement is always less than 10% of body surface area and often just a few lesions are seen.

Other Mucosal Lesions

Other mucosal lesions, seen in major EM may include:
- eye involvement: may cause lacrimation and photophobia
- genital lesions: painful and may result in urinary retention.

Severity Classification of Erythema Multiforme

The extent of involvement of different mucosae is the distinguishing feature between minor and major forms:
- Minor EM:
  - typically affects only one site (mouth alone, or skin or other mucosae)

- rashes are various but are typically 'iris' or 'target' lesions or bullae on the extremities.
- Major EM:
  - about 30% of cases begin with a prodrome, lasting 1 to 2 weeks before the onset of the mucocutaneous manifestations, and often also with flu-like symptoms, sore throat, headache, arthralgias, myalgias or fever
  - widespread lesions appear and affect the mouth, but also other sites such as skin, eyes, genitals, pharynx, larynx and/or oesophagus. Skin involvement may present with bullous and other rashes with epidermal detachment involving less than 10% of the body surface. Ocular changes that resemble those of mucous membrane pemphigoid (dry eyes and symblepharon) may result. Genital changes may include balanitis, urethritis and vulval ulcers.

DIAGNOSIS

A diagnosis of EM can sometimes be difficult to readily establish, as it needs to differentiate from viral stomatitides, recurrent severe aphthosis, pemphigus and the subepithelial immune blistering disorders, e.g. mucous membrane pemphigoid.
- The diagnosis of EM is mainly clinically based on the episodic nature of the lesions, with irregular full-thickness yellow sloughing coalescing ulcers and sparing of the gingivae. The Nikolsky sign is negative. In contrast, aphthae are regular and discrete while the immunobullous disorders are persistent, often affect the gingivae and do not heal without treatment.
- It may be helpful to undertake serological testing for HSV, Epstein-Barr virus (EBV) or *M. pneumoniae*, or other micro-organisms (Table 28.2).
- Biopsy of perilesional tissue, with histological and immunofluorescence examination (to exclude immunobullous diseases), may be helpful. (Fig. 28.4). The histopathology of EM can be varied and immunostaining is not specific — but typically shows:
  - intraepithelial oedema and spongiosis early on
  - satellite cell necrosis (individual eosinophilic necrotic keratinocytes surrounded by lymphocytes)

TABLE 28.2   Initial Investigations for Infective Trigger to Consider in Erythema Multiforme

Investigations

Herpes simplex serology to confirm viral exposure
Epstein Barr virus serology
Coxsackie virus (throat swab and stool sample)
Mycoplasma serology during an acute episode and convalescent serology
Anti-streptolysin titre

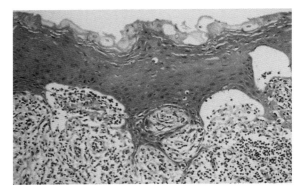

Fig. 28.4 Histopathology of erythema multiforme showing mainly sub-epithelial vesiculation.

- keratinocyte necrosis and dermal inflammation containing eosinophils may occur in drug-related cases
- immune deposits: fibrin and C3 at the epithelial basement membrane zone
- vacuolar degeneration of the junctional zone and severe papillary oedema
- sub- or intraepithelial vesiculation
- increased vascularity
- perivascular lymphocytic infiltrate (CD4$^+$ more than CD8$^+$ T lymphocytes) with a few neutrophils and occasional eosinophils
- perivascular IgM, C3 and fibrin deposits.
  Specific investigations include:
- Herpes simplex serology to establish whether the patient has been exposed to the Herpes Simplex virus.

- Mycoplasma serology.
- An anti-streptolysin titre if a streptococcal infection is a suspected trigger.
- Other infections can be investigated if suspected.

TREATMENT

Spontaneous healing can be slow; up to 3 weeks in minor EM and up to 6 weeks in EM major:
- Patient information is an important aspect of management.
- Early ophthalmologic and dermatological consultations may be needed.
- Precipitating factors, when identified, should be treated, e.g. herpes simplex
- Oral hygiene should be improved with a 0.2% aqueous chlorhexidine mouthwash.
- Antimicrobials may be indicated (Table 28.3):
  - aciclovir or valaciclovir in EM related to the herpes simplex virus
  - tetracycline in EM related to *M. pneumoniae*.
- Patients with minor *EM* often respond to topical corticosteroids, though systemic corticosteroids may also be required.
- Topical corticosteroids are the primary therapeutic agents used to treat ulcerative mucosal lesions, which have an immunologically based aetiology such as EM. Typically, a medium potency corticosteroid such as betamethasone or a higher potency one such as fluocinonide or beclomethasone is required, moving to a super-potent topical corticosteroid, e.g. clobetasol, if the benefit is inadequate. In long-term use, candidosis can arise and thus topical antifungal medication such as miconazole may be prudent.
- Systemic corticosteroids may be needed to reduce the severity and duration of episodes. Prednisolone 25 to 40 mg daily for 3 to 5 days reducing over the following 3 to 7 days may be needed.
- Patients with major *EM* may need admission for hospital care. Supportive care is important and may include IV fluids. A complete blood count, urea and electrolytes, ESR, CRP, liver function tests, and cultures from blood, sputum and erosive areas should be taken. Systemic corticosteroids are helpful in reducing the severity of the episode.

TABLE 28.3   Regimens That Might Be Helpful in Management of Patients Suspected of Having Erythema Multiforme

Regimen	Use in Primary Care (Minor Erythema Multiforme)	Use in Secondary Care or if Recommended (Severe Oral Involvement and/or Extraoral Involvement/Major Erythema Multiforme)[a]
	Topical corticosteroids	Systemic corticosteroids
	Antivirals if suspect herpes simplex trigger	Azathioprine Mycophenolate mofetil Thalidomide
Supportive	Chlorhexidine Benzydamine Diet with little acidic, spicy or citrus content Lidocaine	In-patient care

[a]See text for Stevens-Johnson syndrome/toxic epidermal necrolysis care.

Patients with *Recurrent EM*: If episodes are frequent, e.g. 1 to 2 months, a second-line immunosuppressive agent may be considered, e.g. azathioprine or mycophenolate mofetil. A trial of acyclovir 400 mg twice daily for 6 months may be helpful in those triggered by the herpes simplex virus and continued if this reduces the frequency and severity (see Table 28.3).

FOLLOW-UP OF PATIENTS

Long-term follow-up as shared care is usually appropriate for minor EM.

RECOMMENDED READING

Assier, H., Bastuji-Garin, S., Revuz, J., Roujeau, J.C., 1995. Erythema multiforme with mucous membrane involvement and Stevens-Johnson syndrome are clinically different disorders with distinct causes. Arch. Dermatol. 131, 539.

Auquier-Dunant, A., Mockenhaupt, M., Naldi, L., et al., 2002. Severe cutaneous adverse reactions. Correlations between clinical patterns and causes of erythema multiforme majus, Stevens-Johnson syndrome and toxic epidermal necrolysis: results of an international prospective study. Arch. Dermatol. 138, 1019—1024.

Creamer, D., Walsh, S.A., Dziewulski, P., et al., 2016. UK guidelines for the management of Stevens-Johnson syndrome/toxic epidermal necrolysis in adults 2015. Br. J. Dermatol. 174 (6), 1194—1227.

Roujeau, J.C., 2016. Re-evaluation of 'drug-induced' erythema multiforme in the medical literature. Br. J. Dermatol. 175 (3), 650—651. https://doi.org/10.1111/bjd.14841.

Wetter, D.A., Davis, M.D., 2010. Recurrent erythema multiforme: clinical characteristics, etiologic associations, and treatment in a series of 48 patients at Mayo Clinic, 2000 to 2007. J. Am. Acad. Dermatol. 62, 45.

Stevens-Johnson Syndrome/Toxic Epidermal Necrolysis Spectrum

KEY POINTS
- This spectrum is distinct from erythema multiforme with a much more variable prognosis.
- It is largely triggered by a drug hypersensitivity although there are reports of cases with no drug trigger identified and infection is the presumed cause.
- Stevens-Johnson syndrome (SJS) affects mucous membranes and between 10% and 30% of skin surface area.
- Toxic epidermal necrolysis (TEN) affects mucous membranes and 30% or more skin involvement.
- The prognosis is related to both extent of skin involvement and comorbidities.

INTRODUCTION

Stevens-Johnson syndrome (SJS) and toxic epidermal necrolysis (TEN) form a spectrum that presents with widespread blistering, and potentially other complications such as pneumonia, arthritis, nephritis or myocarditis. It presents with flu-like symptoms such as fever, malaise and upper respiratory tract symptoms followed by an acute macular erythematous rash with bullae. At the more severe end of the spectrum, there may be a separation of large sheets of epidermis from the dermis and extensive blistering and shedding of the skin similar to that seen in large burns. Besides the skin, mucous membranes such as oral, genital, anal, nasal and conjunctival mucosa are frequently involved.

SJS and TEN differ mainly by the extent of skin detachment. SJS affects less than 10% of the skin surface and has an average mortality rate of 1% to 5%, whereas the involvement of 10% to 30% of body surface area is called SJS/TEN overlap. TEN is the most severe form and includes denudation of greater than 30% of surface area and is associated with significant mortality of 30%. Mortality rates can be even higher in older patients and those with a large surface area of epidermal detachment. In those that survive, there may be significant long-term sequelae.

EPIDEMIOLOGY

1 to 2 per million per year.

PREDISPOSING FACTORS

SJS/TEN cases are assumed or identified to be caused by drugs in most cases. NSAIDs, antibiotics and anticonvulsants are the most common triggers, but several drugs are at 'high risk' of inducing TEN/SJS (see Table 29.1).

SJS secondary to drugs shows a strong human leukocyte antigen (HLA) linkage with HLA-A*24:02, HLA-B*44:03 and HLA-Cw*01:02 of the HLA-A, HLA-B and HLA-C genes. There is a strong association between HLA-B*1502 and carbamazepine-induced SJS in Han Chinese and several Asian populations as well as HLA-B*5801 and allopurinol.

PATHOGENESIS

- HLA-restricted presentation of antigens (drugs or their metabolites) to T lymphocytes initiates the immune reactions of SJS/TEN. The manifestation of a dysregulated immune reaction against epithelial cells with the appearance in the epithelium of cytotoxic effector cells mainly activated CD8$^+$ T lymphocytes and macrophages, and neutrophils cause keratinocyte apoptosis leading to satellite cell necrosis and thus sub- and intra-epithelial vesiculation.
- Humoral and cellular components of the innate immune response have been identified in association with SJS/TEN. There is an expansion of major histocompatibility complex class I restricted cytotoxic drug-induced CD8$^+$ lymphocytes

TABLE 29.1 Most Frequently Reported Drugs for Stevens-Johnson Syndrome—Toxic Epidermal Necrolysis
Allopurinol
Carbamazepine
Lamotrigine
Nevirapine
Oxicam NSAIDs
Phenobarbital
Phenytoin
Sulphamethoxazole and other sulpha drugs
Sulfasalazine

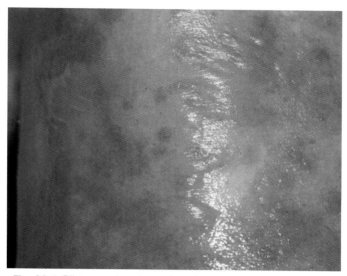

Fig. 29.1 Blisters and erythema in toxic epidermal necrolysis (TEN).

which infiltrate the skin and mucous membranes. Soluble factors including tumour necrosis factor (TNF)-α, interferon (IFN)-γ and inducible nitric oxide synthase may be associated with keratinocyte damage. Fas ligand, perforin and granzyme are implicated in apoptosis with granulysin thought to be the key mediator.

CLINICAL FEATURES

SJS/TEN presents with flu-like symptoms followed within a few days by a mucocutaneous eruption. Ocular and oral symptoms may precede skin involvement.

- The skin is painful followed by the appearance of atypical target lesions or purpuric macules on the upper limbs, trunk and face with subsequent involvement of the lower limbs including the palms and soles. Lesions may become confluent with large areas of denuded skin (Fig. 29.1).
- Patients develop a haemorrhagic mucositis which may extend into the upper and lower airways. The exposed dermis exudes fluid and the loss of skin barrier may lead to skin failure with a high risk of overwhelming infection, ventilatory compromise, profuse diarrhoea and multiorgan failure.

DIAGNOSIS

Diagnosis of SJS/TEN relies mainly on the clinical signs (the Nikolsky sign is often positive), together with a skin biopsy; histopathology shows typical full-thickness epidermal necrolysis (Fig. 29.2). At the milder end of the spectrum, differentiation between erythema multiforme major and SJS can be very difficult but the skin lesions in SJS/TEN are macules or atypical flat target lesions.

TREATMENT

Patients with SJS or TEN require urgent assessment with admission to a burn or intensive care unit if skin loss of greater than 10% body surface area (BSA); prompt withdrawal of the suspected drug (found in 85% cases), fluid and electrolyte

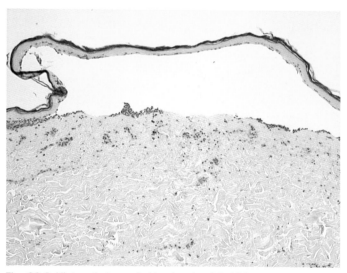

Fig. 29.2 Histopathology of skin showing full thickness epidermal necrosis and a sparse inflammatory cell infiltrate.

replacement and topical wound care. A complete assessment of the patient is needed including completion of a severity score known as SCORTEN which includes the patient's age, presence of a malignancy, heart rate, percentage area of skin detachment, serum urea, glucose and bicarbonate.

No systemic treatment has been established as standard and therefore treatment is primarily symptomatic and supportive and involves a multidisciplinary approach. In the early exudating phase, the use of an air-fluidised bed combined with appropriate skin care is recommended.

Oral ulceration can be so severe combined with upper airways involvement that intubation is required. A multidisciplinary approach is required including ophthalmology to minimise the ocular scarring complications and dermatology.

ORAL CARE

- Daily swabs for microscopy culture and sensitivity (MCS)
- Aqueous chlorhexidine 0.2% mouthwashes may be useful in maintaining oral hygiene
- Regular sweeping of the sulci with a lubricated swab on a stick to avoid synechiae developing.
- Topical combined corticosteroid and if indicated antibiotic or anti-candida treatment may be helpful.

Pain relief is essential. In the conscious patient, analgesic mouth rinses may be helpful.

RECOMMENDED READING

Creamer, D., Walsh, S.A., Dziewulski, P., et al., 2016. U.K. guidelines for the management of Stevens-Johnson syndrome/toxic epidermal necrolysis in adults 2016. Br. J. Dermatol. 174 (6), 1194–1227.

Pemphigoid

KEY POINTS
- Mucous membrane pemphigoid (MMP) is a group of chronic autoimmune diseases affecting mucous membranes +/− skin.
- The autoantibodies are directed against epithelial basement membrane zone (BMZ) proteins. The major antigens are type XVII collagen (BP180) and laminin 332.
- Immune binding deposits result in subepithelial separation.
- Oral lesions include ulcers, blisters and desquamative gingivitis.
- Other mucosae, e.g. conjunctivae, nasopharynx may be involved.
- Diagnosis is achieved by biopsy with immunofluorescence.
- Treatment depends upon severity increasing from topical corticosteroids to tetracycline antibiotics or immune modulation, e.g. dapsone and finally immunosuppressive agents.

INTRODUCTION

Acquired blistering disorders or vesiculobullous disorders include several distinct entities, most of which affect mucous membranes +/− skin (mucocutaneous), while others are predominantly skin diseases. While all are uncommon, pemphigoid and pemphigus are the two that more frequently affect the mouth and are seen in oral medicine clinics, both are autoimmune, long term (chronic) and persistent. Erythema multiforme (see Chapter 28) may also cause blistering and ulceration but is triggered by infection or occasionally drugs and importantly is episodic.

Autoimmune Blistering Diseases May Be Simply Classified by the Level of Blistering

- The subepidermal subset is mediated by autoantibodies that target the epithelial basement membrane zone (BMZ) in a region called the hemidesmosome which links the lowermost keratinocyte in the epithelium, to the underlying corium. It is a highly complex structure composed of an array of interlinking proteins known as anchoring filaments that contribute to the structural strength of the mucosa. Autoantibodies directed against these proteins can produce a range of disorders (Figs 30.1 and 30.2) in which immune deposits at the BMZ result in *subepithelial splitting* of epithelium from the lamina propria. These can be differentiated by immunological and molecular studies.
- The intra-epithelial subsets are mediated by autoantibodies that target the molecules that link one epithelial cell to another resulting in *intraepithelial blistering* (see Chapter 31).

Pemphigoid is the term given to a group of subepithelial immunologically mediated vesiculobullous disorders that affect stratified squamous epithelium and are characterised by damage to at least one of the protein constituents of the BMZ, also known as anchoring filaments. The pemphigoid group may produce similar clinical features (Box 30.1) which include blisters, ulcers and/or desquamative gingivitis.

IgG or IgA autoantibodies may be directed against specific hemidesmosomal antigens such as the major BP antigens and laminin 322, as well as the a6b4 integrin or type VII collagen. All may result in oral lesions but where the mouth is the main site the term 'mucous membrane pemphigoid' (MMP) is used though lesions may also affect other sites such as the ocular, nasopharyngeal, genital or laryngeal mucosae. Patients may have disease limited to a single site, e.g. pure ocular pemphigoid or pure oral pemphigoid, but the majority have a multisite disease.

Mucous Membrane Pemphigoid

MMP is a chronic autoimmune disease affecting the mucous membranes involving stratified squamous epithelia (i.e. the mouth, eyes and upper aerodigestive tract) though it may additionally affect the skin. Scarring is frequent in all but the oral mucosa which is relatively spared.

EPIDEMIOLOGY

- It is a very uncommon disease bordering on rare.
- The onset is usually in the fifth to sixth decades and is approximately twice as common in females.

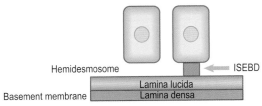

Fig. 30.1 Immune-mediated subepithelial blistering diseases — lesion at basement membrane zone (BMZ). Arrow indicates a level of autoantibody binding.

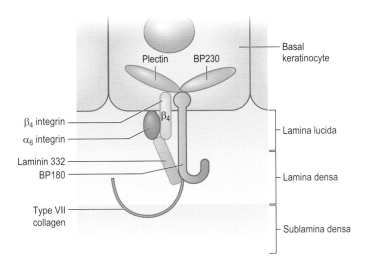

Fig. 30.2 The basement membrane zone is a complex structure containing macromolecules soem of which become autoantigens in pemphigoid.

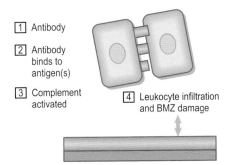

Fig. 30.3 Mucosal pemphigoid pathogenesis.

TABLE 30.1   Main Antigens Implicated in Subepithelial Disorders

Disease	Main antigens
Bullous pemphigoid (skin disease)	BP 230, BP180
Mucous membrane pemphigoid	BP180, laminin 332 (β4 integrin, type VII collagen, BP230 targeted in some patient sera)
Linear IgA disease	Epitopes on BP180
Epidermolysis bullosa acquisita	Type VII collagen

BP, bullous pemphigoid.

- Cytokines and other immune mediators result in the detachment of the basal cells from the BMZ.

CLINICAL FEATURES

The oral lesions in the pemphigoid affect the gingivae, buccal mucosae and palate most frequently. Patients may have pure gingival disease, extra-gingival or both. Clinically, MMP may appear as:
- Bullae or vesicles which are short-lived due to local trauma (Fig. 30.4). These blisters may be blood-filled similar to those of angina bullosa haemorrhagica or clear fluid-filled.
- Persistent irregular ulcers which result from the blisters bursting are typically covered with a yellowish fibrinous slough and have surrounding inflammatory erythema (Fig 30.5). They may resemble ulcerative lichen planus or erythema multiforme.
- Desquamative gingivitis is the most common oral finding and is characterised by erythematous, tender gingiva, usually in a patchy, rather than continuous distribution (Fig. 30.6). The sole involvement of the gingiva is not uncommon and is frequently misdiagnosed as inflammatory periodontal disease. It can also be indistinguishable from LP. There may be erosions and ulcers.
- Scarring is rarely seen in the mouth but may be noted as loss of sulcal depth, buccal or palatal scars. Many affected individuals with MMP will have predominant oral disease, but in some:
  - untreated ocular involvement can lead to blindness mainly due to conjunctival scarring, in-drawing of the

BOX 30.1   Subepithelial Immune-Mediated Vesiculobullous Disorders

- Pemphigoid variants
- Acquired epidermolysis bullosa
- Linear IgA disease
- Chronic bullous dermatosis in childhood

- There is no known geographic incidence.
- A genetic predisposition is suggested by an HLA-DQB1*0301 allele association.
- There is a higher risk of the patient having other autoimmune disorders.
- The precipitating event is unclear though in some may be a stressful life event.
- A few cases are drug-induced.

PATHOGENESIS

MMP is characterised by autoantibody binding at the BMZ, complement activation and subepithelial separation (Fig. 30.3). MMP is characterised immunologically by:
- In vivo bound and circulating autoantibodies to BMZ components, which are typically IgG class +/− IgA (Table 30.1).

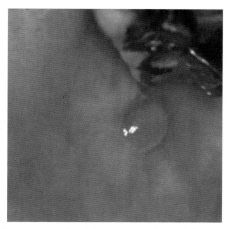

Fig. 30.4 Mucosal pemphigoid may present with blisters, which break to leave erosions.

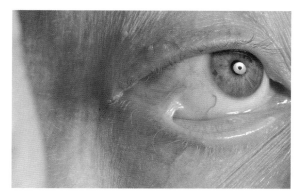

Fig. 30.7 Mucosal pemphigoid may cause ocular disease and scarring.

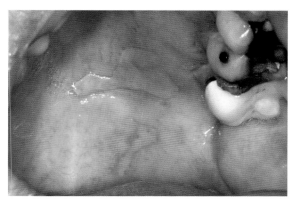

Fig. 30.5 Pemphigoid erosions in the palate.

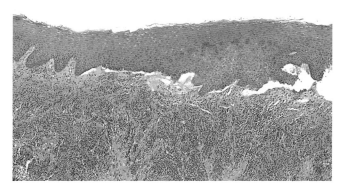

Fig. 30.8 Oral pemphigoid — histopathology showing sub-epithelial split and vesiculation with a mixed inflammatory cell infiltrate.(Courtesy: Professor Edward Odell, King's College London).

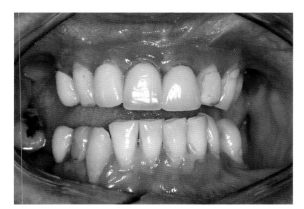

Fig. 30.6 Mucosal pemphigoid commonly presents with desquamative gingivitis.

eyelashes (entropion) and scarring of the cornea. Symblepharon whereby the tarsal and bulbar conjunctiva become tethered is shown (Fig. 30.7).
- nasal lesions may bleed and crust
- genital involvement can be a source of great morbidity
- laryngeal scarring may lead to stenosis
- skin blisters may affect the scalp (leaving hair loss or alopecia) or scarring on other sites.

- In the laminin 332 binding subgroup, there is a possible increased risk of an underlying malignancy, often an adenocarcinoma.

DIAGNOSIS

The pemphigoid variants are indistinguishable one from another clinically and thus a biopsy is needed. A biopsy across the edge of a lesion should be taken for histological examination and, ideally, a separate punch biopsy of perilesional or adjacent normal tissue (in the case of pure DG) is required for direct immunofluorescence. Haematoxylin and eosin staining will demonstrate a sub-epithelial cleft (Fig. 30.8). Direct immunofluorescence microscopy (DIF) detects linear IgG, IgA or C3 along the epithelial BMZ (Fig. 30.9). Indirect immunofluorescence microscopy (IIF) microscopy using patient serum detects epithelial BMZ-binding autoantibodies and can provide both the antibody subclass and titre. Indirect immunofluorescence on a salt-split substrate (a technique that splits the skin in the middle of the BMZ) can distinguish epidermal binding antibodies from dermal binding antibodies. The majority of MMP patients target BP180 and will bind to the roof of the

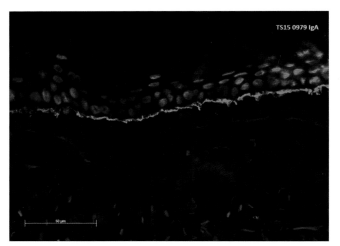

Fig. 30.9 Direct immunofluorescence detects linear IgG, IgA or C3 at the epithelial basement membrane zone.

split. However, those targeting laminin 332 or type VII collagen will bind to the base. ELISA is a newer and more sensitive technique that is able to define antibody specificity more definitively.

DIFFERENTIAL DIAGNOSIS

The oral lesions of pemphigoid should be differentiated from LP, pemphigus vulgaris, erythema multiforme, angina bullosa hae-morrhagica or, occasionally, acquired epidermolysis bullosa.

TREATMENT (SEE ALSO CHAPTERS 4 AND 5)

- Few patients with pemphigoid have spontaneous remission and, thus, treatment is usually indicated (Algorithm 30.1). Patient information is an important aspect of management. Disease activity is important to assess so that treatment effi-cacy can be maintained. Clinical outcome measures such as the Oral Disease Severity Score (ODSS) have been validated for use in MMP. There are non-validated multisite scoring tools available such as the Autoimmune Bullous Severity in-dex (ABSIS) or the MMP disease activity index. However, as patients present primarily with oral and oral ocular lesions, site-specific scoring tools are more sensitive. An International Consensus on MMP categorised patients into 'low-risk' and 'high-risk' groups based upon the site(s) of involvement, with 'low-risk' patients defined as having

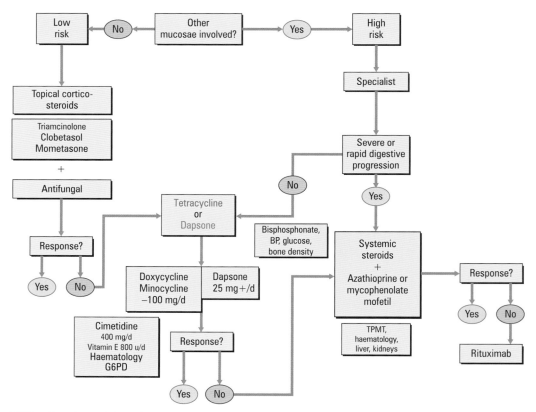

TPMT = thiopurine methyl transferase
BP = blood pressure
G6PD = Glucose 6 phosphate dehydrogenase

Algorithm 30.1 Management of pemphigoid.

only oral mucosal or oral and skin involvement and 'high-risk' patients as having the involvement of the ocular, genital, nasopharyngeal, oesophageal and/or laryngeal mucosae, and requiring more aggressive treatment (see below).

- Ocular manifestations have been reported in up to 70% of patients. In the majority of patients with predominantly oral disease, this may be mild. However, if left untreated, it can lead to blindness and ***thus an ophthalmological consultation is essential.*** Patients with MMP should also be questioned about the presence of other mucosal symptoms, which might indicate genital, nasopharyngeal, oesophageal or laryngeal involvement. Multidisciplinary treatment is indicated for 'high-risk' patients.

Low-Risk Disease

- Patients with oral pemphigoid alone may respond well to topical corticosteroids. Betamethasone as a 1 to 4×/daily mouthwash, fluocinonide or a super-potent topical corticosteroid, e.g. clobetasol as a paste mixed with orabase either applied directly or in a custom-made tray for 15 minutes 3× week can be helpful (Table 5.1). Good oral hygiene should be maintained; chlorhexidine mouthwashes may help. Anti-inflammatory agents, e.g. benzydamine, may also be helpful in the management of oral discomfort.
- For those with the more resistant oral or multisite disease, a stepwise layering of treatments is often required. An immunomodulator such as dapsone, tetracycline or doxycycline +/− nicotinamide might be added. If dapsone is considered, patients should first be screened for their glucose-6-phosphate dehydrogenase level due to the risk of haemolysis if G6PD is low. Monitoring of haemoglobin levels, reticulocyte count and routine bloods during therapy is required to assess for adverse effects including dose-related haemolytic anaemia, methaemoglobinaemia and other idiosyncratic adverse effects such as agranulocytosis and hepatitis (Chapter 5). Dapsone is started at 25 to 50 mg js/day, increasing monthly by up to 100 mg−150 mg depending upon tolerance and response.

High-Risk Disease

- For those with the more resistant oral or multisite disease, a stepwise layering of treatments is often required. If the disease is not controlled then oral prednisolone and an immunosuppressive agent such as azathioprine (checking thiopurine methyl transferase levels first), mycophenolate mofetil or methotrexate may also be required. Finally, for the most resistant cases, IV cyclophosphamide with methyl prednisolone as a monthly infusion, intravenous immunoglobulin infusions or a biological agent such as an anti-CD20 monoclonal antibody may be used.

Complications of Treatment

- Candidosis — topical antifungal medication such as nystatin oral suspension may be prudent if the mouth swab is positive and used for one week per month.
- Adrenal suppression with long-term and/or repeated application of topical or oral prednisolone (Chapter 5).
- Osteoporosis if long-term oral corticosteroids are required. Calcium, vitamin D and a potentially a bisphosphonate may be required.
- Malignancy is a long risk of immunosuppression.

FOLLOW-UP OF PATIENTS

Long-term follow-up in a multidisciplinary team is usually appropriate to ensure a response to treatment, side effects of treatment and changing pattern of disease.

RECOMMENDED READING

Carey, B., Joshi, S., Abdelghani, A., Mee, J., Andiappan, M., Setterfield, J., 2020. The optimal oral biopsy site for diagnosis of mucous membrane pemphigoid and pemphigus vulgaris. Br. J. Dermatol. 182 (3), 747−753. https://doi.org/10.1111/bjd.18032.

Carey, B., Setterfield, J., 2019. Mucous membrane pemphigoid and oral blistering diseases. Clin. Exp. Dermatol. 44 (7), 732−739. https://doi.org/10.1111/ced.13996.

Egami, S., Yamagami, J., Amagai, M., 2020. Autoimmune bullous skin diseases, pemphigus and pemphigoid. J. Allergy Clin. Immunol. 145 (4), 1031−1047.

McParland, H., Ormond, M., Thakrar, P., et al., 2020. An Oral Disease Severity Score validated for use in Mucous Membrane Pemphigoid. Br. J. Dermatol. 183 (1), 78−85. https://doi.org/10.1111/bjd.18566. Epub 2019, Nov 24.

Patient information leaflets. https://bisom.org.uk/wp-content/uploads/2020/02/Mucous-Membrane-Pemphigoid-PIL-October-2019.pdf.

https://www.bad.org.uk/shared/get-file.ashx?id=3421&itemtype=document.

http://www.pemphigus.org/living-with-pemphigus-pemphigoid/pemphigoid/.

Rashid, H., Lamberts, A., Borradori, L., et al., 2021. European Guidelines (S3) on diagnosis and management of mucous membrane pemphigoid, initiated by the European Academy of Dermatology and Venereology—Part I. J. Eur. Acad. Dermatol. Venereol. 35 (9), 1750−1764.

Schmidt, E., Rashid, H., Marzano, A.V., et al., 2021. European Guidelines (S3) on diagnosis and management of mucous membrane pemphigoid, initiated by the European Academy of Dermatology and Venereology—Part II. J. Eur. Acad. Dermatol. Venereol 35, 1926−1948.

Pemphigus

KEY POINTS
- Pemphigus is a group of rare potentially life-threatening chronic autoimmune diseases characterised by intra-epithelial blistering.
- The most common variant is pemphigus vulgaris in which IgG autoantibodies are directed against the intercellular molecules that hold keratinocytes together.
- Autoantibody reactivity results in intra-epithelial splitting (acantholysis).
- Painful blistering and erosions often manifest first in the mouth.
- Diagnosis is confirmed by biopsy and direct immunofluorescence.
- Treatment needs specialist advice and systemic immunomodulation.

INTRODUCTION

Pemphigus is the term for a group of chronic autoimmune diseases characterised by epithelial blistering affecting mucocutaneous surfaces, the term being derived from the Greek (*pemphix* = bubble or blister). Autoantibodies are directed against desmosomes (epithelial adhesion proteins) that bind stratified squamous epithelial cells together and that have a complex protein structure (Fig. 31.1). Variants of pemphigus are each associated with autoantibodies directed against the different desmosome constituents and may bind at different levels within the epithelium. Hence the clinical manifestations may vary (Fig. 31.2).

The main types are:
- Pemphigus vulgaris is the most common variant encountered in patients with oral lesions and is associated with antibodies against desmoglein (Dsg) 3, a constituent of the oral epithelial intercellular adhesion complex. Where the skin is also affected, antibodies target desmoglein 1 (Dsg 1).
- Pemphigus foliaceus is a skin disease and as above, autoantibodies target Dsg 1. Oral lesions are not seen.
- Paraneoplastic pemphigus (PNP) is a rare variant of pemphigus associated with an underlying neoplasm, e.g. lymphoproliferative disorders such as lymphoma, thymoma or the very rare Castleman disease (Chapter 55). Extensive oral and skin lesions are present, and patients are characteristically very unwell.

PEMPHIGUS VULGARIS

Epidemiology
- Pemphigus vulgaris is a rare disease.
- It presents in patients aged 40 to 60 years. There is a slight female preponderance.
- Pemphigus vulgaris predominately occurs in middle-aged and older patients of Ashkenazi Jewish, Asian or Mediterranean descent though it is universal.
- There is a fairly strong genetic background to pemphigus vulgaris, seen in people from the groups above, and an HLA association with HLA DRB1*0402 and DRB1*14 alleles.
- Some cases have been triggered by medications, e.g. antibiotics and antihypertensives (Table 33.99).

Pathogenesis
- Serum antibodies, mainly IgG are directed predominantly against desmosomes in stratified squamous epithelia. Intercellular immune deposits (mainly IgG and C3), are detectable intra-epithelially (Fig. 31.3).
- The antigen-antibody response on epithelial surfaces leads to damage to desmosomal adhesion molecules, particularly Dsg 3. Intracellular signalling pathways are complex but ultimately lead to a reduction of desmosomes and loss of cell–cell contact (acantholysis), and thus intra-epithelial vesiculation (Figs 31.4 and 31.5).
- Since oral epithelium expresses largely Dsg 3, but skin expresses Dsg 1 as well as Dsg 3, damage by antibodies against Dsg 3 results in oral lesions at an early stage, whereas skin integrity is maintained by Dsg 1. However, if Dsg 1 antibodies appear, cutaneous lesions result and when combined oral and skin lesions are present, the disease tends to be more severe (Table 31.1).
- Other autoimmune diseases, such as myasthenia gravis and systemic lupus erythematosus, are occasionally associated.

Clinical Features
Pemphigus vulgaris is the most severe form of pemphigus, and typically runs a chronic course, causing blisters and crusts on

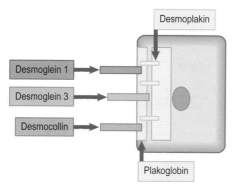

Fig. 31.1 Desmosomal proteins (antigens).

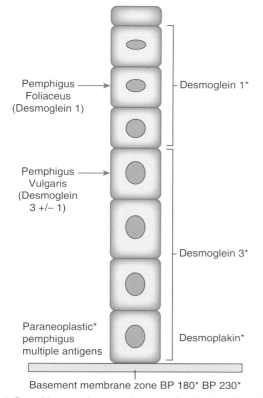

Fig. 31.2 Pemphigus variants and autoantibodies implicated needs modification.

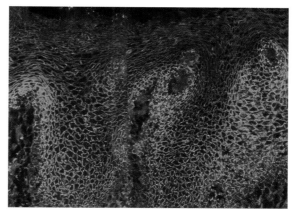

Fig. 31.3 Immunofluorescence in pemphigus showing intercellular binding of IgG directed against Desmoglein 3.

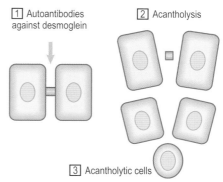

Fig. 31.4 Pathogenesis of pemphigus.

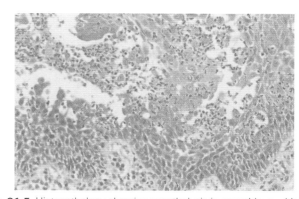

Fig. 31.5 Histopathology showing acantholysis in pemphigus with intra-epithelial vesiculation.

the skin and scalp and also blisters, erosions and ulcers on the mucosae of the:

- mouth
- pharynx
- larynx
- oesophagus
- nose
- conjunctiva
- anogenital region.

Pemphigus vulgaris often begins with very painful blisters in the mouth hence often presenting to the dental surgeon and on the scalp. The blisters are soft and are easily broken and gentle lateral pressure at the edge of the lesion results in extension of

TABLE 31.1 Antibodies to Desmogleins in Pemphigus Vulgaris		
Pemphigus Vulgaris Lesions	Dsg 3	Dsg 1
Mucosal, mainly	+	−
Mucocutaneous	+	+

Dsg, Desmoglein.

the erosion. This is known as the Nikolsky sign. It is a painful procedure and should not be undertaken in clinical practice.

Oral lesions in pemphigus vulgaris:

- are present in almost 100% of patients
- may be an early manifestation (the presenting feature in approximately 70%)
- may be the sole manifestation for a considerable time
- are vesiculobullous, but readily rupture, new bullae developing as the older ones rupture and ulcerate
- form erosions, which are irregular and initially red with a whitish surround (Fig. 31.6), but in sites such as the dorsum of the tongue may develop a white/yellow slough (Fig. 31.7)
- are seen in any mucosal surface of the mouth but frequently:
  - soft palate and posterior hard palate
  - buccal mucosa
  - tongue
  - lips (relatively rarely affected in mucous membrane pemphigoid [MMP])
  - attached gingiva, where lesions usually comprise severe desquamative or erosive gingivitis
  - importantly and in contrast to MMP, lesions heal without scarring though there may be loss of the papillae on the tongue.

In the absence of systemic treatment, oral lesions may be followed by involvement of the skin (Fig. 31.8) or, occasionally, other epithelia, such as the oesophagus, nasopharynx, anogenital sites or conjunctiva.

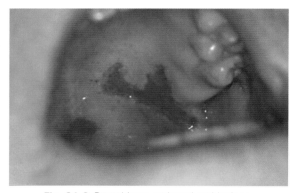

Fig. 31.6 Pemphigus; early red oral lesions.

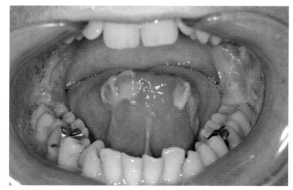

Fig. 31.7 Pemphigus showing widespread oral ulcers on tongue and buccal mucosae.

Diagnosis

- A careful history and physical examination will often provide the diagnosis, but biopsy of perilesional tissue, with histological and immunostaining examination, is essential (Table 31.2).
- Direct immunofluorescence microscopy (DIF) detects IgG and C3 deposits at the epithelial cell surfaces.
- Serum should be collected for titres of circulating anti-Dsg antibodies which may help guide treatment. Serum autoantibodies to Dsg may be detected using both normal human skin and monkey oesophagus. The most sensitive and specific technique, however, is enzyme-linked immunosorbent assay (ELISA). The titre of circulating autoantibodies broadly corresponds to the severity of disease in pemphigus and reduces with successful treatment.
- In the rare PNP, DIF usually reveals deposits at both the epithelial cell surfaces and the epithelial basement membrane zone. In addition to binding to squamous epithelial cell surfaces (e.g. skin, oesophagus substrates), circulating autoantibodies from patients with PNP also label transitional epithelium (e.g. rat bladder).

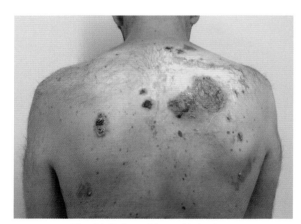

Fig. 31.8 Pemphigus skin lesions.

TABLE 31.2 **Aids That Might Be Helpful in Diagnosis/Prognosis/Management in Some Patients Suspected of Having Pemphigus[a]**	
Initial Management	**Ongoing and Repeated Assessment**
Examine for typical clinical signs	Regular blood monitoring
Dermatological opinion	Repeated ELISA/IIF when
Biopsy and immunofluorescence	considering dose change
ELISA to desmogleins	Disease severity scoring
Full blood picture, renal and liver function	ODSS PDAI
Screening blood tests for immunosuppressive agents	Patient-reported outcome measures
Blood pressure + blood glucose	
DEXA (dual-energy x-ray absorptiometry)	
Clinical photographs	

[a]See text for details and glossary for abbreviations.

Differential Diagnosis

- The differential diagnosis for oral pemphigus includes
  - mucous membrane pemphigoid
  - erythema multiforme
  - pyostomatitis vegetans.

Treatment (see also Chapters 4 and 5)

Before the introduction of corticosteroids, pemphigus vulgaris was potentially fatal — mainly from dehydration or secondary systemic infections. Treatment with potent immunosuppression, particularly if introduced early can result in prolonged remission and may potentially be curative (Table 31.3). Specialist involvement and patient information are vital. The severe oral and multisite disease will require a multidisciplinary team usually led by a dermatologist but additionally including:

- gastroenterologist: to detect possible oesophageal involvement
- ENT for nasopharyngeal lesions
- ophthalmology for conjunctival lesions.

For patients with PNP, there will be additional specialists including the oncology/haematology or others managing the underlying malignancy and potentially a respiratory physician's patients have symptoms or signs suggestive of respiratory difficulty.

Treatment is considered in two phases: induction of remission and maintenance of remission.

Systemic therapy with corticosteroids (e.g. prednisolone 0.5 to 1 mg/kg/day) is usually essential (Table 31.4). Bone protection is required during treatment. Second-line agents are also added early in management to facilitate a gradual reduction in corticosteroid dose (see Table 31.3). About 50% of patients relapse during steroid tapering, and the remainder achieves complete remission off therapy after an average of 3 years of treatment.

The use of an anti-CD20 monoclonal antibody has revolutionised treatment. It has FDA approval for first-line use in moderate and severe PV and similarly in the USA and some European countries. In the UK, it is permitted as a third-line treatment at present after standard immunosuppressive therapies have failed. Many patients go into a prolonged remission and standard immunosuppressive agents can be gradually withdrawn. For recalcitrant pemphigus, intravenous immunoglobulin can be given as a monthly infusion or immunoadsorption can remove considerable amounts of the autoantibodies from the patient with significant and prolonged clinical benefit and minimal adverse effects. The current algorithm for the management of PV is shown in Algorithm 31.1.

Oral care:

- Dental professionals can help achieve and maintain oral health. Oral lesions are often slow to heal, even when cutaneous lesions have resolved. Regular completion of disease severity scores, e.g. oral disease severity score (ODSS) for oral PV or Pemphigus disease activity index for the multisite disease is paramount and inform management.
- Good oral hygiene should be maintained with the help of regular dental hygiene appointments; chlorhexidine or hydrogen peroxide mouthwashes may help.
- Lesions are very painful and anti-inflammatory agents such as benzydamine may help or analgesic gels. Avoid spicy or acidic foods.
- Topical corticosteroids, typically a higher potency one, such as fluocinonide or betamethasone are required as a mouthwash while super-potent topical corticosteroid, e.g. clobetasol mixed with Orabase can be helpful (Table 5.1).

TABLE 31.3 Therapeutic Options

Regimen	Use in Secondary Care (PV With Oral and/or Extraoral Involvement)
	Corticosteroids
	Azathioprine
	Mycophenolate mofetil
	Rituximab
	Intravenous immunoglobulins
	Immunoadsorption
	Cyclophosphamide
Supportive	Benzydamine
	Chlorhexidine
	Diet with little acidic, spicy or citrus content
	Lidocaine

TABLE 31.4 Monitoring Protocol for Patients With Pemphigus on Systemic Corticosteroid Therapy

Daily **Aim to prevent steroid-induced — weight gain, hypertension, infection, bone loss, diabetes**	Maintain weight — reduce sodium and carbohydrate Encourage regular exercise Calcium and vitamin D
Weekly	Oral examination (ODSS) weekly to monthly Blood pressure Record symptoms
Monthly	Titre of desmoglein antibodies between 1 and 3 monthly for the first year Routine blood tests and HbA1c
Baseline and then 1–2 yearly	DEXA scan Asses for use of bisphosphonates for bone protection

ALGO 31.1 An Algorithm for Systemic Treatment

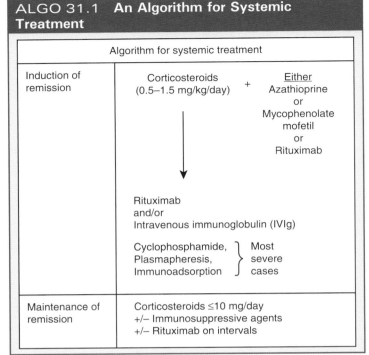

Algorithm for systemic treatment		
Induction of remission	Corticosteroids (0.5–1.5 mg/kg/day) +	Either Azathioprine or Mycophenolate mofetil or Rituximab
	Rituximab and/or Intravenous immunoglobulin (IVIg)	
	Cyclophosphamide, Plasmapheresis, Immunoadsorption	Most severe cases
Maintenance of remission	Corticosteroids ≤10 mg/day +/– Immunosuppressive agents +/– Rituximab on intervals	

FOLLOW-UP OF PATIENTS

Long-term follow-up in secondary care is essential.

RECOMMENDED READING

Patient Information Leaflets

http://www.pemphigus.org/living-with-pemphigus-pemphigoid/ pemphigoid/.

https://www.bad.org.uk/shared/get-file.ashx?id=114&itemtype=document.

https://bisom.org.uk/wp-content/uploads/2020/02/Pemphigus-VulgarisPIL-October-2019.pdf.

Egami, S., Yamagami, J., Amagai, M., 2020. Autoimmune bullous skin diseases, pemphigus and pemphigoid. J. Allergy. Clin. Immunol. https://doi.org/10.1016/j.jaci.2020.02.013.

Murrell, D.F., Peña, S., Joly, P., et al., 2020. Diagnosis and management of pemphigus: recommendations of an international panel of experts. J. Am. Acad. Dermatol. 82 (3), 575–585.e1. https://doi.org/10.1016/j.jaad.2018.02.021.

Harman, K.E., Brown, D., Exton, L.S., et al., 2017. British Association of Dermatologists guidelines for the management of pemphigus vulgaris 2017. Br. J. Dermatol. 177, 1170–1201. Available via: https://doi.org/10.1111/bjd.15930.

Murrell, D.F., Dick, S., Ahmed, A.R., et al., 2008. Consensus statement on definitions of disease, end points and therapeutic response for pemphigus. J. Am. Acad. Dermatol. 58, 1043–1046.

Ormond, M., McParland, H., Donaldson, A.N.A., et al., 2018. An Oral Disease Severity Score (ODSS) validated for use in oral pemphigus vulgaris. Br. J. Dermatol. 3. https://doi.org/10.1111/bjd.16265.

Orofacial Granulomatosis

KEY POINTS
- Granulomatous orofacial swelling is an umbrella term and includes orofacial granulomatosis (idiopathic cases), as well as Crohn disease, sarcoidosis, infections, Melkersson-Rosenthal syndrome and granulomatous vasculitis.
- The largest groups are those with orofacial granulomatosis who usually present with lip swelling.
- Accompanying orofacial lesions may include ulcers, mucosal 'cobble-stoning', mucosal tags, gingival enlargement, facial palsy and perioral erythema and induration.
- Diagnosis is confirmed by biopsy and other investigations.
- Treatment includes topical agents, dietary modification and, if needed, systemic therapy.

INTRODUCTION

The term orofacial granulomatosis (OFG) is a term that should be applied to patients in whom there is no clear underlying cause for the perioral and/or intraoral inflammation. It is an uncommon condition (Fig. 32.1) and often presents with relapsing and remitting lip swelling, which, on biopsy, is granulomatous and is referred to as granulomatous cheilitis. Alongside lip swelling, patients may present with angular stomatitis and/or cracked lips (Fig. 32.2) and periorificial erythema and swelling. Intraorally, there may be ulceration in the sulci, mucosal tags, cobblestoning or gingival hyperplasia. These latter signs may suggest oral Crohn disease and appropriate investigations are essential. Once a diagnosis of Crohn disease or sarcoidosis is made, the patient is then referred to as having oral Crohn disease or oral sarcoid, rather than OFG. However, the perioral or intraoral clinical presentation may be indistinguishable. OFG will be discussed first and then chronic granulomatous swelling for known subgroups will be discussed later.

OROFACIAL GRANULOMATOSIS

Epidemiology
- It is uncommon.

- The onset is usually in adolescents and young adult life and has no known racial predilection.
- Either gender but males may predominate.
- No known geographic incidence.

Predisposing Factors
- Lip and perioral swelling sometimes arise from an adverse reaction to various foods or additives which include cinnamic aldehyde, benzoates, butylated hydroxyinosole or dodecyl gallate (in margarine), or menthol (in peppermint oil).
- There is a strong association with atopy.
- Approximately 10% of cases have or develop, gastrointestinal Crohn disease.
- A small percentage may have sarcoidosis.
- A reaction to antigens (e.g. metals, such as cobalt), paratuberculosis or mycobacterial stress protein mSP65 has been suggested.

Aetiology and Pathogenesis
The cause of OFG is unknown. It is likely to represent a heterogeneous group of disease entities, which each may arise from different combinations of genetic and environmental allergens. A delayed type of hypersensitivity reaction appears to be involved, although the exact antigen inducing the immunological reaction appears to vary in individual patients. The inflammatory response is a Th1-mediated immune response and is associated with non-caseating granulomas in the lamina propria, which appear to cause lymphatic obstruction and lymphoedema, resulting in the clinical swellings (Fig. 32.3).

Clinical Features
OFG presents with:
- Non-tender swelling and enlargement of one or both lips (see Figs 32.1 and 32.2). In the first episode, the swelling typically subsides completely in hours or days, but after recurrent attacks, the swelling may persist, slowly increases in degree and eventually becomes permanent. The lip involved may feel soft, firm or nodular on palpation. Swellings involve, in decreasing order of frequency, the lip and

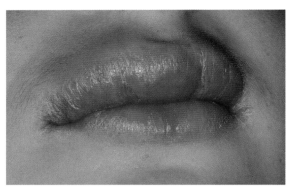

Fig. 32.1 Granulomatous cheilitis — persistent albeit fluctuating painless diffuse swelling.

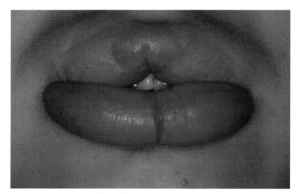

Fig. 32.2 Granulomatous cheilitis.

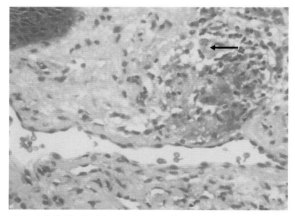

Fig. 32.3 Orofacial granulomatosis; granuloma arrowed.

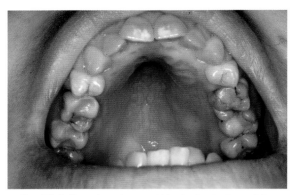

Fig. 32.4 Granulomatous cobblestoning in the palate.

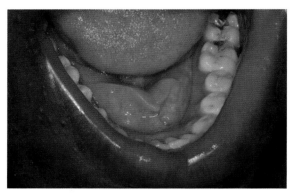

Fig. 32.5 Granulomatous swelling on the floor of mouth ('staghorn sign').

one or both cheeks. Less commonly, lingual, palatal, gingival and buccal swellings also may occur. The forehead, the eyelids or one side of the scalp may be involved as well or in isolation. Skin swelling may or may not be erythematous. The normal lip architecture is eventually chronically altered by the persistence of lymphoedema and non-caseating granulomas in the lamina propria. Once chronicity is established, the enlarged lip appears cracked and fissured, with reddish-brown discolouration and scaling becomes painful and eventually acquires the consistency of firm rubber.

Patients may also present with or develop the following symptoms which may suggest a higher risk of underlying identifiable cause:
- Thickening and folding of the oral mucosa produce a 'cobblestone' type of appearance and mucosal tags (Figs 32.4—32.6). Purple granulomatous enlargements may appear on the gingiva.
- Ulcers may appear: classically involving the buccal sulcus where they appear as linear ulcers, often with granulomatous masses flanking them are more frequently seen in patients with oral Crohn disease.
- In the rare Melkersson-Rosenthal syndrome, also referred to in Chapter 54, patients may present with facial palsy, facial swelling and a fissured tongue. Though intermittent at first, the palsy is a lower motor neurone type and may become permanent. It may be unilateral or bilateral, and partial or complete. It has been reported in association with other conditions including taste disturbance and systemic diseases such as Crohn disease and sarcoidosis. Spontaneous remission occurs in 25% of patients.

Diagnosis

The early attacks of OFG may be impossible to clinically differentiate from angioedema, but the persistence of the

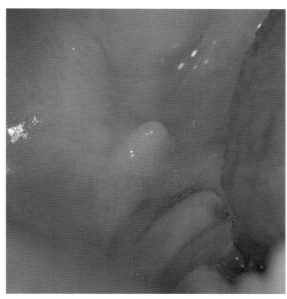

Fig. 32.6 Orofacial granulomatosis mucosal tag.

TABLE 32.1 Investigations That Might Be Helpful in Diagnosis/Prognosis/Management in Some Patients Suspected of Having Orofacial Granulomatosis[a]

In Most Cases	In Some Cases
Gastroenterological opinion	Patch tests
Biopsy	RAST
Full blood picture	TB test
Serum ferritin, vitamin B_{12} and corrected	Elimination diet
Whole blood folate levels	G6PD and TPMT levels
ESR	Blood pressure
SACE	Blood glucose
Chest radiography	DEXA (dual-energy x-ray
Gastrointestinal faecal calprotectin, imaging, endoscopy, biopsy	absorptiometry)

[a]See text for details and glossary for abbreviations.

swelling between attacks should suggest the diagnosis. Similar swelling may also be seen in a range of conditions including:

- Melkersson-Rosenthal syndrome (Chapter 54), Miescher cheilitis (Chapter 54), Crohn disease or sarcoidosis.
- Infections: rare cases of lip or oral swelling related to tuberculosis or leprosy have been reported. Agents such as *Borrelia burgdorferi* have been discounted as causes of OFG.
- Foreign body reactions.
- Rarely, Ascher syndrome, although the swelling of the lip is caused by redundant salivary tissue and is associated with blepharochalasia and present from childhood (see Chapter 54).

The many causes of oedema of the lips make the diagnosis one based on exclusion, clinical signs and histological examination. This is supported by blood tests, radiology, endoscopy and biopsy to differentiate the above (Table 32.1). The lesional biopsy is often indicated but, during the early stages, may show only lymphoedema and perivascular lymphocytic infiltration. However, with time, the infiltrate usually becomes denser and pleomorphic, and small focal granulomas are formed, which in OFG are indistinguishable from those of Crohn disease or sarcoidosis (Fig. 32.3). Salivary and skin microbiology to investigate possible candida or *S. aureus* on the lips. Patch tests and RAST may be indicated to exclude reactions to various foodstuffs or additives. Both standard and urticarial patch testing are used to detect such allergies.

Investigation of the gastrointestinal tract (faecal calprotectin, endoscopy, radiography and biopsy) is mandatory when symptoms suggest bowel involvement to exclude Crohn disease; endoscopic and histologic intestinal abnormalities are common in younger patients even when there are no gastrointestinal symptoms. Sarcoidosis may be investigated by chest radiography and a serum angiotensin-converting enzyme initially and referral as appropriate.

Treatment (see also Chapters 4 and 5)

The principal aims of treatment are to reduce lip swelling thereby improving the cosmetic appearance of the condition and reducing ulceration if present. Using an Oral Disease Severity Score (ODSS) before and after treatment will give an evidence base to the success of treatment.

Reactions to dietary components should be sought and possible provoking substances avoided (Table 32.2). Elimination diets such as a cinnamon and benzoate-free diet should be introduced for a 3-month trial period and has been shown to improve 54% to 78% of patients.

OFG may be an initial manifestation of Crohn disease and so careful surveillance and specialist multidisciplinary care are recommended. Conservative management usually includes topical corticosteroids, intralesional corticosteroid injections (such as low-volume, high-concentrate, extended-release triamcinolone) or topical tacrolimus. Other therapies include short courses of prednisolone, and in patients with underlying Crohn disease treatment with azathioprine, methotrexate, mycophenolate mofetil or anti-TNF alpha agents can be helpful.

In patients with sarcoidosis, appropriate systemic therapy, e.g. hydroxychloroquine may be beneficial.

Cheiloplasty is reserved for severely disfiguring cheilitis and only when the condition is quiescent. Psychological support is important for patients and parents of children with the condition.

TABLE 32.2 Regimens That Might Be Helpful in Management of Patients Suspected of Having Orofacial Granulomatosis

Regimen	Use in Primary Care + Secondary Care	Use in Secondary Care (Severe Oral Involvement and/or Extraoral Involvement)
Orofacial granulomatosis	Dietary modification Topical corticosteroids Topical tacrolimus Treatment of infection	Intralesional corticosteroids Clofazimine Corticosteroids Thalidomide
Sarcoidosis		Hydroxychloroquine Prednisolone
Crohn disease		Azathioprine Infliximab Adalumimab

FOLLOW-UP OF PATIENTS

Long-term follow-up as shared care is usually appropriate.

RECOMMENDED READING

Campbell, H., Escudier, M., Patel, P., et al., 2011. Distinguishing orofacial granulomatosis from Crohn's disease: two separate disease entities? Inflamm. Bowel. Dis. 17, 2109–2115.

Campbell, H., Escudier, M.P., Brostoff, J., et al., 2013. Dietary intervention for oral allergy syndrome as a treatment in orofacial granulomatosis: a new approach? J. Oral Pathol. Med. 42, 517–522.

Fedele, S., Fung, P.P., Bamashmous, N., Petrie, A., Porter, S., 2014. Long-term effectiveness of intralesional triamcinolone acetonide therapy in orofacial granulomatosis: an observational cohort study. Br. J. Dermatol. 170, 794–801.

Hullah, Esther, A., Escudier, Michael, P., 2019. The mouth in inflammatory bowel disease and aspects of orofacial granulomatosis. Periodontology 2000. 80, 61–76.

Complications of Drugs

KEY POINTS
- Drug adverse effects can damage any orofacial tissue.
- Immunosuppressive agents can lead to a range of complications including infection and malignancy.
- Chemotherapy can cause severe mucositis.

INTRODUCTION

A number of medical treatments can result in orofacial complications or diseases.

Therefore, it is important for the clinician to take a comprehensive drug history (including regular prescribed medication, over-the-counter medication, herbal remedies and recreational medicines) and always consider whether a drug may be behind the clinical problem in question. Drugs can sometimes give rise to a range of adverse orofacial manifestations (Table 33.1), particularly salivary changes — notably hyposalivation, but also other features. Amongst the most common and important reactions and drugs implicated are:
- Hyposalivation: antidepressants, antihypertensives, antihistamines and anticholinergics.
- Swelling of gingiva: calcium channel blockers, ciclosporin and phenytoin.
- Swelling of lips/face: ACE inhibitors, aspirin and penicillin.
- Erythema multiforme: allopurinol, barbiturates, nonsteroidal antiinflammatory drugs (NSAIDs) and protease inhibitors.

- Lichenoid lesions: antimalarials, beta-blockers, NSAIDs, phenothiazines and sulphonylureas.
- Ulceration/mucositis: cytotoxic agents (e.g. 5-fluorouracil, doxorubicin and methotrexate), nicorandil, NSAIDs, barbiturates, sulphonamides and tetracyclines.
- Hyperpigmentation: antimalarials, cytotoxic agents, minocycline and zidovudine.
- Bruxism: ecstasy.
- Osteonecrosis: bisphosphonates (BP).

The osteonecrosis resulting from BP known as medication-related osteonecrosis of the jaw (MRONJ); adverse effects from recreational drugs; complications of immunosuppressive medication (see Chapter 34), including opportunistic infections and increased prevalence of dysplastic and malignant lip and oral lesions in immunosuppressed patients, and those using photosensitisers such as antihypertensive drugs are discussed below. Other possible reactions are detailed in Tables 33.2–33.29.

DRUGS RELATED TO SALIVARY GLAND DYSFUNCTION

Hyposalivation

This is a side effect that causes significant morbidity for patients. Drugs are the most common cause of a persistently dry mouth and the list is extensive (see Table 33.2). It is always worth checking each drug specifically as the list will be

TABLE 33.1   Main Adverse Drug Effects in the Orofacial Region

	Effects	Examples	See Table
Salivary changes	Hyposalivation	Tricyclic antidepressants	33.2
	Salivary gland swelling or pain	Antihypertensives	33.4
	Hypersalivation	Anticholinesterases	33.3
Halitosis	Halitosis	Disulfiram	33.5
Mucosal damage	Oral ulceration	Immunosuppressive agents Nicorandil NSAIDs Cytotoxic drugs	33.6
	Candidiasis	Corticosteroids Antibiotics	33.28
	Contact stomatitis	Antibiotics Dentrifices Mouthwashes	33.14
	Lichenoid eruptions	Beta-blockers NSAIDs Phenothiazines Sulphonylureas	33.10
	SJS-TEN	Allopurinol Carbamazepine Barbiturates NSAIDs Protease inhibitors	33.7
	Pemphigoid	Antibiotics	33.8
	Pemphigus	ACE inhibitors	33.9
	Lupus-like (lupoid) disorders	Hydralazine Minocycline	33.11
	Oral mucosal discolouration and pigmentation	Amalgam Antimalarials Minocycline Imatinib	33.12
Cheilitis	Drug induced	Isotretinoin Retinoids	33.13
Swellings	Gingival enlargement	Calcium channel blockers Ciclosporin Phenytoin	33.16
	Angioedema	ACE inhibitors NSAIDs Penicillins	33.15
Neurological	Paraesthesiae	Protease inhibitors	33.18
	Taste acuity loss (hypogeusia) or distortion (dysgeusia)	Antibiotics Antihypertensives	33.17
	Abnormal facial movements	Dopa Metoclopramide Phenothiazines	33.19
	Pain	ACE inhibitors Vinca alkaloids	33.20
	Burning sensation	ACE inhibitors Protease inhibitors	33.21
	Bruxism Trismus	Ecstasy Metoclopramide	33.22

Continued

Tooth	Cleft palate	Alcohol	33.23
		Phenytoin	
	Structural damage	Fluorides	
	Discolouration (Fig. 33.1)	Tetracyclines	33.25
Bone	Osteonecrosis	Bisphosphonates	33.26

NSAIDs, Nonsteroidal antiinflammatory drugs.

TABLE 33.2 Drug-Related Hyposalivation

Drugs Most Commonly Implicated	For Example of Drugs Occasionally Implicated
Antidepressants (serotonin agonists, or noradrenaline and/or serotonin re-uptake blockers)	Diuretics
Alpha receptor antagonists for the treatment of urinary retention	Antihistamines
Diuretics	Antihypertensive agents
Histamine 2 antagonists and proton pump inhibitors	Antimigraine agents
Protease inhibitors	Benzodiazepines, hypnotics, opioids and drugs of abuse
Anticholinergics	Bronchodilators
Antipsychotics such as phenothiazines, lithium	Clonidine
Muscarinic receptor antagonists for the treatment of overactive bladder	Cytotoxics
	Ganglion-blocking agents
	Amphetamines
	Ipratropium
	Leva-dopa

continually updated. Not only is it uncomfortable but patients are at risk of candidal superinfection.

Hypersalivation

See Table 33.3.

DRUGS RELATED TO HALITOSIS

see Table 33.5

DRUGS RELATED TO MUCOSAL DAMAGE

Drugs related to oral ulceration including SJS/TEN, pemphigus and pemphigoid

Oral ulceration is a recognised side effect of medication. Table 33.6 lists those linked to non-specific oral ulcers. The SJS/TEN spectrum (Chapter 29) is almost always associated with underlying drugs and the most frequently encountered are listed in Table 33.7. Avoidance of the drug is essential as the reaction will recur with subsequent exposure. As this spectrum is associated with a significant mortality rate, identification of the offending drug must be a priority. The autoimmune blistering diseases pemphigus vulgaris and bullous pemphigoid are occasionally triggered by drugs Tables 33.8 and 33.9. Discontinuation of the drug is recommended but this is not always followed by resolution of the condition.

Drugs Related to Lichenoid or Lupus-Like Reactions

Drug-induced oral lichenoid reactions are not uncommon, while lupus-like oral reactions are very infrequent. In patients with a temporal association to initiation of drugs listed in Table 33.10, it is important to discuss with the patient and GMP whether it is possible to discontinue treatment for a period of a few weeks at least. A biopsy is sometimes helpful in supporting the likelihood of a drug aetiology.

TABLE 33.3 Drug-Related Hypersalivation

Drugs Most Commonly Implicated	Drugs Occasionally Implicated
Acetylcholinesterases	Alprazolam
Clozapine (Parkinson disease)	Clonazepam
	Diazoxide
	Haloperidol
	Pentoxifylline
	Risperidone
	Rivastigmine

TABLE 33.4 Drug-Related Salivary Gland Swelling or Pain

Drugs Most Commonly Implicated	Drugs Occasionally Implicated
Antihypertensives	Carbimazole
Chlorhexidine	Clonidine
Cytotoxics	Clozapine
Iodides	Ganglion-blocking agents
	Nitrofurantoin

Drugs related to halitosis

TABLE 33.5   Drug-Related Halitosis

Drugs Most Commonly Implicated	Drugs Occasionally Implicated
Drugs causing hyposalivation see table 33.2	Disulfiram aminothiols, antifungals, chemotherapeutic agents, dietary supplements, organosulphur substances.

TABLE 33.6   Drug-Related Oral Ulceration

Drugs Most Commonly Implicated	Drugs Occasionally Implicated
Cytotoxics	Alendronate
Immunosuppressive agents	Aztreonam
Nicorandil	Cocaine
	Mycophenolate mofetil
	Protease inhibitors
	Sulphonamides

TABLE 33.7   Drug-Related Stevens-Johnson Syndrome and Toxic Epidermal Necrolysis

Drugs Most Commonly Implicated	Drugs Occasionally Implicated
Allopurinol	Adalimumab
Anticonvulsants	Bupropion
Carbamazepine	Busulfan
Co-trimoxazole	Cephalosporins
Nonsteroidal antiinflammatory drugs	Clindamycin
Penicillin	Codeine
Phenytoin	Ethambutol
Sulphonamides	Furosemide
	Minoxidil
	Oestrogens
	Progestogens
	Protease inhibitors
	Quinolones
	Rifampicin
	Tetracyclines
	Vancomycin
	Verapamil

TABLE 33.8   Drug-Induced Bullous Pemphigoid

Drugs Most Commonly Implicated	Drugs Occasionally Implicated
Antibiotics	Clonidine
Beta-blockers	
Nonsteroidal antiinflammatory drugs	
Diuretics	
Anti-tumour necrosis factor (TNF)-α	
Dipeptidyl peptidase 4 inhibitors (DPP-4i)	
Immune checkpoint inhibitors targeting programmed cell death receptor 1 (PD-1) and its ligand (PD-L1)	

TABLE 33.9   Drug-Induced Pemphigus

Drugs Most Commonly Implicated	Drugs Occasionally Implicated
Antibiotics: penicillins, cephalosporins, vancomycin	Glibenclamide
Antihypertensive drugs: other angiotensin-converting enzyme inhibitors such as cilazapril, lisinopril, enalapril	Topical application: imiquimod, ketoprofen, neomycin and bacitracin
Piroxicam	
Thiol drugs, including penicillamine, captopril	

In patients with exfoliative cheilitis or an atypical focal lichenoid reaction, patch testing may be performed to establish whether there is a delayed (type 4) hypersensitivity reaction. Drugs that might be implicated are listed in Table 33.13. In addition, an immediate (type 1) hypersensitivity reaction may lead to swelling of the lips, tongue or throat. Relevant drugs include those listed in Table 33.15.

DRUGS RELATED TO SWELLINGS

Angioedema
See Table 33.15

Swellings Associated With Gingival Overgrowth
Drug-induced gingival overgrowth is considered to be multifactorial. It is aggravated by dental plaque and gingival inflammation, and oral hygiene optimisation is essential. However, the fibrogenic response which may be genetically determined as well as the use of drugs that have a negative effect on calcium ion influx across cell membranes, thereby interfering with collagenase function may be relevant.

DRUG-INDUCED NEUROLOGICAL DISTURBANCE

The list of drugs that can affect taste is very extensive and is detailed in a systematic review (see further reading below).

Drugs Related to Mucosal Pigmentation
Oral mucosal pigmentation may be associated with an amalgam tattoo and is usually seen in association with a large restoration close by. The remainder of the drugs listed in Table 33.12 may lead to pigmentation through systemic absorption and may also be associated with skin pigmentation.

DRUGS RELATED TO CHEILITIS

Exfoliative cheilitis can follow certain drugs most frequently the retinoids including isotretinoin prescribed for acne vulgaris and acitretin used in psoriasis. Many other drugs have been described as detailed in Table 33.13.

TABLE 33.10 Drug-Related Lichenoid Reactions

Drugs Most Commonly Implicated	Drugs Occasionally Implicated
Antihypertensives — ACE inhibitors, beta-blockers, nifedipine, methyldopa	Tumour necrosis factor antagonists — infliximab, etanercept and adalimumab
Diuretics — hydrochlorothiazide, frusemide, spironolactone	Imatinib mesylate (tyrosine kinase inhibitor)
Nonsteroidal antiinflammatory drugs (NSAIDs)	Misoprostol (prostaglandin E1 agonist)
Phenothiazine derivatives	Sildenafil citratus (Viagra)
Anticonvulsants — carbamazepine, phenytoin	Vaccines (especially those for herpes zoster and influenza).
Medicines to treat tuberculosis	
Antifungal medication — ketoconazole	
Chemotherapeutic agents — 5-fluorouracil, imatinib	
Antimalarial agents such as hydroxychloroquine	
Sulpha drugs including sulphonylurea hypoglycaemic agents, dapsone, mesalazine, sulfasalazine	
Metals — gold salts	
Others — allopurinol, iodides and radiocontrast media, interferon-α, omeprazole, penicillamine, tetracycline	

TABLE 33.11 Drug-Related Lupus-Like Reactions

Drugs Most Commonly Implicated	Drugs Occasionally Implicated
Hydralazine	Methyldopa
Procainamide	Chlorpromazine
Quinidine	Calcium channel blockers
Isoniazid	Terbinafine
Minocycline	Proton pump inhibitors, e.g. omeprazole
	Ethosuximide
	Griseofulvin
	Phenothiazines
	Phenytoin
	Nonsteroidal antiinflammatory drugs

TABLE 33.12 Drug-Related Oral Mucosal Pigmentation

Drugs Most Commonly Implicated	Drugs Occasionally Implicated
Amalgam	Amlodipine
Antimalarial, e.g. chloroquine or hydroxychloroquine	ACTH
Antibiotics, e.g. minocycline	Amiodarone
Antineoplastic and chemotherapeutic agents, e.g. doxorubicin and hydroxycarbamide	Bismuth
	Imatinib mesylate
Antiviral (e.g. zidovudine)	Iron
Antifungal (e.g. ketoconazole)	Oral contraceptives
Antileprotic (e.g. clofazimine)	

TABLE 33.13 Drug-Related Cheilitis

Drugs Most Commonly Implicated	Drugs Occasionally Implicated
Isotretinoin	Atorvastatin
Acitretin	Busulfan
Protease inhibitors	Clofazimine
Vitamin A	Clomipramine
	Cyanocobalamin
	Methyldopa
	Psoralens
	Streptomycin
	Sulfasalazine
	Tetracycline

TABLE 33.14 Drug-Related Contact Stomatitis (Stomatitis Venenata)

Drugs Most Commonly Implicated	Drugs Occasionally Implicated
Anaesthetics	Cosmetics
Antibiotics	Dental materials
Antiseptics	
Barbiturates	
Dentifrices	
Mouthwashes	
Sulphonamides	
Tetracyclines	

DRUG-INDUCED HARD AND SOFT TISSUE STRUCTURAL ABNORMALITIES

Table 33.23 lists some of the many drugs linked to a risk of cleft lip and palate if taken during the first trimester of pregnancy.

Tooth structure can be damaged in several ways by medication either directly or indirectly by altering the environment, e.g. hyposalivation increasing the sugar content or reducing the pH. These are detailed in Table 33.24.

Drugs may result in loss or alteration of taste. The groups of drugs that commonly lead to these side effects are detailed in Table 33.17 with one or two examples listed only. Many of these, additionally, are reported to cause a dry mouth.

TABLE 33.15   Drug-Related Angio-Oedema

Drugs Most Commonly Implicated	Drugs Occasionally Implicated
ACE inhibitors	Antidepressants
Nonsteroidal antiinflammatory drugs	Bupropion
SSRIs	Clindamycin
COX-2 inhibitors	Droperidol
Angiotensin II antagonists	Statins
Proton pump inhibitors	
Vaccines	
Penicillin	
Sulphonamides	

TABLE 33.16   Drug-Induced Gingival Overgrowth

Drugs Most Commonly Implicated	Drugs Occasionally Implicated
Anticonvulsants, e.g. phenytoin, sodium valproate	Vigabatrin
	Topiramate
Immunosuppressants, e.g. cyclosporin	Tacrolimus, sirolimus
Calcium channel blockers, e.g. nifedipine, amlodipine, felodipine	Verapamil
	Diltiazem
	Amphetamines

TABLE 33.17   Drug-Related Taste Abnormalities

Drugs Most Commonly Implicated	Drugs Occasionally Implicated
Anti-neoplastic agents	Chlorhexidine
Immunomodulating agents	Triamcinolone
Anti-infective agents	Cisplatin
Antihistamine	Enalapril
Antibiotics, e.g. tobramycin, amoxicillin, levofloxacin, clarithromycin	Fluoxetine
	Isotretinoin
Angiotensin-converting enzyme inhibitors	Leva-dopa
Metformin	Phenytoin
Liraglutide	Venlafaxine
Miconazole	
Budesonide	
Sulfasalazine	
Metronidazole	
Protease inhibitors	

TABLE 33.18   Drug-Related Paraesthesia or Hypoaesthesia

Drugs Most Commonly Implicated	Drugs Occasionally Implicated
Acetazolamide (paraesthesia)	Gonadotropin-releasing hormone analogues
Articaine	
Labetalol (paraesthesia)	Hydralazine (paraesthesia)
Protease inhibitors (paraesthesia)	Mefloquine (paraesthesia)
Vincristine (paraesthesia)	Methotrexate (paraesthesia)
	Nitrofurantoin (peripheral neuropathy)
	Prilocaine

TABLE 33.19   Drug-Related Involuntary Facial Movements

Drugs Most Commonly Implicated	Drugs Occasionally Implicated
L-dopa	Carbamazepine
Metoclopramide	Ecstasy
Phenothiazines	Lithium
	Methamphetamine
	Methyldopa
	Phenytoin
	Tricyclic antidepressants

TABLE 33.20   Drug-Related Orofacial Pain

Drugs Most Commonly Implicated	Drugs Occasionally Implicated
ACE inhibitors	Lithium
Nitrites	Penicillins
Vinca alkaloids	Vitamin A

TABLE 33.21   Drug-Related Burning Mouth

Drugs Most Commonly Implicated	Drugs Occasionally Implicated
Cytotoxic drugs	Antidepressants
ACE inhibitors	Clonazepam
Angiotensin receptor blockers	Proton pump inhibitors
Nevirapine	
Efavirenz	

TABLE 33.22   Drug-Related Bruxism or Trismus

Drugs Most Commonly Implicated	Drugs Occasionally Implicated
Ecstasy	Duloxetine
	Fluoxetine
	Metoclopramide
	Tricyclic antidepressants

TABLE 33.23   Drugs Used in Pregnancy That May Induce Cleft Palate

Drugs Most Commonly Implicated	Drugs Occasionally Implicated
Alcohol	Sulfasalazine
Isotretinoin	Naproxen
Anticonvulsants, e.g. phenytoin, topiramate	Corticosteroids
	Methotrexate
Mycophenolate mofetil	Thalidomide
Cocaine	Benzodiazepines
Fluconazole	Anti-retroviral drugs, e.g. efavirenz, nelfinavir, nevirapine and lamivudine
Heroin	

TABLE 33.24 Drugs That May Lead to Tooth Structure Damage

Drug	Examples	Possible Damage to Tooth Structure
Sugar-containing oral (liquid) medication	Various	Caries
Drugs that result in decreased salivary secretion (hyposalivation)	See Table 33.4	Caries
Drugs with a low pH	Aspirin, anti-asthmatic drugs	Erosion
Drugs causing gastro-oesophageal reflux	Theophylline, anticholinergics, progesterone, calcium channel blockers, anti-asthmatics	Erosion
Drugs inducing bruxism	Dopamine agonists, dopamine antagonists, tricyclic antide-pressants, selective serotonin reuptake inhibitors, alcohol, cocaine, amphetamines	Attrition
Drugs used for internal tooth bleaching	Hydrogen peroxide and sodium perborate	Cervical root resorption
Drugs used for the treatment of childhood cancers	Cytotoxic agents	Abnormal dental development
Anticonvulsants	Phenytoin	Abnormal dental development
Fluorides	Any	Fluorosis

TABLE 33.25 Drug-Related Tooth Discoloration

Drugs Most Commonly Implicated	Drugs Occasionally Implicated
Extrinsic	**Extrinsic**
Chlorhexidine mouth rinse	Co-amoxiclav
Fluoride rinses	Clarithromycin
Iron supplements	
Tetracyclines as topical mouth rinse	
Intrinsic	
Fluoride	
Tetracyclines	
Intra-canal, e.g. Ledermix	

A number of topical medicaments result in extrinsic tooth discolouration detailed in Table 33.25. The stain is removable with dentrifices and brushing. Intrinsic widespread tooth discolouration occurs in utero or the first decade during tooth development, e.g. tetracycline antibiotics. Root canal therapy can also introduce localised staining.

MEDICATION-RELATED OSTEONECROSIS OF THE JAW

Medication-related osteonecrosis of the jaw (MRONJ) is defined as exposed necrotic bone or bone that can be probed through an intra-oral or extra-oral fistula, which has been present for more than 8 weeks in patients with a history of treatment with anti-resorptive or anti-angiogenic drugs where there has been no previous history metastatic disease of the jaw or history of radiation therapy. BP are drugs used to prevent and treat osteoporosis, Paget's disease and bone resorption in,

for example, metastatic malignant disease. Bisphosphonates are intravenously used (IV-BPs) for the treatment of hyper-calcaemia of malignancy, as well as the prevention of skeletal-related events (SREs) and reduction of bone pain in cancer patients with osteolytic lesions. They are most commonly used in patients with multiple myeloma, breast, prostate and lung cancers. Oral BPs are used mainly for prophylaxis of osteoporosis, and so are widely prescribed.

Most cases (>90%) of MRONJ have been in patients with cancer who received IV-BPs, in particular, the nitrogen-containing BPs pamidronate and zoledronate, the estimated incidence is 1% (1 case per 100) but the risk from oral BPs is far lower at 0.01% to 0.1% (<1 to 10 cases per 10,000). In addition, nitrogen-containing BPs induce mucosal cell damage and impede wound healing.

Newer anti-resorptive agents such as the RANKL inhibitor monoclonal antibody Denosumab have also been linked to MRONJ; anti-angiogenic agents such as monoclonal antibodies targeting vascular endothelial growth factor (VEGF) receptors such as bevacizumab, tyrosine kinase inhibitors (e.g. sunitinib, sorafenib and pazopanib) or inhibitors of the mammalian target of rapamycin (mTOR) e.g. sirolimus, everolimus and cytotoxic molecules used for chemotherapy may also increase the risk of osteonecrosis of the jaw. Additionally, methotrexate, corticosteroids and thalidomide have also been implicated. The relevant drugs are listed in Table 33.26.

Aetiology and Pathogenesis

BPs act especially by blocking the osteoclast HMG-CoA reductase (mevalonate) path, inhibiting the cell activities, as well as directly inhibiting osteogenesis in bone-healing. BPs remain in bone and exert these effects for many years or even decades. Risk factors for MRONJ include systemic and local factors (Table 33.27), especially tooth extraction.

TABLE 33.26 Drug-Related Osteonecrosis (MRONJ)

Drugs Most Commonly Implicated	Drugs Occasionally Implicated
Bisphosphonates	Methotrexate
Monoclonal antibody, e.g. denosumab	
Vascular endothelial growth factor inhibitors, e.g. bevacizumab	
Tyrosine kinase inhibitors, e.g. sunitib, sorafenib and pazopanib	
Mammalian target of rapamycin inhibitors, e.g. sirolimus, everolimus and temsirolimus	
Fusion protein, e.g. aflibercept	

TABLE 33.27 Local and Systemic Risk Factors for MRONJ

Systemic Risk Factors	Local Risk Factors
Duration of BP exposure	Dental extractions: increase risk at least 16-fold and up to 44-fold
IV administration	
Potent nitrogen-containing BPs (i.e. zoledronate, pamidronate and ibandronate)	Dental trauma
Smoking	Denture wearing: an almost 5-fold increased risk for patients taking zoledronate and also wearing dentures
Diabetes mellitus	
Rheumatoid arthritis and other autoimmune diseases	
CYP2C8 gene diversity or reduced interleukin-17	Periodontal disease: as a risk factor remains controversial
Monoclonal antibody, e.g. denosumab	
Other drugs as in Table 33.26	Other oral infections
Osteomalacia has been implicated	

Clinical Features

MRONJ primarily affects the mandibular alveolar bone/mylohyoid ridge area but other sites can be affected (65% mandible, 28.4% maxilla, 6.5% both mandible and maxilla, 0.1% other locations). Features may include any or all of the following:

- exposed bone
- loose teeth
- foul discharge
- pain
- fistulae
- prolonged jaw pain
- bone enlargement
- gingival swelling
- erythema and ulceration.

Lamina dura sclerosis or loss, and periodontal ligament space widening may be early manifestations. The 2014 American Association of Maxillofacial Surgeons (AAOMS) position paper provided a clinical staging system to describe the severity of MRONJ.

Diagnosis

MRONJ diagnosis is from a history and typical clinical symptoms. Because MRONJ has a variety of appearances on imaging, the diagnosis cannot be made from imaging alone, though periapical and panoramic radiographs serve for initial screening. CT and MRI provide a more comprehensive evaluation. Delineation of the extent of the diseased area by CT may also be helpful for surgical treatment planning. Bone scans can show abnormal radionuclide uptake 10–14 days before radiographic changes are seen on conventional films. Tetracycline bone fluorescence has recently been used to visualise margins of osteonecrosis more precisely. Fluorescence–guided bone resection might improve the surgical therapy of MRONJ.

Management

There is no consensus regarding the optimal management of this condition. The main aims are to:

- eliminate pain
- control infection
- minimise the progression or occurrence of bone necrosis.

Conservative measures result in healing in a significant proportion of patients and comprise the initial approach. It includes antimicrobial mouthwash, antibiotics (if clinically indicated), good oral hygiene and conservative surgical intervention, such as debridement to remove a superficial bone spicule. Most extensive surgical interventions (resection of necrotic bone or soft tissue closure) may be warranted if there are persistent symptoms or impacts on function. There is limited data on the use of non-surgical treatment strategies, including parathyroid hormone (teriparatide), pentoxifylline and vitamin E, low-level laser irradiation and hyperbaric oxygen.

Prevention

Prevention of MRONJ is fundamental since there is no cure, and should include:

- Risk assessment.
- Patient counselling about risks.
- Avoiding elective oral surgery: including extractions or endosseous implant placement or carrying out the treatment well before commencing BPs.
- Preventive measures (dental screening with all dental work done at least 6 weeks before starting BPs). Non-restorable teeth should be extracted. If permitted, initiation of therapy should be delayed until the mucosa has healed or until there is adequate bone healing. These decisions should be made jointly by the treating doctor and dentist. Minor dental procedures with preservation of the root are preferred over total tooth extraction. Conservative restorative dentistry is critical to maintaining functionally sound teeth.
- Modifiable risk factors for MRONJ (e.g. ill-fitting dentures, poorly controlled diabetes and smoking) should be addressed.

IMMUNOSUPPRESSION AND COMPLICATIONS

Immunosuppressive therapy is used to suppress:

- rejection in transplant recipients (bone marrow, kidney, liver, pancreas, heart and heart-lung); these are the most severely immunocompromised patients

- autoimmune disorders
- connective tissue diseases
- some malignant tumours, especially lymphoproliferative neoplasms.

A variety of drugs are used to induce immunosuppression, especially corticosteroids and calcineurin antagonists (such as ciclosporin, tacrolimus and sirolimus). Drugs such as azathioprine, cyclophosphamide and chlorambucil are cytotoxic to a range of cells, including some immunocytes, and are, therefore, also used for immunosuppression. A range of orofacial effects can arise, especially infections and malignant neoplasms. Biologic therapies are also associated with an increased risk of infections (e.g. ant-CD20 Rituximab and anti-TNF therapies).

Infections

Patients on immunosuppressive agents are at risk from oral infections, which may be opportunistic (involving microorganisms that are normally commensal) or may involve exogenous pathogens, and can include:
- Fungal infections:
  - candidiasis (see Chapter 36, Table 33.28)
  - *Aspergillus* spp. may infect the paranasal sinuses, palate or other sites by direct extension and haematogenously. Diagnosis is by demonstration of hyphae in a smear, serology and biopsy. Intravenous amphotericin may be effective
  - mucormycosis (zygomycosis: phycomycosis) is infection by *Mucor* or *Rhizopus* spp., mainly of the paranasal sinuses and nose of immunosuppressed or poorly controlled diabetic or leukaemic patients. Diagnosis is by biopsy and culture: treatment is by control of underlying disease, debridement and intravenous amphotericin mycobacterioses.
- Bacterial infections and mycobacterioses.
- Herpetic infections (Chapter 38).
- Odontogenic infections, which are potentially life-threatening in the immunosuppressed patient, and the broad-spectrum cover is needed (such as penicillin plus gentamicin). Partially erupted third molars are a potential source of infection.

Patients may also be at risk from attempts at treatment; thus, for example, broad-spectrum antibiotics used to control bacterial infections increase the hazard of fungal infections. Patients on ciclosporin and antihypertensive agents are at risk of drug-related gingival swelling from ciclosporin and calcium-channel blockers. The swelling appears to be greater with the combination of ciclosporin—nifedipine than with ciclosporin—amlodipine or ciclosporin only.

Neoplasms

Neoplasms, at least some of which are virally related, may also be a risk in chronic immunosuppression including:
- Kaposi sarcoma
- lymphoproliferative syndromes (post-transplant lymphoproliferative disease: PTLD), which may appear late — even many years after transplantation — and range from hyperplastic-appearing lesions to non-Hodgkin lymphoma or multiple myeloma. Reduction in immunosuppressives can often reverse PTLD. Surgical resection, cytotoxics, anti-CD21 and anti-CD24 antibodies, interferon-alpha and rituximab have been effectively used for treatment of squamous cell carcinomas of the skin and of the lip. Patients must be advised to avoid UV exposure and wear UV protection. They should be screened annually by a dermatologist.

Systemic and potent/super-potent topical corticosteroids have additional risks that need to be mitigated against. These are discussed in Chapter 5.

Checkpoint Inhibitors

PD-1 receptors are present on T cells and act as an 'off-switch' to keep the immune system in check. Cancer cells may have a high concentration of PD-L1 and thus by binding with PD1 on T cells are able to prevent T cell attack. In the last few years, anti-programmed cell death 1 (PD-1) immune checkpoint inhibitors have been developed and are in use. These can cause mucocutaneous side effects resulting from T cell activation. The full side effect profile remains to be fully elucidated, however, dermatologic and oral adverse events are most common. The main oral toxicities of these immune checkpoint inhibitors include:
- Xerostomia
- Dysgeusia
- Lichenoid reactions
- Oral mucositis occurs more rarely.

Treatment requires reduction or discontinuation of the drug and corticosteroids.

RECREATIONAL DRUGS

A range of recreational drugs can impact the orofacial region. Recreational drugs can be taken in various forms and many are absorbed through the lining of the oral mucosa and can be held in the oral cavity, chewed or mixed with other materials and swallowed. Oral health problems that are typically seen with recreational drugs include mucosal dysplasia, xerostomia, periodontal disease, bruxism and taste disturbances. (Table 33.29)

TABLE 33.28 Drug-Related Oral Candidiasis	
Drugs Most Commonly Implicated	**Drugs Occasionally Implicated**
Broad-spectrum antimicrobials	Biologics, e.g. anti-IL17A
Corticosteroids	secukinumab
Cytotoxics	
Drugs causing hyposalivation	
Immunosuppressives	

TABLE 33.29   Maxillofacial Consequences of Use of Specific Recreational Drugs

Drug	Possible Complications
Alcohol	Leukoplakia, carcinoma, tooth erosion, glossitis/oral ulcers/angular stomatitis from malnutrition, sialosis, foetal alcohol syndrome
Amphetamine (e.g. ICE, Speed, crystal meth)	Picking at the face, bruxism, hyposalivation and increased caries incidence 'Meth mouth' is the term given to the neglect and poor oral hygiene seen in methamphetamine users
Barbiturates (downers)	Facial pain, bullous reactions
Betel (betel quid, paan, areca nut, tobacco chewing)	Submucous fibrosis, leukoplakia, carcinoma
Cannabis (marijuana, weed, skunk, hash/hashish synthetic cannabis, e.g. SPICE)	White lesions (burns), hyposalivation, possible leukoplakia, carcinoma
Cocaine (crack cocaine, coke)	Temporarily numbness of lips and tongue, gingival or mucosal erosions, dry mouth, bruxism, dental erosion Caries and periodontal disease, especially acute necrotising gingivitis, are more frequent Cocaine may precipitate cluster headaches Oronasal fistulae
Ecstasy (MDMA, molly)	Tooth clenching, bruxism, TMJ dysfunction, dry mouth, attrition, dental erosion, mucosal burns or ulceration, circumoral paraesthesiae and periodontitis
Khat	Leukoplakia, carcinoma
Nicotine (cigarettes, Shisha, electronic cigarettes)	Due to tobacco: leukoplakia, carcinoma, dry socket, necrotising gingivitis, periodontitis, impaired wound healing and implant success
Opiates (heroin, morphine, methadone)	Hyposalivation
Solvents (glues, aerosols, petrol/gasoline)	Perioral dermatitis

RECOMMENDED READING

Adverse drug effects and reporting service: Available at: https://yellowcard.mhra.gov.uk/.

Dental Medicines Advice Service UK: Available at: https://www.sps.nhs.uk/articles/uk-dental-medicines-advice-service-ukdmas/.

Oral health management of patients at risk of medication-related osteonecrosis of the jaw: Available at: https://www.sdcep.org.uk/published-guidance/medication-related-osteonecrosis-of-the-jaw/.

Medication-related osteonecrosis of the jaw: guidance for the oncology multidisciplinary team. Available at: https://www.rcplondon.ac.uk/guidelines-policy/medication-related-osteonecrosis-jaw-guidance-oncology-multidisciplinary-team.

Rademacher, W.M.H., Aziz, Y., Hielema, A., et al., 2020. Oral adverse effects of drugs: Taste disorders. Oral Dis. 26 (1), 213–223.

Yarom, N., Shapiro, C.L., Peterson, D.E., et al., 2019. Medication-related osteonecrosis of the jaw: MASCC/ISOO/ASCO clinical practice guideline. J. Clin. Oncol. 37 (25), 2270–2290.

34

Transplantation and Graft-Versus-Host Disease

TRANSPLANTATION

Transplantation can result in a range of complications including mucositis, infections and graft-versus-host disease (GVHD). Orofacial complications can follow transplantation of solid organs or bone marrow (human precursor cell transplantation (HPCT) or haematopoietic stem cell transplantation [HSCT]) — largely as a consequence of the immunosuppression used.

Patients who have had organ transplantation are additionally predisposed to:
- oral malignant neoplasms (carcinomas, lymphomas and Kaposi sarcoma)
- food-induced allergic reactions, including transient angioedema
- pyogenic granulomas, commonly affect the gingiva, the lip or the tongue
- mucosal lesions similar to orofacial granulomatosis
- long-standing oral mucosal lesions in solid organ — (liver) transplanted children have been described as multiple spherical nodules on the dorsum of the tongue, which later on displayed a fissured appearance.

Haematopoietic Stem Cell Transplantation

HSCT is increasingly used to treat:
- Haematological malignancies (leukaemias, lymphomas, myelomas and aplastic anaemia) and less commonly:
  - solid malignancies
  - congenital metabolic diseases
  - congenital immune diseases.
  The procedure of HSCT may involve the recipient receiving:
- ablation of bone marrow cells by high-dose CTX with drugs
- total (whole) body irradiation (TBI)
- transfusion of bone marrow aspirate from a donor who has been stimulated with growth factors.
  This regimen results in:
- Profound immunosuppression until the donor bone marrow graft takes and, therefore, patients must be isolated to reduce the risk of infections.

- GVHD which arises in about 60% of cases can produce further immune defects and is potentially lethal.
- Lymphoproliferative syndromes (post-transplant lymphoproliferative disorder [PTLD]) and rarely, lymphomas.

Oral Complications of Haematopoietic Stem Cell Transplantation

Oral complications are common following HSCT and can be a major cause of morbidity from the effects of the underlying disease, chemo- or radiotherapy and immunosuppressant drugs and include:
- GVHD (acute and chronic).
- Mucositis: this typically begins around 5 days post-HSCT, but by around 9 to 14 days post-HSCT basal cells regenerate and it resolves. Mucositis may be ameliorated by the use of glutamine and interleukin-11.
- Ulceration: mainly a consequence of granulocytopenia, this resolves by around 9 to 14 days post-HSCT, when the neutrophils rise greater than 500 cells/mL.
- Infections: superficial infections are frequent and can involve a wide range of microorganisms, mainly:
  - Herpes simplex virus (HSV): about 60% of patients secrete HSV orally within 50 days, and many have lesions, such as ulcers.
  - Cytomegalovirus (CMV): about 60% of patients secrete CMV between days 30 and 150 and lesions, such as ulcers, may result.
  - Varicella-zoster virus (VZV): 40% are infected within 6 months and 80% develop zoster.
  - Epstein–Barr virus (EBV): about 60% secrete EBV and, although uncommon, hairy leukoplakia or lymphoproliferative disease may result.
  - Human papillomaviruses (HPV): can cause extensive warty lesions over the 3 to 8 months post-transplant.
  - Candidiasis: carriage and oral lesions are almost invariable in the absence of prophylactic antifungal therapy.

- Mucormycosis: a rare, but serious complication.
- Bacterial septicaemia is less common, but 25% to 75% of septicaemias arise from the oral cavity involving viridans *Streptococci*, *Enterococci*, *Leptotrichia buccalis* and Gram-negative organisms.
- Hyposalivation.
- Bleeding.
- Dental maldevelopment: most children undergoing HSCT have disturbed tooth development, including missing teeth, shortened roots and arrested root development.
- Malignant neoplasms: most patients develop genetic instability in their oral mucosa and oral malignant disease occasionally arises even after 5 to 10 years after HSCT. In half the cases, the tongue is the primary location. The neoplasms may have more aggressive behaviour, with a poorer prognosis.

GRAFT-VERSUS-HOST DISEASE

GVHD is a major cause of morbidity and mortality in patients following allogeneic HSCT. GVHD refers to multi-organ syndromes of tissue inflammation and/or fibrosis that primarily affects the skin, gastrointestinal tract, liver, lungs and mucosal surfaces. GVHD comprises acute GVHD (aGVHD) and chronic GVHD (cGVHD), Some patients with aGVHD go on to develop cGVHD and in some patients, features of both persist (overlap syndrome) (Table 34.1). The prevalence of GVHD is increasing due to the extension of clinical indications for HSCT treatment and prolonged patient survival. GVHD

TABLE 34.1	Acute and Chronic GVHD
Acute GVHD	**Chronic**
Skin rash GI symptoms: nausea and vomiting Loss of appetite Diarrhoea Cholestatic hepatitis	• A dry, itchy raised rash (erythroderma) or skin thickening, resembling lichen planus) • Loss of skin colour without thickening (vitiligo) • Hardening of skin (scleroderma) may interfere with joint mobility • Hair loss • Nail dystrophy • Oral lesions —lichenoid lesions, erythema, ulceration and mucoceles • Dry mouth • Dry eyes causing irritation and redness • Genital disease, including painful vulval and vaginal ulceration with scarring • Decreased sweating • Liver involvement causing jaundice • Gi disturbance —diarrhoea and weight loss • Lung and GI disorders may occur
Classic: occurs within 100 days	Classic: at least one diagnostic/distinctive manifestation, no time restriction
Persistent/recurrent/late acute: beyond 100 days	Overlap syndrome: features of acute and chronic, no time restriction

GVHD, Graft-versus-host disease.

develops in 40% to 60% of patients following allogeneic HSCT. The oral cavity is rarely affected in aGVHD, but in over 70% of patients with cGVHD, the oral cavity is involved.

GVHD arises when immune cells transplanted from a non-identical donor (graft) into the recipient (host) recognise the host cells as 'foreign', thereby initiating a graft-versus-host reaction. HSCT transfers T lymphocytes which perceive host tissues as antigenically foreign via HLA and other antigens, and mount an immune attack on the host, the transferred T cells producing cytokines, including TNK alpha and IFN-gamma (IFNγ).

aGVHD usually appears within the first 100 days post-transplant. cGVHD usually occurs after 100 days post-HSCT.

Acute Graft-Versus-Host Disease (aGVHD)

Acute GVHD manifests as an inflammatory immune cell infiltrate involving T cells, macrophages, monocytes and neutrophil granulocytes with associated tissue destruction. Innate immunity, impaired tissue repair mechanisms, the transplantation conditioning regimen and gastrointestinal microbiome contribute to the pathophysiology. aGVHD affects mainly the liver, gastrointestinal tract and mucocutaneous tissues, and can be lethal. Skin lesions are often the earliest visible sign of the disease. Prophylactic immunosuppressive therapy using corticosteroids and ciclosporin is usually used for the first 100 days post-HSCT. The oral manifestations of aGVHD are difficult or impossible to differentiate from chemotherapy-induced mucositis and consist of:

- Painful mucosal desquamation and ulceration. Erythema and ulceration are most pronounced at 7 to 11 days after HSCT and may be associated with obvious infection. Small white lesions affect the buccal and lingual mucosa early on but are clear by day 14. The ventral surface of the tongue, buccal and labial mucosa and gingiva may be affected.
- Cheilitis.
- Hyposalivation; most significant in the first 14 days after transplantation and is a consequence of drug treatment and/or irradiation.
- Infections; candidiasis, HSV stomatitis (occasionally zoster), CMV, protozoal and Gram-positive bacterial infections.
- Purpura and bleeding.

The severity of aGVHD is graded from I to IV depending on the combination of the degree of involvement of the skin, liver and the GI tract. aGVHD is treated with high-dose immunosuppressive therapy.

Chronic Graft-Versus-Host Disease cGVHD)

Chronic GVHD is severe and involves multiple organs, mainly the skin, gastrointestinal tract, lungs, eyes and in 80% of cases, the mouth. The pathogenesis of cGVHD is complex and involves early inflammation and tissue injury, chronic inflammation, and aberrant tissue repair and fibrosis. The oral lesions are painful and limit food and drink intake and present as:

- lichenoid lesions (Fig. 34.1)
- hyperkeratotic plaques

- generalised mucosal erythema
- ulceration
- mucoceles of minor salivary glands.
  Other problems include:
- hyposalivation
- taste abnormalities
- infections, especially candidiasis
- sclerodermatous changes manifesting with restriction of mouth opening and loss of elasticity of the lips and restricted tongue movement
- drug-induced gingival swelling, e.g. ciclosporin (Fig. 34.2).

The National Institute of Health (NIH) cGVHD Task Force developed a scoring system for cGVHD which includes three types of oral manifestations (erythema, lichenoid and ulcers) which can be graded in three activity levels (mild, moderate and severe) (see Table 34.2).

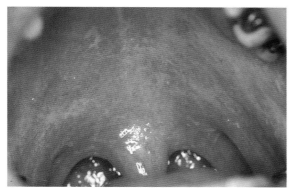

Fig. 34.1 Lichenoid lesions in graft-versus-host disease.

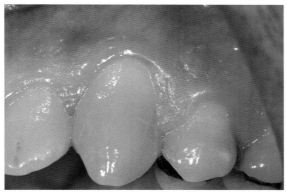

Fig. 34.2 Very early lesions of ciclosporin-induced gingival swelling appeared on the interdental papilla.

Diagnosis of Graft-Versus-Host Disease

Diagnosis is from the history and clinical features and a mucosal or labial salivary gland biopsy, which shows mononuclear cell infiltrates. Histopathological findings of oral mucosal cGVHD include lichenoid interface inflammation, leukocyte exocytosis and keratinocyte apoptosis.

Management of Graft-Versus-Host Disease

The aim of treatment is to alleviate symptoms to allow normal oral function. Topical treatment is the same for aGVHD and cGVHD. Treatment is based on disease severity. For mild cGVHD, topical treatment rather than systemic therapy is recommended to avoid adverse effects and complications of systemic immunosuppressive therapy. For more severe cGVHD, systemic therapy includes corticosteroids with or without ciclosporin, sirolimus, tacrolimus, mycophenolate mofetil, ruxolitinib, ibrutinib, imatinib or rituximab. Non-pharmacologic approaches include extracorporeal photopheresis.

Management of oral lesions:
- Maintenance of oral hygiene and dentition
  - topical fluoride
  - dietary advice
  - non-alcoholic chlorhexidine mouthwash
  - neutral-pH toothpaste with a soft toothbrush.
- Pain relief with topical anaesthetic agents such as lidocaine or benzydamine hydrochloride mouthwash or spray.
- Topical corticosteroids can be applied as solutions, gels, creams or ointments several times a day. Intralesional injections of corticosteroids (e.g. triamcinolone acetonide) for localised persistent ulcers are helpful. Calcineurin inhibitors such as tacrolimus ointment (available as 0.03% and 0.1%). Tacrolimus is also available as a mouthwash and may be used for intraoral involvement.
- Xerostomia
  - Oral lubricants and saliva replacements and stimulants, e.g. sugar-free gum, artificial saliva sprays and gels and pastilles.
  - Pilocarpine 5mg three to four times daily; or cevimeline 15 to 30 mg two to three times daily.
- In patients with sclerotic disease, physiotherapy exercises daily to improve the flexibility of the perioral tissues.
- Topical and systemic antifungal therapy to treat candidiasis.
- There is limited data that low-level laser therapy, CO_2 laser therapy and phototherapy are effective in treating oral cGVHD lesions.

TABLE 34.2			**Scoring of Oral Chronic GVHD Lesions**						
Erythema	None	0	Mild or moderate erythema (<25%)	1	Moderate (≥25%) or severe (≤25%) erythema	2	Severe erythema (≥25%)	3
Lichenoid	None	0	Lichen-like changes (<25%)	1	Lichen-like changes (25%–50%)	2	Lichen-like changes (>50%)	3
Ulcers	None	0			Ulcers involving (≤20%)	3	Severe ulcerations (>20%)	6
Total score for all mucosal changes								

- Patients should be screened regularly as the risk for developing oral cancer is seven times higher in long-term survivors of allogeneic HSCT, with the risk increasing the longer the time since transplantation. The average time for oral cancer development following HSCT is 6 to 8 years.

RECOMMENDED READING

Albuquerque, R., Khan, Z., Poveda, A., et al., 2016. Management of oral graft vs host disease with topical agents: a systematic review. Med. Oral. 211, e72—e81.

Bassim, C.W., Fassil, H., Mays, J.W., et al., 2014. Validation of the National Institutes of Health chronic GVHD Oral Mucosal Score using component-specific measures. Bone Marrow Transplant. 49 (1), 116—121.

Fall-Dickson, J.M., Pavletic, S.Z., Mays, J.W., Schubert, M.M., 2019. Oral Complications of Chronic Graft-Versus-Host Disease. J. Natl. Cancer Inst. Monogr. 2019 (53), lgz007.

Treister, N., Duncan, C., Cutler, C., Lehmann, L., 2012. How we treat oral chronic graft-versus-host disease. Blood. 120 (17), 3407—3418.

35

Oral Manifestations of Disorders of Specific Systems

This chapter annotates the orofacial manifestations of disorders of specific biological systems.

BOX 35.1 Cardiovascular Diseases

Angina Pectoris
- Pain referred to jaw rarely
- Ulceration caused by nicorandil

Anticoagulants
- Bleeding tendency

Giant Cell Arteritis (Cranial or Temporal Arteritis)
- Pain usually over the temple
- Rarely, tongue pain or ischaemic necrosis

Hereditary Haemorrhagic Telangiectasia
- Telangiectasias that may bleed profusely

Hypertension (Problems Caused by Some Anti-Hypertensive Agents)
- Dry mouth
- Gingival swelling (nifedipine)
- Lichenoid lesions (methyldopa, ACE inhibitors)
- Angioedema (ACE inhibitors)
- Burning mouth (ACE inhibitors)
- Taste changes (Ca channel blockers, B blockers, diuretics)

Ischaemic Heart Disease
- Arterial calcifications on orthopantomogram
- Possibly periodontitis

Polyarteritis Nodosa
- Ulcers

Shunts: Right to Left (e.g. Fallot Tetralogy)
- Cyanosis
- Delayed tooth eruption

BOX 35.2 Connective Tissue Diseases

Any Connective Tissue Disease
- Sjögren syndrome
- Lymph node enlargement
- Facial sensory loss

Ehlers–Danlos Syndrome
- Temporomandibular joint hypermobility
- Pulp stones
- Periodontitis rarely

Felty Syndrome
- Temporomandibular arthritis
- Sjögren syndrome
- Drug reactions (e.g. lichenoid)
- Ulcers

Lupus Erythematosus
- White lesions, lesions resembling lichen-planus
- Ulcers
- Sjögren syndrome

Mixed Connective Tissue Disease
- Ulceration
- Pain
- Sjögren syndrome

Rheumatoid Arthritis
- Temporomandibular arthritis
- Sjögren syndrome
- Drug reactions (e.g. lichenoid)

Still Syndrome
- Temporomandibular arthritis
- Sjögren syndrome
- Ankylosis

BOX 35.2   Connective Tissue Diseases—cont'd

Systemic Sclerosis
- Stiffness of lips, tongue, etc.
- Trismus
- Telangiectasia
- Sjögren syndrome
- Periodontal ligament widened on radiography
- Mandibular resorption

BOX 35.3   Endocrine Conditions

Acromegaly
- Spaced teeth
- Mandibular prognathism
- Macroglossia

Diabetes Mellitus
- Periodontal disease, accelerated
- Hyposalivation
- Candidiasis
- Sialosis
- Lichen planus
- Burning mouth symptoms
- Taste alterations

Gigantism
- Spaced teeth
- Mandibular prognathism
- Macroglossia
- Megadontia

Hyperparathyroidism
- Giant cell granulomas
- Loss of lamina dura
- Osteitis fibrosa cystica, rarely

Hypoadrenocorticism (e.g. Addison disease)
- Mucosal hyperpigmentation

Hypoparathyroidism (Congenital)
- Dental hypoplasia
- May be chronic candidosis if there is an associated immune defect

Hypopituitarism (Congenital)
- Microdontia
- Retarded tooth eruption

Hypothyroidism (Congenital)
- Macroglossia
- Retarded tooth eruption

Menopause
- Osteoporosis

Precocious Puberty
- Accelerated tooth eruption (fibrous dysplasia in Albright syndrome)

Pregnancy
- Gingivitis
- Epulis

BOX 35.4   Gastrointestinal Disorders

Chronic Pancreatitis
- Sialosis
- IgG4 disease

Coeliac Disease
- Ulcers
- Glossitis
- Angular stomatitis
- Dental hypoplasia in severely affected children

Crohn Disease
- Facial or lip swelling
- Mucosal tags
- Gingival hyperplasia
- Cobblestoning of mucosa
- Mucogingivitis
- Ulcers
- Glossitis
- Angular stomatitis
- Cervical lymphadenopathy

Ulcerative Colitis
- Pyostomatitis vegetans
- Aphthous ulceration

Cystic Fibrosis
- Salivary gland swelling

Gardner Syndrome (Familial Colonic Polyps)
- Osteomas

Gastric Regurgitation
- Tooth erosion
- Halitosis

Malabsorption Syndromes
- Ulcers
- Glossitis
- Angular stomatitis
- Sialosis

Patterson–Kelly Syndrome
- Oral cancer

Pancreatic Cancer
- Periodontitis

Pernicious Anaemia
- Ulcers
- Glossitis
- Angular stomatitis

Peutz–Jeghers Syndrome (Small Intestinal Polyps)
- Melanosis

BOX 35.5   Haematological Disorders and Immune Defects

Aplastic Anaemia
- Ulcers
- Bleeding tendency

Graft-Versus-Host Disease
- Lichenoid lesions
- Dry mouth

Haematinic—Iron, Folic Acid or Vitamin B$_{12}$ Deficiency
- Burning mouth sensation
- Glossitis
- Ulcers
- Angular cheilitis

Haemolytic Disease of the Newborn
- Pigmentation
- Rarely, enamel defects

Haemopoietic Stem Cell Transplantation
- Ulcers
- Mucositis
- Hyposalivation
- Graft-versus-host disease (see Chapter 34)

Hypereosinophilic Syndrome
- Ulceration

Hypoplasminogenaemia
- Gingival swelling and ulceration

Leukaemia
- Infections
- Ulcers
- Bleeding tendency
- Gingival swelling in myelomonocytic leukaemia
- Cervical lymph node enlargement
- Labial sensory loss

Leucocyte Defects
- Infections, especially herpetic and candidal
- Ulcers

Lymphoma
- Infections
- Ulcers
- Swelling
- Cervical lymph node enlargement

Multiple Myeloma
- Bone pain
- Tooth mobility
- Amyloid

Myelodysplastic Syndrome
- Ulcers
- Labial sensory changes

Sickle Cell Anaemia
- Jaw deformities caused by marrow expansion
- Rarely, osteomyelitis or pain

Thalassaemia Major
- Jaw deformities caused by marrow expansion

Thrombocytopenia
- Bleeding tendency
- Purpura

Immune defects
- See Box 35.7 for HIV

Ataxia Telangiectasia
- Recurrent sinusitis
- Ulceration
- Facial and oral telangiectasia
- Cervical lymphomas
- Mask-like facial expression

Chédiak—Higashi Syndrome
- Cervical lymph node enlargement
- Ulceration
- Periodontitis

Chronic Benign Neutropenia
- Ulceration
- Severe periodontitis

Chronic Granulomatous Disease
- Cervical lymph node enlargement and suppuration
- Candidosis (including CMC)
- Enamel hypoplasia
- Acute gingivitis
- Ulceration

Cyclic Neutropenia
- Ulceration
- Severe periodontitis
- Eczematous lesions of the face

Common Variable Immunodeficiency
- Recurrent sinusitis
- Candidosis (including CMC)

DiGeorge Syndrome (CATCH22)
- Abnormal facies
- Candidosis (including CMC)
- Viral infections
- Bifid uvula
- Dental hypoplasia

Haim—Munk Syndrome
- Periodontitis

Hereditary Angioedema
- Swellings of face, mouth and pharynx

Job syndrome
- Abnormal facies
- Mucocutaneous candidiasis

Lazy Leucocyte Syndrome
- Periodontitis
- Candidiasis (including CMC)

BOX 35.5 Haematological Disorders and Immune Defects—cont'd

Papillon—Lefevre Syndrome
- Periodontitis

Selective IgA Deficiency
- Tonsillar hyperplasia
- Ulceration
- Viral infections
- Parotitis

Severe Combined Immunodeficiency (SCID)
- Candidiasis (including CMC)
- Viral infections
- Ulceration

- Absent tonsils
- Recurrent sinusitis

Sex-Linked Agammaglobulinaemia
- Cervical lymph node enlargement
- Ulceration
- Recurrent sinusitis
- Absent tonsils

Wiskott—Aldrich Syndrome
- Candidiasis
- Viral infections
- Purpura

BOX 35.6 Immunological Disorders

See also connective tissue disorders and skin diseases.

Angioedema
- Facial swelling

Behçet Syndrome
- Ulcers

Graft-Versus-Host Disease
- Lichenoid lesions
- Sicca syndrome
- Infections
- Mucoceles
- Squamous cell carcinoma

Kawasaki Disease (Mucocutaneous Lymph Node Syndrome)
- Cervical lymph node enlargement
- Sore tongue
- Cheilitis

Langerhans Histiocytoses (Histiocytosis X)
- Loosening of teeth
- Jaw radiolucencies

Myasthenia Gravis and Other Myopathies
- Facial weakness
- Lingual weakness
- Dysarthria

Reiter Syndrome (Reactive Arthritis)
- Ulcers
- Lesions like erythema migrans

Sarcoidosis
- Hyposalivation
- Salivary gland swelling
- Heerfordt syndrome (parotid swelling, lacrimal swelling, facial palsy)
- Sjögren syndrome
- Oral swellings

Sweet Syndrome
- Ulcers

Wegener Granulomatosis
- Gingival swelling/strawberry gingivitis
- Ulcers

BOX 35.7 Infectious Diseases: Oral Manifestations

Aspergillosis
- Antral infections

Candidiasis
- White lesions
- Red lesions
- Angular stomatitis

Cat-Scratch Disease
- Lymph node enlargement

Coxsackie Viruses
- Ulcers in herpangina and hand, foot and mouth disease

Cryptococcosis
- Ulcers

Cytomegalovirus
- Ulcers
- Sialadenitis

ECHO viruses
- Ulcers in herpangina and in hand, foot and mouth disease

Epstein—Barr Virus (in Infectious Mononucleosis)
- Sore throat
- Tonsillar exudate
- Palatal petechiae
- Cervical lymph node enlargement
- Ulcers
- Lymphoma
- Sialadenitis
- Recurrent parotitis, possibly in children
- Facial palsy

Gonorrhoea
- Pharyngitis
- Gingivitis
- Temporomandibular arthritis

Hepatitis C (see Chapter 37)
Herpes Simplex
- Ulcers in primary infection
- Gingivitis in primary infection
- Vesicles on lips in recurrence (rarely, oral ulcers)
- Lymph node enlargement
- Facial palsy
- Erythema multiforme

Herpes Zoster-Varicella
- Ulcers in chickenpox, or zoster of trigeminal maxillary or mandibular divisions
- Pain in maxillary or mandibular zoster
- Facial palsy in Ramsay—Hunt syndrome of zoster of the geniculate ganglion

Human Herpesvirus-8
- Kaposi sarcoma

Histoplasmosis
- Ulcers

HIV (Human Immunodeficiency Virus Causing AIDS)
- Lymph node enlargement
- Infections, particularly herpetic and candidal
- Ulcers
- Kaposi sarcoma
- Lymphoma
- Hairy leukoplakia
- Parotitis
- Hyposalivation
- Periodontitis
- Cranial nerve lesions
- Purpura

Leprosy
- Cranial nerve palsies

Lyme disease
- Facial palsy
- Facial sensory loss
- Facial pain

Measles
- Koplik's spots

Mucormycosis
- Antral infections

Mumps
- Salivary gland swelling

Papilloma Viruses
- Warts
- Papillomas
- Condyloma acuminata
- Focal epithelial hyperplasia

Paracoccidioidomycosis
- Ulcers

Rubella
- Palatal petechiae
- Dental hypoplasia in congenital rubella

Syphilis
- Chancre
- Mucous patches
- Condyloma lata
- Ulcers
- Gumma
- Leukoplakia
- Lymph node enlargement
- Hutchinson teeth in congenital syphilis
- Pain from neurosyphilis

Toxoplasmosis
- Cervical lymph node enlargement

Tuberculosis (Including Atypical Mycobacteria)
- Ulcers rarely
- Cervical lymph node enlargement

BOX 35.8   Liver Disorders

Alcoholic Cirrhosis
- Bleeding tendency
- Sialosis

Biliary Atresia
- Dental hypoplasia
- Pigmented teeth

Chronic Active Hepatitis
- Lichen planus

Hepatitis C
- Salivary swelling and hyposalivation
- Lichen planus

Jaundice
- Bleeding tendency
- Jaundice

Kernicterus
- Dental hypoplasia
- Pigmented teeth

Primary Biliary Cirrhosis
- Sjögren syndrome
- Lichen planus

Transplants
- Infections
- Neoplasms
- Gingival swelling

BOX 35.9   Metabolic Disorders

Amyloidosis
- Macroglossia
- Purpura
- Salivary swelling
- Hyposalivation

Erythropoietic Porphyria
- Reddish teeth
- Bullae/erosions
- Dental hypoplasia

Folic Acid Deficiency
- Burning mouth
- Ulcers
- Glossitis
- Angular cheilitis

Haemochromatosis
- Salivary swelling
- Hyposalivation

Hypophosphataemia
- Dental hypoplasia
- Large pulp chambers

Hypophosphatasia
- Loosening and loss of teeth (hypoplastic cementum)

Iron Deficiency
- Burning mouth
- Ulcers
- Glossitis
- Angular cheilitis

Lesch–Nyhan Syndrome (Congenital Hyperuricaemia)
- Self-mutilation

Mucopolysaccharidosis
- Spaced teeth
- Retarded tooth eruption
- Temporomandibular joint anomalies
- Enamel defects
- Cystic lesions

Neimann–Pick Disease
- Retarded tooth eruption
- Loosening of teeth
- Mucosal pigmentation

Rickets (Vitamin D Dependent)
- Dental hypoplasia
- Large pulp chambers

Scurvy
- Gingival swelling
- Purpura
- Ulcers

Tangier Disease
- Orange tonsillar deposits

Trimethylaminuria
- Halitosis

Vitamin B_{12} Deficiency
- Burning mouth
- Ulcers
- Glossitis
- Angular cheilitis

BOX 35.10 Neurological Disorders

Alzheimer Disease
- Hyposalivation
- Impaired oral hygiene

Bulbar Palsy
- Fasciculation of tongue

Cerebral Palsy
- Spastic tongue
- Dysarthria
- Attrition
- Drooling

Cerebrovascular Disease
- Facial palsy
- Facial sensory loss
- Drooling

Choreoathetosis
- Green staining of teeth in kernicterus

Disseminated Sclerosis
- Pain
- Sensory loss
- Facial palsy
- Taste changes

Down Syndrome
- Delayed tooth eruption
- Macroglossia
- Scrotal tongue
- Maxillary hypoplasia
- Anterior open bite
- Hypodontia

- Periodontal disease
- Cheilitis
- Drooling

Dysautonomias
- Drooling or dry mouth

Epilepsy
- Trauma to teeth/jaws/mucosa
- Gingival swelling if on phenytoin

Facial Palsy
- Palsy and poor natural cleansing of mouth on the same side

Neurosyphilis
- Pain rarely
- Dysarthria
- Tremor of tongue

Parkinsonism
- Drooling
- Tremor of tongue

Riley–Day Syndrome
- Self-mutilation
- Prominent fungiform papillae
- Salivary swelling
- Sialorrhoea/drooling

Stroke
- Periodontitis

Trigeminal Neuralgia
- Pain

BOX 35.11 Mental Health Disorders

Any Disorder
- Pain
- Impaired oral hygiene
- Periodontal disease
- Caries

Anorexia Nervosa
- Tooth erosion
- Sialosis

Anxiety States
- Dry mouth
- Cheek biting
- Bruxism

Bulimia
- Tooth erosion

Depression, Hypochondriasis and Various Psychoses
- Dry mouth

- Discharges
- Pain
- Disturbed taste
- Disturbed sensation
- Artefactual ulcers
- Exfoliative cheilitis
- Bruxism
- Burning mouth

Drug Abuse
- Oral burns
- Bruxism
- Oral neglect
- HIV/AIDS

Munchausen Syndrome
- Self-mutilation
- Feigned dental disease

BOX 35.12   Genitourinary Disorders

Chronic Kidney Disease
- Hyposalivation
- Halitosis/taste disturbance
- Leukoplakia
- Dental hypoplasia in children
- Renal osteodystrophy
- Bleeding tendency
- Angioedema

Dialysis
- Hyposalivation
- Sialadenitis

Nephrotic Syndrome
- Dental hypoplasia

Post-Renal Transplantation
- Infections, particularly herpetic and candidiasis
- Bleeding tendency
- Gingival swelling if on ciclosporin or nifedipine
- Leukoplakia and carcinoma

Renal Rickets (Vitamin D Resistant)
- Delayed tooth eruption
- Dental hypoplasia
- Enlarged pulp

Urethroplasty
- Postoperative complications from oral mucosal grafting

BOX 35.13   Respiratory Disorders

Asthma
- Candidiasis
- Caries

Bronchiectasis
- Dry mouth
- Malodour

Chronic Obstructive Airways Diseases
- Cyanosis

Kartagener Syndrome
- Sinusitis

Pneumonia
- Periodontitis

BOX 35.14   Skeletal Disorders

Cherubism
- Jaw swellings

Cleidocranial Dysostosis (Dysplasia)
- Delayed tooth eruption
- Multiple supernumerary teeth
- Dentigerous cysts
- Short tooth roots

Craniofacial Dysostosis (Crouzon Syndrome)
- Maxillary hypoplasia
- Cleft palate

Fibrous Dysplasia
- Expansive jaw lesions

Mandibulofacial Dysostosis (Treacher–Collins Syndrome)
- Cleft palate
- Mandibular hypoplasia

Osteogenesis Imperfecta
- Dentinogenesis imperfecta in some

Osteopetrosis (Albers–Schonberg Disease)
- Cranial neuropathies
- Delayed tooth eruption
- Osteomyelitis after tooth extractions

Osteoporosis
- Jaw osteoporosis
- Bisphosphonate osteochemonecrosis

Paget Disease
- Expansive jaw lesions
- Hypercementosis
- Osteomyelitis rarely after tooth extractions
- Post-extraction bleeding

BOX 35.15 Skin Diseases

Acanthosis Nigricans
- Papillomas

Chronic Bullous Disease in Childhood
- Ulcers
- Blisters, rarely
- Desquamative gingivitis

Chronic Mucocutaneous Candidosis
- Chronic candidiasis

Darier Disease
- White lesions

Dermatitis Herpetiformis
- Ulcers
- Blisters, rarely
- Desquamative gingivitis

Ectodermal Dysplasia
- Hypodontia
- Dental anomalies (peg-shaped teeth)
- Hyposalivation

Ellis–van Creveld Syndrome (Chondroectodermal Dysplasia)
- Multiple fraeni
- Short roots
- Hypodontia

Epidermolysis Bullosa
- Blisters
- Erosions
- Scarring
- Dental hypoplasia
- Oral squamous cell carcinoma

Erythema Multiforme
- Ulcers
- Blood-stained crusting of lips

Lichen Planus
- White lesions
- Red lesions
- Erosions
- Desquamative gingivitis

Linear IgA Disease
- Ulcers
- Blisters, rarely
- Desquamative gingivitis

Pemphigoid
- Blisters
- Ulcers
- Desquamative gingivitis

Pemphigus
- Ulcers
- Blisters, rarely
- Desquamative gingivitis

Psoriasis
- White lesions
- Lesions like erythema migrans

Toxic Epidermal Necrolysis
- Ulcers

RECOMMENDED READING

Porter, S.R., Mercadante, V., Fedele, S., 2017. Oral manifestations of systemic disease. Br. Dent. J. 223 (9), 683–691.

Yeoh, S.C., Hua, H., Yepes, J.F., Peterson, D.E., 2018. Oral manifestations of systemic diseases and their treatments. In: Farah, C., Balasubramaniam, R., McCullough, M. (Eds.), Contemporary Oral Medicine. Springer, Cham.

Oral and Maxillofacial Infections

36

Candidiasis and Other Fungal Infections

KEY POINTS

- *Candida* species are common mouth commensals.
- *Candida* proliferates if the local ecology changes or if immune defences fall.
- Candidiasis manifests with red or white lesions and soreness.
- Specific-related conditions such as denture stomatitis and angular cheilitis are common.
- Treatment includes correcting the local ecological factors, and/or improving immune defences, together with antifungal medication.
- Other fungal infections are rare and usually only seen in a severely immunocompromised patient.

CANDIDIASIS

INTRODUCTION

At least 70% of the normal population carry the fungus *Candida albicans* as a normal oral commensal mainly on the posterior dorsum of the tongue (without any disease) and are therefore termed 'Candida carriers'. It is usually transmitted from mother to baby at birth. This opportunistic pathogen can grow in several different morphological forms. The commensal form is a unicellular budding yeast whereas the pathogenic form is true hyphae with parallel-side wall infection with *Candida* (usually *C. albicans*) known as candidiasis, or candidosis, is seen mainly in people who are immunocompromised, e.g. HIV infected patients, transplant recipients, chemotherapy patients and low-birth-weight babies; candidiasis is thus called a 'disease of the diseased'. *Candida* typically colonises mucocutaneous surfaces and causes only superficial infections but in

immunocompromised patients, candidiasis is commonly oropharyngeal and can be a portal for entry into deeper tissues and invasive candidiasis.

AETIOLOGY

Host defences against *Candida* species include the following:
- Oral epithelium: a physical barrier.
- Microbial interactions: competition and inhibition by the oral flora.
- Salivary non-immune defences: mechanical cleansing plays a major role, but other factors include salivary antimicrobial proteins (AMPs):
  - glycoproteins antigenically similar to blood group antigens — affect adherence to mucosa.
- Secretions in breast milk, e.g.
  - lactoferrin: is antifungal and antibacterial due to the binding of iron or altering yeast cell wall permeability
  - lactoperoxidase: is anticandidal via multiple factors (H_2O_2 and halides).
- Components of the innate immune system including
  - lysozyme (muramidase) which can damage *Candida*, stimulate phagocytosis and agglutinate *Candida*
  - histatins
  - β-defensin 2 (skin-antimicrobial peptide 1).
  - antileukoprotease (ALP)
  - histidine-rich polypeptides
  - calprotectin.
- T cells and phagocytes. The full expression of phagocyte effectiveness is dependent on augmentation by cytokines

synthesised or induced by T cells, such as lymphokines and interferon-γ (IFN-γ). Polymorphonuclear leukocytes (PMNL) and macrophages phagocytose and produce cytokines, such as myeloperoxidase, tumour necrosis factor (TNF), IFN-γ, nitric oxide and granulocyte-macrophage colony-stimulating factor (GM-CSF).

- Salivary sIgA antibodies: which aggregate *Candida* organisms and/or prevent adherence.

PATHOGENESIS

- *C. albicans* can switch frequently and reversibly between several variants, heritable, phenotypes associated with changes in micromorphology, physiology and virulence ('colony switching').
- *C. albicans* adhere to the oral epithelial surface via extracellular polymeric materials, including mannoprotein and adhesins.
- Adhesins, such as hyphal wall protein 1 (HWP1), originating from the yeast cell surface, appear important in making hyphal forms adhere more strongly than do yeast forms.
- Hyphae invade the superficial epithelium and penetrate, via enzymes such as the phospholipases, lysophospholipases and aspartyl proteinase (secretory aspartyl proteinases; SAP) (Fig. 36.1) as far as the stratum spinosum.
- Epithelial endocytic pathways are key innate immune mechanisms in host defence. Defective endolysosomal maturation may partially explain the inability of oral epithelial cells to kill *C. albicans*.
- *C. albicans* invades oral epithelial cells by inducing its own endocytosis by the adhesin and invasin Als3 and gains access to epithelial vacuolar compartments. *C. albicans* is internalised by oral epithelial cells through actin-dependent clathrin-mediated endocytosis and is taken into vacuolar compartments immediately following its internalisation. *Candida*-containing endosomes transiently acquire early endosomal marker EEA1, but show marked defects in the acquisition of late endosomal marker LAMP1 and lysosomal marker cathepsin D.
- The innate immune system is a first-line defence and involves pattern recognition receptors such as Toll-like receptors and C-type lectin-receptors that not only induce innate immune responses but also modulate cellular and humoral adaptive immunity.
- Interleukin (IL)-12: a cytokine family which includes IL-12, IL-23, IL-27 and IL-35 — links to both innate and adaptive immunity systems. An essential component of the response that leads to the generation of Th1-type cytokine responses and protection activity against disseminated candidiasis.
- CD4 T-cells are crucial in the regulation of immunity and inflammation; Th1/2, helper cells, together with Th17 and Treg cells are important.
- Th17 and release IL-17 (which recruits neutrophils), IL-21 (which stimulates CD8 or NK cells) and IL-22, the latter stimulating epithelial cells to produce proteins with antimicrobial activity against *Candida*.

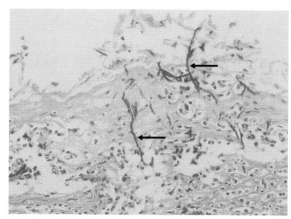

Fig. 36.1 Candidal hyphae stained with periodic acid—Schiff, seen penetrating the epithelium.

- Fungal pattern-recognition receptors such as C-type lectin receptors trigger protective Th17 responses which play the predominant role against mucosal candidiasis. IL-17A and IL-17 F are essential for mucocutaneous immunity against *C. albicans*
- Dectin-1, a C-type lectin that recognises 1,3-beta-glucans from fungi, including *Candida*, is involved in the initiation of the immune response against fungi. Patients bearing the Y238X polymorphism in the DECTIN-1 gene are more likely to be colonised with *Candida* species, compared with patients bearing wild-type DECTIN-1.
- Oral epithelial cells orchestrate an innate response to *C. albicans* via NF-κB and a biphasic MAPK response.
- Activation of NF-κB and the first MAPK response, constituting c-Jun activation, is due to fungal cell wall recognition while the second MAPK phase, constituting MKP1 and c-Fos activation, depends upon hypha formation and fungal burdens — and correlates with the pro-inflammatory responses.
- Activation of the kallikrein—kinin system and other factors result in an inflammatory response in the connective tissue comprising lymphocytes, plasma cells and other leukocytes.
- PMNL migrate into the epithelium in defensive mode, but candidal cell-wall mannans and glycans may impair PMNL chemotaxis, phagocytosis, respiratory burst, T lymphocyte reactivity and the macrophage secretion of TNF.
- Defective cell-mediated immune responses are commonly associated with mucocutaneous *Candida* infections.

CLINICAL FEATURES

Candidiasis; (candidosis) is the state when *Candida species* cause lesions or symptoms:
- The most dominant oral *Candida* species, in decreasing order of frequency, are:
  - *C. albicans*
  - *C. tropicalis*
  - *C. glabrata*
  - *C. parapsilosis*

- *C. krusei*
- other *Candida* species.
- *C. albicans* is the only common cause of oral fungal or yeast infection. It accounts for more than 70% of cases. *C. albicans* can be differentiated serologically into A and B serotypes, equally distributed in healthy individuals, but there is a significant shift to type B in immunocompromised patients.
- Species other than *C. albicans* (especially *C. krusei*) are increasingly seen, especially in persons with compromised immunity. In HIV disease, for example, *C. dubliniensis* and *C. geotrichium* may appear.
- Antifungal resistance is an increasingly serious clinical reality.
- Symptomatic oral candidiasis presents as mainly:
  - white lesions, in which hyphal forms are common: these include thrush, candidal leukoplakia and chronic mucocutaneous candidiasis (CMC)
  - red lesions, in which yeast forms predominate: these include denture-related stomatitis, median rhomboid glossitis (MRG) and erythematous candidiasis. These may be symptomless, although antibiotic stomatitis and angular cheilitis, in particular, can cause soreness.
- Factors that can increase the liability of oral candidiasis are shown in Box 36.1. Candidiasis may also affect:
  - pharynx, oesophagus and rarely lungs, or elsewhere
  - anogenital region: candidiasis can also be sexually transmitted
  - skin and nails.

By tradition, the most frequently adopted classification of oral candidiasis according to clinical phenotypes is:
- acute pseudomembranous (thrush)
- atrophic acute (e.g. post antibiotics) or chronic (e.g. denture stomatitis)
- chronic hyperplastic, which was further subdivided into four groups based on localisation patterns and endocrine involvement as follows: chronic oral candidiasis (*Candida* leukoplakia); candidiasis endocrinopathy syndrome; chronic localised mucocutaneous candidiasis; and chronic diffuse candidiasis. MRG is also considered to be a form of chronic hyperplastic candidiasis
- erythematous.

A newer classification (Box 36.2) categorises candidiasis into:
- primary candidiasis, which is confined to oral and perioral tissues
- secondary candidiasis which is distributed in other parts of the body as well as the oral cavity.

DIAGNOSIS OF CANDIDIASIS

Diagnosis can, if necessary, be supported by:
- identification of blastospores and pseudohyphae in stained smears from a lesion
- culture, usually on Sabouraud or dextrose Sabouraud medium. Normal salivary counts per mL are up to 2000 cfu/mL but can be greater than 10,000 cfu/mL in infection

BOX 36.1 Factors Predisposing to Oral Candidiasis

Local factors influencing oral immunity or ecology, include:
- hyposalivation
- smoking
- broad-spectrum antimicrobials
- corticosteroids
- dental appliances or local factors such as piercings
- irradiation involving the mouth or the salivary glands
- local alteration of the mucosal barrier, e.g. oral lichen planus

Systemic immune defects, such as those caused by:
- extremes of age
- malnutrition
- cytotoxic chemotherapy
- immune T-cell defects, especially HIV infection, leukaemias, lymphomas and cancer, and leukocyte defects, such as in diabetes and immunosuppressant drugs
- anaemia

- PCR studies — mainly for detection of invasive candidiasis
- biopsy and histology stained by periodic acid–Schiff (PAS) in hyperplastic candidiasis.

However, the diagnosis of candidiasis in most instances is clinical and investigations can be complicated by the facts that:
- over 70% of the population are carriers any attempt at quantification of *Candida* is affected by the time of sampling and the way in which the specimen is handled. Salivary counts are generally more useful than swabs, except for swabs of dentures in chronic atrophic candidiasis. Since oral candidiasis is often associated with nutritional deficiencies or blood dyscrasias, estimates of haemoglobin, white blood cell counts, corrected whole blood folate, vitamin B_{12} and serum ferritin can be important.

Tests of immune function are indicated mainly in HIV disease or CMC.

Since some endocrine disorders may be associated with CMC, tests of thyroid, parathyroid and adrenocortical function are warranted in selected individuals (Table 36.1).

BOX 36.2 Classification of Oral Candidiasis

Primary oral candidiasis (group I)
- Acute: pseudomembranous, erythematous
- Chronic: pseudomembranous, erythematous
- *Candida*-associated lesions

Secondary oral candidiasis (group II)
- Denture-related stomatitis, angular stomatitis, median rhomboid glossitis
- Oral manifestations of systemic mucocutaneous candidiasis (due to diseases such as thymic aplasia and candidiasis endocrinopathy syndrome)
- Hyperplastic plaque-like, nodular

TREATMENT OF CANDIDIASIS

Few patients have spontaneous remission unless the condition is solely related to, for example, the use of an antimicrobial, or a topical corticosteroid, and thus, in other cases, treatment is often indicated (Table 36.2). Often, in the treatment of fungal infections, attention to the underlying cause will avoid the need for prolonged or repeated courses of treatment. Intermittent or prolonged topical antifungal treatment may be necessary where the underlying cause is unavoidable or incurable. Treatment includes the following measures:

- Avoid or reduce smoking.
- Treat any local predisposing cause, such as hyposalivation.
- Improve oral hygiene; chlorhexidine also has some anticandidal activity.
- Antifungals:
  - topical antifungal agents are useful for most lesions restricted to the oral cavity and are available as suspensions, tablets, gels and creams. Oral suspensions, gels or liquids are useful for patients with a dry mouth who may have difficulty in dissolving tablets. Available preparations include nystatin oral suspension and miconazole gel or tablets (intended for topical use), and systemic azoles (used as 'swish and swallow'). Fluconazole, itraconazole and posaconazole are available as suspensions effective against oropharyngeal candidiasis, and voriconazole as a liquid. In resource-poor areas, gentian violet is often used; a solution at a concentration of 0.00165% does not stain the oral mucosa, is stable and still possesses potent antifungal activity
  - systemic antifungals are increasingly used, especially fluconazole
  - fluconazole-resistant *Candida* may respond to itraconazole, voriconazole or posaconazole.

  See also the relevant clinical presentations described below.

Prophylaxis of Candidiasis

In patients with severe immunosuppression, prevention of colonisation and infection is the goal because the oropharyngeal

TABLE 36.2 Regimens That Might Be Helpful in Management of Patient Suspected of Having Candidiasis

Regimen	Use in Primary or Secondary Care
Beneficial	Nystatin Miconazole Fluconazole Itraconazole
Potentially beneficial	Chlorhexidine Yoghurt Probiotics Sodium iodide Ciclopirox Gentian violet
Systemic treatments for resistant candida	Caspofungin Posaconazole Voriconazole
Supportive	Smoking cessation ART in HIV infection Benzydamine Diet with little acidic, spicy or citrus content Lidocaine

region may be the primary source of initial colonisation and allow the subsequent spread of the infection.

Those in greatest need of such prophylactic antifungals include patients:

- with HIV disease
- receiving cancer chemotherapy
- on immunosuppressive therapy
- on prolonged antibiotic therapy.

CLINICAL PRESENTATIONS OF CANDIDIASIS

The most common form of oral candidiasis is denture-related stomatitis, and sometimes this is complicated by angular stomatitis, again often a *Candida*-related lesion. However, most clinicians are more aware of acute pseudomembranous candidiasis ('thrush'), which is not uncommon in neonates, but was rare in older persons before the advent of immunosuppressive therapies and HIV/AIDS. The latter has also highlighted the other red, or erythematous, forms of oral candidiasis.

The various types are now discussed in more detail.

WHITE FORMS OF CANDIDIASIS

Acute Pseudomembranous Candidiasis

Thrush is the common title for acute pseudomembranous candidiasis and is so termed because the white flecks resemble the appearance of the breast of the bird of that name.

TABLE 36.1 Investigations That Might Be Helpful in Diagnosis/Prognosis/Management in Some Patients Suspected of Having Candidiasis (Candidiasis)[a]

In Most Cases	In Some Cases
Culture and sensitivity	Biopsy
Full blood picture	Serum ferritin, vitamin B$_{12}$ and corrected whole blood folate levels
HbA1c	ESR
Detailed review of topical or systemic medication	CRP
	CD4 counts
	Saliva production (mL/min)

[a]See text for details and glossary for abbreviations.

Epidemiology

- Neonates, who are otherwise healthy but have yet to develop immunity to *Candida* species, may develop thrush, but it is otherwise uncommon in healthy individuals of any age. It is far more common in immunocompromised persons; thrush is a 'disease of the diseased'.
- Can occur at any age.
- It can occur in either gender.
- Candidiasis is seen worldwide.

Predisposing Factors

Predisposing factors include changes in local or systemic immunity in the mouth. Thrush in most patients is related to antibiotic or corticosteroid use, or hyposalivation. However, if these local factors cannot be identified, the systemic disease should be suspected — mainly immune defects, such as in terminally ill patients, leukaemia and other malignancies, HIV disease and patients on immunosuppressive treatment.

Aetiology and Pathogenesis

Thrush is mainly caused by *C. albicans* but, in infants, *C. parapsilosis* is frequently found. The highest incidence of thrush amongst cancer patients is seen in head neck cancers, where most infections are caused by *C. albicans* but one-third of patients harbour non-*C. albicans* strains such as *C. krusei* or *C. glabrata,* which are often more resistant to antifungal agents.

The plaques in oral thrush are made up of necrotic material, *Candida* and desquamated parakeratotic epithelia. Oedema and micro-abscesses containing PMNL are found in the outer layers of the epithelium, while the deeper parts show acanthosis and sometimes even dysplasia.

Clinical Features

Thrush is classically an acute infection, but it may persist for many months or even years in patients using corticosteroids topically or by aerosol, in HIV-infected individuals, and other immunocompromised patients.

Thrush is characterised by:
- white papules on the surface of the oral mucosa. These may form confluent plaques that resemble milk curds (Fig. 36.2). These can be wiped off with gauze to reveal a raw, erythematous and sometimes bleeding base

- complications, which may sometimes be lesions of the mucosa of the upper respiratory tract and the oesophagus, a combination particularly prevalent in HIV-infected patients.

Diagnosis

The diagnosis of thrush is usually clinical and straightforward, but it has been over-diagnosed in the past. In immunosuppressed patients, a Gram-stained smear should be taken to distinguish it from the thrush-like plaques produced by opportunistic bacteria. Hyphae seem to indicate that the *Candida* are acting as pathogens.

Treatment

Possible predisposing causes should be looked for and dealt with, if possible. Topical polyene antifungals such as nystatin, or imidazoles such as miconazole or fluconazole are often indicated (Chapter 5). With the increasing use of antimycotic therapy, especially in HIV disease, there is a shift towards antifungal-resistant *C. albicans*, as well as the appearance of novel species, such as *C. dubliniensis*, but also towards other species, such as *C. glabrata* and *C. krusei.*

Follow-Up of Patients

Long-term follow-up as shared care is usually appropriate.

Chronic Hyperplastic Candidiasis

Chronic hyperplastic candidiasis or candidal leukoplakia is a persistent white or speckled red/white lesion (Fig. 36.3), characterised histologically by parakeratosis and chronic intra-epithelial inflammation with fungal hyphae invading the superficial layers of the epithelium. The epithelium of some leukoplakias is invaded by *Candida* hyphae, but it is unclear whether the yeasts are secondary invaders or are causally involved in the development or transformation of leukoplakia. The cellular changes often include hyperplasia, but cellular atypia, mild or severe dysplasia and ultimately in situ or invasive carcinoma may arise.

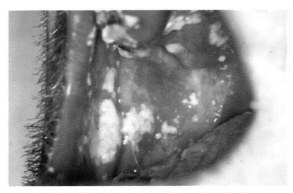

Fig. 36.2 Thrush showing white and red lesions.

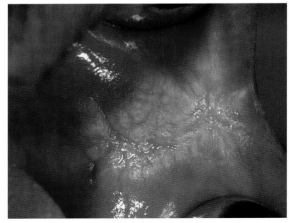

Fig. 36.3 Chronic hyperplastic candidiasis, in a typical location.

Epidemiology

- It is uncommon.
- It is found in adults.
- It can occur in either gender.
- It can be found worldwide.

Predisposing Factors, Aetiology and Pathogenesis

C. albicans is the species by far the most commonly isolated from candidal leukoplakia, and it may be predisposed to in a minority of patients by:

- smoking
- iron and folate deficiencies
- defective cell-mediated immunity
- blood group secretor status (blood Group O (non-ABH secretors) more likely to carry candida).

The *Candida* biotypes associated with leukoplakias differ from those isolated from normal oral cavities and those from non-homogeneous leukoplakias such as candidal leukoplakia have higher nitrosation potentials, which might indicate a possible role of specific types in the malignant transformation of these leukoplakias.

Clinical Features

Candidal leukoplakias are chronic, discrete raised lesions that vary from small, palpable, translucent, whitish areas to large, dense, opaque plaques, hard and rough to the touch (plaque-like lesions) and are non-homogeneous 'speckled' leukoplakias in up to 50%.

Candidal leukoplakias usually occur on the buccal mucosa on one or both sides, mainly just inside the commissure (see Fig. 36.3), less often on the tongue dorsum.

Diagnosis

Candidal leukoplakias can be indistinguishable from other leukoplakias except by biopsy when *Candida* hyphae can be seen after staining with PAS. Candidal leukoplakia should, therefore, be biopsied both to:

- distinguish it from other non-candidal lesions
- examine for dysplasia.

Treatment

From 9% to 40% of candidal leukoplakias may develop into carcinomas. Factors influencing the prognosis may include:

- risk factors, such as tobacco and alcohol use
- whether the lesion is speckled (more dangerous) or homogeneous
- the presence (more dangerous) and degree of epithelial dysplasia
- the management adopted.
  In order to improve the prognosis:
- tobacco and alcohol habits should be stopped
- antifungals should be used. The lesions of candidal leukoplakia may prove poorly responsive to polyene antifungal drugs and, in some cases, respond only to systemic fluconazole or itraconazole
- excision is indicated if there is more than mild dysplasia

- the patient should be fully informed about the condition and reviewed regularly.

Follow-Up of Patients

Long-term follow-up as shared care is usually appropriate.

Chronic Mucocutaneous Candidiasis

In many patients with persistent oral candidiasis, no local cause or underlying defect can be identified. However, in general, the more severe the candidiasis and the more widespread the sites involved, the greater the likelihood that an underlying immunological defect (particularly of cell-mediated immunity) can be identified.

CMC is not a specific condition, but rather a phenotypic presentation of a spectrum of immunologic (e.g. candidiasis thymoma, endocrinologic (candidiasis-endrocrinopathy syndrome) and autoimmune disorders.

Patients who lack broad T-cell immunity (e.g. those with severe combined immune deficiency syndrome (SCID) or DiGeorge syndrome [CATCH 22]) or patients with severely impaired T-cell function (e.g. patients with HIV/AIDS) are also susceptible to chronic candidal infections but are not usually included in CMC.

CMC is the term given to a heterogeneous group of rare syndromes, sometimes familial in which there is persistent *mucocutaneous* candidiasis and, to a lesser extent, other infections such as HPV infections. An underlying immune defect is present that responds poorly to even prolonged topical antifungal treatment.

CMC is associated with a defect in cell-mediated immunity that may either be limited to *Candida* antigens or be part of a more general immune defect. Some forms are due to the autosomal recessive deficiency in the cytokine receptor, interleukin-17 receptor A (IL-17RA), others to autosomal dominant deficiency of the cytokine IL-17 F. Others have a defect of cytokine production (interleukin-2 and IFN-γ) in response to candidal and some bacterial antigens, with reduced Th1 lymphocyte function and enhanced Th2 activity (and increased interleukin-6).

Clinical Features

Patients with CMC suffer from chronic candidiasis caused mainly by *C. albicans*, with irremovable whitish patches and deep fissures on the tongue and often the palate as the most common oral manifestations but patients may also have candidal infections of other mucosae, skin and nails. Repeated courses of azole antifungals have led to microevolution and point mutations and the development of azole-resistant isolates. Alternative *Candida* treatment options, other than azoles — such as chlorhexidine, should therefore be considered.

Oral carcinomas have developed in some patients with CMC.

Autoimmune polyendocrinopathy-candidiasis (APEC) is a group of rare autosomal recessive diseases, which may involve autoimmune hormonal hypofunction affecting the thyroid, parathyroids, gonads and/or pancreas.

Hyper-IgE syndrome (HIES/Job syndrome) is a rare congenital immunodeficiency characterised by mutations in signal transducer and activator of transcription 3, leading to defects in IL-6 and IL-23, and hence Th17 defects. HIES patients develop mucocutaneous candidiasis.

Specialist care is indicated.

RED (ERYTHEMATOUS) FORMS OF CANDIDIASIS/ ATROPHIC CANDIDIASIS

Erythematous or atrophic candidiasis may be seen in
- denture-related stomatitis
- angular cheilitis
- antibiotic- or steroid-induced stomatitis
- HIV infection — it may develop de novo, may precede pseudomembranous candidiasis, or may arise as a consequence of persistent acute pseudomembranous candidiasis when the pseudomembranes are shed. Sometimes in MRG.

Denture-Related Stomatitis

Denture-related stomatitis (chronic atrophic candidiasis) consists of mild inflammation and erythema of the mucosa beneath a dental appliance, usually a complete upper denture. It is asymptomatic and is typically seen under the maxillary denture. Candida predominate on the denture rather than the palate. Patients may additionally have symptomatic angular cheilitis also due to candida overgrowth. Treatment includes correcting the local ecological factors and improving appliance hygiene, together with antifungal medication.

Epidemiology

- Common; in some studies of institutionalised older denture-wearing patients, figures as high as 70% have been found, but it is overall considerably less common in normal healthy subjects.
- This is a disease mainly of the middle-aged or older.
- It is slightly more prevalent in women than men.
- This is seen worldwide.

Predisposing Factors

Main factor
- dental appliance wearing (mainly maxillary dentures), especially when worn throughout the night, or with a dry mouth.

Occasional factors
- smoking
- diabetes or a high carbohydrate diet.
- hyposalivation.
- haematinic deficiencies are a rare underlying factor.
- HIV.

Factors that are usually *not* significant include:
- allergy to the dental material (if it were, denture-related stomatitis would affect mucosae other than just that beneath the appliance)
- trauma; the condition is more common beneath maxillary dentures than mandibular dentures, yet trauma is more common under the latter
- pharmacological agents.

Aetiology and Pathogenesis

Dentures and other appliances can produce a number of ecological changes, including the accumulation of microbial plaque (bacteria and/or yeasts) on or within the fitting surface of the denture and the underlying mucosa. Histological examination of the soft tissue beneath dentures has shown proliferative or degenerative responses with reduced keratinisation and thinner epithelium.

Fungi, such as *Candida*, are isolated in up to 90% of persons with denture-related stomatitis, also referred to as 'Candida-associated denture stomatitis', 'denture-induced candidiasis' or 'chronic atrophic candidiasis'. The most frequently isolated organism is *C. albicans*. In some persons, the cause appears to be related to a non-specific plaque, which undergoes sequential development and is finally colonised by *Candida* organisms. Although there is no increased aspartyl proteinase production from the *Candida* involved, the decreased salivary flow and a low pH under the denture probably result in a high *Candida* enzymatic activity, which can cause mucosal inflammation.

Candida, however, are not the only microorganisms associated with denture-related stomatitis; occasionally, bacterial infection is responsible, or mechanical irritation has a role.

It is not yet clear why only some denture-wearers develop denture stomatitis, since most patients with denture-related stomatitis appear otherwise healthy and they have no serious cell-mediated immune defects, but they may sometimes be deficient in migration-inhibition factor (MIF) and may have overactive suppressor T cells or other T lymphocyte or phagocyte defects.

Clinical Features

The characteristic presenting features of denture-related stomatitis are:
- An absence of symptoms. The former term 'denture sore mouth' was a misnomer.
- Chronic erythema and oedema of the mucosa that contacts the fitting surface of the denture, usually a complete upper denture (the denture-bearing area); the mucosa below lower dentures is rarely involved (Figs 36.4 and 36.5).
- Complications may include:
  - angular stomatitis, and rarely
  - papillary hyperplasia in the vault of the palate (idiopathic papillary epithelial hyperplasia (IPEH), which usually needs to be surgically removed before the appliance is replaced or relined).

Classification

Denture-related stomatitis has been classified into three clinical types (Newton types), increasing in severity (Table 36.3).

Diagnosis

This is a clinical diagnosis.

A full blood picture, haematinic assays and smears for fungal hyphae and culture may be warranted (Table 36.4). If there is angular stomatitis, or other oral or systemic lesions, or a suspicion of an immunocompromising condition, then diabetes and HIV, in particular, should be excluded.

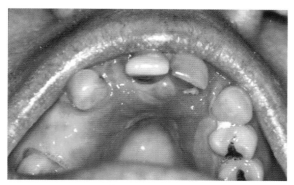

Fig. 36.4 Denture-related stomatitis.

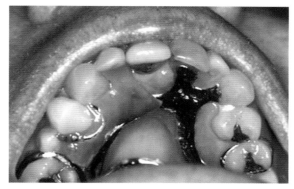

Fig. 36.5 Denture-related stomatitis (denture in situ; same patient as in Fig. 36.4).

Treatment

Patient information is probably the most important aspect of management.

- Any underlying systemic disease should be treated where possible.
- Smoking cessation is important.
- The denture or other appliance fitting surface and plaque is usually harbouring *C. albicans*. Scrupulous appliance hygiene is mandatory, with a daily thorough brushing. The appliance should be removed from the mouth overnight and as much as possible at other times (see Fig. 36.4), while the denture is cleaned and disinfected. This can be achieved by microwave irradiation for 3 minutes at 650 W with the appliance immersed in 200 mL of water. Disinfection can also be achieved using an inexpensive option of 10% acetic acid (vinegar) or an antiseptic denture cleanser and storing the appliance in it overnight. Suitable antiseptic solutions include chlorhexidine or dilute sodium hypochlorite (10 drops of household bleach in a 500 mL container filled with tap water). Hypochlorite, however, can turn chrome cobalt dentures black. Many other cleansers are available (alkaline peroxides, alkaline hypochlorites, acids, yeast lytic enzymes), proteolytic enzymes, tea tree oil (*Melaleuca alternifolia*) and *Punica granatum* (dwarf pomegranate).
- The mucosal infection is eradicated by brushing the palate and using antifungals for 4 weeks (Table 36.5), with the denture

removed from the mouth and being disinfected as frequently as possible. Antifungal agents (e.g. miconazole gel) should also be applied to the tissue-contacting surface of the appliance before every re-insertion. Effective topical antifungals include nystatin suspension, miconazole gel or mucoadhesive tablets, fluconazole suspension or topical ketoconazole if available,

TABLE 36.3 Newton Classification of Denture-Related Stomatitis		
Type	**Definition**	**Comment**
1	Localised simple inflammation or a pinpoint hyperaemia	Early lesion usually
2	Erythematous or generalised simple type presenting as more diffuse erythema involving a part of, or the entire, denture-covered mucosa	Common type
3	Granular type (inflammatory papillary hyperplasia) commonly involving the central part of the hard palate and the alveolar ridge	Uncommon

TABLE 36.4 Investigations That Might Be Helpful in Diagnosis/Prognosis/Management in Some Patients Suspected of Having Denture-Related Stomatitis[a]	
In Most Cases	**In Rare Cases**
Full blood picture	ESR
Serum ferritin, vitamin B_{12} and corrected whole blood folate levels	HIV test
Blood glucose	
Culture and sensitivity	

[a]See text for details and glossary for abbreviations.

TABLE 36.5 Regimens That Might Be Helpful in Management of Patient Suspected of Having Denture-Related Stomatitis	
Regimen	**Use in Primary or Secondary Care**
Beneficial	Nystatin
	Miconazole
	Fluconazole
	Itraconazole
Supportive	Chlorhexidine
	Dental appliance hygiene
	Smoking cessation
	Probiotics
	Yoghurt

which can be administered concurrently with an oral antiseptic with antifungal activity — such as chlorhexidine. Lacquer or tissue conditioners containing antifungals are also effective.

Studies of sensitivity to antifungal agents have shown that isolates from different strains are sensitive to nystatin but less sensitive to miconazole and fluconazole.

Follow-Up of Patients

Long-term follow-up in primary care is usually appropriate.

Angular Cheilitis (Angular Stomatitis)

Introduction

Angular cheilitis is a chronic inflammatory lesion affecting usually both commissures (Fig. 36.6). Most cases are seen in people with denture-related stomatitis and are related to candida.

Epidemiology

- Angular cheilitis is common.
- It occurs mostly in adults, particularly the older age group.
- It occurs in both males and females.
- No known geographic incidence.

Predisposing Factors

Angular cheilitis is most often chronic, and due to infective and/or mechanical causes. It is predisposed by what are known as the '3Ds' (Fig. 36.7):

- Dental appliance or denture-wearing, denture-related stomatitis and disorders that predispose to candidiasis: including dry mouth and tobacco smoking.
- Deficiency states, such as:
  - deficiency anaemias
  - iron deficiency
  - hypovitaminoses (especially B)
  - malabsorption states (e.g. Crohn disease) or eating disorders
  - possibly zinc deficiency, but only rarely
  - immune defects, such as Down syndrome, HIV infection, diabetes (Figs 36.8 and 36.9), cancer, immunosuppression and eating disorders.
- Disorders where the lip-anatomical relationships are changed — such as when the vertical dimension of occlusion is reduced, or where lips are enlarged, such as in orofacial granulomatosis, Crohn disease and Down syndrome.

Aetiology

A number of factors (infective, mechanical, nutritional or immunological) may be implicated alone or in combination.

- Most angular cheilitis is seen in older patients who are wearing a complete maxillary denture beneath which is denture-related stomatitis. Infective agents, mainly *C. albicans* or *Staphylococcus aureus*, can be isolated in up to 54% of lesions. *C. albicans* is most commonly isolated and is typically carried in the saliva.
- Mechanical factors may play a part. As a consequence of ageing, the upper lip overhangs the lower at the angles of the mouth, producing a fold that keeps a small area of skin macerated.

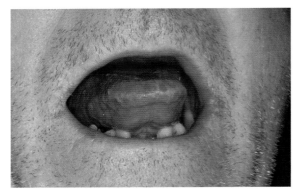

Fig. 36.8 Angular cheilitis in diabetes.

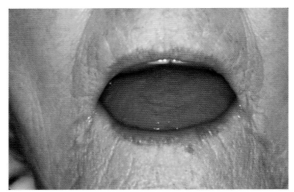

Fig. 36.6 Angular cheilitis — typical bilateral lesions.

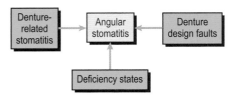

Fig. 36.7 Pathogenesis of angular cheilitis.

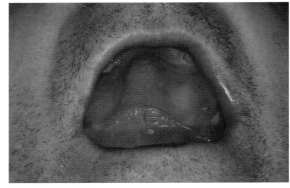

Fig. 36.9 Chronic atrophic candidiasis, same patient as shown in Fig. 36.8.

- Nutritional deficiencies that may underlie some cases include deficiency of haematinics (iron, folate, vitamin B_{12}) or of immunity (which can lead to the proliferation of *Candida* species and other micro-organisms).
- Dry mouth also predisposes to candidiasis.
- Immunodeficiency such as in diabetes, Down syndrome, HIV disease or immunosuppression may result in angular cheilitis associated with candidiasis.

Clinical Features

- The common complaints are soreness, erythema and fissuring affecting the angles of the mouth. Typically, the condition persists or recurs. Atrophy, erythema, ulceration, crusting and scaling may be seen. Lesions occasionally extend beyond the vermilion border onto the skin in the form of linear furrows or fissures radiating from the angle of the mouth (rhagades), mainly in the more severe forms, especially in denture wearers. An eczematous dermatitis may extend onto the cheek or chin as an infective eczematoid reaction or as a reaction to topical medicaments. In long-standing lesions, suppuration and granulation tissue may develop. Commonly, there is also associated denture-related stomatitis. Rarely, there is also commissural candida-related leukoplakia intraorally.

Diagnosis

- This is usually a clinical diagnosis, made by clinical examination. Maceration of the commissural epithelium can also be brought about by habitual licking or by sucking on objects, but this is not true angular cheilitis and the erythema usually extends well beyond the commissural areas and vermilion. Intraoral inspection in angular cheilitis may reveal palatal erythema caused by associated denture-related stomatitis, usually due to candidosis. An underlying nutritional deficiency may be revealed by a depapillated tongue (glossitis) in iron deficiency, a depapillated glossy red tongue in folate deficiency or a reddish-purple depapillated tongue in vitamin B deficiency. Angular cheilitis, if accompanied by systemic features such as diarrhoea and non-specific oral ulcerations, most commonly of the tongue and buccal mucosa, may suggest Crohn disease, HIV infection or zinc deficiency.
- In all cases of angular cheilitis in wearers of dental appliances, Candida should be sought not only in the lesions but also from the appliance-fitting surface. The skin lesions should also be swabbed. Microbial cultures and a haematological workup (blood picture, and assays of levels of serum iron/ferritin, serum vitamin B_{12} and corrected red blood cell folate) are indicated when systemic involvement is suspected. Diagnosis is often supported by investigations, especially if there are associated lesions such as ulceration and/or glossitis (Table 36.6).

TABLE 36.6 Investigations That Might Be Helpful in Diagnosis/Prognosis/Management in Some Patients Suspected of Having Angular Cheilitis (Angular Stomatitis)[a]

In Most Cases	In Some Cases
Full blood picture	Swab for culture and sensitivity
Serum ferritin, vitamin B_{12} and corrected whole blood folate levels	Serum zinc
ESR	Serology for infections (HIV, syphilis)
Blood glucose	

TABLE 36.7 Regimens That Might Be Helpful in Management of Patient Suspected of Having Angular Cheilitis

Regimen	Use in Primary and Secondary Care
Beneficial	Miconazole Fucidin
Supportive	Treat related denture stomatitis

Treatment

Management of angular cheilitis is sometimes difficult and therapy may need to be prolonged (Table 36.7):

- Tobacco habits should be stopped.
- Underlying systemic disease must be investigated and treated: a course of oral iron and vitamin B supplements may be helpful in such cases.
- If the infection is the cause of angular cheilitis, treatment will only be effective if the infection is treated. A permanent cure can be achieved only by eliminating candidiasis as well as the growth of Candida beneath, and in, the denture-fitting surface. Recurrence of angular cheilitis must be prevented, by eliminating organisms from their reservoir on the denture, so the dentures should be kept out of the mouth at night and disinfected in a candidacidal solution, such as hypochlorite. Denture-related stomatitis should be treated with an antifungal. Miconazole oral gel has some gram-positive bacteriostatic action, but there is a high relapse rate unless treatment is prolonged. Miconazole is absorbed systemically and may occasionally potentiate the action of warfarin, phenytoin and the sulphonylureas. In patients taking these drugs, nystatin (as oral suspension) should, therefore, be tried first.
- Angular cheilitis should be treated with a topical antifungal (e.g. miconazole). Staphylococcus infection can be cleared with topical antibiotics, such as fusidic acid (Fucidin) ointment or cream used at least four times daily. Mixed

infections of Candida and Staphylococcus respond best to topical miconazole. Miconazole plus hydrocortisone cream, Fucidin plus hydrocortisone cream, clotrimazole plus hydrocortisone cream, nystatin plus hydrocortisone cream, are other choices.

- Mechanical predisposing factors should be corrected. A change in dentures may be necessary; new dentures that restore facial contour may help. In rare intractable cases, surgery or, occasionally, collagen or silicone or other filler injections may be useful in trying to restore normal lip commissural anatomy.

Antibiotic or Steroid-Induced Stomatitis

Epidemiology

- It is uncommon.
- It can occur at any age.
- It can occur in either gender.
- It has no known geographic incidence.

Predisposing Factors

Acute oral candidiasis may complicate corticosteroid or antibiotic therapy, particularly with long-term, broad-spectrum antimicrobials, such as tetracycline.

Clinical Features

There is widespread erythema and soreness of the oral mucosa, sometimes, also with thrush.

Diagnosis

This is a clinical diagnosis, but if the aetiology is not absolutely clear, a blood picture and smears for fungal hyphae and culture may be helpful management.

Treatment

- The causal drug should be stopped if possible.
- Tobacco habits should be stopped.
- Antifungals are indicated. However, the lesions may prove poorly responsive to the polyene antifungal drugs and, therefore, an azole is preferred. Some cases respond only to systemic fluconazole or itraconazole (Chapter 5).

Follow-Up of Patients

Long-term follow-up is rarely required.

Median Rhomboid Glossitis

MRG, or glossal central papillary atrophy, is a depapillated rhomboidal area in the centre line of the dorsum of the tongue, just anterior to the sulcus terminalis (Fig. 36.10).

Epidemiology

- It is uncommon.

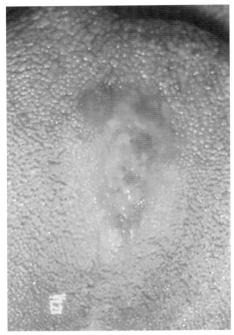

Fig. 36.10 Median rhomboid glossitis.

- It can occur at any age.
- It can occur in either gender.
- It has no known geographic incidence.

Predisposing Factors

Candida species colonise mainly the posterior dorsum of the tongue, even in healthy patients, but MRG is predisposed by:
- smoking
- denture wearing
- corticosteroid sprays/inhalers
- HIV infection.

Aetiology and Pathogenesis

Formerly thought to be caused by persistence of the embryonic tuberculum impar, this lesion is now thought to be related to candidiasis because:
- culture frequently shows *Candida*, although often in a mixed bacterial/fungal microflora
- histopathologically, candidal hyphae infiltrate the superficial layers of the parakeratotic epithelium and a neutrophil infiltrate occupies the epithelium, with elongated hyperplastic rete ridges (pseudoepitheliomatous hyperplasia), and lymphocyte infiltration in the corium. Thus, there can be a trap for the unwary, since the lesion may be mistaken for a cancer clinically (Fig. 36.11) and the histopathology is of pseudo-epitheliomatous hyperplasia — it also mimics cancer.

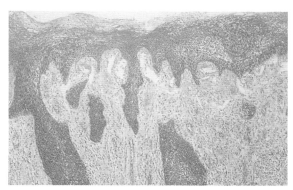

Fig. 36.11 Median rhomboid glossitis, showing the histopathological appearance of pseudoepitheliomatous hyperplasia that may lead to confusion with carcinoma.

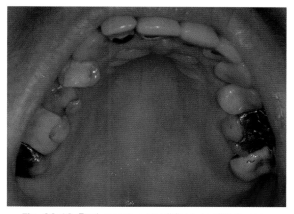

Fig. 36.12 Erythematous candidiasis in HIV disease.

Clinical Features

MRG is only rarely sore but is more usually detected incidentally by the patient or dentist. It is characterised by:

- an area of papillary atrophy, which is usually flat, reddish or red and white, or occasionally white. It is elliptical or rhomboidal in shape, symmetrically placed centrally at the midline of the tongue, just anterior to the circumvallate papillae (see Fig. 36.10)
- occasionally by a hyperplastic or even lobulated exophytic appearance.

Diagnosis

MRG is usually a clinical diagnosis. The biopsy is indicated if there is any concern it could be a neoplasm; histology shows irregular epithelial hyperplasia, which resembles, but is not, a carcinoma (because of the pseudoepitheliomatous hyperplasia) (see Fig. 36.11).

Rarely, is there a need for a blood picture, smears for fungal hyphae or culture.

Treatment (see also Chapters 4 and 5)

- Tobacco habits should be stopped.
- Antifungals are indicated. However, the lesions may prove poorly responsive to the polyene antifungal drugs, and some cases respond only to systemic azoles (Chapter 5).

Follow-Up of Patients

Long-term follow-up as shared care is usually appropriate.

Erythematous Candidiasis in HIV Disease

Epidemiology

- It is uncommon.
- It can occur at any age.

- It can occur in either gender.
- It has no known geographic incidence.

Predisposing Factors

- The immunological defect.
- Smoking.
- Corticosteroid therapy.
- Broad-spectrum antibiotic therapy.
- Hyposalivation (from HIV-salivary gland disease, antiretroviral agents or other agents which have this effect) (Chapter 33).

Clinical Features

- The clinical presentation is of irregular erythematous macules and/or patches, generally on the dorsum of the tongue, palate or buccal mucosa.
- Lesions are often seen in the central palate and are sometimes termed 'thumbprint lesions' (Fig. 36.12).
- Lesions on the dorsum of the tongue present as glossitis or depapillated areas.
- There can be an associated angular stomatitis.

Diagnosis

This is a clinical diagnosis; a biopsy is only rarely indicated. Occasionally there is a need for smears or culture.

Treatment (see also Chapters 4 and 5)

- Tobacco habits should be stopped.
- Antiretroviral treatment.
- Candidiasis in HIV disease may prove poorly responsive to polyene antifungal drugs, so systemic fluconazole is usually indicated (Chapter 5).

Follow-Up of Patients

Long-term follow-up by a specialist is usually appropriate.

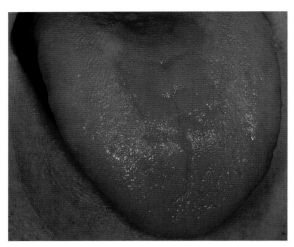

Fig. 36.13 Multifocal candidiasis: lingual lesion.

CHRONIC MULTIFOCAL ORAL CANDIDIASIS

In a minority of apparently healthy individuals, chronic red and/or white candidal infection may be seen in multiple oral sites, without other mucosal or skin candidiasis; this is termed 'chronic multifocal oral candidiasis' (Fig. 36.13). Diagnostic criteria include:

- lesions of greater than 1 month duration
- an absence of predisposing medical conditions. It excludes patients who have received radiotherapy or drugs of the following types: antibiotics, anti-inflammatory or immuno-suppressive drugs, cytotoxic or psychotropic agents.

Epidemiology

- It is uncommon.
- Adults usually; most of the patients are in their fifth or sixth decade.
- Most patients are males.
- No known geographical incidence.

Predisposing Factors

Tobacco smoking is a known risk factor.

Clinical Features

Various combinations can be seen, including:

- retro-commissural leukoplakia, which is the most constant component

- angular cheilitis, which is unilateral or bilateral and encountered mainly in denture-wearers
- median rhomboid or erythematous glossitis
- palatal red irregular patches.

Diagnosis

This is a clinical diagnosis. A blood picture, smears for fungal hyphae and culture may help management.

Treatment (see also Chapters 4 and 5)

- Tobacco habits should be stopped.
- Antifungals are indicated. However, the lesions may prove poorly responsive to the polyene antifungal drugs and some cases respond only to systemic fluconazole (Chapter 5).

Follow-Up of Patients

Long-term follow-up by a specialist is usually appropriate.

OTHER ORAL FUNGAL INFECTIONS

While candidiasis is the most common superficial fungal infection routinely encountered in the oral cavity, deep fungal infections can also occur intraorally. Associated risk factors include immunodeficiency, use of immunosuppressive/immuno-modulatory, organ transplantation or chemotherapeutic agents. The most frequent deep fungal infection is aspergillosis. However, deep fungal infections which are observed in areas other than in oral tissue are indicators of systemic or disseminated infections. These are summarised in Table 36.8.

DIAGNOSIS

Recommended sampling methods for oral mycosis are the collection of whole saliva, rinsing sample, scraping over lesion/smear, moistened swab, imprint impression, blister fluid or pus/inflammatory material from the active lesion. The moistened swab method is best suited for the oral fungal lesions that occur on the mucous membrane, lip, circumoral skin and tongue. A prosthodontic impression, swab or smear is the best sampling method in denture stomatitis cases.

FUNGAL INFECTIONS ASSOCIATED WITH SARS-COV-2 (COVID-19)

The COVID-19 infection has had a major world impact since March 2020. As a consequence of systemic antibiotics, systemic corticosteroids and severe illness requiring intensive care,

TABLE 36.8 Additional Oral Fungal Infections

Species	Predisposing Factors	Clinical Features	Treatment
Aspergillus *Aspergillus fumigatus*, followed by *Aspergillus flavus*, *Aspergillus niger* and *Aspergillus terreus*	Second most frequent oral mycosis. Opportunistic infection of immunosuppressed and bone marrow transplantation patients. The organism invades vascular tissue, leading to thrombosis and infarction. Three forms: invasive (highly lethal), non-invasive (aspergilloma) and destructive non-invasive forms.	Life-threatening complications in immunocompromised. Primary aspergillosis may occur in the paranasal sinuses, larynx, eyes, ears or oral cavity. Oral aspergillosis is typically characterised by black or yellow necrotic tissue on an ulcer base over the palate or in the posterior tongue. Inhalation of *Aspergillus* spores can lead to both upper and/or lower respiratory infection resulting in pulmonary aspergillosis.	Surgical management plays a significant role in treating invasive aspergillosis. Systemic medication is also essential for invasive aspergillosis. amphotericin B (AMB), voriconazole, itraconazole and caspofungin.
Cryptococcus *Cryptococcus neoformans*	Cryptococcosis — an invasive infection that affects the lungs with later meningitis. Commonly observed in both immune-competent and suppressed patients. Infection acquired by the inhalation of infectious aerosols. Most frequent in HIV infection.	Deep fungal infection characterised by invasive characteristics and is often associated with morbidity and mortality. Most frequent sites for cutaneous cryptococcosis are the face, neck and scalp. Oral lesions are extremely rare but do occur in opportunistic conditions, e.g. mucosal surface ulceration, nodules or granuloma formation. May resemble carcinoma.	Fluconazole 400 mg for 6 months to 1 year. HIV-associated meningeal infection has recommended guidelines.
Histoplasmosis *Histoplasmosis capsulatum*	Deep fungal infection that affects pulmonary tissue or mucocutaneous areas.	The mucocutaneous form of histoplasmosis may produce ulcerative, erosive lesions with firm rolled borders on the tongue, palate and/or buccal mucosa (mimicking a malignancy). Oral lesions are frequently identified in cases with disseminated histoplasmosis and in acute pulmonary histoplasmosis. Oral lesions appear as solitary painful or painless ulcerations with a duration of several weeks.	Itraconazole in mild-to-moderate disease. Moderately/severe AMB therapy.
Blastomycosis *Blastomyces dermatitidis*	Blastomycosis is an endemic fungal infection reported in the Mississippi and Ohio River basins.	Disseminated blastomycosis affects the oral cavity and is characterised by ulcerated indurated an elevated margin. Most commonly affects the pulmonary, cutaneous, osseous, genitourinary and central nervous system tissues.	Acute and mild cases may resolve spontaneously. Pulmonary blastomycosis (mild/moderate cases) oral itraconazole. Severe cases or immunosuppressed amphotericin B
Mucormycosis *Rhizopus, Mucor, Cunninghamella, Rhizomucor, Saksenaea, Apophysomyces* or *Lichtheimia*	Mucormycosis is a deep fungal infection that occurs in acute and aggressive forms. Primarily affects immunocompromised, transplant patients or those with haematological malignancies or poorly controlled diabetes.	Oral mucormycosis occurs in paranasal sinuses or nasal areas and leads to palatal necrosis and/or ulceration.	Both medication and surgical management strategies. Amphotericin B (liposomal) is the most commonly used drug.
Geotrichosis *Geotrichum candidum*	Geotrichosis — uncommon opportunistic oral fungal infection usually in the immunocompromised.	Resembles pseudomembranous form of oral candidiasis and characterised by a white, pseudomembranous appearance, palatal ulcerations or villous hyperplastic areas. Oral ulceration is common.	As for candidiasis.
Rhinosporidiosis *Rhinosporidium seeberi*	Sporadic infection resulting from traumatic inoculation leads to chronic granulomatous disease.	Hyperplastic verrucous lesions with hypervascularity most commonly seen on the soft palate, nasopharynx and oropharynx.	Surgical removal.

patients have been at increased risk of candidiasis usually secondary to *C. albicans*.

RECOMMENDED READING

British HIV Association guidelines on the management of opportunistic infection in people living with HIV, 2021. The clinical management of Candidiasis 2019. HIV Med. 22 (1), 73.

Coronado-Castellote, L., Jimenez-Soriano, Y., 2013. Clinical and microbiological diagnosis of oral candidiasis. J. Clin. Exp. Dent. 5, e279—e286.

Garcia-Cuesta, C., Sarrion-Pérez, M.G., Bagán, J.V., 2014. Current treatment of oral candidiasis: A literature review. J. Clin. Exp. Dent. 6 (5), e576—e582.

Lynch, D.P., 1994. Oral candidiasis. History, classification, and clinical presentation. Oral Surg. Oral Med. Oral Pathol. 78, 189—193.

Pankhurst, C.L., 2013. Candidiasis (oropharyngeal). BMJ Clin. Evid. 2013, 1304.

Pappas, P.G., Kauffman, C.A., Andes, D.R., et al., 2016. Clinical practice guideline for the management of candidiasis: 2016 update by the Infectious Diseases Society of America. Clin. Infect. Dis. 62, e1—e50.

Viral Infections: An Overview

KEY POINTS
- Both RNA and DNA viral species can inhabit the oral cavity.
- Viruses can infect different oral tissues including epithelial cells, lymphocytes, macrophages, neural tissues and salivary glands.
- Some effects are local to the oral cavity and others have systemic manifestations.
- Systemic therapy is usually needed to treat oral viral infections.
- Dental healthcare workers can be at risk of infection from transmissible oral viruses.

INTRODUCTION

Viruses are unique since, unlike bacteria and fungi, they need a host cell to replicate and survive. Both DNA and RNA viruses can infect the oral tissues and they may cause acute, chronic or latent infections. Viruses can also be associated with malignancies, either via chronic inflammation or DNA damage (e.g. Epstein–Barr virus [EBV] and oncogenic strains of human papillomavirus [HPV]). A wide spectrum of viruses can affect the oral cavity. The majority of viral infections affecting the orofacial region are self-limiting in otherwise healthy individuals. Virus infections can affect both keratinised and non-keratinised epithelium, in contrast to aphthous ulceration (Fig. 37.1). Atypical presentations with systemic complications are more likely to occur in immunocompromised hosts (e.g. herpes infections).

Dental healthcare workers (HCWs) including nurses and hygienists are at risk from several of these viruses including coronaviruses. The most common relevant viruses to the orofacial region include the HSV and HPV virus families.

However, there are several other systemic viral infections that can present with oral and orofacial manifestations (Table 37.1).

HERPES GROUP OF VIRUSES (SEE CHAPTER 38)

Herpes viruses are the most common infections in the oral cavity, and perhaps the most widely pathogenic. There are eight sub-types of Herpes viruses which span three subfamilies (α, β, γ). α herpes viruses include herpes simplex viruses (HSV1 and HSV2) causing herpetic stomatitis and varicella virus (VZV) causing shingles and chickenpox. β herpes viruses include Cytomegalovirus which may cause some salivary infections. γ herpes viruses include EBV which causes infectious mononucleosis, and may be associated with nasopharyngeal carcinoma, lymphomas and hairy leukoplakia (Chapter 39). HHV8 is associated with Kaposi sarcoma (see Chapter 39).

HEPATITIS VIRUS

Hepatitis viruses cause acute or chronic inflammation of the liver (hepatitis). Hepatitis is defined as acute if it resolves within 6 months, and chronic if it lasts longer than 6 months. Chronic hepatitis may progress to scarring of the liver (cirrhosis), liver failure and liver cancer.

There are five main clinical types:
- hepatitis A (HAV)
- hepatitis B (HBV)
- hepatitis C (HCV)
- hepatitis D (HDV)
- hepatitis E (HEV).

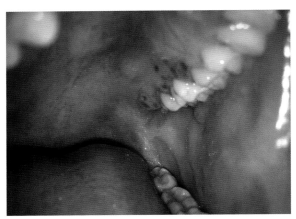

Fig. 37.1 Herpetic-like ulceration involving the left palate showing multiple small ulcers infecting keratinised mucosa.

TABLE 37.1 Main Virus Species Causing Oral Manifestations
Herpes group of viruses (Chapter 38)
Human Papillomaviruses
Coxsackie virus
Hepatitis virus
Epstein–Barr virus (Chapter 38)
Human immunodeficiency virus (Chapter 39)
Coronaviruses
Other viruses with orofacial manifestations
Congenital and neonatal viral infections

The five have different modes of transmission, severity and geographic distribution. Hepatitis A and E are mainly spread by contaminated food and water. Hepatitis B is mainly sexually transmitted, but may also be passed from mother to baby during pregnancy or childbirth and spread through infected blood. Hepatitis C is commonly spread through infected blood, such as may occur during needle sharing by intravenous drug users. An association with oral lichen planus has been reported in some countries. Hepatitis D can only infect people already infected with hepatitis B.

Out of the five, types B and C lead to chronic disease, causing liver cirrhosis, cancer (hepatocellular carcinoma) and death. Some people with hepatitis have no symptoms, whereas others develop jaundice, vomiting, tiredness, abdominal pain and diarrhoea with associated loss of weight.

Hepatitis A, B and D are preventable with immunisation and due to the established risk of infection from patients carrying hepatitis viruses, all dental HCW should be immunised.

According to the World Health Organization (WHO), it is estimated that over 260 million people globally live with HBV and about 75 million with chronic HCV infection.

HAV infection:
- Can lead to mild to severe illness.
- Is transmitted through contaminated food and water or from an infected individual (faecal–oral route).
- The majority of infected individuals recover completely after a short illness, with immunity lasting lifelong and mortality reported within a small group.

HBV infection:
- Is highly contagious.
- Presents as either an acute or a chronic disease.
- Transmitted through contact with blood or other body fluids and vertical transmission from an infected mother to a child.
- Chronic infection can lead to liver cirrhosis and hepatocellular carcinoma.
- Several antiviral medications including tenofovir, lamivudine, emtricitabine, adefovir and entecavir are effective in treating HBV.
- Once a person develops HBV, there is no cure.
- Is generally diagnosed via serologic testing.
- The best mode of prevention is through effective vaccination against HBV.

HCV generally:
- Presents as a chronic disease with varying degrees of disease severity, including cirrhosis and liver cancer.
- Is highly infectious.
- Can be transmitted through a very small quantity of infected blood.
- Main mode of HCV transmission is through injecting drug use, accidental exposure, unsafe conditions in healthcare practices and transfusion of infected blood.
- Diagnosis is by testing for anti-HCV antibodies.
- Chronic HCV infection can lead to cirrhosis and hepatocellular carcinoma.

Management: A liver ultrasound is generally the screening test of choice. Patients with active HCV should be managed by antiviral medications, which are curative. There are no effective HCV vaccines available at present.

HDV:
- Requires HBV for its replication, hence it occurs as a super-infection.
- Transmission is through infected blood, body fluids and rarely vertical transmission from mother to child.
- HDV can be treated with interferon-based regimens.
- The best prevention is a vaccination for HBV as there is no vaccine for HDV.

HEV:
- Is a highly infectious virus that can lead to serious illness and death.
- The main mode of transmission is via faecally contaminated water.
- It has been recorded globally and commonly in Southeast Asia.
- Pregnant women are at a particularly high risk of complications from HEV.
- There is no generally available vaccine to date.

Orofacial Manifestations and Considerations

Hepatitis viruses cause serious liver damage and its consequences, especially susceptibility to bleeding and contraindications of certain drugs. There are several physical signs of end-stage liver disease, including icterus or yellowing of the oral mucous membranes, due to jaundice.

Sialadenosis and sialadenitis affecting the parotid glands are common. Halitosis, cheilitis, atrophic tongue, xerostomia and perioral rash have also been reported. A close relationship between oral lichen planus with HCV in some parts of the world has been documented.

CORONAVIRUSES

Coronaviruses are enveloped single-stranded RNA viruses that cause a variety of infections in both humans and animals. The virus is named because of its crown-like appearance on electron microscopy, first identified in 1964 at St Thomas Hospital in London. Two genera of coronavirus, α and β, infect humans. Alpha coronaviruses are one of the causes of the common cold. Beta coronaviruses include several important human pathogens, including the Middle East respiratory syndrome coronavirus (MERS-CoV) and severe acute respiratory syndrome coronaviruses (SARS-CoV-1 and SARS-CoV-2).

MERS-CoV

A novel zoonotic infection that likely originated from camels, was first identified in 2012 in Saudi Arabia. Patients with MERS-CoV typically present with a respiratory tract infection that can progress to pneumonia and death in up to one-third of patients. Human-to-human transmission is thought to be limited.

SARS-CoV-1

A zoonotic infection that may have originated from palm civets, was first identified in Guandong Province in China in 2003. Patients with SARS-CoV-1 also typically present with an influenza-like illness that can progress to pneumonia and death in approximately 15% of patients. Like MERS-CoV, human-to-human transmission is thought to be limited with adequate infection control precautions. There are no current cases of SARS-CoV-1 infections. However, it has re-emerged four times since 2003. It can infect salivary glands.

SARS-CoV-2

Is a zoonotic virus that likely originated in bats in Wuhan, China at the end of 2019. By the end of 2021, over 250 million people worldwide had been infected with SARS-CoV-2 with over 5 million deaths. Coronavirus disease 2019 (COVID-19) is the name of the clinical syndrome for patients infected with SARS-CoV-2. Patients with COVID-19 often present with influenza-like illness symptoms, with fevers, cough, fatigue and myalgia. However, other presentations include anosmia, dysgeusia and diarrhoea. However, a substantial proportion of patients may have no symptoms at all.

The virus is primarily transmitted via large respiratory droplets. Aerosols and surfaces are other potential additional sources of transmission. The live virus can be detected in aerosols and very high numbers in saliva in the first 10 days of infection. Transmission of SARS-CoV-2 is substantially reduced by wearing masks including from patients to HCWs. Pre-procedural antiviral mouthwashes (e.g. 0.23% povidone-iodine or cetyl pyridinium chloride) appear to be effective in reducing risk and continue to be recommended by the ADA during procedures in the nose, throat, oropharynx and respiratory tract.

Pathogenicity

- The incubation period is up to 14 days.
- The virus spike protein binds to the receptor-binding domain of the cellular receptor angiotensin-converting enzyme 2 (ACE2), which is distributed throughout the respiratory tract, the ducts of salivary glands and the conjunctiva.
- Age is easily the highest risk factor for morbidity and mortality, over obesity, diabetes and immunosuppression.

Diagnosis

The current gold standard for diagnosing COVID-19 is RT-PCR for SARS-CoV-2 RNA. Lateral flow tests can give false negatives, and RT-PCR can give false positives since a dead virus is recognised as well as a live virus. A single negative test should not rule out the disease in symptomatic patients. The sensitivity and specificity of these tests vary depending on the manufacturer.

Antibody tests can confirm exposure to SARS-CoV-2 but since the protective level of antibodies is unclear, does not necessarily indicate immunity from further infection.

Oral Manifestations

As has been found with HIV, early infection with SARS-CoV-2 can give rise to oral ulcers of a vesicular type, usually on the buccal and labial mucosa. Dysgeusia is common, often aligned with anosmia and possibly related to heavy SARS-CoV-2 infection of the minor and major salivary glands. Reported manifestations include taste impairment, oral mucosal changes (petechiae, ulcers, plaque-like lesions, reactivation of HSV1, desquamative gingivitis) parotiditis and dry mouth. The mucosal lesions occur mainly on the tongue, palate and labial mucosa.

Vaccines Against SARS-CoV-2

Since the beginning of the worldwide pandemic in early 2020, over 100 new vaccines have been developed worldwide with the objective of producing long-lived protective immunity. These fall into four main groups (Table 37.2):
- inactivated viral product vaccines
- protein-based vaccines
- viral vector vaccines
- genetic vaccines.

The advantage of these technologies is the possibility of large-scale production. Antibody titres to SARS-CoV-2 vaccines seem to be relatively short-lived compared with other

TABLE 37.2	Current Vaccines Against SARS-CoV-2 Virus	
Vaccine Type	**Nature**	**Administration**
Inactivated vaccines	Produced by harvesting viruses or products from cell culture	Usually administered intramuscularly
Recombinant protein vaccines	Can be divided into recombinant spike-protein-based vaccines, recombinant RBD (part of the spike protein)-based vaccines and virus-like particle (VLP)-based vaccines	Usually administered intramuscularly
Viral vector vaccines	Non-pathogenic viruses, mainly adenoviruses, are modified to carry SARS-CoV-2 genes, including the whole spike protein	Replication of the virus in host cells exposes the host to coronavirus viral proteins
Genetic vaccines, mRNA or DNA	mRNA specific for a spike or other SARS-CoV-2 antigens are injected into muscle cells and the protein is expressed for a short period sufficient to induce an immune response	Alternatively, plasmid viral DNA can be produced at a large scale in bacteria containing expression promoters and the gene that encodes the spike protein

viral vaccines, and the minimum protective titre is also unclear. Thus, booster immunisations have been accepted as required after a double vaccination to ensure longer-lasting protection.

Monoclonal antibodies against COVID-19 are not preventative measures like vaccines, but treatments. They are laboratory-made monoclonal antibodies that mimic those produced naturally or by vaccines. The monoclonal antibodies are usually directed against the spike proteins.

COXSACKIE VIRUSES

There are a large number of coxsackie viruses but only a few which regularly colonise the oral cavity. Two major clinical oral diseases caused by coxsackie viruses are hand, foot and mouth disease and herpangina. Less common is acute lymphonodular pharyngitis.

Hand, Foot and Mouth Disease

Hand, foot and mouth disease (HFMD) is a common viral and exanthematous illness, typically affecting infants and children between 3 and 10 years of age. Whole families can be infected and the disease can occur more than once. Coxsackie virus group A type 16 (CoxA16) is the main pathogen and usually an alternative to or joins in prevalence with enterovirus 71 (EV71) causing hand, foot and mouth disease. The infection can also be caused by many other strains of coxsackie virus.

HFMD:

- Occurs most commonly in the summer and small epidemics are frequently reported among schoolchildren or those attending nurseries, or in families.
- Transmission usually takes place via the faecal-oral route or respiratory inhalation of infected droplets.
- The incubation period is 3 to 7 days and the disease is most contagious in the first week of illness.
- Presentation is usually with fever, reduced appetite, sore throat and malaise.
- Vesicles and oral ulcers are usually 2 to 7 mm in size and vary in number from 1 to 30 (Fig. 37.2).
- Affects mainly the buccal mucosa, labial mucosa and tongue but any site of the oral mucosa can be involved.

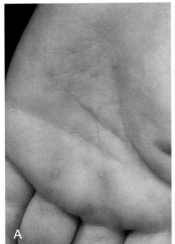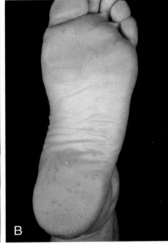

Fig. 37.2 Hand, foot and mouth disease coxsackie A6 infection showing erythematous lesions on (A) palm of hand (B) soles of feet.

- Lasts about 1 week and has no notable long-lasting consequences.

Following the appearance of oral lesions, the palms of the hand and soles of the feet are usually affected. The vesicles or small blisters with an erythematous base appear at the distal flexor aspect of the fingers or toes.

The diagnosis is typically based upon the clinical picture, and treatment is mainly supportive via hydration, topical, or systemic analgesics and antipyretics (e.g. paracetamol or ibuprofen).

Herpangina

- Herpangina is caused by a type A coxsackie group viral infection.
- Characteristically, there are numerous small vesicles, particularly the soft palate and fauces area which rupture quickly to give rise to shallow and painful ulcers (Fig. 37.3).
- Most frequent in children and often spreads among them.
- The virus is transmitted via saliva or occasionally by the oro-faecal route.
- Symptoms arise 2 to 10 days following exposure to the virus and resolve 7 to 10 days later.

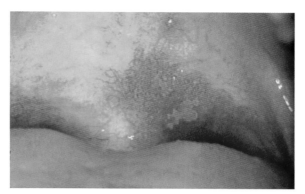

Fig. 37.3 Herpangina: irregular ulceration of soft palate area formed by coalescing ulcers caused by coxsackie virus.

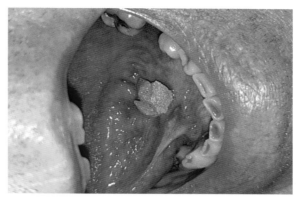

Fig. 37.4 Human papillomavirus-induced warty type lesion under the tongue.

- Clinical features: fever, sore throat, headache, dysphagia, and malaise.
- Diagnosis: the diagnosis is usually clinical, while therapy is directed towards ensuring adequate hydration, appropriate analgesia and antipyretics.

Acute Lymphonodular Pharyngitis

- Comprised of small numbers of discrete white to yellow papules on the uvula, soft palate, palatoglossal folds and posterior pharyngeal wall.
- Caused by coxsackie virus A10.
- Typically affects children and young adults.
- Has an incubation period of about 5 days.
- Gives rise to symptoms of sore throat, pyrexia, mild headache and anorexia.
- Oral lesions 2 to 3 days after onset of the systemic features.
- The lesions usually regress in about 10 days without any blistering or ulceration.
- Therapy is to reduce any pyrexia and ensure adequate hydration.

OTHER VIRUSES WITH OROFACIAL MANIFESTATIONS

Human Papillomaviruses

HPV are DNA viruses with approximately 200 different subtypes. They cause a wide range of usually benign skin or squamous mucosal lesions:
- can primarily infect the skin (dermatotrophic) or mucosa (mucosotrophic)
- can also be classified as oncogenic (i.e. cancer-causing) and non-oncogenic
- skin lesions include plantar warts, flat warts, genital condyloma acuminate
- oral lesions include papillomas, multifocal epithelial hyperplasia.

HPV is typically transmitted by direct contact with an infected lesion. Oral lesions may arise as a result of biting a wart of the skin. Similarly, oral or genital condyloma may arise as a consequence of oral sex. It has been claimed that transmission via oral fluids or food utensils may account for the acquisition of multifocal epithelial hyperplasia.

Clinical presentation
- The most common oral HPV lesions are squamous papillomas (SP).
- These manifest as small frond-like projections resulting in a lesion with a rough or cauliflower-like surface (Fig. 37.4).
- HPV 6 and HPV 11 are the most commonly isolated genotypes.
- Condyloma acuminata — warts possibly acquired sexually.
- HPV types 2, 6 and 11 are the most commonly isolated genotypes of condyloma acuminata.

The diagnosis of HPV-related warts is confirmed by histopathology. Viral proteins can be identified by immunohistochemistry. Treatment: SP removal either via scalpel surgery or laser surgery incorporating a rim of normal mucosa in the excisional biopsy.

Multifocal Epithelial Hyperplasia (Sometimes Termed Heck Disease)
It is:
- More common in children and adolescents than in adults in most examined populations.
- Occur only on oral mucosa, mainly lower lip and buccal mucosa.
- Multiple soft, flat or rounded elevated nodules.
- Are asymptomatic, persist for several years and regress spontaneously.
- Multifocal epithelial hyperplasia is rare and tends to occur in certain ethnic and racial groups (e.g. Inuit Indians, Eskimos).
- Many HPV genotypes have been detected in MEH lesions although types 13 and 32 are the most commonly associated types, representing 75% to 100% of the isolated HPV.
- The clustering of MEH in socioeconomically deprived groups and ethnically related cohorts suggest that both acquired and genetic factors may underlie the transmission and acquisition of causative HPV genotypes.

Oncogenic types of HPV are now recognised as a cause of some squamous cell carcinoma, particularly of the posterior tongue, tonsillar area and upper pharynx. HPV-related oropharyngeal squamous cell carcinoma (OPSCC) seems to be distinct from head and neck carcinomas associated with tobacco and alcohol intake, although recent evidence suggests that HPV may be an exacerbating factor in most head and neck cancers.

- Patients tend to be male, under 50 years of age and have no history of notable tobacco and/or alcohol use.
- Outcomes of treatment of HPV-related OPSCC appear better (80% survival at 5 years) than oropharyngeal cancer due to alcohol and tobacco (40% to 50% 5-year survival rate).
- The incidence of HPV-positive OPSCC has climbed greatly in the past 30 years.
- OPSCC are HPV 16 and sometimes HPV 18 positive (HPV 16 dominant genotype in cervical cancer).
- There is no convincing evidence that the virus is acquired via orogenital or oroanal contact.
- Vaccination in both boys and girls against the oncogenic types of HPV (particularly 16 and 18) is being undertaken across many countries.
- Vaccination appears to have markedly reduced the incidence of cervical carcinomas. Given the strong association between HPV 16 and oral cancers, it is hoped that similar reductions in oral cancers may occur.

Rubella

Rubella virus (RV) is transmitted via respiratory droplets. Vertical transmission from an infected mother can occur transplacentally during the first semester of pregnancy and can cause congenital rubella syndrome (malformations, premature birth or spontaneous abortion in severe cases).

- Rubella has an incubation period of 2 to 3 weeks.
- Cutaneous rash develops, usually on the face that gradually evolves on all cutaneous surfaces.
- Clinical symptoms: cervical lymphadenopathy and headache, low-grade fever, malaise and mild conjunctivitis.
- Oral lesions can arise in about 20% of affected individuals as dark-red macules or petechiae (Forchheimer sign) on the soft palate (at the same time as skin rash).
- Clinical features in congenital rubella syndrome: infants may include developmental delay, microcephaly, intellectual disability and seizures.
- Immunisation markedly reduces the risk of rubella infection.
- Passive immunity can be provided by the administration of human anti-rubella immunoglobulin.

Measles

Measles is caused by the Rubeola virus which is a paramyxovirus. It is:
- Transmitted via person-to-person contact as well as airborne spread.
- Highly contagious and continued yearly multiple outbreaks occur worldwide.
- A leading worldwide cause of death in unvaccinated children less than 5 years of age.
- Can result in neurologic, pulmonary and gastrointestinal complications.

- Koplik spots are the peculiar spots present on the buccal mucosa and are considered a diagnostic/pathognomic feature of measles/rubeola in the pre-eruptive stage.
- Prevented by vaccination and there is no specific anti-viral therapy.
- Has an incubation of 7 to 14 days.
- Clinical features include Koplik spots, rash (maculopapular), conjunctivitis, runny nose, cough, fever, malaise and anorexia.
- Diagnose from clinical features; a rising antibody titre is confirmatory.
- Management is symptomatic.

VIRAL INFECTIONS OF THE SALIVARY GLANDS

Salivary glands appear to be particularly susceptible to viral infections. The best known are mumps, HIV-salivary gland disease and coronaviruses, although claims of virus involvement in SS and other conditions have been made.

Mumps

Mumps is an acute self-limiting disease of salivary glands caused by the mumps virus, an RNA paramyxovirus.
   The virus is:
- Transmitted via the droplet route mainly in 5- to 16-year-olds.
- Patients are infectious about 48 h before the onset of the salivary gland swelling and for a further 9 to 10 days.
- The infection has an incubation period of 15 to 21 days.
- Vaccination is effective and has reduced the incidence.
- Clinical signs: initial pyrexia followed by swelling of one or both parotid glands with cervical lymphadenopathy.
- The submandibular glands, and rarely the sublingual glands can become involved.
- Salivary gland swelling diminishes after about 9 days.
   Systemic manifestations include short-term orchitis (infection of the testicles, often unilateral) which can arise 4 to 5 days after the onset of parotid enlargement, causing local pain. Viral meningitis can occur giving rise to headaches and photophobia even in the absence of any parotid enlargement.

HIV Salivary Gland Disease (HIVSGD) (see also Chapter 39)

Salivary gland manifestations can arise in up to 30% of children with untreated HIV infection (less common in adults).
- Symptoms include parotid gland swelling and in a proportion of cases hyposalivation.
- Histologically there are cystic-like spaces develop in the glands with CD8+ cell infiltration.
- HIVSGD is associated with the small DNA tumourvirus BK polyomavirus (BKPyV).
- Infection with other viruses may occur.

INFECTION CONTROL PRINCIPLES FOR VIRUSES (AND OTHER INFECTIVE AGENTS)

Potential exposure to hepatitis, SARS or other viruses in an oral health practice may include needle sticks or other sharps injury, contact with potentially infectious body fluids and exposure to mucus membranes. Depending on the nature of the exposure, baseline serologic data may be obtained from both the patient and the dental HCW. Exposed HCWs should be monitored closely after exposure and, depending on the nature of the exposure, postexposure prophylaxis (PEP) may be ordered. There have been many instances of transmission of hepatitis B from dentists to patients.

Protection of the Dental Team

Transmission of viruses in a clinical setting from patient to dental HCWs can be reduced by following simple steps:
- All dental HCWs should receive routine vaccines for viral illnesses, including hepatitis B and SARS-CoV-2.
- Dental HCWs should always follow standard infection control procedures when caring for patients.
- Third, dental HCWs should report any occupational exposures and follow local PEP guidelines to minimise the chance of acquiring a viral infection from a patient.
- Appropriate diagnosis of oral viral infections is critical, especially to distinguish it from other infections, as some of them may well have the potential to turn sinister.
- An infected healthcare professional must avoid patient care during the infectious stages until free of detectable antigen.

Dentistry is classified as one of the highest-risk professions for transmitting COVID-19. Until further research on COVID-19 transmission dynamics in dental settings is performed, dentists should wear the following personal protective equipment:
- FFP3 (Europe) or N95 (USA) respirator
- disposable gown
- gloves
- eye protection (goggles or face shield).

In case of the unavailability of FFP3 respirators (99.95% filtration of 0.3 μ particles), N95 (95% filtration of 0.3 μ particles) or FFP2 (94% filtration of 0.3 μ particles) masks were considered to provide enough protection provided that they are face-fit tested for the specific user.

Current (2022) evidence-based treatments for COVID-19 include remdesivir and dexamethasone.

RECOMMENDED READING

Demicheli, V., Rivetti, A., Debalini, M.G., Di Pietrantonj, C., 2012. Vaccines for measles, mumps and rubella in children. Cochrane Database Syst. Rev. 2012 (2), CD004407. https://doi.org/10.1002/14651858.CD004407.pub3. Update in: Cochrane Database Syst. Rev. 2020 Apr 20;4:CD004407.

Li, P., Chen, Y., Tang, A., Gao, F., Yan, J.B., 2021. Seroprevalence of coxsackievirus A16 antibody among people of various age groups: a systematic review and meta-analysis. Arch. Public. Health 79 (1), 166. https://doi.org/10.1186/s13690-021-00688-z.

Syrjänen, S., Lodi, G., von Bültzingslöwen, I., et al., 2011. Human papillomaviruses in oral carcinoma and oral potentially malignant disorders: a systematic review. Oral. Dis. 17 (Suppl. 1), 58−72.

Walekhwa, A.W., Ntaro, M., Kawungezi, P.C., et al., 2021. Measles outbreak in Western Uganda: a case-control study. BMC. Infect. Dis. 21 (1), 596. https://doi.org/10.1186/s12879-021-06213-5.

Herpesvirus Infections

KEY POINTS

- Herpesviruses are DNA viruses that can be transmitted in body fluids such as saliva, contracted in early life, characterised by latency and reactivated during immunosuppression.
- There are eight sub-types of herpes viruses which span three subfamilies (α, β, γ):
  - α herpes viruses include herpes simplex viruses (HSV1 and HSV2) and varicella-zoster virus (VZV) herpes simplex virus (HSV) causes primary herpetic stomatitis and recurrent herpes labialis or intraoral recurrences. Herpes zoster VZV causes chickenpox and shingles
  - β herpes viruses include cytomegalovirus (CMV) which may cause some salivary infections.
  - γ herpes viruses include Epstein—Barr virus (EBV) which causes infectious mononucleosis and may be associated with nasopharyngeal carcinoma, lymphomas and hairy leukoplakia. HHV8 is associated with Kaposi sarcoma.
- A range of anti-herpes virus drugs is now available.

- transmitted in saliva and other secretions
- characterised by latency and a variable reproductive cycle
- reactivated during immunosuppression — when they are associated with more severe and protracted disorders, particularly in HIV infection, in cancer patients and those immunosuppressed after organ grafts.

Herpesviruses and the orofacial disorders with which they may be associated are shown in Table 38.1. Some herpesviruses can cause malignant tumours (i.e. are *oncogenic*).

HERPES SIMPLEX VIRUS INFECTIONS

The term 'herpes' is often used loosely to refer to infections with HSV, a ubiquitous virus that commonly produces lesions in the mouth, oropharynx and ano-genital region. Oral or oropharyngeal infections are mainly caused by HSV-1, while ano-genital infections are mainly caused by HSV-2.

INTRODUCTION

Herpesviruses (from Greek *herpein* = to creep) are DNA viruses that are mostly:
- contracted in early life

PRIMARY HERPES SIMPLEX VIRUS INFECTIONS

Primary oral infection is often subclinical between the ages of 2 and 4 years and is a common cause of 'teething'. Herpetic stomatitis (gingivostomatitis) is:

TABLE 38.1 Herpesvirus Infections and Their Known Possible Oral Sequelae

Subfamily	Herpesvirus	Abbreviation	Typical Primary Infection	Common Clinical Oral Sequelae	Other Known Possible Sequelae, Particularly in Immunocompromised Patients
α	Herpes simplex	HSV-1	Stomatitis	Herpes labialis	Ulcers Erythema multiforme Bell palsy
α	Herpes simplex	HSV-2	Anogenital herpes	Recurrent herpes	Ulcers
α	Herpes varicella-zoster	VZV	Chickenpox	Zoster	Jaw necrosis
γ	Epstein—Barr virus	EBV	Glandular fever	Sore throat Fatigue	Hairy leukoplakia Lymphomas Nasopharyngeal carcinoma
β	Cytomegalovirus	CMV	Glandular fever	?	Ulcers
β	Human herpesvirus-6	HHV-6A HHV-6B	Exanthem subitum	None known	Chronic fatigue syndrome Associated with multiple sclerosis and Alzheimer disease. Reactivation in transplant recipients: encephalitis, bone marrow suppression and pneumonitis
β	Human herpesvirus-7	HHV-7	Exanthem subitum, pityriasis rosea	None known	Neurological manifestations and transplant complications
γ	Human herpesvirus-8	HHV-8 or KSHV (Kaposi sarcoma herpesvirus)	Rash	Kaposi sarcoma	Castleman disease Primary effusion lymphoma

- the primary clinical infection with HSV
- usually caused by HSV-1
- seen mainly in children
- may be seen in older patients when it is sometimes due to HSV-2 and is transmitted sexually.

It is important to remember that primary HSV-1 may also cause throat, facial skin, eye and central nervous system infections with a wide differential diagnosis.

Epidemiology
- Primary oral HSV is a common, universal infection more frequent in under-developed areas of the world.
- About 67% of the world population under the age of 50 has HSV-1.
- It is seen mainly in children and adolescents and affects both sexes equally.
- It is more frequently encountered when children are in a crowded environment.
- Oropharyngeal herpes is seen mainly in adolescents and recurrent HSV is seen mainly in adults.

Predisposing Factors
- Close contact with infected individuals. HSV is contracted from infected saliva or other body fluids with an incubation period of 2 to 12 days.
- HSV-1 can cause oral or oropharyngeal infection, usually via infection from saliva.

- HSV-2 can cause oropharyngeal infection, usually via sexual contact. It is most frequent amongst female prostitutes (75%) and men who have sex with men (80%). HSV-1 genital infection is less common and usually less severe than HSV-2 infection.
- Neonatal HSV infections contracted during vaginal delivery from an infected mother, are potentially dangerous as they may lead to disseminated involvement and encephalitis, and often leave neurological sequelae.
- Patients with immune defects are liable to severe and/or protracted and/or disseminated HSV infections.

Aetiology and Pathogenesis
- HSV must contact mucosae or abraded skin to initiate infection.
- HSV surface glycoproteins mediate cell attachment and penetration.
- HSV is neuroinvasive and neurotoxic and infects neurones of dorsal root and autonomic ganglia.
- HSV remains latent thereafter in the ganglion, usually the trigeminal ganglion, but can be reactivated and result in clinical recrudescence (see below).
- *Primary* infection is when a susceptible (non-immune) individual develops the infection.
- *Recurrent* infection occurs when an individual who has contracted either HSV-1 or HSV-2 develops reactivated latent virus.

- HSV is also implicated in Bell's palsy (see Chapter 48), erythema multiforme (see Chapter 28), herpetic encephalitis and Alzheimer disease.

Clinical Features

Some 50% of primary HSV infections are subclinical but the main features of clinical disease are:

- High fever and/or malaise. The fever subsides after 3 to 5 days and recovery is usually complete within 2 weeks.
- The mouth or oropharynx is sore (herpetic stomatitis); this may explain some instances of 'teething'.
- A single episode of oral vesicles, which may be widespread, and break down to leave oral ulcers. These are initially pinpoint, but fuse to produce irregular painful ulcers (Fig. 38.1).
- Gingival oedema, erythema and ulceration.
- Often drooling and there may be skin lesion in contact with infected saliva.
- The cervical lymph nodes may be enlarged and tender. Usually, several nodes in the anterior triangle of the neck (especially the jugulodigastric nodes) are enlarged but the posterior triangle and nodes elsewhere are not enlarged, unless there are systemic complications or lesions in other sites.
- There is no hepatosplenomegaly, unless there are systemic complications or lesions elsewhere.

Diagnosis

- Diagnosis is largely clinical.
- Herpetic stomatitis should be differentiated from other causes of mouth ulcers (see Chapter 6), especially acute necrotising ulcerative gingivitis (ANUG), herpangina, hand, foot and mouth disease, chickenpox and shingles, erythema multiforme and rarely leukaemia. A full blood picture is warranted.
- Viral studies which are occasionally used for diagnosis include (Table 38.2):
  - polymerase chain reaction detection of HSV-DNA: sensitive and rapid, but expensive
  - Antibody detection of HSV antigens (direct fluorescent antibody; DFA): sensitive and rapid serology for detection of a rising titre of serum antibodies; confirmatory, but only gives the diagnosis retrospectively; conventional

TABLE 38.2   Investigations That Might Be Helpful in Diagnosis/Prognosis/Management in Some Patients Suspected of Having Herpesvirus Infections[a]

In Most Cases	In Some Cases
Full blood picture	Serum ferritin, vitamin B_{12} and corrected whole blood folate levels
	ESR
	HSV, VZV, HIV, EBV, CMV, HHV8 serology, direct fluorescent immunostaining or PCR

[a]See text for details and glossary for abbreviations.

enzyme-linked immunosorbent assays (ELISA) for serum antibodies have poor sensitivity and specificity, while newer assays based on gG-1 HSV glycoproteins are comparable with Western blot assays.

- Culture: takes days to give a result
- Electron microscopy: not always available
- Smears for viral damaged cells: now rarely used.

Treatment (see also Chapters 4 and 5)

Although patients eventually have spontaneous remission, treatment is indicated particularly to reduce fever and control pain (Table 38.3). Patient information is an important aspect of management:

- Pregnant women and neonates must receive urgent specialist care. HSV infection in pregnancy can cause foetal disorders ranging from minor issues to death, herpes being one of the peri-natal infections causing the so-called TORCH syndrome or complex (toxoplasmosis; rubella; CMV; herpes).
- Adequate fluid intake is important, especially in children.
- Antipyretics/analgesics, such as paracetamol help relieve pain and fever.
- A soft bland diet may be needed, as the mouth can be very sore.
- Local antiseptics (0.2% aqueous chlorhexidine mouthwashes) may aid in the resolution of the lesions.
- Antivirals may be effective if used systemically within 5 days of symptoms, though they do not reduce the frequency of

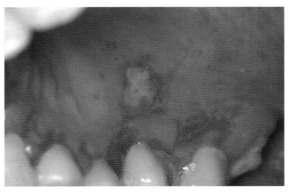

Fig. 38.1 Herpetic stomatitis; ulcers in the palate.

TABLE 38.3   Regimens That Might Be Helpful in Management of Patient Suspected of Having Herpetic Stomatitis

Regimen	Use in primary or secondary care[a]
Beneficial	Aciclovir, valaciclovir or famciclovir
Supportive	Adequate hydration
	Benzydamine
	Chlorhexidine
	Diet with little acidic, spicy or citrus content
	Lidocaine
	Paracetamol, ibuprofen

[a]Specialist care for neonates, pregnant or immunocompromised people.

subsequent recurrences: 200 mg aciclovir tablets five times daily, or sugar-free oral suspension (200 mg/5 mL) five times daily or valaciclovir or famciclovir.
- Aciclovir must be used systemically with care in pregnancy, older patients, renal disease or when infused (Chapter 5). Systemic antivirals are useful especially in neonates, pregnancy and immunocompromised patients; but all such patients should be seen by a specialist.

Follow-Up of Patients
Long-term follow-up is rarely required.

RECURRENT HERPES SIMPLEX VIRUS INFECTIONS
Epidemiology
- Up to 15% of the population have recurrent HSV-1 infections. — usually, lip lesions (herpes labialis). Approximately 30% with primary HSV-1 will develop a recurrent infection. Occurs mainly in adults.
- Both genders are affected.
- Herpes labialis is the most common form of recurrence and is seen mainly in sunny climes.
- Recurrent HSV may recur at the site of initial inoculation or in the distribution of the associated nerves.
- Asymptomatic shedding may occur for a week before and after visible infection. It may also occur in asymptomatic individuals.

Predisposing Factors
Reactivating factors include:
- sunlight
- fever, such as caused by upper respiratory tract infection (hence herpes labialis is often termed 'cold' sores)
- trauma
- immunosuppression
- stress
- hormonal changes.

Aetiology and Pathogenesis
HSV-1 is latent in the trigeminal ganglion after primary infection. The virus can be reactivated, is shed into saliva, and there may be clinical recrudescence, recurrently, to produce herpes labialis or, occasionally, intraoral ulceration. Lesions may also occur in the peri-oral or peri-nasal skin. Patients may secrete virus for or may be asymptomatic shedders.

Clinical Features
- Features of recurrent herpes labialis are lip lesions at the mucocutaneous junction (Fig. 38.2).
- Lesions may be preceded (hours to a few days) by pain, burning, tingling or itching, and begin as macules that rapidly become papular, then vesicular for about 48 hours, then become pustular, and scab within 72 to 96 hours and heal without scarring.

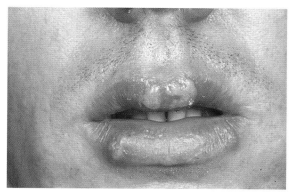

Fig. 38.2 Herpes labialis.

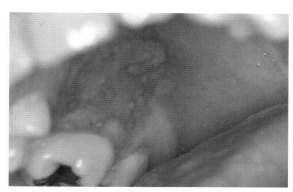

Fig. 38.3 Recurrent intraoral herpes.

- Widespread recalcitrant lesions may appear in immuno-compromised patients.
- Features of recurrent intraoral herpes include:
  - In apparently healthy patients: a small crop of ulcers over the greater palatine foramen, following a palatal local anaesthetic injection, presumably because of the trauma (Fig. 38.3). This can mimic zoster.
  - In immunocompromised patients: chronic, often dendritic, ulcers, frequently on the tongue dorsum.
  - In patients with severe facial eczema, where they develop herpes labialis or are asymptomatic viral shedders. Eczema herpeticum may occur with a widespread vesicular lesion on the skin. Herpetic keratoconjunctivitis is a serious risk and ophthalmological review is urgent.

Diagnosis
- Differential diagnosis of herpes labialis is mainly from zoster, impetigo or carcinoma (rarely). Diagnosis is largely clinical, although viral studies are used very occasionally.
- Diagnosis of recurrent intraoral herpes in healthy patients is mainly from zoster. Diagnosis is largely clinical and viral studies are used very occasionally.
- Diagnosis of recurrent intraoral herpes in immune-compromised patients can be difficult since the lesions can mimic many other causes of oral ulceration. Clinical diagnosis tends to underestimate the frequency of these lesions

and viral studies may be needed, particularly as there may be co-infection with other agents such as CMV.

Treatment (see also Chapters 4 and 5)

- Patient information is an important aspect of management.
- Patients should avoid any triggers they have identified. For example, if sunlight is a trigger, they should use a good quality sunblock. Once a lesion appears, most patients will have spontaneous remission within 7 to 10 days, but the condition is both uncomfortable and unsightly, and, thus, early treatment is indicated.
- Antivirals will achieve maximum benefit only if given in the prodrome or early in the disease (Chapter 5), and may be indicated in herpes labialis especially in:
  - patients who have severe, widespread or persistent lesions
  - immunocompromised persons.
- Lip lesions in healthy patients may be minimised with topical penciclovir 1% cream or aciclovir 5% cream applied from the prodrome, every 2 hours whilst awake (Chapter 5; Table 38.4). Penciclovir may be marginally the more effective.
- Lip lesions in immunocompromised patients may require systemic aciclovir or other antivirals, such as valaciclovir or famciclovir (the precursor of penciclovir).
- Recurrent intraoral herpes in healthy patients can be managed with symptomatic treatment with a soft diet and adequate fluid intake, antipyretics/analgesics (paracetamol, ibuprofen) and local antiseptics (0.2% aqueous chlorhexidine mouthwashes). Systemic aciclovir or other antivirals, such as valaciclovir or famciclovir may be indicated for persistent lesions.
- Recurrent intraoral herpes in immunocompromised patients is difficult to manage and systemic aciclovir or other antivirals may well be needed. A soft diet and adequate fluid intake, antipyretics/analgesics (paracetamol elixir) and local antiseptics (0.2% aqueous chlorhexidine mouthwashes) may help. Antiviral resistance is becoming a significant problem for immunocompromised persons, especially those with a severe immune defect.

- Other therapies tried for recurrent herpes are shown in Table 38.4.
- There is insufficient evidence to support the use of many other preparations including echinacea, eleuthero, zinc or aloe vera.
- Reliably effective anti-herpes vaccines are not currently available.

Follow-Up of Patients

For healthy patients, no follow-up is required.

HERPES VARICELLA-ZOSTER VIRUS INFECTIONS

Primary Varicella-Zoster Virus Infections

Chickenpox (varicella) is the primary infection with the virus.

Epidemiology

- Chickenpox is common.
- It mainly occurs in children.
- Both sexes are affected.
- No known geographic incidence, it occurs worldwide.

Predisposing Factors

Chickenpox is highly contagious and VZV is readily spread by droplets.

Aetiology

After this primary infection, the virus remains latent in the dorsal root ganglia.

Clinical Features

- The incubation period is 10 to 21 days.
- Some 50% of VZV infections are subclinical.
- Clinical features include:
  - rash: often very prominent and seen mainly on the face and trunk; consists of itchy papules then vesicles, pustules and scabs, in crops
  - fever
  - malaise

TABLE 38.4	Regimens That Might Be Helpful in Management of Patient Suspected of Having Recurrent Herpes Simplex Lesions	
Regimen	Use in primary care (herpes labialis)	Use in secondary care (severe oral involvement and/or extraoral involvement), or immunocompromised
Beneficial	Topical penciclovir or aciclovir	Systemic aciclovir, valaciclovir or famciclovir
Likely to be beneficial	Protective hydrocolloid patches	
Unproven effectiveness	Monolaurin L-lysine, aspirin Lemon balm Topical zinc Liquorice root cream Tea tree oil Urea	
Supportive	Lip balm	

- irritability
- anorexia
- mouth lesions are common and may precede skin lesions: they start as white oval vesicles often on the buccal mucosa or palate that rupture to form ulcers. The gingivae are not usually affected.
- cervical lymphadenitis.
- Infection in adults may be more severe occasionally leading to pneumonia or encephalitis.

Diagnosis

The diagnosis is on clinical grounds. A rising antibody titre is confirmatory. Differentiation is from other mouth ulcers, especially herpes simplex and other viral infections. Viral PCR can distinguish VZV but is rarely indicated.

Treatment (see also Chapters 4 and 5; Table 38.5)

- Patient information is an important aspect of management.
- Most patients will have spontaneous remission within 1 week to 10 days.
- Symptomatic care is important (see Chapter 4).
- Antivirals are rarely indicated.
- Neonates and pregnant women should receive specialist care and are usually treated with antivirals. Immunocompromised patients should receive specialist care and are usually treated with antivirals and immune globulin.

Prevention of Varicella-Zoster Virus infections

A live-attenuated VZV vaccine is available.

Follow-Up of Patients

Long-term follow-Up is rarely required.

Recurrent Varicella-Zoster Virus Infections

Recurrence of VZV, which has been latent in dorsal root ganglia, causes zoster or shingles. The word 'zoster' comes from the Greek for 'belt', since the lesion occurs in a belt-like distribution.

Epidemiology

- Zoster is uncommon.
- It occurs mainly in older adults and immunocompromised patients.
- Both sexes are affected.
- It is universal.

Predisposing and Protective Factors

- Zoster mainly affects the older, or immune-compromised patients, such as in HIV infection, leukaemia or cancer. Zoster has become a fairly common feature in HIV-infected patients treated with HAART.
- Fresh fruit appears to be associated with a reduced risk of developing zoster.

Aetiology and Pathogenesis

- Reactivation of VZV latent in sensory ganglia.

TABLE 38.5 Regimens That Might Be Helpful in Management of Patient Suspected of Having Chickenpox

Regimen	Use in primary or secondary care[a]
Likely to be beneficial but rarely indicated	Aciclovir or valaciclovir or famciclovir orally or parenterally
Supportive	Adequate hydration
	Benzydamine
	Diet with little acidic, spicy or citrus content
	Lidocaine
	Paracetamol

[a]Specialist care for neonates, pregnant or immunocompromised people.

Clinical Features

- The main features are pain and a rash in one dermatome (the area of skin and mucosa supplied by a sensory nerve). While herpes zoster in children is often painless, in older people, the disease tends to be more severe. Early or late in the disease, a rash is absent (and in zoster sine herpete).
- Most zoster is seen in the thoracic region; 30% is in the trigeminal region.
- Pain occurs before, with and after the rash.
- Rash is unilateral vesiculating then scabbing in dermatome (Fig. 38.4).
- Mouth ulcers are seen in maxillary or mandibular zoster only:
  - mandibular zoster: ipsilateral on buccal and lingual mucosa
  - maxillary: ipsilateral on palate and vestibule.
- Reactivation within the geniculate ganglion (Ramsay Hunt syndrome) is characterised by otitis externa, a unilateral lower motor neurone palsy of the facial nerve, ulceration of the soft palate and anterior 2/3 of the tongue unilaterally.
- Post-herpetic neuralgia (PHN; see Chapter 43) is the condition when the pain persists long after the rash has healed.

Diagnosis

Diagnosis is clinical; differentiation from toothache and other causes of ulcers, especially HSV, is important.

Treatment (see also Chapters 4 and 5)

- Antivirals given within 72 hours of the onset of zoster inhibit VZV replication, may help pain and healing and can reduce the severity and duration of zoster – and minimise PHN (Table 38.6) with minimal side effects, but antivirals do not reliably prevent PHN. Antiviral treatment is recommended for all immunocompetent patients over 50 years of age. 800 mg JS aciclovir tablets five times daily, or sugar-free oral suspension, for 7 days, or valaciclovir 1000 mg three times daily for 7 days JS, or famciclovir 500 mg three times daily for 7 days are useful JS. The addition of systemic corticosteroids may be beneficial in reducing PHN in patients over 50. In ophthalmic zoster, valaciclovir 1000 mg three times

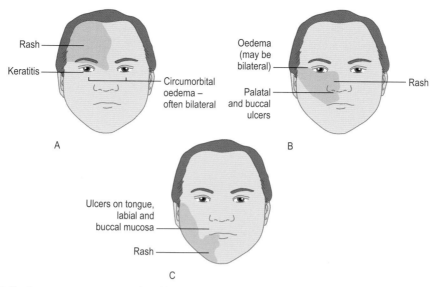

Fig. 38.4 Zoster can cause severe pain, skin rash and mucosal ulceration in any of the three divisions of the trigeminal nerve (A, ophthalmic; B, maxillary; C, mandibular divisions of trigeminal nerve).

TABLE 38.6	Regimens That Might Be Helpful in Management of Patient Suspected of Having Zoster	
Regimen	Use in primary care	Use in secondary care (severe oral involvement and/or extraoral involvement) or immunocompromised
Likely to be beneficial	Aciclovir, valaciclovir For post-herpetic neuralgia Systemic-gabapentinoids Opioids Tricyclic antidepressants	Aciclovir, valaciclovir or famciclovir orally or parenterally Systemic-gabapentinoids Opioids Tricyclic antidepressants Intrathecal methylprednisolone
Supportive	Post-herpetic neuralgia Topical-lidocaine patches or capsaicin	

daily is indicated JS, and an ophthalmological opinion, since there can be corneal ulceration.

- Immunocompromised patients should receive specialist care and are usually treated with antivirals and immune globulin.
- Analgesics are also needed. The evidence base supports the oral use of tricyclic antidepressants, certain opioids and gabapentinoids in PHN. Topical therapy with lidocaine patches and capsaicin is similarly supported. Intrathecal administration of methylprednisolone appears to be effective, but its safety requires further evaluation.

Follow-Up of Patients

Most patients make a complete recovery and do not require long-term follow-up.

EPSTEIN—BARR VIRUS INFECTION

EBV is a ubiquitous virus that commonly produces 'glandular fever', 'infectious mononucleosis' or 'mono', often with lesions in the mouth and oropharynx. It is also associated with oral hairy leukoplakia (Chapter 39), a number of malignancies of the head and neck including oropharyngeal carcinoma and some lymphomas.

INFECTIOUS MONONUCLEOSIS

Epidemiology

- EBV infection is common among young adults (especially students) and is often subclinical. By adulthood, 90% to 95% of people have been infected.
- Both sexes are affected.
- It is universal.

Predisposing Factors

- Close contact with infected individuals, predisposes to EBV infection, which appears to be spread by close oral contact, such as kissing ('the kissing disease').
- EBV is found in pharyngeal epithelium and appears in the saliva of patients with infectious mononucleosis for several months after apparent recovery.

- EBV is contracted from infected saliva or other body fluids after an incubation period of approximately 20 to 40 days.
- EBV is contracted earlier in resource-poor persons than in resource-rich persons.
- Patients with immune defects are liable to severe and/or protracted infections or EBV may be reactivated, leading to viral shedding, recurrence of infectious mononucleosis or, rarely, producing lymphoproliferative disease.

Clinical Features

The clinical features of EBV infection are as follows:
- A glandular fever syndrome termed 'infectious mononucleosis' which includes mainly:
  - lymphadenopathy
  - sore throat
  - fever
  - headache
  - malaise/severe lethargy.
  - Rashes including rashes of a non-allergic nature affecting the extensor surfaces of the limbs in patients taking ampicillin or amoxicillin with infectious mononucleosis or lymphatic leukaemia.
  - May develop hepatosplenomegaly.

Recovery can take weeks or months and the virus thereafter remains latent in pharyngeal and/or salivary epithelial cells. Particular features predominate in some patients:
- The anginose type of infectious mononucleosis (sore-throat type) is characterised by a sore oedematous throat with soft palate petechiae and a whitish exudate on the tonsils. Pharyngeal oedema may threaten the airway.
- The glandular type of infectious mononucleosis is characterised mainly by general lymph node enlargement and splenomegaly.
- The febrile type of infectious mononucleosis is characterised mainly by fever.

Complications

Complications are rare but may include:
- autoimmune haemolysis (and cold agglutinins)
- CNS involvement (meningitis, encephalitis, etc.)
- erythema multiforme
- hepatomegaly or hepatitis
- jaundice (from hepatic involvement or haemolysis)
- pericarditis or myocarditis
- pneumonitis
- splenic rupture
- thrombocytopenia.
  EBV is also implicated in:
- hairy leukoplakia
- chronic infection, which may cause persistent malaise
- Burkitt and some other lymphomas
- post-transplantation lymphoproliferative disorder
- nasopharyngeal carcinoma.

Diagnosis

- Differentiation from other glandular fever syndromes caused by CMV, HHV-6, HIV or *Toxoplasma* infection is important.
- Investigations are indicated: characteristics of infectious mononucleosis are:
  - mononucleosis: large numbers of atypical mononuclear cells in the blood.
- Serological changes such as heterophile antibodies (human antibodies which agglutinate animal (sheep and horse) erythrocytes and are detectable by the Paul–Bunell (Paul–Bunell–Davidson) or monospot tests) and antibodies to EBV viral capsid antigen (VCA). IgM anti-EBV reflects a current infection.
- Abnormal liver function tests.

Treatment (see also Chapters 4 and 5)

- Treatment is aimed at easing the symptoms, and can usually be done at home with rest, fluids, over-the-counter medications and analgesia/antipyretic such as paracetamol or NSAIDs. Serious complications are rare but contact sports and heavy physical activity should be banned, to avoid splenic rupture.
- No specific reliably effective antiviral treatment is available (Table 38.7). Valaciclovir may be helpful in complicated mononucleosis.
- Systemic corticosteroids are required if there is pharyngeal oedema severe enough to hazard the airway.

Follow-Up of Patients

Long-term follow-up as shared care may be appropriate in patients with complications. However, most will recover fully with no follow-up required.

CYTOMEGALOVIRUS INFECTION

CMV is a ubiquitous herpesvirus that infects most persons at some time during their lives and thereafter remains latent. It has been termed the 'salivary gland inclusion virus' since there are inclusion bodies seen histopathologically in the salivary glands of infected people. These strikingly enlarged cells (the property of 'cytomegaly', from which CMV acquires its name) contain intranuclear inclusions that have the histopathological appearance of owl's eyes. CMV affects especially the CNS and arguably causes the most morbidity and mortality of all herpesviruses.

Epidemiology

- It is common, especially in children in resource-poor conditions but is also seen in adolescents and adults in resource-rich conditions.
- Infection is often subclinical.
- Both sexes are affected.

TABLE 38.7 Regimens That Might be Helpful in Management of Patient Suspected of Having Infectious Mononucleosis (IM)

Regimen	Use in primary care	Use in secondary care (severe oral involvement and/or extraoral involvement)
Likely to be beneficial		Systemic corticosteroids if the airway is threatened, or there is haemolysis or thrombocytopenia
		Valaciclovir in complicated i.m.
Supportive	Adequate hydration	
	Benzydamine	
	Diet with little acidic, spicy or citrus content	
	Lidocaine	
	Paracetamol	

Predisposing Factors

- Close contact with infected individuals predisposes to infection.
- CMV can also be transmitted via saliva, blood, sexually and transplacentally, and in transplantation.
- CMV is contracted from infected saliva, urine, semen or other body fluids after an incubation period of approximately 20 to 40 days.
- Patients with immune defects are liable to severe and/or protracted infections, or CMV may be reactivated.

Clinical Features

- While the majority of perinatally infected infants are asymptomatic, 30% may develop hearing impairment, transplacental CMV infection may cause abortion, learning disability or other defects, and the affected child excretes CMV in urine for months or years after birth and is a major reservoir of the virus.
- CMV infection in normal children or adults is usually asymptomatic.
- CMV infection in some otherwise apparently healthy children and adults causes the CMV mononucleosis syndrome ('infectious lymphocytosis') of headache, back and abdominal pain, sore throat, fever and atypical lymphocytosis, but with a negative Paul—Bunell test.
- Immunocompromised patients may be infected with CMV, or latent CMV may be reactivated. In these patients, CMV acts as an opportunistic infection and may cause various clinical syndromes with viral dissemination leading to multiple organ system involvements, the most important clinical manifestations consisting of CMV pneumonitis, GI disease and retinitis. They also excrete the virus in body fluids.
- The long-term health consequences of CMV infection may include atherosclerosis, immunosenescence and an increased risk of malignancy.

Diagnosis

- Differentiation from other glandular fever syndromes caused by EBV, HHV-6, HIV or *Toxoplasma* infection is important.
- Virus isolation and serology may be of value in the diagnosis.

Treatment (see also Chapters 4 and 5)

Treatment is usually symptomatic in the immunocompetent patient. Immunocompromised patients, however, require specialist care. Valaciclovir may prevent CMV infections and valganciclovir may treat them in immunocompromised patients.

Follow-Up of Patients

Long-term follow-up in secondary care is usually appropriate for immunocompromised patients.

OTHER HUMAN HERPESVIRUSES

- HHV-6 has two subtypes:
  - HHV-6A has been detected in patients with multiple sclerosis and Alzheimer disease.
  - HHV-6B is usually associated with a rash in children (exanthem subitum also known as Roseola infantum, but reactivation has also been implicated in some cases of drug-induced hypersensitivity syndromes (DRESS), manifesting with lymphadenopathy.
- HHV-6 may be reactivated in organ transplant patients.
- HHV-7 may be associated with skin rashes and, if reactivated, with neurological manifestations in transplant patients.
- HHV-8 (now termed Kaposi sarcoma herpesvirus [KSHV]) is transmitted mainly sexually and is strongly associated mainly with Kaposi sarcoma (Chapter 39).

RECOMMENDED READING

Arduino, P.G., Porter, S.R., 2008. Herpes simplex virus type 1 infection: overview on relevant clinico-pathological features. J. Oral. Pathol. Med. 37 (2), 107—121.

Crimi, S., Fiorillo, L., Bianchi, A., D'Amico, C., Amoroso, G., Gorassini, F., 2019. Herpes virus, oral clinical signs and QoL: systematic review of recent data. Viruses. 11 (5), 463.

Fatahzadeh, M., Schwartz, R.A., 2007. Human herpes simplex virus infections: epidemiology, pathogenesis, symptomatology, diagnosis, and management. J. Am. Acad. Dermatol. 57 (5), 737—763.

Moomaw, M.D., Cornea, P., Rathbun, R.C., Wendel, K.A., 2003. Review of antiviral therapy for herpes labialis, genital herpes and herpes zoster. Expert Rev. Anti. Infect. Ther. 1 (2), 283—295.

Ordoñez, G., Vales, O., Pineda, B., Rodríguez, K., Pane, C., Sotelo, J., 2020. The presence of herpes simplex-1 and varicella zoster viruses is not related with clinical outcome of Bell's Palsy. Virology 549, 85—88.

Woo, S.B., Challacombe, S.J., 2007. Management of recurrent oral herpes simplex infections. Oral Surg. Oral Med. Oral Pathol. Oral Radiol. Endod. 103 (Suppl), S12.e1—S12.e18.

Human Immunodeficiency Virus Infection

KEY POINTS

- Human immunodeficiency virus (HIV) is a lethal retrovirus infection transmitted by blood and body fluids.
- HIV damages a subset of cells (CD4$^+$ cells) leading to severe T-helper cell immune defects.
- Defences against fungi, viruses, mycobacteria and parasites are especially impaired.
- Clinical disease (HIV disease) manifests after a long latency — with tumours, infections and other features.
- Common manifestations are Kaposi sarcoma and lymphomas; infections with herpesviruses and papillomaviruses, candidiasis and cryptococcosis, tuberculosis, and toxoplasmosis.
- Acquired immune deficiency syndrome (AIDS) is the term used when the CD4 T lymphocyte count falls less than 200 cells/mL and the patient is HIV antibody positive.
- Antiretroviral therapy (ART) can successfully prolong life in HIV/AIDS but can cause cardiac and other adverse effects.
- There is no cure and no vaccine currently exists for HIV.

INTRODUCTION

Human immunodeficiency viruses (HIV) infection is a potentially lethal condition and approximately 40 million people have died worldwide since the beginning of the HIV pandemic. Infection with the RNA retroviruses known as HIV — produces HIV infection where the virus targets and damages CD4$^+$ T lymphocytes (T helper cells), thus causing decreases in CD4$^+$ cells and thus HIV disease and ultimately the acquired immune deficiency syndrome (AIDS). In healthy people aged 5 years and older, with normally functioning immune systems, the CD4$^+$ T-cell counts usually range from 500 to 1500 cells/mL.

These immunocytes are crucial to host defences against fungi, viruses, mycobacteria and parasites and thus, HIV and lowered CD4 counts are predisposed to infection with these microbiota in particular. Infections with other clinical signs and HIV antibody positive are termed 'HIV disease'. This then progresses over time to AIDS, defined as a CD4$^+$ T-lymphocyte count at or less than 200 cells/mL in the presence of HIV infection (antibody positive). In the untreated, premature death follows (Figs. 39.1 and 39.2) though current antiretroviral treatment (ART) has transformed expectations to a normal lifespan.

Epidemiology

- AIDS was first recognised in the USA in the early 1980s in the male gay populations, although the infection has subsequently been recognised to have existed in Africa some decades before then, at least in the 1950s. Over 60% of the world's people living with HIV are in Africa. The epidemic has spread worldwide in all sections of the community, largely in resource-poor groups so that, in the developing world HIV/AIDS is a leading cause of death in young people. The rate of new infections (adults and children) is approximately 5000 **a day.** HIV therapy has had a global impact, with AIDS-related deaths decreasing by 33% since 2015. The majority of the world's HIV is in low- and middle- resource countries and social determinants are

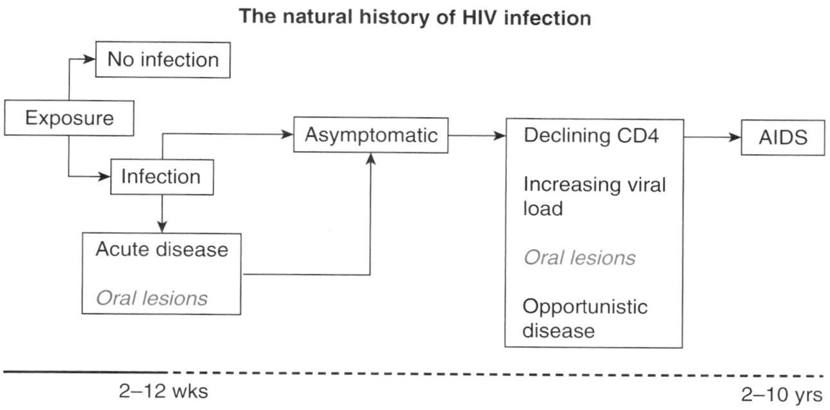

The natural history of HIV infection

Fig. 39.1 Development of HIV/AIDS natural history of HIV infection.

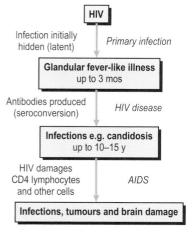

Fig. 39.2 Natural history of HIV infection.

strongly related. Many people living with HIV, or at risk for HIV, still do not have access to prevention, care or treatment.

- Worldwide, sexually active adults continue to be the age group mainly affected and the predominant route of transmission is heterosexual. In developed countries, men who have sex with men (MSM) are a major cohort. The number of cases in older adults is rising with increasing longevity and in children continues to rise, largely through the increasing prevalence of infection in pregnant females.
- Worldwide more females than males are living with HIV though the difference in gender affected by HIV is small.
- The HIV epidemic:
  - appears to have originated from an epicentre in sub-Saharan Africa, probably Zaire and Cameroon
  - about 40 million people worldwide are living with HIV
  - worldwide has spread mainly via heterosexual sex, although the incidence is still especially high in MSM
  - rate of increase has slowed in most parts of the developed world
  - the World prevalence of HIV is about 0.23% but is over 0.3% in Southeast Asia, Latin America, North America

and Eastern Europe and with a particularly high prevalence in the Caribbean (1.1%) and sub-Saharan Africa (5.5%).

- Is not infrequently accompanied by infection with other blood-borne agents (e.g. hepatitis viruses) and/or tuberculosis which is increasingly multidrug resistant (MDR-TB).

PREDISPOSING FACTORS AND TRANSMISSION

HIV is present in tissues and body fluids (including blood and saliva) of HIV-infected persons, transmitted mostly where the viral load is high and transmitted:

- Most commonly by unprotected sexual intercourse with an infected person. The risk of transmission via various sexual practices varies; anal intercourse is more risky than vaginal, and genital intercourse is riskier than oral sex.
- Readily through sharing needles and/or syringes (primarily for recreational drug injection).
- Sometimes to babies born to HIV-infected women, before or during birth — or through breastfeeding after birth. HIV does not cross the placenta.
- Less commonly (and now very rarely in countries where blood is screened for HIV), through transfusions of infected blood or blood clotting factors, or transplants.
- Rarely in the healthcare setting, by being stuck with needles or other sharps containing HIV-infected blood (needlestick injuries). Transmission via the eyes of splashed infected blood has been reported.
- Rarely by saliva, presumably because of protection from anti-viral factors in saliva including:
  - secretory leukocyte protease 1 (SLP1)
  - peroxidases
  - lactoferrin
  - human beta defensins (HBD-2 and 3)
  - high molecular weight glycoproteins.

Barrier precautions are highly effective at preventing transmission in all social and work situations, except for needlestick injuries. For HIV-uninfected patients, pre-exposure prophylaxis (PrEP) using antiretroviral medications prevents new infections in those at greatest risk.

Following an occupational exposure (e.g. sharps or mucosal splash) from an HIV-positive case with an unknown or detectable HIV viral load, post-exposure prophylaxis (PEP) is routinely offered to reduce the risk of HIV transmission. PEP should be initiated as soon as possible after exposure, preferably within 24 hours.

AETIOLOGY AND PATHOGENESIS

- There are two main HIV viruses responsible for HIV infection and several strains of each, but little difference between them in terms of pathogenesis, manifestations of infection, treatment or prognosis:
  - HIV-1 is by far the most common worldwide
  - HIV-2 has spread from West Africa mainly.
- Most HIV infections are initiated at mucosal sites, including the oral mucosa. HIV RNA, proviral DNA and infected cells are detected in the oral mucosa and saliva of infected individuals. It appears that oral epithelium can be infected by HIV, but is not a site of replication. HIV exposure through oral sex appears sufficient to induce systemic HIV-specific $CD4^+$ and $CD8^+$ T-cell immune responses in some uninfected individuals. Serum neutralising anti-HIV-1 activity also develops and may be protective, as well as be evidence of exposure.
- Infection with HIV infects cells with CD4 receptors. Though these are largely $CD4^+$ T-helper lymphocytes, brain glial cells are also $CD4^+$ and thus become dysfunctional and die. The declining CD4 cell count thus can result not only in progressive immune deficiency but also in encephalopathy and dementia.
- CD4 is the primary receptor for HIV gp120, while **either CXCR4 or CCR5** can act as coreceptors. A small percentage of the population appears to have genetically modified coreceptors and are thus resistant to HIV infection.
- As T-cell-mediated immune protection diminishes, patients become predisposed to infection with fungi, viruses, mycobacteria and parasites.
- Infections arise from commensal organisms (i.e. organisms that in the immunocompetent host cause no or little obvious harm) which become opportunistic pathogens, or from exogenous pathogens.
- Opportunistic pathogens include Candida species and other fungi, and some herpesviruses — especially herpes simplex virus (HSV), varicella-zoster virus (VZV), Epstein—Barr virus (EBV), cytomegalovirus (CMV) and human herpesvirus-8 (HHV-8). Some viruses may cause neoplasms; HHV-8 causes Kaposi sarcoma (KS), EBV causes lymphomas and some human papillomaviruses (HPV) may cause cervical, anal and oropharyngeal carcinomas.
- Exogenous pathogens encountered depend on the environment but include especially some mycoses such as *Pneumocystis carinii (jiroveci)*, cryptococcus and histoplasmosis; tuberculosis and atypical mycobacteria, such as *Mycobacterium avium-intercellulare*; as well as parasites including cryptosporidia, *Toxoplasma gondii* and Leishmania.

CLINICAL FEATURES

Acute HIV Infection

Acute HIV infection passes unrecognised in the majority since features are so non-specific. In one-third to one-half of those infected, during the 4- to 7-week period of rapid viral replication immediately following exposure, there can be fever, malaise, lymphadenopathy, myalgia and other features closely mimicking glandular fever. Rarely, some individuals may present with oral ulceration. Seroconversion and a broad HIV-1 specific immune response occur, usually within 30 to 50 days. High levels of HIV RNA are present in the blood.

Continuing HIV Infection

Following acute infection, HIV remains within the body, unlike many other infections that the host can combat. There follows an asymptomatic and variable period, often for years, when the virus appears latent but where there appears to be a balance between viral replication in $CD4^+$ cells and the immune response. There is a massive viraemia with wide dissemination of HIV in the blood to lymphoid organs, but the resulting immune response only partially suppresses HIV, and some virus survives, leading to the gradual loss of $CD4^+$ T cells and progressive deterioration of immune function. There may be persistent generalised lymphadenopathy (PGL).

HIV Disease

HIV disease (symptomatic HIV infection) manifests as the $CD4^+$ T cell count progressively declines over a period which may extend over 5 to 15 years or more, and the person starts to manifest:

- Infections: the most important infections are *P. carinii* pneumonia (PCP), candidiasis (Fig. 39.3), cryptococcosis, herpesviruses (especially HSV, VZV, EBV and CMV) and parasites, such as toxoplasmosis and leishmaniasis. Tuberculosis is common in HIV-infected persons, especially in developing countries, in whom it may involve mycobacteria resistant to a range of antitubercular drugs (multi-drug-resistant tuberculosis: MDR-TB).
- Neoplasms: which include KS associated with KSHV (Chapter 38; Fig. 39.4), lymphomas associated with EBV, and cervical or anal carcinomas associated with HPV.

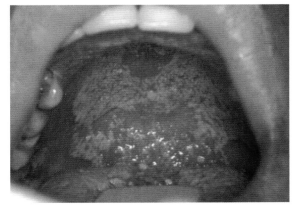

Fig. 39.3 Pseudomembranous candidiasis in HIV/AIDS.

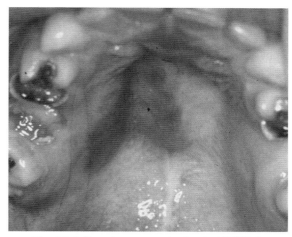

Fig. 39.4 Kaposi sarcoma of palate in HIV/AIDS.

- Oral hairy leucoplakia associated with EBV.
- Neuropsychiatric disease: which may include dementia and other cerebral syndromes. A degenerative neurological condition characterised by loss of coordination, mood swings, loss of inhibitions and widespread cognitive dysfunction, is the most common CNS complication.
- General deterioration with anorexia, diarrhoea, wasting ('slim disease'), premature ageing and autoimmune phenomena, such as thrombocytopaenia.

AIDS

AIDS is the most severe manifestation of HIV infection. The US Centers for Disease Control and Prevention (CDC) list numerous opportunistic infections and neoplasms that, in the presence of HIV infection, constitute an AIDS diagnosis. These criteria include a CD4$^+$ T-cell count ≤200 cells/mL in the presence of HIV infection (HIV antibody positive) (summarised in Table 39.1) and clinical conditions associated with HIV infection in the untreated, as follows:
- Category A: (HIV infection)
  - asymptomatic HIV infection
  - PGL
  - acute (primary) HIV infection with accompanying illness or history of acute HIV infection.
- Category B: (HIV disease)
  - bacillary angiomatosis (epithelioid angiomatosis)
  - candidiasis, oropharyngeal (thrush)
  - candidiasis, vulvovaginal
  - cervical dysplasia
  - constitutional symptoms, such as fever (38.5°C) or diarrhoea
  - oral hairy leukoplakia
  - herpes zoster (shingles)
  - idiopathic thrombocytopaenic purpura
  - listeriosis
  - pelvic inflammatory disease
  - peripheral neuropathy.
- Category C: (AIDS)
  - candidiasis, bronchi, trachea or lungs

TABLE 39.1 CDC Classification of HIV and AIDS

CD4 Count (Cells/mL) (Category)	Acute HIV Infection, Asymptomatic or PGL (A)	Symptoms and Signs of Progressive HIV Infection, Not AIDS (B)	AIDS (C)
≥500 (1)	A1	B1	C1
200–499 (2)	A2	B2	C2
<200 (3)	A3	B3	C3

AIDS, Acquired immune deficiency syndrome; *HIV,* human immunodeficiency viruses; *PGL,* persistent generalised lymphadenopathy.

- candidiasis, oesophageal
- cervical cancer, invasive
- coccidioidomycosis, disseminated or extrapulmonary
- cryptococcosis, extrapulmonary
- cryptosporidiosis, chronic intestinal
- CMV disease
- CMV retinitis
- encephalopathy, HIV related
- herpes simplex: chronic ulcer(s); or bronchitis, pneumonitis or esophagitis
- histoplasmosis, disseminated or extrapulmonary
- isosporiasis, chronic intestinal
- Kaposi Sarcoma (KS)
- lymphoma, Burkitt
- lymphoma, immunoblastic
- lymphoma, primary, of brain
- *M. avium* complex or *M. kansasii,* disseminated or extrapulmonary
- *Mycobacterium tuberculosis,* any site (pulmonary or extrapulmonary)
- *Mycobacterium,* other species, disseminated or extrapulmonary
- *P. carinii* (now *jiroveci*) pneumonia (PCP)
- pneumonia, recurrent
- progressive multifocal leukoencephalopathy
- *Salmonella septicaemia,* recurrent
- toxoplasmosis of brain
- wasting syndrome due to HIV ('slim disease').

Prognosis

The prognosis of HIV/AIDS if untreated has almost invariably been poor and death, although there are rare patients with genetically modified coreceptors CCR5 or CXCR4 who show remarkable resistance. Newer antiretroviral agents have transformed the prognosis so now HIV affected people can survive for many years with an expectation of a nearly normal lifespan.

DIAGNOSIS OF HIV INFECTION

Considerable compassion is required in explaining the diagnosis of such a serious infection as HIV since it impacts virtually all aspects of the person's life as well as that of their family and others. Confidentiality must be maintained at all times and the patient's consent and views always sought, including when considering informing other healthcare workers of any details about the person involved. There must always be appropriate counselling:

- HIV testing is discussed in Chapter 3. HIV infection at the very early stage may manifest no detectable antibody production and thus, at this time, the test for serum HIV antibodies alone (serotesting) can be falsely negative. Early HIV infection is characterised by markedly elevated HIV RNA levels detectable by the reverse transcriptase-polymerase chain reaction (RT-PCR) test. The p24 antigen is a viral core protein that appears in the blood as the viral RNA level rises following HIV infection. The p24 antigen test, also available as a combination HIV antibody/p24 antigen test, shortens the window period between HIV acquisition and a positive test. Anyone newly diagnosed with HIV infection should undergo testing for other sexually transmitted infections.

MANAGEMENT OF HIV DISEASE

Few, if any, patients have spontaneous remission and thus treatment is almost invariably indicated although, in rare cases, the disease progresses very slowly and may only at a very late-stage manifest with serious complications. Patient information is an important aspect of management.

There has been remarkable progress in improving the quality and duration of life of HIV-infected persons because of:
- better education of patients and health professionals
- better recognition of opportunistic disease processes
- better therapy for acute and chronic complications
- the introduction of effective chemoprophylaxis; trimethoprim-sulphamethoxazole in particular reduces not only the incidence of PCP but also toxoplasmosis and bacterial infections
- the development of a range of antiretroviral therapies (ARTs) and their use now in early infection. Protease inhibitors are used together with reverse transcriptase inhibitors (see Chapter 5) which has significantly reduced the incidence of most infections and extended life substantially. However, some infections, such as herpes zoster and HPV-induced warts have increased. However, many drugs are liable to fairly severe adverse reactions and, perhaps more significantly, viral resistance has arisen (see Chapter 33). Combination antiretroviral therapy (CART) has increased life expectancy but also cardiac complications and drug adverse effects may cause more morbidity than AIDS. Effective and safe vaccines against HIV, however, are not yet available, partly due to the very high mutation rate of HIV.

IMMUNE RECONSTITUTION INFLAMMATORY SYNDROME

The immune reconstitution inflammatory syndrome (IRIS) is a paradoxical immunoinflammatory reaction brought about by

improved immune status following ART which can be serious, even fatal. IRIS initiation and progression seem to be linked to a sudden increased CD4$^+$ T-helper and CD8$^+$ T-suppressor cell count and reduction in T-regs, with exaggerated cytokine release following the introduction of ART. Though rare, AIDS patients are more at risk if they are put on ART for the first time, or if they have recently been treated for an opportunistic infection. IRIS manifests with features that often resemble an AIDS-defining illness such as a rapid increase in the size of a KS over 2 to 3 weeks, before then reducing in size.

Clinical Features

The clinical presentation of IRIS is usually atypical. The manifestations depend on the triggering antigen, which can be an infective agent (viable or nonviable), a host antigen or a tumour antigen. The range of common conditions that can occur or be exacerbated in IRIS are shown in Table 39.2; oral lesions are discussed below.

Diagnosis

IRIS lesions may have atypical presentations, but the diagnosis is usually made by astute clinicians, aware of the possibility of IRIS when the clinical condition worsens rather than improves as expected after the initiation of ART.

Treatment

Most IRIS is self-limiting, but since a few cases can be overwhelming and even life-threatening, early recognition is important. Treatment is usually to continue the anti-HIV regimen and to give antimicrobials to treat infections and systemic corticosteroids to temporarily suppress the inflammatory process.

OROFACIAL LESIONS IN HIV/AIDS

Oral features of HIV/AIDS reflect the T-cell immune defect and are, thus, mainly the consequence of fungal or viral or sometimes mycobacterial or parasitic infections (Tables 39.1–39.3 and Box 39.1):
- The most common are candidiasis and hairy leukoplakia (HL). Necrotising gingivitis, accelerated periodontitis, KS,

TABLE 39.2   Manifestations of Immune Reconstitution Syndrome

Known Infections	Other Conditions
Cryptococcus	Aphthous-like ulcers
Cytomegalovirus	Castleman disease (Chapter 54)
Hepatitis viruses	Eosinophilic folliculitis
Herpes simplex virus lesions	Graves disease
Herpes zoster	Leprosy
Histoplasmosis	Myopathy
Kaposi sarcoma herpesvirus (HHV8/ KSHV)	Non-Hodgkin lymphoma (NHL)
Mycobacterium avium	Progressive multifocal leukoencephalopathy
Papillomavirus	Sarcoidosis
Pneumocystis carinii	Systemic lupus erythematosus
Tuberculosis	(SLE)

TABLE 39.3 Orofacial Lesions in HIV/AIDS

Type of Disorder		Examples	Manifestations
Infection	Viral	Herpes simplex	Ulceration
		Herpes varicella zoster	Ulceration and pain
		Cytomegalovirus	Ulceration
		Epstein–Barr virus	Ulceration, lymphoma, hairy leukoplakia
		Kaposi sarcoma herpesvirus (KSHV), HHV8	Kaposi sarcoma
		Human papillomaviruses	Papillomas or warts
		Molluscum contagiosum	Papules
	Fungal	*Candida*	White or red lesions, ulceration or lump
		Cryptococcus neoformans	
		Geotrichium candidum	
		Histoplasma capsulatum	
		Mucoracea	
		Aspergillus	
	Bacterial	*Mycobacterium tuberculosis*	Ulceration or lump
		Non-tuberculous mycobacteria	
		Escherichia coli	
		Klebsiella pneumoniae	
		Actinomyces israelii	
		Bartonella (Rochalimaea) henselae and *quintana*	Epithelioid angiomatosis
		Periodontal flora	See text
	Protozoal	Leishmania	Ulceration or lump
Autoimmune		Aphthous-like ulcers	
		HIV salivary gland disease	
		Thrombocytopaenia	
Other		Facial palsy	
		Trigeminal neuralgia	
		Taste disturbance	
		Exfoliative cheilitis	
		Hyperpigmentation	

AIDS, Acquired immune deficiency syndrome; *HIV*, human immunodeficiency viruses.

lymphomas, salivary gland disease, ulcers of various infective aetiologies and other lesions may also be seen.
- These oral diseases have a number of common features, namely that generally they are:
  - not absolutely specific for HIV/AIDS, but are more a manifestation of the immune defect; thus, similar lesions can be seen in other immune defects
  - generally more likely to manifest as the CD4 cell count falls to low levels
  - more likely to be seen where the oral hygiene is poor
  - more likely where there is also malnutrition
  - more likely if the patient smokes tobacco
  - often controlled, at least temporarily, by antiretroviral treatment (however, some lesions — such as zoster and warts — have increased since the advent of ART; see below).

Oral lesions may:
- indicate HIV infection that is previously undiagnosed
- be used in staging and therapy decisions
- cause the patient pain or aesthetic problems

- increase the liability for HIV transmission.

HIV-Related Oral Candidiasis

Oral levels of *Candida albicans* and other yeasts are increased in HIV infection, and infection is common. Oral candidiasis is:
- the most common opportunistic infection in HIV-infected persons
- often the initial manifestation of symptomatic HIV infection
- seen at some point in at least 90% of HIV-infected patients
- seen in all groups at risk, especially HIV-infected intravenous drug users.

Oral candidiasis is related to:
- the immune defect; in general, the frequency of isolation of *Candida* species increases with increasing severity of HIV disease and with lower CD4 and/or CD4/CD8 ratios. T cells from HIV-infected patients also produce low interferon (IFN)-gamma, and there is a non-protective Th0/Th2 response to *C. albicans* antigen

BOX 39.1   Classification of Oral Lesions in HIV Disease

Group I: Lesions Strongly Associated With HIV Infection
- Candidiasis:
  - erythematous
  - hyperplastic
  - pseudomembranous (thrush)
- Hairy leukoplakia (EBV)
- HIV gingivitis
- Necrotising ulcerative gingivitis
- Necrotising ulcerative periodontitis
- Kaposi sarcoma
- Non-Hodgkin lymphoma

Group II: Lesions Less Commonly Associated With HIV Infection
- Atypical ulceration (oropharyngeal)
- Idiopathic thrombocytopaenic purpura
- Salivary gland diseases:
  - hyposalivation
  - unilateral or bilateral swelling of major salivary glands
- Viral infections (other than EBV):
  - cytomegalovirus
  - herpes simplex virus
  - human papillomavirus (warty-like lesions): condyloma acuminatum, focal epithelial hyperplasia and verruca vulgaris
  - varicella-zoster virus: herpes zoster and varicella

Group III: Lesions Possibly Associated With HIV Infection
- A miscellany of rare diseases

- C. albicans from HIV+ people show greater adhesion to epithelial cells and thus may contribute to the establishment of candidiasis
- hyposalivation and other salivary changes in HIV infection, such as reduced calprotectin, IgA, lactoferrin and anti-Candida antibodies
- smoking
- antimicrobial use.

Aetiology and Pathogenesis
- Yeasts colonise the mouths of about 85% of HIV-infected persons.
- CD4 lymphocytes are deficient in the cellular infiltrate of candidal lesions in HIV infection. Salivary histatin-5 concentrations are also significantly lower.
- C. albicans causes greater than 85% of oral candidiasis, but Candida dubliniensis species are increased in HIV.
- The strain of Candida usually remains constant. Recurrence is usually caused by a persistent strain, but occasionally a different strain appears and there may be sexual reinfection.
- C. albicans isolates from HIV-infected persons may show increased:
  - adherence to oral epithelial cells
  - hyphal formation with epithelial invasion
  - aspartyl proteinase secretion

- resistance to antifungal drugs, especially amphotericin, itraconazole and fluconazole, even despite no previous exposure.
- C. albicans serotypes change with the progression of HIV disease from the A predominant biotype to serotype B, although the latter is found especially in homosexual men, irrespective of their HIV serostatus.
- Serotype B in particular appears resistant to fluconazole, although itraconazole, voriconazole and posaconazole may still be active.
- About 15% of candidiasis in HIV disease is due to non-albicans species, including:
  - C. dubliniensis
  - Candida kruseii
  - Candida tropicalis
  - Candida parapsilosis
  - Candida lambica
  - Candida kefyr
  - Candida geotrichium
  - Torulopsis glabrata
  - Saccharomyces cerevisiae.
- Infections with non-albicans species are increasing, coincident with the increasing use of prolonged antifungal therapy.
- C. krusei and T. glabrata particularly are becoming a problem since they are less likely to respond to fluconazole.
- New organisms, such as C. dubliniensis, related to C. albicans, have appeared, and at present remain largely fluconazole-sensitive.
- Up to 25% of HIV-infected patients with candidiasis have the infection by C. albicans plus other species (in contrast to usual single-species infection).

Clinical Features

Thrush (pseudomembranous candidiasis) is one of the most obvious oral lesions in HIV infection and tends to be associated with lower CD4 counts, typically less than 200 cells/mL (see Fig. 39.3).

Other types of candidiasis may also be seen, especially:
- erythematous; this form of candidiasis may be a common early oral manifestation of HIV infection and presents as pink or red macular lesions, typically on both the palate and dorsum of the tongue as contact lesions (Fig. 39.5)
- angular stomatitis (cheilitis)
- median rhomboid glossitis
- hyperplastic candidiasis.

Diagnosis

This is mainly clinical, supported by investigations discussed in Chapter 36.

Treatment (see also Chapters 4 and 5)

Early treatment of oral candidiasis in HIV disease is warranted, not only because of the discomfort but also because foci may act as reservoirs for spreading, particularly to the oesophagus:
- Predisposing factors, such as smoking and hyposalivation should be managed first.

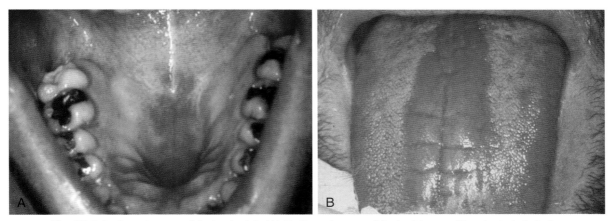

Fig. 39.5 Erythematous candidiasis of palate (A); Erythematous candidiasis of tongue (B).; a typical site is the vault of the palate in a 'thumbprint' pattern.

- ART which includes protease inhibitor treatment appears to inhibit candidiasis infection.
- Antifungals; topical therapy of candidiasis with gentian violet, nystatin or clotrimazole is often successful initially within about 14 days, but relapses are common and these agents are not always palatable or accepted by children. Failures are mainly attributable to underlying immunodeficiency and poor patient compliance due to:
  - polypharmacy
  - gastrointestinal upset
  - unpalatable taste of some agents
  - drug intolerance.
- Topical chlorhexidine is typically of minimal significant benefit in candidiasis but triclosan may be beneficial. Gentian violet rinse can be effective.
- Antifungal prophylaxis should also be considered. A regime of intermittent antifungal therapy of 1 week in four, especially with polyenes may keep candida levels low. Antifungal resistance to azoles is now a significant clinical problem in HIV-infected persons, even in patients who have received no fluconazole, since resistance may be transferred, and fluconazole-resistant species may be transmitted between patients. Risk factors include:
  - severe immune defect
  - previous fluconazole use, especially intermittent or low-dose therapy. Fortunately, in fluconazole-resistant candidiasis, amphotericin, ketoconazole, itraconazole, voriconazole and posaconazole may remain clinically effective. Therapy in fluconazole-resistant cases, therefore, includes topical amphotericin/nystatin or ketoconazole (400 mg/day) or itraconazole (200 to 400 mg/day). Voriconazole, posaconazole or caspofungin may be indicated in recalcitrant cases.

Hairy Leukoplakia

HL are bilateral, corrugated (or 'hairy') white lesions usually seen on the sides of the tongue mainly in HIV/AIDS and rarely in other immunocompromised states.

HL:

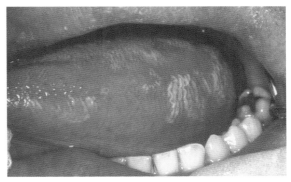

Fig. 39.6 Hairy leukoplakia is typically symptomless and bilateral on sides of tongue.

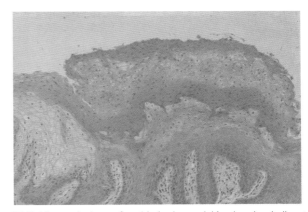

Fig. 39.7 Histopathology of oral hairy leucoplakia showing koilocytosis and irregular keratinisation of epithelial cells.

- is associated with EBV
- typically affects the lateral margins of the tongue (Figs 39.6 and 39.7)
- produces white lesions that are not removed by wiping with a gauze
- is not known to be premalignant
- is a predictor of a bad prognosis.

Diagnosis is largely clinical, supported by proof of EBV and usually HIV testing. Biopsy or treatment is not often required, but the condition often resolves with aciclovir or other agents active against EBV, or with antiretroviral agents.

Kaposi Sarcoma

Kaposi sarcoma:

- arises from endothelial cells
- is transmitted sexually, especially in MSM, and seen rarely in HIV-infected children or haemophiliacs
- is caused by HHV8 (KSHV), which is transmitted sexually, often as a co-infection with HIV. Like all herpesviruses, this is a DNA virus which remains latent after infection. It is found in saliva
- presents initially as asymptomatic red, blue or purple macules or swellings
- progresses to papules, nodules or ulcers and may become painful
- is most common around the face (especially on the nose) and mouth
- occurs especially in the hard palate or the gingivae (see Fig. 39.4)
- may reflect KS elsewhere in the body.

Diagnosis of KS must be supported by biopsy examination), since a clinically and histologically similar but distinct lesion caused by the bacterium *Bartonella (Rochalimaea) henselae* or *quintana* can cause a lesion, epithelioid angiomatosis, that responds well to antibiotics. Management of oral KS is often with intralesional injections of vinblastine, or systemic chemotherapy. KS responds badly to irradiation. ART has significantly improved the management of orofacial KS associated with AIDS.

Rapidly progressive facial lymphoedema developing concurrently with, or immediately after rapid enlargement of oral KS may herald impending demise.

Lymphomas

Lymphomas are seen increasingly in AIDS and are often:

- non-Hodgkin lymphomas (NHL)
- part of widespread disease
- seen in the tongue or maxillary gingivae/fauces (Fig. 39.8)
- lymphomas occurring more specifically in HIV-positive patients are usually of B cell or plasmablastic cell origin. In Africa, a significant proportion are Burkitt lymphomas. Plasmablastic lymphoma (PBL) is an aggressive variant of diffuse large B-cell lymphoma but lacks CD20 expression. There is a good early response of lymphomas to chemotherapy, but high relapse rates and poor prognosis, though better overall survival compared with patients with extraoral lymphomas
- associated with EBV (NHL) or KSHV (PBLs)
- fairly resistant to therapy.

Diagnosis must be confirmed by biopsy examination. Management is with chemotherapy.

Gingival and Periodontal Diseases

Necrotising ulcerative gingivitis (Fig. 39.9) and necrotising ulcerative periodontitis (Fig. 39.10) can be features of HIV infection, and typically these:

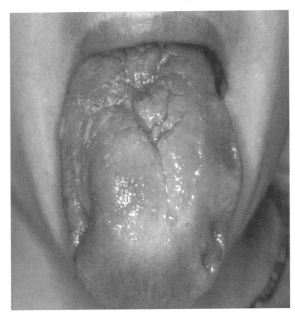

Fig. 39.8 Lymphoma in HIV/AIDS, causing tongue swelling and indentation of teeth.

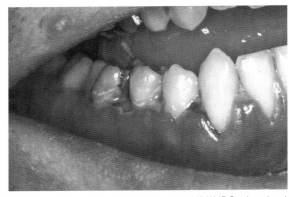

Fig. 39.9 Necrotising ulcerative gingivitis in HIV/AIDS, showing loss of interdental papillae.

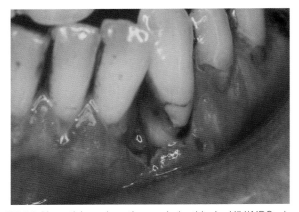

Fig. 39.10 Necrotising ulcerative periodontitis in HIV/AIDS showing deep pockets extending to bone.

- occur disproportionately to the level of oral hygiene and plaque control
- are painful
- are localised
- cause rapid alveolar bone loss.

Diagnosis is clinical. The possibility of HIV/AIDS is heightened where there are additional suggestive lesions or where there is a clear high risk of HIV infection, such as in an intravenous drug user. Management is with improved oral hygiene, debridement, chlorhexidine and sometimes metronidazole.

In addition, the rate of progression of chronic inflammatory periodontal disease appears to be increased in HIV infection.

Mouth Ulceration

Mouth ulcers may appear in HIV disease, but are, of course, common lesions in many non-HIV-infected persons. Ulcers may be unrelated to the HIV infection or may be related to HIV, especially if non-recurrent or of relatively recent onset. Differential diagnosis includes:

- aphthous-type ulcers up to 10 mm in diameter
- neoplasms, such as KS or lymphoma
- opportunistic pathogens, such as the herpesviruses (herpes simplex, varicella-zoster, EBV, CMV), fungi (e.g. histoplasmosis or cryptococcosis), mycobacteria (e.g. tuberculosis or non-tuberculous mycobacteria [NTM]) or protozoa (e.g. leishmaniasis)
- drug use.

Ulcers may be part of widespread diseases, such as disseminated CMV infection, disseminated cryptococcosis or disseminated lymphoma, and thus the advice of a physician can be helpful if not mandatory. Diagnosis can be difficult and biopsy with microbial DNA studies may well be indicated. The history is important.

Management depends on the diagnosis, but chlorhexidine and topical analgesics can be helpful. Antimicrobials or other specific therapies are often indicated to control the lesions, depending on the cause. Granulocyte colony-stimulating factors or thalidomide may be helpful in aphthous-like ulceration (Chapter 5).

Salivary Conditions

- Parotitis, enlarged parotids and/or hyposalivation (HIV-salivary gland disease; HIV-SGD) are seen particularly in HIV-infected children. HIV-SGD, a hallmark of diffuse infiltrative lymphocytosis syndrome may have a BK virus pathogenesis and cells may be CD8$^+$. Cystic salivary lesions are common.
- Factors significantly associated with both hyposalivation and xerostomia include; sex, age, stage of HIV infection, systemic disease, concurrent candidiasis and medication use.

Other Orofacial Lesions

A wide spectrum of other orofacial lesions can be seen in HIV/AIDS, including the following:

- Cervical lymph node enlargement, as part of PGL.

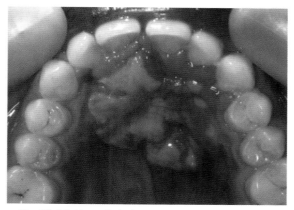
Fig. 39.11 Herpetic lesions in HIV infection on palate.

- Chronic sinusitis, which may be related to bacterial or, increasingly, fungal pathogens, such as aspergillosis or zygomycosis.
- HSV infections (see Fig. 39.10).
- HPV infections, in particular, genital warts (condyloma acuminata) in or around the mouth (Fig. 39.11). Persistent HPV infection is very frequent in HIV-positive MSM and these seem to have more frequent penile and oral HPV-associated diseases. Concurrent oral and anogenital HPV infection appears to be uncommon. Two manifestations of HPV that may be on the rise are HPV-32-associated oral warts and HPV-16-associated oral cancers.
- Cranial neuropathies, such as facial palsy, pain or sensory loss.

Orofacial Consequences of Antiretroviral Therapy (see also Chapters 5, 33)

Use of ART may long-term be associated with:
- reduced risks of having orofacial pain
- reduced prevalence of candidiasis, oral hairy leucoplakia, NUG, NUP
- increased risk of having oral warts, hyposalivation, erythema multiforme, toxic epidermal necrolysis, lichenoid reactions and exfoliative cheilitis. HPV-associated oral warts have a prevalence of 0.5% in the general population, up to 5% in persons living with HIV and in up to 23% of those ART
- IRIS and orofacial lesions: especially candidiasis but also herpes labialis, necrotising periodontitis, HL, zoster, KS and HPV lesions. Other oral lesions in IRIS of uncertain aetiopathogenesis include parotid swelling, hyposalivation and ulceration.

RECOMMENDED READING

https://www.cdc.gov/hiv/basics/whatishiv.html
https://www.who.int/health-topics/hiv-aids#tab=tab_1
Palfreeman, A., Sullivan, A., Rayment, M., et al., 2020. British HIV Association/British Association for Sexual Health and HIV/British Infection Association Adult HIV Testing Guidelines 2020. HIV. Med. 21 (Suppl. 6), 1–26.
Tappuni, A.R., 2020. The global changing pattern of the oral manifestations of HIV. Oral. Dis. 26 (Suppl. 1), 22–27.

Bacterial Infections

KEY POINTS
- Viral, fungal and bacterial infections of the oral mucosa are common.
- Infections secondary to systemic disease or medical therapy are frequently seen.
- Bacterial infections can be odontogenic or non-odontogenic in origin.
- Bacterial infections can arise from commensal flora (intrinsic) or extrinsic sources.
- Intrinsic bacterial infections include wound infections, odontogenic infections and actinomycosis.
- Extrinsic infections include sexually transmitted diseases, tuberculosis and possibly noma.

BACKGROUND

Many oral bacterial infections are secondary to changes in the oral environment by immunosuppressives and other immunomodulating drugs, many are associated with systemic disease (see Chapter 34) and many are associated with hyposalivation (see Chapter 20). Fungal infections are addressed in Chapter 36 and viral infections in Chapter 37. Bacterial infections are also common in oral medicine and can be primarily odontogenic, or non-odontogenic, the latter associated with the same fungal and viral risk factors as above, but others direct infections of the oral cavity with or without concurrent systemic disease.

Extrinsic bacterial infections are where the origin of the bacterial infection is outside the normal microbiome, intrinsic where the infection is caused by otherwise commensal bacteria invading host tissues, and iatrogenic where the infections are secondary to drugs prescribed for medical conditions which are immunosuppressive or cause changes in the oral environment, such as hyposalivation. The nature of the infection in some diseases such as noma remains unclear

ENDOGENOUS INFECTIONS

Opportunistic or secondary infections are frequently seen in the practice of oral Table 40.1 medicine. Candidiasis (Chapter 36) and herpesvirus infections (Chapter 38) are common in immuno-compromised patients, or those treated with agents causing hyposalivation, antimicrobials, and some topical corticosteroid and other agents. Tuberculosis (see below) is an increasing issue in immunocompromised people, and people on immunosuppressive drugs including those treated with biological agents (Chapter 5). The blood-borne agents such as hepatitis viruses, HIV, syphilis and prions should not be transmitted if standard infection control procedures are implemented. Hospital-acquired infections have thus far not been a major issue in oral medicine

Actinomycosis

Actinomyces species are anaerobic commensals in the mouth and gut and rarely cause infection of the pelvis and mouth. Risk factors for acquiring head and neck actinomycosis include poor oral hygiene; local tissue damage by trauma, recent surgery or irradiation; Infection is:

TABLE 40.1 **Endogenous (Intrinsic) Oral Bacterial Infections**

Iatrogenic-induced infections
Actinomycosis
Acute necrotising ulcerative gingivitis
Bacterial sialadenitis
Wound infections
Odontogenic infections
Noma (cancrum oris, gangrenous stomatitis)

- Caused by *Actinomyces israelii*, usually below the mandibular angle (not lymph nodes) and may follow jaw fracture or tooth extraction.
- The infection can slowly erode through facial planes and develop chronic sinus tracts.
- Infections are thought to occur due to muscular injury, which allows *A. israelii* to penetrate and grow in an anaerobic environment.
- Most cases are diagnosed when aspirates or a biopsy reveals classic gram-positive filamentous bacteria with or without so-called 'sulphur granules'.
- Granules are composed of a protein–polysaccharide complex which have become mineralised.
- Drainage and prolonged therapy, usually with penicillin, are indicated.

Acute (or Chronic) Necrotising Ulcerative Gingivitis
Necrotising ulcerative gingivitis (NUG) is:

- A non-contagious anaerobic gingival infection associated with overwhelming proliferation of *Borrelia vincentii* and fusiform bacteria.
- Predisposing factors include smoking, viral respiratory infections and immune defects, such as in HIV/AIDS.
- Uncommon, except in resource-poor groups, this typically affects adolescents and young adults, especially in institutions, armed forces, etc., or people with HIV/AIDS.
- It becomes chronic in HIV and is known as NUG (Chapter 39).

Characteristic features include severe gingival soreness, profuse bleeding, halitosis and a bad taste. Interdental papillae are ulcerated with necrotic slough. Malaise, fever and/or cervical lymph node enlargement (unlike herpetic stomatitis) are rare. Cancrum oris (noma) is a very rare complication, usually in debilitated children (see below).

Diagnosis is usually clinical. Smear for fusospirochaetal bacteria and leukocytes; blood picture occasionally. Differentiate from acute leukaemia or herpetic stomatitis. Managed by oral debridement, metronidazole (penicillin if pregnant) and oral hygiene.

Bacterial sialadenitis

is a retrograde infection of the salivary glands usually following irreversible hyposalivation. This may follow irradiation and cytostatic drugs which, with poor general health, renders cancer patients liable to ascending infective (bacterial) sialadenitis. Usually caused by *Streptococcus viridans* species and *Staphylococcus aureus* (often penicillin-resistant), ascending from the oral cavity. The management of sialadenitis often means hospitalisation of the patient and includes:

- analgesia and prompt treatment with amoxicillin (flucloxacillin or amoxicillin/clavulanate if staphylococci and not allergic to penicillin; erythromycin or azithromycin in penicillin allergy)
- surgical drainage if there is fluctuation
- hydration.

Bacterial sialadenitis may also occur in severe Sjogren syndrome due to hyposalivation and is usually accompanied by mucositis and angular cheilitis involving *S. aureus*.

Wound infection

can produce significant pain, swelling, restricted function and poor cosmetic results and will likely prolong hospitalisation. Infections are most likely:). The diagnosis of infection is usually as, at about 3 to 7 days after an operation, the wound appears inflamed, swollen and tender. There may be pus and pyrexia. Causative organisms are members of the oral flora, normally commensal and include *S. viridans*.

Dry socket (alveolar osteitis) is a local osteomyelitis caused by commensal bacteria usually *Streptococci* and *Bacteroides* but sometimes *Staphylococcus*. It is painful and associated mainly with wisdom teeth extraction. It occurs when the expected blood clot at the site fails to develop or is dislodged or dissolves before the wound has healed. Local antiseptics and analgesics are helpful.

Staphylococci frequently cause secondary infections of wounds or herpes infections. Some key infections caused by *Staphylococcus* and *Streptococcus* species are summarised in Table 40.2.

Odontogenic infections

can be potentially life-threatening in the immunosuppressed patient, and a broad-spectrum cover is needed (such as penicillin plus gentamicin). Partially erupted third molars are a potential source of infection.

Patients may also be at risk from attempts at treatment; thus, for example, broad-spectrum antibiotics used to control bacterial infections increase the hazard of fungal infections. Patients are

TABLE 40.2	Bacterial Species and Prions Implicated in Oral Infections	
Bacteria	**Various**	**Wound Infections**
	Staphylococcus aureus	Implicated in some cases of angular cheilitis, sialadenitis, osteomyelitis, lymphadenitis and other infections
	Methicillin-resistant *S. aureus* (MRSA)	May be community- (CA-MRSA) or hospital-acquired (HA-MRSA)
	Vancomycin-resistant *S. aureus* (VRSA)	May also be resistant to meropenem and imipenem
	Mycobacterium tuberculosis and non-tuberculous mycobacterioses	A serious issue in immunocompromised people Implicated in some cases of ulceration and cervical lymphadenopathy
Prions	Creutzfeldt-Jakob and new variant Creutzfeldt-Jakob disease	Infectious agent composed of a protein in a misfolded form, highly resistant to sterilisation

TABLE 40.3 Extrinsic (Exogenous) Infections of the Head and Neck Region

Sexually transmitted infections
Tuberculosis
Noma (cancrum oris, gangrenous stomatitis)
Impetigo contagiosa
Erysipelas

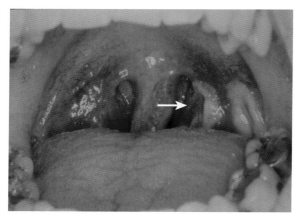

Fig. 40.1 Gonorrhoea infection showing pseudomembranes in the fauces area.

often on ciclosporin and antihypertensive agents and are at risk of drug-related gingival swelling from ciclosporin and calcium channel blockers (Chapter 33). The swelling appears to be greater with the combination of ciclosporin-nifedipine than with ciclosporin-amlodipine or ciclosporin only.

EXTRINSIC (EXOGENOUS) INFECTIONS OF THE HEAD AND NECK REGION

The main extrinsic infections affecting the head and neck are summarised in Table 40.3.

SEXUALLY TRANSMITTED INFECTIONS — BACTERIAL (STI)

Three main sexually transmitted infections have oral medicine implications: Chlamydia, gonorrhoea and syphilis.

Chlamydia

- Caused by *Chlamydia trachomatis*, an obligate intracellular gram-negative bacterium.
- Very common worldwide STI.
- Acquired via vaginal, anal or oral sex with an infected partner.
- Commonly causes genital infections in the cervix, urethra or epididymis.
- Extragenital infections commonly present as pharyngitis and conjunctivitis.

Diagnosis

C. trachomatis is generally diagnosed via nucleic acid amplification testing (NAAT) on cervical, ureteral, oral and rectal smears. Clinical features:

- Oral infections are often asymptomatic, but fever and lymphadenopathy may occur.
- Tonsillar infections typically manifest as erythema with small punctuate lesions.
- Lesions may also occur uncommonly in other locations in the mouth and are described as being erythematous, pustular, erosive or ulcerated.
- Doxycycline and azithromycin are the preferred antibiotics for treatment.

Gonorrhoea

- Caused by *Neisseria gonorrhoea*, a gram-negative diplococcus.
- Gonorrhoea is extremely prevalent, easily transmitted and mainly genital.

- Annual global incidence over 80 million, thus a significant public health concern.
- Peak incidence occurs in the 15- to 30-year age group, particularly in singles and individuals of lower socioeconomic status.
- Infection in the mouth is uncommon or rarely recognised since gonococci are not able to invade epithelium, either mucosal or skin.
- Infection can occur easily in the presence of inflammation or breaches of the mucosa.
- Pharyngitis or infection of fauces may occur after orogenital or oroanal contact (Fig. 40.1).
- Swab for culture and sensitivity.
- Treat with amoxicillin or ciprofloxacin.

Syphilis

A sexually transmitted infection caused by *Treponema pallidum* increasing globally. Four main clinical presentations are:

- *Congenital syphilis*: this manifests with frontal bossing, saddle nose, Hutchinson notched incisors, Moon or mulberry molars, corneal keratitis and hard palate defects rhagades. Learning disability, interstitial keratitis, deafness, sabre tibiae and Clutton joints may be seen (Chapter 54).
- *Acquired syphilis*: predominantly an infection of the sexually promiscuous (prostitutes, men who have sex with men). Diagnosis is by a direct smear of primary and secondary stage lesions. Serology becomes positive late in the primary stage. Penicillin by injection (or erythromycin or tetracycline). Incubation period is 9 to 90 days.
- *Primary syphilis (Hunterian or hard chancre)*: this is a small papule which develops into a large painless indurated ulcer, with regional lymphadenitis. (Fig. 40.2) A chancre heals spontaneously in 1 to 2 months. Rare on the lip (upper) or intraorally — usually the tongue. *T. pallidum* in smear (dark-field examination). Serology is positive late in this stage. Differentiate from trauma, herpes labialis, pyogenic granuloma and carcinoma.

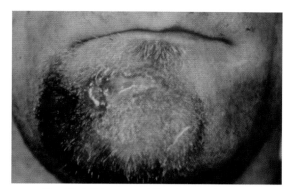

Fig. 40.2 Primary syphilic ulcer on the chin.

- *Secondary syphilis*: oral lesions include mucous patches, split papules or snail-track ulcers, which are highly infectious. Rash (coppery coloured typically on palms and soles), condylomata lata and generalised lymph node enlargement can also be present. Approximately 15% of patients with primary syphilis will present with highly infectious intraoral chancres.
- *Tertiary syphilis*: this may cause glossitis (leukoplakia) and gumma (usually midline in the palate or tongue). These are non-infectious, but may be associated with cardiovascular complications (aortic aneurysm) or neurosyphilis (tabes dorsalis, general paralysis of the insane, Argyll—Robinson pupils).

OTHER IMPORTANT INFECTIONS

Impetigo Contagiosa

A highly contagious skin infection with streptococci (group A). Uncommon, and seen mainly in underprivileged children (aged 2 to 6 years), lesions spread by touch to several areas. Clinical features include papules which change into vesicles surrounded by erythema then multiple pustules with golden crusts. Regional lymphadenitis is sometimes seen, but systemic symptoms are rare. Diagnosis is clinical together with a culture of pus. On lips, herpes labialis is the prime differential diagnosis, but other vesiculobullous diseases should also be excluded (Fig. 40.3). Management is with antibiotics. If there is no systemic toxicity, use chlortetracycline cream. If there are systemic symptoms, oral flucloxacillin should be used. *S. aureus* phage type 71 causes bullous impetigo, a severe form with fever.

Erysipelas

Erysipelas is a superficial skin infection:
- Characterised clinically by a sharply demarcated erythematous patch.
- Usually caused by betahemolytic streptococci (usually group A or group G) sometimes with *S. aureus* or gram-negative bacteria.
- Entry through breaches of the skin secondary to trauma or another skin disease.
- Mainly occurs in older adults.

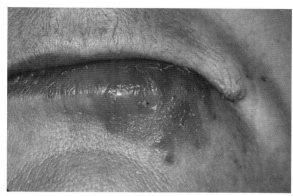

Fig. 40.3 Secondary Staphylococcus infection of a herpetic lesion of the lower lip causing impetigo appearance.

- Probably as a result of predisposing co-morbidities such as venous insufficiency, impaired lymphatic drainage, immunosuppression, diabetes, obesity, corticosteroid therapy and chemotherapy.

Noma

(cancrum oris; gangrenous stomatitis, fusospirochetal gangrene, stomatitis gangrenosa) is a rapidly progressive and often fatal infection of the mouth and face. Predominantly affects children between the ages of two and six years old in the least developed countries around the world, especially in Africa where there are dedicated noma hospitals. Noma may follow acute ulcerative gingivitis in malnourished, debilitated or severely immunocompromised patients. *Fusobacterium necrophorum* and *Prevotella intermedia* appear important bacterial pathogens in this disease process, interacting with one or more other bacterial organisms (including *Treponema denticola*, *Treponema vincentii*, *Porphyromonas gingivalis*, *Tannerella forsythia*, *S. aureus* and certain species of viridans *Streptococci*). Bone viruses have also been implicated. The isolation from human noma lesions of *F. necrophorum*, a pathogen primarily associated with animal diseases, may have important etiologic and animal transmission implications. Antibiotic therapy and antiseptic use can help arrest the infection. However, the severely affected and disfigured tissues require surgery.

Predisposing factors which have been associated include:
- malnutrition
- vitamin deficiency (particularly vitamin A and vitamin B)
- living in proximity to livestock
- contaminated drinking water
- immunodeficiency
- poor oral hygiene
- recent acute necrotising ulcerative gingivitis, measles, malaria or severe diarrhoea.

Clinical features: rapidly spreading necrosis penetrates the buccal mucosa, leading to gangrene and an orocutaneous fistula and scarring (Fig. 40.4).

Diagnosis is clinical; an immune defect should always be excluded.

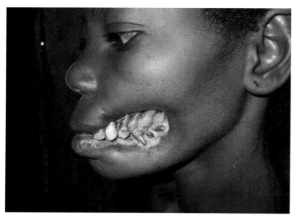

Fig. 40.4 Noma (cancrum oris) in a young African girl causing severe facial disfigurement. (Courtesy of Dr T Hodgson)

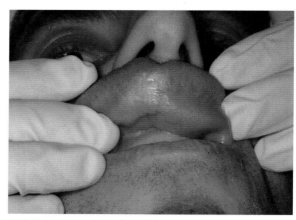

Fig. 40.5 Tuberculous infection of the upper lip in a patient with pulmonary TB. (Ilyas S, et al., 2002. *HIV Med.* 3, 283–286.)

Management includes improving nutrition, systemic antibiotics (clindamycin, penicillin, tetracyclines or metronidazole) and plastic surgery.

Tuberculosis

Infection with mycobacteria, usually *Mycobacterium tuberculosis*, but rarely atypical mycobacteria, e.g. *M. avium-intracellulare*, *M. scrofulaceum* and *M. kansasii*, especially in HIV *infection*. Individuals acquire TB by inhaling airborne particles from other infected people and thus unimmunised dental care professionals are at risk. TB is a major global killer (prevalence of over 10 million cases) but is now less common in developed countries. Despite being a preventable and curable disease, 1.5 million people die from TB each year — making it the world's top infectious killer. TB is usually pulmonary and seen mainly in immuno-compromised groups including alcoholics, diabetics, patients with immune defects (including HIV infection) and certain racial groups (e.g. Asian). TB proliferates inside of alveolar macrophages which migrate to local lymph nodes and form 'ghon focuses' which can be seen *on chest radiographs.*

- Clinical features may include a single chronic ulcer on the dorsum of the tongue or palate associated with (post-primary) pulmonary infection or firm swelling of the affected lips) Fig. 40.5).

- Diagnosis is confirmed by biopsy, sputum culture, tuberculin testing and chest radiography.
- Management is with combination chemotherapy. Treatment is started with three drugs in combination in order to minimise the emergence of bacterial resistance and is then continued with two or more antibiotics, usually from the following: rifampicin, isoniazid, ethambutol or streptomycin.
- Chemotherapy is usually an effective treatment, but must be given for prolonged periods and, if chemotherapy is less than adequate, bacterial resistance readily develops.
- Multi-drug resistance (MDR) and highly resistant strains (X DR-TB) are increasing in HIV/AIDS.
- TB can remain dormant for decades (latent TB) and be reactivated in immuno-deficiency.

RECOMMENDED READING

Irani, S., 2017. Orofacial bacterial infectious diseases: an update. J. Int. Soc. Prev. Community Dent. 7 (Suppl. 2), S61–S67.

Saini, M., Brizuela, M., 2021. Bacterial Infections of the Oral Mucosa. StatPearls Publishing, Treasure Island, Florida.

Speiser, S., Langridge, B., Birkl, M.M., Kubiena, H., Rodgers, W., 2021. Update on Noma: systematic review on classification, outcomes and follow-up of patients undergoing reconstructive surgery after Noma disease. BMJ Open. 11 (8), e046303. https://doi.org/10.1136/bmjopen-2020-046303.

Orofacial Pain and Sensory/Motor Disturbances

41

Pain: An Overview

KEY POINTS

- Pain is defined as an unpleasant sensory and emotional experience associated with actual or potential tissue damage or described in terms of such damage.
- Stimulation of pain receptors (nociceptors) begins the pathway of recognition of pain.
- Modulation, either enhancing or inhibiting nociception, is crucial to pain perception.
- Nociception is the physiological process of activation of specialised neural pathways, specifically by tissue damaging or potentially damaging stimuli.
- Prostaglandins stimulate nerves at the site of injury and can cause inflammation and fever.
- Cytokines can trigger pain by promoting inflammation.

INTRODUCTION

Pain in the head, face, mouth or teeth is the most common reason that patients consult their dental professionals.

Pain is defined as an unpleasant sensory and emotional experience associated with actual or potential tissue damage or described in terms of such damage. Pain relation with tissue damage may not be constant and it is often associated with affective and cognitive responses.

The pain pathway starts at nociceptors and is transmitted via sensory nerves, the spinal cord dorsal horn, midbrain, thalamus and hypothalamus eventually to be perceived in the brain in the cerebral cortex (somatosensory and limbic) (Fig. 41.1).

Modulation, either enhancing or inhibiting nociception, is also crucial to pain perception.

The initial steps relate to the neurochemical signals of actual or impending tissue damage (nociceptive stimuli); nociception is the physiological process of activation of specialised neural pathways, specifically by tissue damaging or potentially damaging stimuli. These include injury, which releases algogenic substances or tissue autocoids, such as bradykinin and prostaglandins from damaged cells, platelets or mast cells. Prostaglandins stimulate nerves at the site of injury and can cause inflammation and fever. Cytokines can trigger pain by promoting inflammation. Injuries also release peptides (tachykinins) (such as substance P [SP] and neurokinin A) which play a role in pain responses by activating pain receptors (nociceptors). SP acts on mast cells to release histamine and on vessels to release bradykinin. Other relevant small peptides found in nervous tissue, function as synaptic neurotransmitters and include:

- inhibitory neuropeptides: somatostatin, enkephalins
- calcitonin gene-related peptide (CGRP), vasoactive intestinal polypeptide (VIP), cholecystokinin, neuropeptide Y.

Other small peptides act in a paracrine fashion as diffusible hormones that affect many neurones over a great distance (neurohormones like endorphins and enkephalins — natural painkillers).

OROFACIAL PAIN

Most orofacial pain (probably over 95%) arises from diseases of the teeth and is termed 'odontogenic' (Fig. 41.2). There are also non-odontogenic causes that can be of organic origin (neurological, vascular or referred) or non-organic (psychogenic or

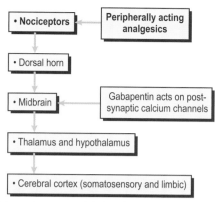

Fig. 41.1 Pain pathway: modulation by peripherally acting analgesics and gabapentin.

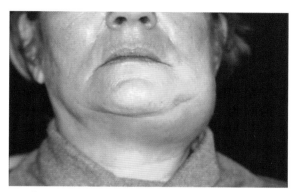

Fig. 41.2 Dental abscess; most orofacial pain is of odontogenic origin.

BOX 41.1   Main Causes of Orofacial Pain

- Local
- Vascular
- Referred
- Neurological
- Idiopathic

BOX 41.2   Differential Diagnosis: List of Causes of Orofacial Pain

Local Disorders
- Teeth and supporting tissues
- Jaws
- Maxillary antrum
- Salivary glands
- Nose and pharynx
- Eyes

Vascular Disorders
- Migraine
- Giant cell arteritis
- Neuralgia-inducing cavitational osteonecrosis (NICO)

Neurological Disorders
- Classical trigeminal neuralgia
- Malignant neoplasms affecting the trigeminal nerve
- Glossopharyngeal neuralgia
- Herpes zoster (including post-herpetic neuralgia)
- Multiple (disseminated) sclerosis
- Post-stroke pain
- Paroxysmal hemicrania
- Trigeminal autonomic cephalalgias

Idiopathic Causes
- Persistent idiopathic facial pain
- Burning mouth syndrome
- Temporomandibular disorder

Referred Pain
- Sinuses
- Eyes
- Ears
- Neck
- Nasopharynx
- Chest
- Cardiac (including angina)
- Respiratory (including lung cancer)

BOX 41.3   Assessment of Head and Neck Pain

Site
Onset
Character
Radiation
Associations
Time course
Exacerbating/relieving factor
Severity

'functional'). Most orofacial pain and most recurrent headaches (tension-type, migraine and cluster headaches) are not life-threatening, but these conditions can interfere with the quality of life.

The causes of orofacial pain (local, vascular, referred, neurological, psychogenic) can be remembered from the mnemonic; 'let veterans read news papers' (Boxes 41.1 and 41.2).

DIAGNOSIS OF PAIN

The most important means of diagnosis of orofacial pain is the history. Indeed, there are no investigations available to prove that the patient is suffering pain, or the severity of it.

In order to differentiate the widely disparate causes, it is essential to determine key points about the pain (Box 41.3): which can be remembered by the acronym 'SOCRATES'.

- **Site:** valuable information can be obtained by watching the patient when asked if the pain is localised or diffuse. For example, patients frequently point with one finger when describing trigeminal neuralgia, but persistent (atypical) idiopathic facial pain (PIFP) is much more diffuse and may radiate.

- **Onset:** the average duration of each episode may help diagnosis. For example, pain from exposed dentine is fairly transient, lasting only for seconds, while the pain from pulpitis lasts for a longer period. Trigeminal neuralgia is a brief lancinating pain lasting up to about 5 seconds, migrainous neuralgia lasts 30 to 45 minutes, migraine lasts hours or days, while PIFP is persistent.
- **Character:** patients should be asked about the severity and whether the pain is 'sharp', 'dull', 'aching', 'throbbing' or 'shooting'. Trigeminal neuralgia is sharp and shooting (lancinating); odontogenic pain often throbbing; giant cell arteritis is 'burning' while PIFP is typically dull.
- **Radiation:** is the pain referred elsewhere?
- **Associated features:** some types of pain may be associated with other features that are helpful diagnostically. These include a swollen face in dental abscess, nausea and vomiting in migraine, a history of nasal stuffiness or lacrimation in migrainous neuralgia, or a number of other complaints such as dry mouth, bad taste, irritable bowel syndrome, back pain, etc., in some patients with PIFP.
- **Time course:** determine whether the pain occurs at specific times. A pain diary can help. For example, the pain of sinusitis is often aggravated by lying down, while periodic migrainous neuralgia frequently disturbs the patient's sleep at a specific time each night, around 2.00 a.m. The pain of temporomandibular disorder (TMD; temporomandibular joint pain—dysfunction syndrome) may be more severe on waking whereas PIFP tends to worsen through the day.
- **Exacerbating and relieving factors:** ask if any factors influence the pain. For example, the temperature often aggravates dental pain, touching a trigger zone may precipitate trigeminal neuralgia attacks, stress may worsen PIFP and alcohol may induce migrainous neuralgia episodes. Exercise may induce cardiac anginal pain referred to the mouth. It may be necessary to resort to leading questions, asking about the effects of temperature, biting, posture, analgesics, alcohol, etc.
- **Severity:** ask the patient to rate the pain severity on a scale of zero (no pain) to 10 (most severe pain that the patient has experienced), or ask them to mark this on a line divided into 10 equal sections (visual analogue scale) or use an assessment instrument such as the McGill pain questionnaire. These help assess the severity, accepting always that it is subjective, and may also be useful in monitoring the response to treatment. Disturbance of the normal sleep pattern by pain is also useful in assessing the severity.

Thus, the answers to a series of features may be needed, including:
- Previous history
- Character:
  - dull
  - throbbing
  - lancinating
  - burning sensation
  - interferes with sleep

- shooting
- aching
- pins and needles
- stabbing
- sharp
- tender
- electric shock
- cramping.
- Provoking or relieving factors:
  - food (hot/cold/sweet) worse on biting/pressure on teeth
  - prolonged chewing
  - wide mouth opening/yawning
  - worse with exercise
  - talking
  - stooping/bending
  - lying down
  - swallowing
  - tooth brushing
  - shaving
  - cold/wind
  - fatigue/tiredness
  - stress/tension
  - noise/light/smell
  - diet
  - alcohol.
- Other features:
  - ocular or nasal symptoms
  - neurological signs or symptoms
  - nausea/vomiting
  - relieved by analgesics/drugs
  - weight loss
  - temporomandibular click
  - trismus
  - otalgia/tinnitus/fullness in the ear.

LOCAL CAUSES OF OROFACIAL PAIN

Most orofacial pain is related to dental disease — odontogenic causes.

Dentinal Pain

Pain originating in dentine:
- is sharp and deep
- is usually evoked by an external stimulus (normally food and drinks which are hot, cold, sweet, sour or, sometimes, salty). Although extreme changes in temperature (e.g. hot soup followed by ice cream) may cause pain in intact, non-diseased teeth, pain evoked by natural stimuli usually indicates a hyperalgesic state of the tooth
- usually subsides within a few seconds of withdrawal of stimulus
- may be poorly localised, often only to an approximate area within two to three teeth adjacent to the affected tooth. Sometimes, the patient is unable to distinguish whether the pain originates from the lower or the upper jaw. Pain

from affected posterior teeth is more difficult to localise than that from anterior teeth. However, patients rarely make localisation errors across the midline.

Pulpal Pain

Checking that the pulp is vital using a pulp vitality tester may be indicated. Pain associated with pulp disease:

- is spontaneous: pain may be described by patients in different ways, and a continuous dull ache can periodically be exacerbated (by stimulation or spontaneously) for short (minutes) or long (hours) periods. The pain of pulpitis is frequently discontinuous and abates spontaneously; the precise explanation for such abatement is not clear
- is strong, and can be excruciating for many minutes
- is often throbbing
- may increase and throb when the patient lies down
- may wake the patient from sleep
- is typically exacerbated by temperature change and pressure on a carious lesion
- outlasts the stimulus (unlike stimulus-induced dentinal pain)
- is poorly localised, particularly when the pain becomes more intense
- tends to radiate or refer to the ipsilateral ear, temple and cheek, but does not cross the midline.

Periodontal Pain

Pain originating in the periodontium:

- is more readily localised than is pulpal pain. The improved ability to localise the source of pain may be attributed to the proprioceptive and mechano-receptive sensibility of the periodontium that is lacking in the pulp. However, although localisation of the affected tooth is often precise, in up to half of the cases, the pain is diffuse and radiates into the jaw on the affected side
- may be less severe than pulpal pain
- is often associated with tenderness to pressure on the affected teeth
- is usually not aggravated by heat or cold.

Acute Periapical Periodontitis

Pain associated with acute periapical inflammation:

- is spontaneous in onset
- is moderate to severe in intensity
- persists for long periods of time (hours)
- is exacerbated by biting on the tooth and, in more advanced cases, even by closing the mouth and bringing the affected tooth gently into contact with the opposing teeth. In these cases, the tooth feels 'high' (extruded) and is very sensitive to touch
- has often been preceded by pulpal pain
- is usually better tolerated than the paroxysmal and excruciating pain of pulpitis
- is usually precisely localised and the patient is able to indicate the affected tooth. During the examination, the affected tooth is located readily by means of tooth percussion

- is usually associated with a non-vital tooth
- is usually associated with tenderness to palpation in the periapical buccal vestibular area
- may be associated with swelling of the face, caused by oedema and cellulitis or sometimes connected with fever and malaise. Usually, when the face swells, the pain diminishes in intensity due to rupture of the pus through the periosteum of the bone around the affected tooth and the consequent decrease in pressure of the tooth apex.

Lateral Periodontal Abscess

- The pain is similar to that of acute periapical periodontitis, though often less severe, and is well localised and with swelling and redness of the gingiva.
- The swelling is usually located more gingivally than in the case of an acute periapical lesion.
- The tooth pulp is usually vital.
- The affected tooth is sensitive to percussion and is often mobile and slightly extruded, and there is a deep periodontal pocket. Probing the pocket may cause pus exudation and subsequent relief from pain.

Food Impaction

The cause of food impaction is usually a faulty contact between the teeth because of caries or poor restorations. Examination shows a faulty contact between two teeth and often food trapped between these teeth; the gingival papilla is tender to touch and bleeds easily.

Food impaction interdentally can cause:

- localised pain that develops between or in two adjacent teeth after meals, especially when food is fibrous (e.g. meat)
- pain associated with a feeling of pressure and discomfort, which may gradually disappear until being evoked again at the next meal, or may be relieved immediately by removing the impacted food
- the adjacent teeth to be sensitive to percussion
- oral malodour.

Cracked Tooth

The examination may fail to elicit the cause of pain. Cracks may be revealed by biting on rubber or a Tooth Sloth or Fracfinder, by fibre optic or blue light illumination or by staining with, for example, disclosing solution. Teeth can crack under trauma and can give rise to pain, which is:

- severe
- worse on biting
- often precipitated by hot or cold.

Pericoronitis

Acute pericoronal infections are common and are related to incompletely erupted teeth partially covered by flaps of gingival tissue (operculum), particularly lower third molars. Pain is spontaneous and is often exacerbated by closing the mouth. In more severe cases, pain may be aggravated by swallowing, and there may be trismus and, occasionally, fever, lymphadenopathy and malaise. Examination shows an operculum that is acutely inflamed, red and oedematous. Frequently, an opposing upper tooth indents or ulcerates the oedematous operculum.

Acute Necrotising Gingivitis

Examination shows necrosis and ulceration of the gingival papilla with different degrees of marginal gingival destruction. Similar features but with more intense pain may be seen in necrotising periodontitis in HIV/AIDS. Acute necrotising gingivitis may cause:

- soreness and pain. In the early stages, some patients may complain of a feeling of tightness around the teeth. Pain is fairly well localised to the affected areas
- profuse gingival bleeding
- halitosis
- metallic taste, sometimes
- fever and malaise, sometimes.

MUCOSAL PAIN

Pain from oral mucosal lesions can be either localised or diffuse. Localised pain is usually associated with an erosion or ulcer. Diffuse pain may be associated with widespread infection, mucosal atrophy or erosion, a systemic underlying deficiency disease or other factors, and is usually described as 'soreness' or sometimes 'burning'. Mucosal pain may be aggravated mechanically by touch, or by sour, spicy, salty or hot foods.

Other Local Causes of Orofacial Pain

Jaws

Pain from the jaws can be caused by acute infection, malignancies, Paget disease and direct trauma. Lesions such as cysts, retained roots and impacted teeth are usually painless unless associated with infection or fracture of the jaw. Odontogenic and other benign tumours of the bone do not normally produce pain, but malignant tumours usually produce deep, boring pain, sometimes associated with paraesthesia, hypoaesthesia or anaesthesia. Radiation therapy or bisphosphonate may result in severe pain due to infection associated with osteonecrosis.

Temporomandibular Joint

Pain from the temporomandibular joint (Chapter 42) may result from dysfunction, trauma, acute or chronic inflammation, or primary or secondary malignant tumours. An examination may reveal that the masticatory muscles are tender to palpation or occasionally the joint is swollen and warm to touch or tender to palpation via the external auditory meatus. Pain from the temporomandibular joint:

- is usually dull
- is usually caused by muscle spasms. Nociceptors may be triggered by the release of substances such as cytokines (interleukin-1 and IL-6, and tumour necrosis factor), lactic acid, potassium ions, prostaglandin E2, bradykinin, leukotriene B4, serotonin, neuropeptides such as SP, neuropeptide Y, CGRP or somatostatin
- is usually poorly localised

- may radiate widely
- is usually intensified by the movement of the mandible
- may be associated with trismus because of the spasm in the masticatory muscles.

Salivary Glands

Examination usually reveals the salivary gland swollen and sensitive to palpation. In acute parotitis, mouth-opening causes severe pain, and thus there is a degree of trismus. Salivary flow from the affected gland is usually reduced. Pain may be associated with fever and malaise. In children, the most common cause is mumps. In adults, pain from salivary glands results usually from blockage of a salivary duct by calculus or a mucus plug, or sialadenitis, when pus may exude from the duct orifice. Pain from salivary gland disorders:

- is localised to the affected gland
- may be quite severe
- may be intensified by increased salivation, such as before and with meals — the pain may wane in the minutes/hours following such salivary stimulation.

Sinuses and Pharynx

A disease of the paranasal sinuses and nasopharynx can cause oral and/or facial pain. In acute sinusitis, there has usually been a preceding 'cold' followed by local pain and tenderness (but not swelling) and radio-opacity of the affected sinuses, sometimes with an obvious fluid level. Transillumination from a light in the oral cavity may show a fluid level. With maxillary sinusitis, pain may be felt in related upper molars and premolars, any of which may be tender to percussion. The pain of ethmoidal or sphenoidal sinusitis is deep in the nose. Pain in any type of acute sinusitis may be aggravated by a change of position of the head.

Tumours of the sinuses or nasopharynx can also cause facial pain. These tumours are often carcinomas that infiltrate various branches of the trigeminal nerve and can remain undetected until too late. Nasopharyngeal carcinoma often presents late, with facial pain, paraesthesia, ipsilateral deafness and/or cervical lymph node enlargement (Trotter syndrome).

Pressure on the Mental Nerve

Rarely, pain is caused by pressure from a denture on the nerve, which comes to lie on the crest of the ridge as the alveolar bone is resorbed in the edentulous mandible. Either the denture should be relieved from the area or, occasionally, it is necessary to re-site the nerve surgically.

VASCULAR CAUSES OF OROFACIAL PAIN

Disorders in which the most obvious organic feature is vascular dilatation or constriction cause orofacial pain. The pain is usually obviously in the face or head rather than in the mouth, but occasionally can involve both, and can be difficult to differentiate from other causes of orofacial pain (Table 41.1). Migraine and giant cell arteritis are discussed in Chapter 45.

TABLE 41.1   Differential Diagnosis of Oral Pain

Source of Pain	Character	Exacerbating Factors	Localisation	Associated With	Pain Provoked by	Radiography
Dental						
Dentinal	Evoked, does not outlast	Hot/cold, sweet/sour	Poor	Caries, defective restorations, exposed dentine	Hot/cold, probing dentine	May show interproximal caries, defective restorations
Pulpal	Severe, intermittent, throbbing	Hot/cold, sometimes biting	Poor	Deep caries, extensive restoration	Hot/cold, probing, sometimes percussion	May show deep caries or deep restoration
Periodontal						
Periapical	For hours at same intensity; deep, boring	Biting	Good	Periapical swelling and redness, tooth mobility	Percussion, palpation of periapical area	Periapical views may show periapical changes
Lateral	For hours at same level, boring	Biting	Good	Periodontal, boring, deep pockets with pus exuding, tooth mobility	Percussion, palpation of periodontal area	Useful when x-rayed with probe inserted into pocket
Gingival	Pressing, annoying	Food impaction, toothbrushing	Good	Acute gingival inflammation	Touch, percussion	Not applicable
Mucosal						
Mucosal	Burning, sharp	Sour, sharp and hot food	Good	Erosive or ulcerative lesions, redness	Palpation	Not applicable

CAUSES OF REFERRED OROFACIAL PAIN

Pain may occasionally be referred to the mouth, face or jaws from any pathology affecting the trigeminal nerve and from the following:

- Sinuses.
- Eyes: pain from the eyes can arise from disorders of refraction, retrobulbar neuritis (e.g. in disseminated sclerosis) or glaucoma (raised intraocular pressure), and can radiate to the orbit or frontal region.
- Ears: middle-ear disease may cause headaches. Conversely, oral disease not infrequently causes pain referred to the ear, particularly from lesions of the posterior tongue. The classic picture is an older man with undiagnosed tongue cancer who complains of earache.
- Neck: cervical vertebral disease, especially cervical spondylosis, very occasionally causes pain referred to the face.
- Pharynx: carcinoma of the pharynx may cause facial pain.
- Oesophagus: pain plus sialorrhoea may result from oesophageal lesions.
- Styloid process (stylalgia): eagle syndrome, a rare disorder due to an elongated styloid process, may cause pain on chewing, swallowing or turning the head.
- Heart, in patients with angina: the latter pain usually affects the mandible, is initiated by exercise (especially in the cold) and abates quickly on rest.

- Lungs: orofacial pain emanating from lung cancer is a well-recognised entity and has been misdiagnosed as temporomandibular joint pain or idiopathic facial pain.

Neurological (Neuropathic) Causes of Orofacial Pain

Sensory innervation of the mouth, face and scalp depends on the trigeminal nerve so that the disease affecting this nerve can cause orofacial pain or, indeed, sensory loss — sometimes with serious implications.

FACIAL NEURALGIA CAUSED BY TUMOURS OR OTHER LESIONS

Any lesion affecting the trigeminal nerve, whether it be traumatic, cerebrovascular disease, disseminated sclerosis, infections such as HIV/AIDS or Lyme disease, inflammatory or neoplastic (e.g. a nasopharyngeal or antral carcinoma), may cause pain, often with physical signs, such as facial sensory or motor impairment.

Trigeminal Neuralgias

Disorder of the trigeminal nerve that consists of episodes of unilateral intense, stabbing, electric shock-like pain that is abrupt in onset and termination in the areas of the face supplied by one or more divisions of the trigeminal nerve (see Chapter 43).

Trigeminal Autonomic Cephalgias

Trigeminal autonomic cephalgias (TACs) are strictly unilateral headaches characterised by episodic, stereotypic attacks and, often prominent, cranial autonomic symptoms, such as lacrimation, conjunctival injection and/or rhinorrhoea. There are discussed in Chapter 45.

Glossopharyngeal and postherpetic neuralgias may also cause orofacial pain.

IDIOPATHIC CAUSES OF OROFACIAL PAIN

The mouth and perioral soft tissues have among the richest sensory innervation in the body. Furthermore, a large part of the sensory homunculus on the cerebral cortex receives information from orofacial structures. Right from infancy, the mouth is concerned intimately with the psychological development of the individual, and disorders of structures, such as the lips, teeth and oral mucosa can hold enormous emotional significance. A number of idiopathic orofacial conditions exist including:
- PIFP
- TMD
- burning mouth syndrome
- atypical odontalgia.

These orofacial pain conditions share a number of features:
- Constant chronic discomfort or pain.
- Pain often of a dull boring or burning type.
- Pain that is poorly localised (it may cross the midline to involve the other side or may move elsewhere).
- Pain that rarely wakens the patient from sleep; however, sleep disturbances are common.
- Total lack of objective signs of organic disease.
- All investigations are also negative.
- The majority of patients are female.
- Often recent adverse 'life events', such as bereavement or family illness.
- Often other chronic pain conditions such as headaches, chronic back or neck pain, irritable bowel syndrome or dysmenorrhoea (Table 41.2).
- A cure is uncommon in most, yet few of those suffering seem to try or persist in using medication.

Medically unexplained symptoms (MUS) are commonplace in, from 50% in primary care to 15% in hospital outpatients, especially manifesting as chest pain, dyspnoea, dizziness or headache. The reasons for MUS may include the following:
- Possible links between neurohumoral mechanisms and altered CNS function.
- The heightening of bodily sensations (lowered pain threshold) as a consequence of physiological processes, such as autonomic arousal, muscle tension, hyperventilation or inactivity.

TABLE 41.2 Medically Unexplained Symptoms — Pain at Various Body Sites

System	Examples
Chest	Tietze syndrome
Gastrointestinal	Irritable bowel syndrome
Musculoskeletal	Low back pain
Ear, nose and throat	Dysphagia (globus hystericus)
Orofacial	Idiopathic facial pain/oral dysaesthesia

- Misattribution of normal sensations to serious physical disorders.

Multiple pains and other complaints may occur simultaneously or sequentially, and relief is rarely found (or admitted). Patients may bring diaries of their symptoms to emphasise their problem. Occasional patients quite deliberately induce painful oral lesions, and some have Munchausen syndrome, where they behave in such a fashion as to appear to want operative intervention.

DIAGNOSIS OF OROFACIAL PAIN

The cause of orofacial pain is established mainly from the history and examination findings, but it is important to consider the usefulness of additional investigations, particularly imaging of the head and neck, using MRI or CT (Algorithms 41.1–41.3). It is important not to miss detecting serious organic diseases (Tables 41.1–41.4).

TREATMENT OF OROFACIAL PAIN (SEE ALSO CHAPTERS 4 AND 5)

Pain is the most important symptom suggestive of orofacial disease, but the absence of pain does not exclude organic disease and the presence of pain does not necessarily mean organic disease. There is also considerable individual variation in response to pain, and the threshold is lowered by tiredness and psychological and other factors:
- Simple analgesics, such as NSAIDs, should be used initially, before embarking on more potent preparations. Chronic pain requires regular analgesia (not just as required). Details are given in Chapter 5.
- Anticonvulsants may help in neuropathic pain (neuralgias).
- Opioids may help in cancer and mucositis pain.
- Antidepressants may help.
It is important also:
- where possible, to identify and treat the cause of pain
- to relieve factors that lower the pain threshold (fatigue, anxiety and depression)
- to avoid polypharmacy.

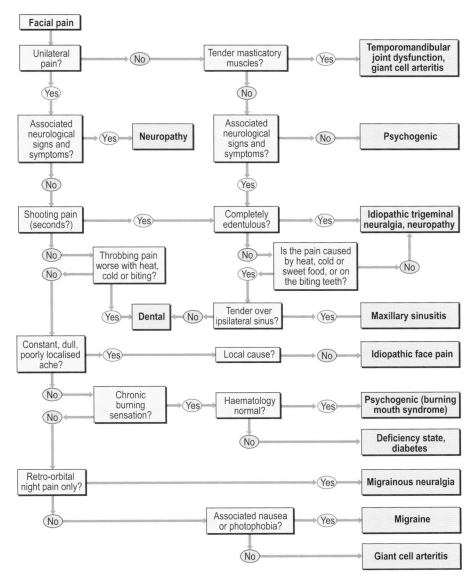

Algorithm 41.1 Diagnosis of facial pain.

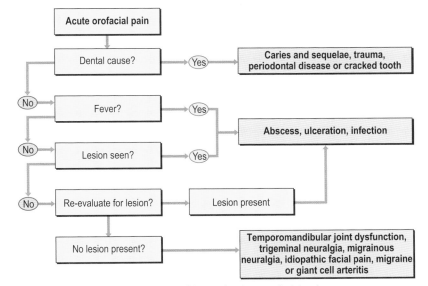

Algorithm 41.2 Diagnosis of acute facial pain.

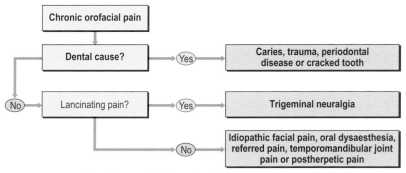

Algorithm 41.3 Diagnosis of chronic orofacial pain.

TABLE 41.3   Characteristics of Important Types of Facial Pain

	Temporomandibular Disorder (TMJ Pain-Dysfunction)	Migraine	Persistent Idiopathic Facial Pain	Classic Trigeminal Neuralgia	Giant Cell Arteritis
Age (years)	15–30	Any	30–50	50	60–80
Gender	F > M	F > M	F > M	F > M	F > M
Site	Unilateral Temporal Jaw Ear	Any, especially supraorbital	± Bilateral, maxilla	Unilateral, mandible or maxilla	Temple
Associated features	Click Limited movements	± Photophobia ± nausea ± vomiting	± Depression	—	Polymyalgia
Character	Dull	Throbbing	Dull	Lancinating	Burning
Duration	Weeks to months	Hours (usually daytime)	Continual	Brief (seconds)	Hours
Precipitating factors	Trauma	± Foods	None	Trigger areas	None
Relieving factors	Rest	Sumatriptan, clonidine; ergot derivatives	Antidepressants	Carbamazepine	Corticosteroids

TABLE 41.4   Investigations That Might Be Helpful in Diagnosis/Prognosis/Management in Some Patients With Orofacial Pain[a]

In Most Cases	In Some Cases
Tooth vitality testing	Neurological opinion
Radiography	Nasendoscopy
	MRI of head
	Blood pressure
	ESR
	Temporal artery biopsy
	Psychological assessment

[a]See text for details and glossary for abbreviations.

Frey Syndrome

Frey syndrome (auriculotemporal syndrome, see Chapter 54) is a paroxysmal burning pain, usually in the temporal area or in front of the ear, associated with flushing and sweating on eating, which often follows parotid surgery and appears to be due to abnormal reinnervation.

RECOMMENDED READING

Barmherzig, R., Kingston, W., 2019. Occipital neuralgia and cervicogenic headache: diagnosis and management. Curr. Neurol. Neurosci. Rep. 19 (5), 20.

Dworkin, R.H., O'Connor, A.B., Audette, J., et al., 2010. Recommendations for the pharmacological management of neuropathic pain: an overview and literature update. Mayo Clin. Proc. 85 (3 Suppl), S3–14.

Mogil, J.S., 2012. Pain genetics: past, present and future. Trends Genet. 28 (6), 258–266.

Temporomandibular Disorder

> **KEY POINTS**
> - Temporomandibular disorder (TMD) refers to pain and dysfunction involving the masticatory muscles and the temporomandibular joints (TMJs).
> - The condition affects young people mainly, typically teenagers or young adults. Women are affected more frequently than men.
> - The aetiology is multifactorial.
> - Diagnosis is mainly clinical.
> - A biopsychosocial illness model is recommended in the treatment of TMD pain.

INTRODUCTION

The temporomandibular joints (TMJs) are complex joints that need to work in concert, are essential for mastication, and are probably the most used joints in the body. Temporomandibular disorder (TMJ pain—dysfunction syndrome; myofascial pain dysfunction, facial arthromyalgia, mandibular dysfunction) refers to pain and dysfunction involving the masticatory muscles and the TMJs. It may present with pain in the face and preauricular area, limitations in jaw movement and noise from the TMJs during jaw movements.

TMD is the most common orofacial complaint and also one of the most controversial areas in dentistry in terms of suggested aetiopathogenesis, diagnosis and management.

EPIDEMIOLOGY

- The prevalence is at least 12% of the general population, but these symptoms have been reported at some time by up to 88%.
- The condition affects women more frequently than men and is most common in young adults, typically teenagers and up to 20 to 30 years of age.
- No known geographic incidence.
- Aetiology is multifactorial.

AETIOLOGY AND PATHOGENESIS

TMD is a complex musculoskeletal disorder of multifactorial aetiology. Several risk factors predispose or precipitate TMD-pain, including biological factors, trauma, occlusal changes, parafunctional habits and psychosocial factors (e.g. stress, catastrophising and mood). Patients suffering from TMD pain commonly have comorbid pain conditions such as headache, neck pain and back pain. Many patients with fibromyalgia also exhibit TMD pain. Injuries, prolonged mouth opening and parafunctional habits are other possible causes. The relationship between dental occlusion and TMD is controversial. Patients with TMD show higher levels of stress, anxiety, depression and pain catastrophising.

The origin of pain in TMD has traditionally been attributed to increased contraction and increased muscle tension affecting the muscles of mastication (mainly the temporalis, masseter and pterygoid muscles) as a psychological response to stress that becomes chronic.

Peripheral mechanisms are likely to play a role in the onset of TMD, whereas central factors such as central sensitisation of second-order neurons, as well as genetic predisposition, prolong the pain.

The aetiology is multifactorial.

Trauma

Trauma which is obvious, including from road accidents, sports injuries, fights and dental treatment or extractions is common and can occasionally be followed by TMD.

TMD can also be secondary to microtrauma and subsequent muscle hyperactivity. Microtrauma can result from prolonged mouth opening, as in dental treatment sessions, general anaesthesia, choir singing, wind instrument playing or parafunctional habit, such as day-time jaw clenching or night-time tooth grinding (bruxism), and habits, such as tongue thrusting, fingernail biting and pen-chewing.

Trauma can result in muscle spasms or hyperactivity.

Muscle Hyperactivity

Psychological stress can also cause muscle hyperactivity. Muscle hyperactivity has been demonstrated in TMD patients during activities, such as school examinations and watching horror films.

Fifty to seventy percent of patients (twice as common as controls) have experienced stressful life events in the 6 months before onset. These problems concerning work, money, health, loss and interpersonal relationships probably have a causative role by inducing anxiety, which then produces increased jaw muscle activity.

Depression and sleep deprivation are important risk indicators.

Occlusion

Abnormalities in the dental occlusion are controversial as a cause of TMD. There is no neurophysiological evidence to support a primary aetiological role for the occlusion in TMD and many people with gross malocclusions have no TMJ dysfunction. There is no significant difference in the incidence of occlusal abnormalities between TMD patients and control subjects, nor is there any evidence for a relationship between orthodontic treatment (or the wearing of orthodontic headgear) and TMD.

Hormonal

As the condition is more common in females, some studies have suggested that female sex hormones, such as oestrogen, are involved in pain modulation.

CLINICAL FEATURES

The signs and symptoms are highly variable but can include pain, limited range of movement and TMJ sounds:

- **Pain in the joint and/or surrounding muscles and elsewhere:** the main site is usually preauricular, but can radiate to the back of the mouth, down the neck, up to the temple or behind the ear. Pain may occur at an early stage or sometimes after the onset of clicking or stiffness of the jaw. It may range from a vague dull ache to an acute pain. Myalgia is the most common TMD pain and occurs in approximately 80% of patients. Patients with a night-time clenching or grinding habit (bruxism) may awake with joint pain which abates during the day. The symptoms of individuals who clench or grind during working hours tend to worsen towards the evening, and sometimes have a psychogenic basis. The pain may be aggravated by chewing or other jaw movements. The masseters, temporalis and pterygoid muscles may be tender to palpation, but there is no detectable swelling. Sometimes the pain is more clearly sited in a single jaw muscle, and sometimes trigger points can be located. The pain is often aggravated by chewing, yawning or talking. Some patients may also complain of tension-type headaches, neck aches, lower back pain and depression and anxiety.
- **Jaw locking or limitation of movement:** limitation of opening may be intermittent, with jaw 'locking'. There may be deviation of the jaw to the affected side on attempted opening with variable jaw deviation or locking, but rarely severe trismus. If there is reduced mouth opening, this often suggests bilateral disease. Limitation may be more obvious on awakening, especially after nocturnal grinding. In some others, the limitation increases throughout the day.
- **Recurrent clicking in the TMJ:** clicking occurs either on attempted mouth opening or closing. Often the click allows the completion of that phase of mandibular movement. Sometimes clicking ceases and the jaw locks either open or closed. Clicks are not diagnostic since they are common in normal TMJs.
- **Joint diseases:** Osteoarthritis or rheumatoid arthritis are degenerative joint diseases. A grating noise (crepitus) may signify intra-articular arthritic change, and there may be crepitus at any point of jaw movement, especially with lateral movements.

DIAGNOSIS

Diagnosis of TMD is mainly on clinical grounds but it is crucial to exclude organic disease in the TMJ or elsewhere and referred to the area (Table 42.1). Pain and tenderness on palpation of the muscles of mastication and TMJ are the most common clinical signs and often coexist.

Self-rating assessments for psychological factors may be helpful. The occlusion and any dental appliances should also be assessed. There are several diagnostic systems for TMD (Table 42.2). The Diagnostic Criteria for TMD (DC/TMD), a revised version of the RDC/TMD, comprises two domains, a physical Axis I (diagnosis) and a psychosocial Axis II (psychosocial assessment). The graded chronic pain scale and hospital anxiety and depression scale are helpful tools for psychosocial assessment.

Imaging

Any osseous changes in organic TMJ disease, such as osteoarthritis or rheumatoid arthritis are unlikely, in the absence of long-standing disease, to be revealed by imaging. Indeed, radiographic changes are uncommon and the condylar position as seen on radiography is unreliable for diagnosis and does not indicate disc displacement. Imaging is rarely indicated but MRI, CT, CBCT or OPG can be helpful if there are:

TABLE 42.1   **Aids That Might Be Helpful in Diagnosis/Prognosis/Management in Some Patients Suspected of Having Temporomandibular Disorder[a]**

In Most Cases	In Some Cases
—	Radiography (OPG)
	CT/MRI
	Full blood picture
	ESR
	ANA
	RF

[a]See text for details and glossary for abbreviations.

TABLE 42.2 International Classification of Orofacial Pain (ICOP) Diagnostic Criteria for Primary Temporomandibular Joint Pain

A. Pain in and/or in front of the ear(s), fulfilling criteria B—D

B. Occurring in one or more episodes,[1] or unremitting

C. Both of the following:

1. Confirmation on examination of location in the area(s) of one or both temporomandibular joint(s).

2. Provoked by either or both of: (a) palpation of and/or around the lateral pole(s) of the mandibular condyle(s), (b) maximum unassisted or assisted jaw opening, right or left lateral and/or protrusive movement(s).

D. Modified[2] by jaw movement, function or parafunction (e.g. tooth-grinding or clenching).

E. Not better accounted for by another ICOP diagnosis.

[1]Episodes may be single or recurrent within any day, each lasting at least 30 min and with a total duration within the day of at least 2 h.
[2]Pain may be increased or decreased.

- a history of trauma
- significant limitation of movement, change in occlusion or a mandibular shift
- sensory or motor alteration
- a real possibility of organic joint or other disease.

TREATMENT

Patient information is an important aspect of management. TMD appears not to lead to long-term joint damage and some patients have spontaneous remission: thus, treatment is not always indicated. There is no indication, for example, for attempting treatment for TMJ clicks that are otherwise symptomless. However, in persons who complain of pain, treatment may be worthwhile (Table 42.3). The aims of treatment are to control immediate pain, lower psychological stress (reassure) and eliminate TMJ damage.

There is a wide range of treatments offered for TMD, including physical, medical, psychological and surgical approaches but conservative approaches are typically successful. The level of placebo response and the response from reassurance is impressive, and conservative measures are at least partially successful in up to 90% — usually within 6 months.

- Conservative measures include rest, massage, heat and cold compresses, avoidance of trauma, wide opening and abnormal habits and remedial jaw exercises to control discomfort. Jaw exercises may improve coordination, relax and strengthen the muscles.
- Plastic splints on the occlusal surfaces (occlusal splints) may reduce joint loading, eliminate faulty occlusal interferences, protect the teeth from wear due to bruxism and provide cognitive awareness of damaging oral habits and engender a placebo effect (Fig. 42.1).
- Medical therapy includes:
  - analgesics (NSAIDs); topical NSAIDs may help: ibuprofen gel (5% or 10%)

TABLE 42.3 Regimens That Might Be Helpful in Management of Patient Suspected of Having Temporomandibular Disorder

Regimen	Use in Primary or Secondary Care
Conservative measures	Reassurance Rest Massage Heat and cold compresses Avoidance of trauma, wide opening and abnormal habits Jaw exercises Occlusal splint (overlay appliance)
Medical approaches	Analgesics (NSAIDs); topical NSAIDs may help: ibuprofen gel (5% or 10%) Muscle relaxants[a] (e.g. benzodiazepines (clonazepam 0.25 mg/day, temazepam 10 mg or baclofen 10 mg three times daily) — controversial Antidepressants[a] (e.g. tricyclics) — as indicated from psychological assessment
Surgical approaches	Arthroscopy Arthroplasty Joint replacement

[a]Should only be used with specialist care and in chronic cases unresponsive to simple measures

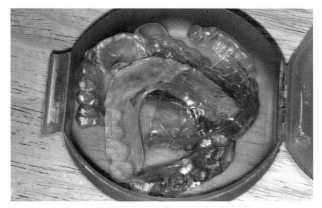

Fig. 42.1 Splints for temporomandibular pain-dysfunction syndrome.

- muscle relaxants (e.g. benzodiazepines [clonazepam 0.25 mg/day, temazepam 10 mg] or baclofen 10 mg three times daily) — controversial
- antidepressants (e.g. tricyclics) - as indicated by psychological assessment
- intra-articular injections (triamcinolone or hyaluronate).
- Behavioural therapies are an essential part of management and include education, cognitive behavioural therapy (CBT), self-care programs at home after instruction, and relaxation techniques such as meditation and yoga.
- Acupuncture may be helpful in TMD patients with myalgia.
- There is no evidence that occlusal adjustments (grinding on teeth) are more or less effective than a placebo in the treatment of TMD pain.

- Surgical approaches are only appropriate in selected cases (such as in those with obvious intra-articular pathology) and include arthroscopic procedures.

Follow-Up of Patients

Long-term follow-up in primary care is usually appropriate.

RECOMMENDED READING

Mujakperuo, H.R., Watson, M., Morrison, R., et al., 2010. Pharmacological interventions for pain in patients with temporomandibular disorders. Cochrane. Database. Syst. Rev. 10, CD004715.

Rajapakse, N., Ahmed, A., Sidebottom, J., 2017. Current thinking about the management of dysfunction of the temporomandibular joint: a review. Br. J. Oral. Maxillofac. Surg. 55 (4), 351–356.

Schiffman, E., Ohrbach, R., Truelove, E., et al., 2014. Diagnostic criteria for temporomandibular disorders (DC/TMD) for clinical and research applications: Recommendations of the International RDC/TMD consortium network* and orofacial pain special interest group. J. Oral. Facial. Pain. Headache 28, 6–27.

Slade, G.D., Ohrbach, R., Greenspan, J.D., et al., 2016. Painful temporomandibular disorder: decade of discovery from OPPERA studies. J. Dent. Res. 95, 1084–1092.

Written, illustrated instructions for examination of the TMJ are available at http:// www.rdc-tmdinternational.org

Trigeminal and Other Neuralgias

KEY POINTS
- Trigeminal neuralgia (TN) is characterised by touch-evoked unilateral brief shock-like, stabbing, intense paroxysmal pain in one or more divisions of the trigeminal nerve. TN is divided into classical TN and secondary TN.
  - TN is one of the most severe pains known.
  - Pain is sometimes triggered by touching areas or by certain daily activities, such as eating, talking, washing the face, shaving or cleaning the teeth.
  - There is no neurological deficit.
  - Organic causes of neuralgia must be excluded by history, physical examination and special investigations.
  - First-line therapy is medical with an anticonvulsant, such as carbamazepine.
  - Surgical/ablative therapies are reserved for recalcitrant TN.

INTRODUCTION

Trigeminal neuralgia (TN) is a disorder of the trigeminal nerve that consists of episodes of unilateral intense, stabbing, electric shock-like pain that is abrupt in onset and termination in the areas of the face supplied by one or more divisions of the trigeminal nerve. TN is not fatal, but it is universally considered to be one of the most painful afflictions known.

Sensory innervation of the mouth, face and scalp depends on the trigeminal (fifth cranial) nerve (Figs 43.1 and 43.2), so that disease affecting this nerve can cause not only orofacial pain but also sensory loss, or, indeed, both, sometimes with serious implications.

TN may occur in tumours of the trigeminal nerve (e.g. neuroma), with lesions affecting the trigeminal nerve at the cerebellopontine angle and in disseminated sclerosis or cerebral neoplasms, and these cases are termed secondary or symptomatic TN (STN), when there may be detectable physical signs — initially a reduced corneal reflex, progressing to trigeminal sensory loss. TN, however, much more frequently has no *clinically obvious* neurological cause (termed classical TN, CTN) and is then usually ascribed to pressure on the trigeminal nerve from an adjacent but atherosclerotic artery.

CLASSICAL TRIGEMINAL NEURALGIA

This is also known as idiopathic ITN, benign paroxysmal TN, TN and tic douloureux.

Epidemiology

- Uncommon, probably about 4 cases per 100,000 population, although CTN is the most common neurological cause of facial pain.
- The average age of onset is 53 years in classical TN and 43 years in secondary TN.
  - It is slightly more common in women.
  - There is no known geographic incidence.
  - No predisposing factors have been identified for classical TN.

Aetiology and Pathogenesis

CTN is caused by demyelination of primary sensory trigeminal afferents in the root entry zone. Demyelination results in neuronal discharge. In a significant proportion of the patients, the demyelination is caused by a neurovascular conflict (typically the superior cerebellar artery) resulting in morphological changes of the trigeminal nerve such as distortion, dislocation, distension, indentation, flattening or atrophy. There are also other unknown aetiological factors since only half of the CTN patients have morphological changes.

STN is severe orofacial pain suggestive of TN, but an organic cause is detectable. STN is usually seen in younger people and/or sometimes with physical signs, such as facial sensory or motor impairment, and can result from cerebrovascular disease, multiple sclerosis, infections such as HIV infection, space-occupying lesions such as neoplasms or aneurysms, or lesions that may irritate the trigeminal nerve roots along the pons, or the tracts more centrally in the CNS. In

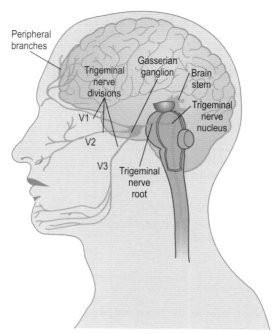

Fig. 43.1 Trigeminal nerve anatomy.

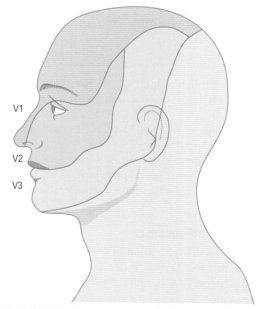

Fig. 43.2 Trigeminal nerve sensory distribution by dermatomes.

STN, the pathophysiological mechanism is likely the same as in CTN but is dependent on the specific structural lesion. For example, an MS plaque may affect the trigeminal root, or a space-occupying lesion located in the cerebellopontine angle such as epidermoid tumour, meningioma, arteriovenous malformation or aneurysm.

Clinical Features

In both CTN and STN, the pain is unilateral and follows the sensory distribution of cranial nerve V, typically radiating to the maxillary (V2) or mandibular (V3) area (see Fig. 43.2). TN has the following main characteristics:

- Pain is restricted to one or more divisions of the trigeminal nerve.
- TN most frequently affects V2 and/or V3 division and the right side is slightly more often affected than the left side. Bilateral TN is very rare in classical TN and should raise suspicion of STN.
- Abrupt in onset and typically lasts only a few seconds (2 minutes at maximum).
- Pain may arise spontaneously but can be triggered by innocuous mechanical stimuli or movements such as eating, talking, washing the face, shaving or cleaning the teeth.
- May experience additional continuous pain in the same distribution and same period as the paroxysmal pain (TN with concomitant continuous pain).
- Electric shock-like, shooting, stabbing or sharp in quality.
- No clinically evident neurological deficit.
- Usually entirely asymptomatic between paroxysms, but some patients experience a dull ache at other times.
- Attacks are stereotyped in the individual patient.
- There is no neurological deficit in CTN, but STN needs to be excluded by history, physical examination, imaging and special investigations, when necessary. There is also an increased risk of cerebrovascular events in patients with TN, so blood pressure assessment is indicated.
- Many patients experience a refractory period after a paroxysmal attack where new attacks cannot be elicited.
- TN patients may have autonomic symptoms. Important differential diagnoses include trigeminal autonomic cephalgias.

Diagnosis

The diagnosis of TN is primarily based on patient history, as there is no definitive diagnostic test. An MRI brain should be undertaken early in the work-up to exclude tumours or multiple sclerosis. Trigeminal sensory testing is important to elicit deficits, bilateral involvement of the trigeminal nerve, and abnormal trigeminal reflexes associated with an increased risk of STN (Algorithm 43.1):

- History.
- Examination, including careful neurological assessment, especially of the cranial nerves — particularly the trigeminal nerve and those closely related to the trigeminal (i.e. cranial nerves VI, VII and VIII). Patients with CTN should have a completely unremarkable neurological examination. Sensory changes on neurological examination are suggestive of underlying pathology (i.e. symptomatic TN).
- Investigations (Table 43.1):
  - imaging: intra-oral x-rays if pain appears to be of dental origin, MRI or CT to exclude cerebral space-occupying or demyelinating lesions. Many specialists recommend elective MRI for all patients to exclude an uncommon mass lesion or aberrant vessel compressing the trigeminal nerve roots, or demyelination, and it is mandatory if any atypical features or neurological features are present, and in patients under 50 years. MRI should always

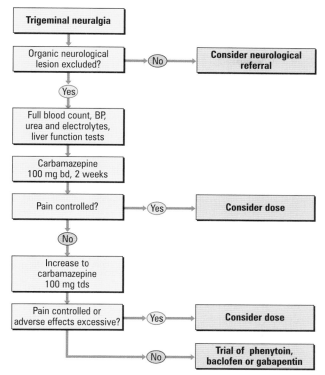

Algorithm 43.1 Trigeminal neuralgia management.

TABLE 43.1 Investigations That Might be Helpful in Diagnosis/Prognosis/Management in Some Patients Suspected of Having Trigeminal Neuralgia[a]

In Most Cases	In Some Cases
Neurosurgical opinion	Dental radiography
MRI/CT	Serum ferritin, vitamin B_{12} and
Full blood picture[b]	corrected whole blood folate levels
Blood pressure[b]	Serology (Lyme disease, HIV)
Urea and electrolytes[b]	ANA
Liver function tests[b]	ESR
	HLA-B1502, if Asian/Chinese

[a]See text for details and glossary for abbreviations.
[b]For monitoring carbamazepine adverse effects.

be performed prior to surgery or other therapeutic procedures to exclude secondary causes such as tumours.
- blood tests: liver and kidney function.

Generally, CTN is diagnosed from the typical history, a negative neurological exam, a negative MRI and investigations, together with a positive response to a trial of the anticonvulsant carbamazepine.

Treatment

- Patient information is an important aspect of management.
- Patients with TN are best seen at an early stage by a specialist in order to confirm the diagnosis and initiate treatment.

TABLE 43.2 Regimens That Might be Helpful in Management of Patients Suspected of Having Trigeminal Neuralgia

Regimen	Use in Primary Care	Use in Secondary Care (Intractable Pain)
Beneficial	Carbamazepine Oxcarbazepine	Microvascular decompression Gamma knife radiofrequency thermocoagulation of trigeminal Gasserian ganglion
Likely to be beneficial	Lamotrigine Baclofen Gabapentin Pregabalin	
Unproven effectiveness	Acupuncture Neurostimulation	

- CTN is often an intermittent disease with apparent remissions for months or years, but recurrence is common and very often the pain spreads to involve a wider area over time and the intervals between episodes tend to shorten. Few patients have spontaneous remission. Thus, active treatment is usually indicated (Table 43.2), typically being medication. Pain relief is the goal of therapy.

Medical Treatment

Medical treatment is successful for greater than 80% of patients, the preferred treatments being anticonvulsant drugs or muscle relaxants. Treatment recommendations are generally the same in CTN and STN. Carbamazepine or oxcarbazepine (better tolerability) are recommended as first-line treatments. Carbamazepine, a sodium channel blocker, is the first-choice anticonvulsant in most instances and prevents attacks of neuralgia in 60% of patients.

It is not an analgesic and, if given when an attack starts, will not relieve the pain; rather it must be given continuously prophylactically for long periods. It is typically given in 100 mg doses twice daily initially, then three times daily, increasing by 100 mg every 3 days to a maximum of 1200 mg/day. Most patients respond to 200 to 400 mg carbamazepine three times daily.

It must be used carefully and under strict medical surveillance, and never in patients who are HLA-B1502, if Asian/Chinese because of the risk of erythema multiforme.

It is contraindicated in pregnancy as it is teratogenic. The dose should be increased to control the pain, while at the same time avoiding adverse effects.

Carbamazepine may cause adverse effects in up to one-third of patients, which include mainly:
- somnolence
- drowsiness
- dizziness
- rash
- tremor

- ataxia
- headache
- gastrointestinal effects
- facial dyskinesias
- folate deficiency.

It can cause other less common, but potentially serious, adverse effects, including:

- rashes, sometimes severe and exfoliative, though rarely life-threatening
- pancytopenia or rarely leucopenia, which is idiosyncratic but typically occurs within the first 3 months of treatment. Monitoring of patients should include:
- balance (disturbed – ataxia): this tends to be the feature that limits the dose of carbamazepine
- blood pressure (may increase): patients must have a baseline test and then blood pressure estimations for 3 months, then six times monthly
- blood tests: electrolytes (sodium levels may be reduced – hyponatraemia); liver function (may be impaired); bone marrow function (red and white cells and/or platelets may be depressed), folate levels
- may interact with cimetidine and isoniazid, potentiates lithium and interferes with oral contraceptives.

Combination treatment should be considered when carbamazepine or oxcarbazepine cannot reach full dosage because of intolerable side effects. The synergistic combination of carbamazepine with lamotrigine, pregabalin, gabapentin or baclofen may provide relief. These agents may be used as monotherapy. Long-acting local analgesic injections as peripheral blocks (e.g. mepivacaine) may be of additional value.

If these regimens fail to control TN, a neurosurgical opinion is necessary. Table 43.2.

Some patients report having reduced or relieved pain by means of alternative medical therapies, such as acupuncture, chiropractic adjustment, self-hypnosis or meditation.

For patients refractory to medical treatments, or where adverse effects are intolerable, surgery may be needed.

Neurosurgical Treatment

Gasserian ganglion percutaneous techniques, gamma knife surgery and microvascular decompression (MVD) are the most promising options, but patients may elect to try peripheral surgery first:

- Peripheral surgery: which involves deliberately interrupting nerve conduction in a division or branch of the trigeminal nerve and may bring temporary relief of analgesia for some months and without permanent anaesthesia. These procedures include:
  - injections, usually of long-acting analgesics such as ropivacaine, or streptomycin, alcohol or glycerol, around the mandibular or infraorbital foramen
  - local cryosurgery

  - chemical peripheral neurectomy of a trigeminal nerve division, using alcohol or phenol
  - radiofrequency thermocoagulation
- Intracranial surgery: Open surgical procedures include posterior cranial fossa procedures, which are successful in providing instant and prolonged pain relief, but with possible morbidity and even mortality. In medically refractory patients, with a neurovascular conflict, MVD is the first choice treatment.
  - MVD involves repositioning the artery that compresses the trigeminal nerve as it emerges from the brain stem. It gives the longest duration of being pain-free and provides significant pain relief in 73% of patients after five years. Minor complications including new aching or burning pain or sensory loss occur in 2% to 7%. Major complications such as major cranial nerve dysfunction (2%), stroke (0.3%) and death (0.2%) are rare.
  - Percutaneous approaches to trigeminal gangliolysis by heating, compressing, or chemicals are considered to have less associated risk and less cost than open procedures. They can be done by inserting a needle into the skull through the face. Radiofrequency ablation is the most commonly performed of these procedures. Percutaneous Fogarty balloon microcompression (PBM) and percutaneous retrogasserian glycerol rhizotomy (PRGR) are also used. Pain is exchanged for anaesthesia (and, therefore, a risk of damage to the cornea) and, sometimes, continuous anaesthesia, but with pain (anaesthesia dolorosa).
  - Stereotactic gamma knife radiosurgery: Here the target is the trigeminal root, which is lesioned by convergent beams of radiation. It is the least invasive treatment, with the fewest adverse effects. It often takes 6 weeks or more to be considered successful.
  - Neurostimulation is a relatively new treatment option, though there are few studies available to define its role in the management of TN.

Follow-Up of Patients

Long-term follow-up as shared care is usually appropriate. If the patient has already had surgical intervention, secondary care is more appropriate.

TRIGEMINAL AUTONOMIC CEPHALALGIAS

See Chapter 45.

OTHER NEURALGIAS

Glossopharyngeal Neuralgia

Glossopharyngeal neuralgia is much less common than TN. The pain is of a similar nature, but affects the throat and ear, and is typically triggered by swallowing or coughing. Occasionally, glossopharyngeal neuralgia is secondary to lesions (often tumours) in the posterior cranial fossa or jugular foramen (jugular foramen syndrome) and there are then often lesions of the vagus (X) and accessory (XI) nerves. Carbamazepine is usually a less effective treatment than for TN and adequate relief of pain can be difficult.

Herpetic and Post-Herpetic Neuralgia

Herpes zoster (shingles) is often preceded and accompanied by neuralgia. Neuralgia may also persist after the rash has resolved. Pain in the trigeminal region may follow an attack of zoster, especially in older patients. In half of those patients, the pain resolves within 2 months but in others, it may continue for up to 2 years or longer. Post-herpetic neuralgia is defined by the International Headache Society as pain developing during the acute phase of herpes zoster and persisting greater than 6 months thereafter. Spontaneous improvement may follow, however, after about 18 to 36 months in some patients.

Post-herpetic neuralgia causes continuous burning pain that may be so intolerable that suicide can become a risk. Few analgesics relieve post-herpetic neuralgia, and treatment is difficult, but there may be relief using gabapentin, antidepressants (amitriptyline), carbamazepine, topical capsaicin 0.025% or lidocaine, transcutaneous electrical nerve stimulation (TENS — which increases beta-endorphin and met-enkephalin).

In acute zoster, a regimen of valaciclovir 1000 mg three times a day for 7 days plus gabapentin at an initial dose of 300 mg/day may be effective in ameliorating zoster and reducing post-herpetic neuralgia.

RECOMMENDED READING

Bendtsen, L., Zakrzewska, J.M., Abbott, J., et al., 2019. European Academy of Neurology guideline on trigeminal neuralgia. Eur. J. Neurol. 26 (6), 831–849.

Guidelines for the Management of Trigeminal Neuralgia 2021. Royal College of Surgeons of England. Available at: https://www.rcseng.ac.uk/dental-faculties/fds/publications-guidelines/clinical-guidelines/.

44

Persistent Idiopathic Facial Pain

> **KEY POINTS**
> - Persistent idiopathic facial pain (PIFP) is a chronic orofacial discomfort or pain disorder recurring daily for more than 2 h per day over more than 3 months, in the absence of a clinical neurological deficit.
> - PIFP is the current terminology for atypical facial pain.
> - The pain is poorly localised; persists for much or all of the day, and is often of a deep, dull, boring or burning character.
> - There are often multiple oral and/or other complaints and consultations.
> - Cognitive behavioural therapy or psychoactive medication may be needed.

INTRODUCTION

Persistent idiopathic facial pain (PIFP) is described as a persistent facial and/or oral pain, with varying presentations but recurring daily for more than 2 hours per day over more than 3 months, in the absence of clinical neurological deficit. The pain cannot be attributed to any pathological process. It is a diagnosis that can be difficult to make since it is reached only by the exclusion of organic disease. The current theory is that PIFP is a disproportionate reaction to a mild injury, but the exact pathophysiology is still unknown.

Atypical odontalgia (AO), a term that should no longer be used, is included as a subtype of PIFP. AO is a neuropathic syndrome and it has been widely referred to as 'phantom toothache'.

EPIDEMIOLOGY

- PIFP is rare. PIFP may account for up to 20% of the patient population in orofacial pain clinics.
- Mean age of onset is in the mid-40s.
- Most patients are female.
- There are no geographic factors implicated.
- There are often recent adverse life events, such as bereavement or family illness and/or dental or oral interventive procedures.

AETIOLOGY AND PATHOGENESIS

The mouth and para-oral tissues have among the richest sensory innervation in the body. Furthermore, a large part of the sensory homunculus on the cerebral cortex receives information from orofacial structures. PIFP is considered a neuropathic pain syndrome. Studies show increased neuronal excitability at the brainstem level, disturbed inhibitory function of the prefrontal cortex and alterations in the dopamine systems associated with pain transmission and modulation. Sensory changes consistent with neuropathy or neuropathic pain have also been shown. Positron emission tomography in persons with PIFP shows enhanced cerebral activity, suggesting an enhanced alerting mechanism in response to peripheral stimuli. Psychiatric and psychosocial disability have often been associated with PIFP, in particular anxiety and depression.

CLINICAL FEATURES

- Onset is often associated with minor surgical or other invasive dental procedures either as the initiating event or as an attempt to manage the pain.
- The location of the pain is unrelated to the anatomical distribution of trigeminal nerve innervation, poorly localised and sometimes crosses the midline to involve the other side or moves to another site. Usually unilateral but may be bilateral in up to 40%.
- The pain is long-lasting (years) and often of a deep, dull, boring or burning type, persisting for much or all of the day, but does not wake the patient from sleep. There are few, if any, periods of remission.
- Patients rarely use analgesics to try and control the pain.
- Anxiety and depression are common, and pain may be aggravated by emotional stress.
- Objective signs are lacking.
- Investigations are normal.
- Response to treatment is poor.

- May coexist with other chronic orofacial pain or headache syndromes.
- There are often multiple oral and/or other complaints, such as:
  - dry mouth
  - bad taste
  - headaches
  - chronic back pain
  - irritable bowel syndrome
  - dysmenorrhoea.
- The pain may lead patients to seek dental intervention but to little avail. Patients may seek conservative dentistry, but this is rarely helpful — often rather to the contrary. The saga of pain may lead the clinician eventually to undertake endodontics or exodontics.
- There is a high level of utilisation of healthcare services. There have often already been multiple consultations and unsuccessful attempts at treatment. Many sufferers persist in blaming organic diseases (or the clinician!) for their pain.

DIAGNOSIS

Making this diagnosis is not simple and follows a process of elimination of other potential causes of orofacial pain. PIFP occurs in the trigeminal nerve territory, and the pain may sometimes be as severe as trigeminal neuralgia, but it is usually different in severity, character and distribution. PIFP is usually diffuse, persistent, burning, aching, dull or crushing, whereas trigeminal neuralgia is characterised by quick episodes of jabbing or lancinating pain in a division of the trigeminal nerve.

An effort should be made to exclude all pathology. Examination of at least the mouth, perioral structures and cranial nerves, and imaging (tooth/jaw/sinus/skull radiography, MRI/CT scan with particular attention to the skull base) to exclude organic diseases, such as space-occupying or demyelinating diseases, are important. MRI scan of the head has a better yield than CT because of its better resolution of the brain stem and cranial nerves. PIFP is diagnosed when the clinician has exhausted all possible alternatives.

The findings on clinical examination in patients with IFP include:
- no erythema, tenderness or swelling in the area
- no obvious odontogenic or other local cause for the pain
- total lack of objective physical (including neurological) signs.

Investigation findings include (Table 44.1):
- all imaging studies are negative
- all blood investigations are normal.

PIFP is a clinical diagnosis, only made after careful dental and otolaryngologic evaluation, and other tests rule out organic causes.

TREATMENT

Few patients with PIFP have spontaneous remission and thus treatment is indicated. The approach to management should consider the patient's beliefs about pain and the impact of the

TABLE 44.1 Investigations That Might Be Helpful in Diagnosis/Prognosis/Management in Patients Suspected of Having Atypical (Idiopathic) Facial Pain[a]

In Most Cases	In Some Cases
Tooth/jaw/sinus/skull radiography	Full blood picture
MRI/CT	Serum ferritin, vitamin B_{12} and corrected whole blood folate levels
	ESR
	Serology (Lyme disease)
	ANA
	Psychological assessment
	Neurological opinion

[a]See text for details and glossary for abbreviations.

TABLE 44.2 Regimens That Might Be Helpful in Management of Patients Suspected of Having Persistent Idiopathic (Atypical) Facial Pain

Regimen	Use in Primary or Secondary Care
Beneficial	Patient education
	Cognitive behavioural therapy
Likely to be beneficial	Amitriptyline
	Venlafaxine
	Fluoxetine
	Duloxetine
	Gabapentin
	Nortriptyline
Emerging therapies	Pulsed radiofrequency of sphenopalatine ganglion
	Repetitive transcranial magnetic stimulation
	Hypnosis

pain disorder on their quality of life (Table 44.2). A multidisciplinary approach is needed for the management of PIFP.
- Patient education on the condition is a very important aspect of management.
- The patient should be discouraged from any further invasive interventions such as restorative treatment, endodontia or exodontia since these are rarely successful. Any active dental or oral surgical treatment, in the absence of any specific indication, should be avoided.
- A specialist referral may be appropriate.
- Considering the chronicity and distress that result, behavioural interventions such as cognitive behavioural therapy may be indicated.

The clinician should clearly acknowledge the reality of the patient's symptoms and distress and never attempt to trivialise or dismiss them. Goal setting which includes helping the patient cope with symptoms rather than attempting any impossible cure is an important aspect of management. Clinicians should avoid repeat examinations or investigations at subsequent appointments since this only serves to reinforce illness behaviour and health fears.

Pharmacological treatment with antidepressants, antiepileptic or other drugs can also be tried (see Table 44.2). A trial of an antidepressant may be appropriate, explaining that this is being used to treat the symptoms rather than any depression and that antidepressants have been shown in controlled trials to be effective for this problem, even in non-depressed persons. The pain reduction achieved with antidepressants exceeds that produced by placebos. Amitriptyline is the primary choice starting at 10 mg at night, given as tablets or solution, increasing if needed by 10 mg each week to 50 mg. It is important to trial antidepressants for a sufficient duration (e.g. 6 to 12 weeks) before determining whether the medication is not effective. Trials on duloxetine, venlafaxine and anticonvulsants have shown beneficial effects. Surgery is rarely appropriate for the treatment of PIFP. Pulsed radiofrequency treatment of the sphenopalatine ganglion has been reportedly effective. High frequency repetitive transcranial magnetic stimulation (rTMS) is a promising new therapy in patients with neuropathic orofacial pain. Hypnosis might also be a promising approach. A conservative, multidisciplinary approach is recommended.

FOLLOW-UP OF PATIENTS

Long-term follow-up as shared care is usually appropriate.

RECOMMENDED READING

Benoliel, R., Gaul, C., 2017. Persistent idiopathic facial pain. Cephalalgia. 37 (7), 680—691.

Maarbjerg, S., Wolfram, F., Heinskou, T.B., Rochat, P., Gozalov, A., Brennum, J., Olesen, J., Bendtsen, L., 2017. Persistent idiopathic facial pain — a prospective systematic study of clinical characteristics and neuroanatomical findings at 3.0 Tesla MRI. Cephalalgia. 37 (13), 1231—1240.

Zakrzewska, J.M., 2016. Chronic/persistent idiopathic facial pain. Neurosurg. Clin. N. Am. 27 (3), 345—351.

Headache

KEY POINTS
- Headache is defined as a pain in the region above the orbitomeatal line.
- Headache disorders are common.
- Tension-type headache (TTH) and migraine are the most common types of headaches affecting the population.
- 'Red flag' features should increase suspicion of a dangerous underlying aetiology and prompt further brain imaging.

EPIDEMIOLOGY

- Headache disorders are common.
- The lifetime prevalence of any headache is estimated to be 93% in men and 99% in women.
- Tension-type headache (TTH) and migraine are the most common headache disorders. The lifetime prevalence of TTH is 30% to 78%. Migraine affects up to 12% of the population. Trigeminal autonomic cephalalgias (TACs) are relatively rare (1%), while cluster headache has a prevalence of 0.09% to 0.32%.
- Prevalence of migraine is highest in North America and Western Europe.
- Migraines typically occur in early adult life and decline in the 40s and 50s.

INTRODUCTION

The International Headache Society (IHS) has a classification of headache referred to as the International Classification of Headache Disorders, Third Edition (ICHD-3). It divides headaches into primary and secondary headaches, along with cranial neuralgias and other facial pain conditions. TTH and migraine are the most common types of headaches. TTH is more prevalent than migraine.

Obtaining a thorough history is important to focus the clinical examination and determine if further investigations are required. The aim of the history and examination is to exclude underlying pathology and assess for secondary causes of headache. The history should include:
- Onset — age of onset
- Timing — duration of a single episode, frequency, clinical course, sudden/gradual
- Location
- Frequency, intensity and duration of the attack
- Number of headache days per month
- Unilateral/bilateral
- Character
- Precipitating factors/exacerbating factors — altered sleep-wake cycle, physical activity, stress, food or alcohol, fluctuations in hormone levels, lying down or standing up, recent trauma
- Relieving factors
- Radiation
- Associated symptoms — presence or absence of aura and prodrome, nausea/vomiting, photopsia, photophobia, neck stiffness, seizures, visual disturbances, lacrimation, rhinorrhoea, allodynia
- Response to previous treatments
- Family history
- History of trauma
- Severity/impact on quality of life/disability — days off work/school.
  The clinical examination should include:
- Blood pressure and pulse
- Palpation of the head, neck and shoulders
- Assessment of temporal and neck arteries
- Examination of the cervical spine and neck muscles
- Neurologic examination: assessment of mental status, cranial nerve examination, fundoscopy, and motor, reflex, cerebellar (coordination) and sensory tests
- Examination of the teeth and oral cavity.

There are no routine recommended lab tests for headaches. Thyroid abnormalities, anaemia or electrolyte abnormalities may contribute to a headache disorder. In older patients, ESR and CRP may be appropriate to evaluate for vasculitis and giant cell arteritis (GCA).

The following features indicate those who are **unlikely** to have a serious underlying cause for headache:
- Typical features of primary headaches
- Prior history of similar headache
- Absence of neurologic findings
- No sudden change in usual headache pattern
- No new or concerning findings on history or examination
- Typical headache pattern
- No red flags for headaches

Imaging is often not required in these cases.

'Red flag' features (Table 45.1) that should increase suspicion of a dangerous underlying headache can be summarised using the mnemonic 'SNOOP10':
- **S**ystemic symptoms — fever, weight loss, stiff neck
- **N**eurological symptoms or abnormal signs — cognitive impairment, impaired consciousness, personality change
- **O**nset — sudden, abrupt, thunderclap
- **O**lder — new-onset and progressive headache, above 50 years of age
- 10 '**P**'
  - Pattern change (increased frequency) or recent onset of new headache
  - Papilloedema
  - Precipitating factors (Valsalva, sneezing, coughing, exercise, etc.)
  - Positional aggravation (orthostatic headache)
  - Progressive headache and atypical presentations, headaches not responding to treatment
  - Pregnancy or puerperium

- Painful eye with autonomic features
- Post-traumatic onset of headache
- Pathology such as HIV, cancer and head trauma
- Painkiller (analgesic) overuse (medication overuse headache) or new drug at onset of headache.

Any of these findings should prompt further brain imaging with magnetic resonance imaging (MRI) or computed tomography (CT).

Additional tests may be indicated depending on the underlying cause:
- Lumbar puncture — for suspected meningitis, inflammatory process, malignancy, subarachnoid haemorrhage
- Electroencephalogram (EEG) — for any form of suspected seizures
- Temporal artery biopsy — if GCA is suspected.

MIGRAINE

Migraine is a chronic, genetically determined, episodic, recurrent headache disorder with attacks lasting 4 to 72 hours. It is most common in those aged 30 to 39 and more frequent in women. Migraine is in most instances inherited.

The headaches are often unilateral, pulsating in quality, moderate to severe in intensity, aggravated by physical activity (such as walking) and associated with nausea and/or vomiting, photophobia and phonophobia (sensitivity to light or noise).

Migraines with aura are characterised by recurrent attacks, of unilateral fully reversible visual, sensory or other central nervous system symptoms (speech and/or language, motor, brainstem, retinal) that usually develop gradually and are usually followed by headache and associated migraine symptoms. Migraine with aura occurs in approximately 15% to 30% of cases. Some patients may experience aura without headache.

Risk factors include
- a positive family history
- motion sickness in childhood
- increased caffeine intake
- female sex, menstruation
- obesity (also associated with an increased frequency and severity)
- stress
- sleep disturbance
- visual stimuli
- weather changes
- nitrates
- fasting
- wine
- high altitude
- overuse of headache medications.

The old vascular theory of migraine, which attributed aura to constriction and headache to reflex dilation of cranial blood vessels, has been discredited. Current evidence suggests the brain is hyperexcitable to a variety of stimuli. Neurogenic inflammation of first-division trigeminal sensory neurons that innervate large vessels and meninges of the brain result in headache. When activated, the trigeminal neurons release

TABLE 45.1	Red Flag Features That Should Increase Suspicion of a Dangerous Underlying Headache (SNOOP10)
Systemic symptoms — fever, weight loss, stiff neck	
Neurological symptoms or abnormal signs — cognitive impairment, impaired consciousness, personality change	
Onset — sudden, abrupt, thunderclap	
Older — new-onset and progressive headache, >50 years of age	
10 'P'	
Pattern change (increased frequency) or recent onset of new headache	
Papilloedema	
Precipitating factors (Valsalva, sneezing, coughing, exercise, etc.)	
Positional aggravation (orthostatic headache)	
Progressive headache and atypical presentations, headaches not responding to treatment	
Pregnancy or puerperium	
Painful eye with autonomic features	
Post-traumatic onset of headache	
Pathology such as HIV, cancer, head trauma	
Painkiller (analgesic) overuse (medication overuse headache) or new drug at onset of headache	

substances (substance P, calcitonin gene-related peptide and neurokinin A) that cause vasodilation, plasma protein extravasation into surrounding tissue, and platelet activation. Aura is caused by neuronal dysfunction.

A typical migraine attack progresses through four phases: the prodrome, the aura, the headache and the postdrome.

- **Prodrome** — 24 to 48 hours prior to the onset of headache. Symptoms include increased yawning, irritability, food cravings and low mood.
- **Aura** — duration no longer than one hour and complete reversibility. Most often visual, but can also be auditory, verbal, somatosensory (e.g. pain, paraesthesia) or motor (e.g. jerking) disturbances.
- **Headache** — often unilateral, throbbing or pulsatile, may be accompanied by nausea +/− vomiting, photophobia or phonophobia. Headache can last 4 hours to several days and often resolve in sleep.
- **Postdrome** — patients often feel drained or exhausted.

The diagnosis is based on the history and clinical examination (Table 45.2). No laboratory tests or imaging studies are required.

Treatment

Treatment involves:
- identification and avoidance of triggers
- medication to treat the acute attack and to prevent future attacks.

For mild to moderate migraine attacks not associated with vomiting or severe nausea, monotherapy nonsteroidal antiinflammatory drugs (NSAIDs) or paracetamol may be an effective initial treatment. If unresponsive, the combination of an NSAID with a 5HT1 agonist (triptan) may be effective. The combination of paracetamol and an anti-emetic is equivalent in efficacy to oral sumatriptan with fewer adverse effects.

For moderate to severe migraine attacks, a triptan or combination therapy of NSAIDs or triptans (e.g. sumatriptan and ibuprofen) can be used. Combining treatment improves the efficacy of acute treatment. Ergotamine is approved for the acute treatment of migraine.

Prophylactic treatment is indicated if the headaches occur more than 2 days per week, are long-lasting or impact on quality of life. The main drug treatments used for the prevention of migraine are:
- anticonvulsants (e.g. valproate and topiramate)
- tricyclic antidepressants (e.g. amitriptyline)
- beta-blockers (e.g. propranolol).

Non-pharmacological therapy may be beneficial including relaxation techniques, acupuncture and cognitive behavioural therapy. Botulinum toxin type A has been found to reduce migraine attacks and improve quality of life.

TENSION-TYPE-HEADACHE

TTH is very common and may co-exist with migraine. The exact mechanisms of TTH are not known but peripheral pain mechanisms most likely play a role. Episodes of headache are typically generalised throughout the head, often bilateral,

TABLE 45.2 The ICHD-3 Diagnostic Criteria for Migraine

Migraine without aura:
(A) At least five attacks fulfilling criteria B through D
(B) Headache attacks lasting 4—72 h (untreated or unsuccessfully treated)
(C) Headache has at least two of the following characteristics:
- Unilateral location
- Pulsating quality
- Moderate or severe pain intensity
- Aggravation by or causing avoidance of routine physical activity (e.g. walking or climbing stairs)
(D) During headache at least one of the following:
- Nausea, vomiting or both
- Photophobia and phonophobia
(E) Not better accounted for by another ICHD-3 diagnosis
Migraine with aura:
(A) At least two attacks fulfilling criteria B and C
(B) One or more of the following fully reversible aura symptoms:
- Visual
- Sensory
- Speech and/or language
- Motor
- Brainstem
- Retinal
(C) At least three of the following six characteristics:
- At least one aura symptom spreads gradually over ≥5 min
- Two or more symptoms occur in succession
- Each individual aura symptom lasts 5—60 min
- At least one aura symptom is unilateral
- At least one aura symptom is positive[a]
- The aura is accompanied, or followed within 60 min, by a headache
(D) Not better accounted for by another ICHD-3 diagnosis

ICHD-3, International Classification of Headache Disorder, Third Edition.
[a]Scintillations and pins and needles are examples of positive symptoms.

pressure-like or tightening in quality. The pain can last from minutes to days. It is not exacerbated by physical activity. There is no associated nausea.

TRIGEMINAL AUTONOMIC CEPHALALGIAS

TACs are a group of relatively rare headache disorders characterised by moderate to severe, short-lived pain in the trigeminal distribution with unilateral autonomic features (Table 45.3).

1. Cluster Headache

Cluster headache is very rare. Age at onset is usually 20 to 40 years with men affected three times more often than women. It is characterised by attacks of severe, strictly unilateral pain

TABLE 45.3 **Clinical Features of Trigeminal Autonomic Cephalalgias and Hemicrania Continua**

	Cluster Headache	Paroxysmal Hemicrania	SUNCT	Hemicrania Continua
Pain type	Stabbing, boring	Throbbing, boring, stabbing	Burning, stabbing, sharp	Throbbing, sharp, pressure
Pain severity	Severe	Severe	Severe	Baseline: mild, moderate or severe Exacerbations: severe
Pain site	Orbit, temple	Orbit, temple	Periorbital	Orbit, temple, hemicranial
Attack frequency	1/alternate day–8/day	1–40/day (>5/day for more than half the time)	3–200/day	Daily and continuous
Duration of attack	15–180 minutes	2–30 minutes	5–240 seconds	Continuous
Autonomic features	Yes	Yes	Yes	Yes
Alcohol trigger	Yes	One-fifth	No	Yes
Abortive treatment	Sumatriptan injection Sumatriptan intranasal Oxygen	None**	None**	Indomethacin
First-line prophylactic therapy	Verapamil	Indomethacin	Lamotrigine	Indomethacin

which is orbital, supraorbital or temporal. Attacks last 15 to 180 minutes and occur once every other day to eight times a day, with intervals of no headache between attacks. Attacks may occur at the same time of the day. The pain is associated with autonomic signs or symptoms on the side of the pain such as ipsilateral conjunctival injection, tearing, nasal congestion, rhinorrhoea, forehead and facial sweating, miosis +/− ptosis, eyelid oedema and/or a sense of restlessness or agitation.

Treatment: For acute attacks, treat with 100% oxygen for 20 minutes or triptans (e.g. subcutaneous or intranasal sumatriptan).

2. Paroxysmal Hemicrania

Characterised by attacks of severe, strictly unilateral pain which is orbital, supraorbital +/− temporal and lasts 2 to 30 minutes. There is no gender predominance with onset in adulthood. Attacks occur several times a day, often greater than 5 per day. The attacks are usually associated with ipsilateral conjunctival injection +/− tearing, nasal congestion +/− rhinorrhoea, forehead and facial sweating, miosis +/− ptosis and eyelid oedema.

Treatment: Patients respond to indomethacin. The starting dose for adults is 75 mg daily in three divided doses (25 mg three times daily). The dose should be increased to 150 mg daily (50 mg three times daily) if there is an incomplete response after 3 days. The dose may need to be further increased to 225 mg daily (75 mg three times daily) for 10 days for partial responders.

3. Short-Lasting Unilateral Neuralgiform Headache Attacks

Two subtypes are recognised: Short-lasting unilateral neuralgiform headache attacks with conjunctival injection and tearing (SUNCT) and short lasting unilateral neuralgiform headache attacks with cranial autonomic symptoms (SUNA).

Characterised by attacks of moderate or severe, strictly unilateral head pain which is orbital, supraorbital, temporal and/or other trigeminal distribution. The attacks last 1 to 600 seconds as single stabs, a series of stabs or in a saw-tooth pattern.

Attacks occur at least once a day. The episode is usually associated with autonomic symptoms or signs on the same side of the pain such as conjunctival injection +/− tearing, nasal congestion +/− rhinorrhoea, eyelid oedema, forehead and facial sweating or forehead and facial flushing, the sensation of fullness in the ear, miosis +/− ptosis.

In contrast to trigeminal neuralgia, SUNCT and SUNA can be triggered without a refractory period after each attack.

Treatment: Lamotrigine is used as an initial preventive therapy, starting at 25 mg daily for 2 weeks, then increasing to 50 mg daily for 2 weeks. The dose may be further titrated as tolerated.

HEMICRANIA CONTINUA

Persistent (>3 months), strictly unilateral headache, associated with ipsilateral conjunctival injection +/− tearing, nasal congestion +/− rhinorrhoea, forehead and facial sweating, miosis +/− ptosis and eyelid oedema, with a sense of restlessness or agitation.

Treatment: The headache responds to indomethacin.

HEADACHE ATTRIBUTED TO GIANT CELL ARTERITIS

GCA should be considered in patients greater than 50 years with new-onset or worsening headaches. If untreated, permanent blindness may occur due to anterior ischaemic optic neuropathy. Patients with GCA are at risk of cerebral ischaemic events and dementia. The headache features are varied, but may be associated with jaw claudication, muscle pain and scalp tenderness.

Diagnosis: Temporal artery biopsy is the diagnostic procedure of choice. Serial sections should be sampled because the temporal artery may appear uninvolved in some areas (skip lesions).

Treatment: It commonly improves or resolves within 3 days of high-dose corticosteroid treatment.

HEADACHE ATTRIBUTED TO TEMPOROMANDIBULAR DISORDER

This headache is caused by a disorder involving elements of the temporomandibular joint(s), muscles of mastication +/− associated structures on one or both sides. The headache is usually most prominent in the temporal region(s), preauricular area(s) and/or masseter muscle(s) and aggravated by jaw movement, function (such as chewing) and parafunctional habit. It is provoked by palpation of the temporalis muscle or passive movement of the jaw.

Treatment: Treatment of the temporomandibular disorder (see Chapter 42).

RECOMMENDED READING

1. www.ihs-headache.org/en/resources/guidelines/.
2. www.ichd-3.org/.
3. www.bash.org.uk.
4. www.nice.org.uk/guidance/cg150.

Burning Mouth Syndrome

> **KEY POINTS**
> - Burning mouth syndrome (BMS) is the term used when symptoms, usually described as a burning sensation, exist in the absence of clinically identifiable oral mucosal disease when a medical or dental cause has been excluded.
> - BMS is defined as 'an intraoral burning or dysaesthetic sensation, recurring daily for more than 2 hours per day over more than 3 months, without clinically evident causative lesions'.
> - BMS is seen predominantly in postmenopausal women.
> - BMS most frequently affects the tongue, with persistent discomfort but can affect other intraoral sites.
> - Treatment of primary BMS is difficult.

INTRODUCTION

A burning sensation in the mouth may be a primary condition, or secondary to identifiable causes (Fig. 46.1). Burning mouth syndrome (BMS) — also known as oral dysaesthesia, glossodynia or stomatodynia — is the term used when symptoms, usually described as a burning sensation, exist in the absence of clinically identifiable oral mucosal disease when a medical or dental cause has been excluded. The International Headache Society defines BMS as an 'intraoral burning or dysaesthetic sensation, recurring daily for more than 2 hours per day over more than 3 months, without clinically evident causative lesions'.

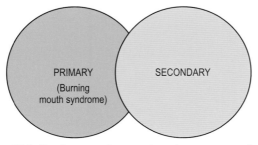

Fig. 46.1 Burning sensation may be primary or secondary.

EPIDEMIOLOGY

- BMS is seen especially in middle-aged or older patients. It is most frequent in postmenopausal women, with a general population prevalence of around 1%.
- BMS is seen in women in a ratio of about 10:1.
- BMS is seen worldwide.

PREDISPOSING FACTORS, AETIOLOGY AND PATHOGENESIS

- There is consistent evidence for neuropathic alterations in primary BMS. Damage to peripheral small nerve fibres can produce a burning sensation and may result from deficiency, endocrine disorders, viral infection and Sjogren syndrome. Tongue biopsies have shown a lower density of small fibres in symptomatic areas suggesting damage of peripheral small fibres as a possible cause. Nerve growth factor (NGF) peptide and tryptase activity appear significantly and persistently raised in saliva in BMS. It can also follow damage to the cauda tympani nerve.
- In Parkinson disease, 40% of patients report burning mouth. The reduction in dopamine in the nigrostriatal neurons and the putamen in primary BMS patients found by positron emission tomography (PET) studies are similar to PET findings in early Parkinson disease.
- The predisposition of BMS in peri-/postmenopausal females has suggested dysfunction of the hypothalamus-pituitary-gonadal (HPG) axis may play a role.
- There is a high prevalence of psychiatric symptoms and/or disorders in BMS: Anxiety, depression, somatisation, cancer phobia and insomnia are the most common diagnoses seen in this patient group.

CLINICAL FEATURES

BMS most frequently affects the tongue, especially its tip and anterior two thirds but it can also affect the anterior palate or, less commonly, the lips or gingivae. Usually, symptoms are bilateral and symmetrical. Symptoms of BMS vary from

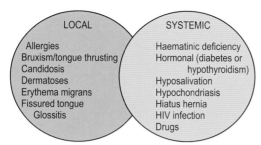

Fig. 46.2 Burning sensation may have local or systemic causes.

occurring mildly with occasional symptoms-free days, to unremitting constant burning. The pain tends to be worse as the day progresses. Dry mouth and dysgeusia (altered taste perception) are also frequently described. Frequent comorbid conditions include depression and anxiety, chronic fatigue and gastrointestinal symptoms.

The symptoms are variable and may be:
- moderately severe (visual analogue scale 5 to 8)

- relieved by eating and drinking, in contrast to pain caused by organic lesions, which is typically aggravated by eating
- persistent though fluctuating in severity, but do not disturb sleep
- prolonged.

Patients uncommonly use analgesics to try to control the symptoms. There may be changes in sleep patterns and mood and there have often already been multiple consultations and attempts at treatment.

DIAGNOSIS

BMS is the diagnosis when all organic causes have been excluded, investigations are all negative, and examination shows no:
- clinically detectable signs of mucosal disease
- tenderness or swelling of the tongue or affected area
- neurological or other objective signs.

Defined clinical conditions that must be excluded, since they can also present with a burning sensation, including (Fig. 46.2) (see Algorithm 46.1):

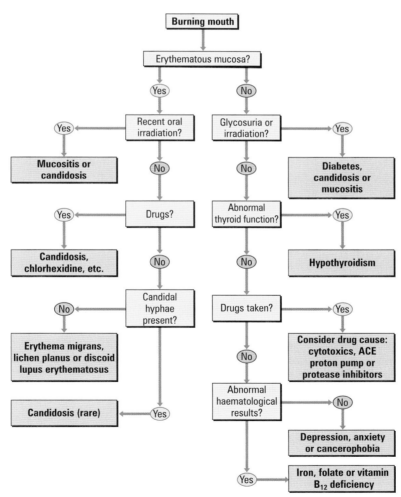

Algorithm 46.1 Burning mouth syndrome: diagnosis.

- **A**llergies (e.g. denture allergy)
- **B**ruxism/tongue thrusting/restricted tongue space from poor denture construction
- **C**andidosis
- **D**ermatoses such as lichen planus, **d**ry mouth (Sjogren syndrome), **d**iabetes and **d**rugs (cytotoxics, angiotensin-converting enzyme [ACE] inhibitors, clonazepam, antidepressants, hormone replacement therapy (HRT), proton pump inhibitors (PPIs) or protease inhibitors (PIs), **d**eficiencies (iron, zinc, vitamin B_{12} or folic acid)
- **E**rythema migrans (geographic tongue)
- **F**issured tongue
- **G**lossitis such as caused by haematinic (iron, folic acid or vitamin B) deficiency in about 30%
- **H**ormonal disorders (such as diabetes and hypothyroidism).

Investigations indicated may include psychological screening using, for example, the hospital anxiety and depression scale (HADS), and laboratory screening (Table 46.1) in order to exclude:

- Anaemia, vitamin, iron or trace element (zinc) deficiency
- Diabetes
- Hypothyroidism
- Hyposalivation (salivary flow rates)
- Candidosis (oral rinse).

TREATMENT

- Few patients have spontaneous remission in the short term, and thus treatment is usually indicated (Fig. 46.3); BMS may be controlled by neuropathic drugs. Patient information is an important aspect of management and often reassurance is very helpful in alleviating anxiety from the outset.
- Active dental or oral surgical treatment, or attempts at 'hormone replacement', in the absence of any specific indication, should be avoided. Attention to factors such as haematinic deficiencies may occasionally be indicated.
- Patients should avoid anything that aggravates symptoms, such as sparkling wines, citrus drinks and spices.
- It is important to clearly acknowledge the reality of the patient's symptoms and distress and never to trivialise or dismiss them.

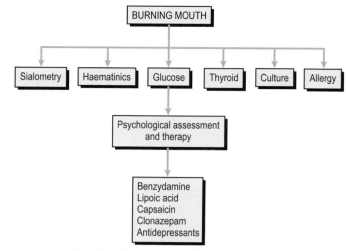

Fig. 46.3 Management of burning sensation.

- Set goals, which include helping the patient cope with the symptoms, rather than attempting an impossible cure.
- Do not repeat examinations or investigations at subsequent appointments, since this only serves to reinforce illness behaviour and health fears.
- Cognitive—behavioural therapy or a specialist referral may be indicated.
- Some patients respond to medication — for example to:
  - topical medication: benzydamine rinse or spray; capsaicin cream 0.025% (Zacin) or a clonazepam tablet 0.5 mg sucked for 2 minutes before discarding
  - mouth wetting agents (for BMS patients with hyposalivation)
  - α-lipoic acid systemically
  - HRT
- Antidepressants in low doses (Table 46.2) have shown in controlled trials to be effective for BMS, whether or not the patient is depressed.

TABLE 46.1 Investigations That Might Be Helpful in Diagnosis/Prognosis/Management in Some Patients Suspected of Having Burning Mouth Syndrome (Oral Dysaesthesia)[a]

In Most Cases	In Some Cases
Full blood picture	Allergy testing
Serum ferritin, vitamin B_{12} and folate levels	Culture and sensitivity
ESR	Psychological assessment
Sialometry	
Thyroid function tests	
HbA1c	
Zinc	

[a]See text for details and glossary for abbreviations.

TABLE 46.2 Regimens That Might Be Helpful in Management of Patient Suspected of Having Burning Mouth Syndrome

Regimen	Use in Primary Care
Likely to be beneficial	Cognitive behavioural therapy
	Topical capsaicin
	Topical clonazepam
	Gabapentin
	Antidepressants (amitriptyline, nortriptyline, dosulepin, doxepin, fluoxetine, venlafaxine)
Unproven effectiveness	Alpha-lipoic acid
	Hormone replacement
Supportive	Benzydamine
	Diet with little acidic, spicy or citrus content
	Lidocaine
	Mouth wetting agents

FOLLOW-UP OF PATIENTS

Long-term follow-up in primary care, or shared care is usually appropriate.

RECOMMENDED READING

Ariyawardana, A., Chmieliauskaite, M., Farag, A.M., et al., 2019. World Workshop on Oral Medicine VII: burning mouth syndrome: a systematic review of disease definitions and diagnostic criteria utilized in randomized clinical trials. Oral. Dis. 25 (Suppl 1), 141–156.

Feller, L., Fourie, J., Bouckaert, M., et al., 2017. Burning mouth syndrome: aetiopathogenesis and principles of management. Pain. Res. Manag. 1926269.

Galli, F., Lodi, G., Sardella, A., Vegni, E., 2017. Role of psychological factors in burning mouth syndrome: a systematic review and meta-analysis. Cephalalgia. 37, 265.

Lauria, G., Majorana, A., Borgna, M., et al., 2005. Trigeminal small-fiber sensory neuropathy causes burning mouth syndrome. Pain. 115, 332.

McMillan, R., Forssell, H., Buchanan, J.A., Glenny, A.M., Weldon, J.C., Zakrzewska, J.M., 2016. Interventions for treating burning mouth syndrome. Cochrane Database Syst. Rev. 11, CD002779.

47

Sensory and Motor Changes

INTRODUCTION

Sensory, motor or autonomic neuropathies may affect the orofacial region. The main orofacial sensory and motor lesions are shown in Table 47.1.

Sensory changes most frequently follow nerve damage from trauma. Weakness of the facial muscles is most commonly seen in neurological disorders and presents with paralysis (palsy) but is also seen in primary muscle disease and neuromuscular junction disorders. In these cases, it is then usually symmetrical. The uncommon causes include myasthenia gravis, dystrophia myotonica and facioscapulohumeral dystrophy.

SENSORY CHANGES

Normal facial sensation, mediated by the trigeminal nerve, is important to protect the skin, mucosae and especially the cornea of the eye from damage. Facial sensory changes can be caused by lesions of a sensory branch of the trigeminal nerve or the central connections (Fig. 47.1). Sensory loss is categorised as: may lead to sensory awareness that is:
- anaesthesia: complete inability to perceive pain, temperature, touch or vibration
- hypoaesthesia: reduced ability to perceive pain, temperature, touch or vibration
- paraesthesia: abnormal sensation without a stimulus, often 'pins and needles', tingling or burning — and may arise during recovery from nerve damage
- hyperaesthesia: abnormal increase in sensitivity to stimuli
- analgesia: complete insensitivity to painful stimuli.

Sensory defects may lead to unrecognised damage from trauma or burns and are occasionally associated with hyperaesthesia.

AETIOLOGY AND PATHOGENESIS

Causes of lesions affecting the trigeminal nerve are shown in Box 47.1.

Extracranial Causes

Extracranial causes of facial sensory loss are most common and include damage to the trigeminal nerve. Lesions in the peripheral nerve usually present as hypoaesthesia, or anaesthesia. Lesions involving single nerves cause disturbance in the sensory distribution of the nerve.

Trauma

This is the usual cause of sensory loss, especially after orthognathic or cancer surgery. Ipsilateral hypoaesthesia or anaesthesia usually results. If the nerves are stretched or compressed (neuropraxia), there is often only hypoaesthesia, and recovery of sensation is speedy, typically within days. However, if the nerves are severed (neurotmesis), anaesthesia is profound and recovery is delayed for months, often accompanied by paraesthesia or hyperaesthesia. Recovery is sometimes not complete: repair may be indicated.
- Trauma to the mandibular division can have a variety of causes:
  - inferior alveolar local analgesic injections
  - fractures of the mandibular body or angle
  - surgery (particularly surgical extraction of lower third molars, osteotomies or jaw resections) or even endodontics or implants.
- Trauma to the mental nerve can have a variety of causes:
- operations in the region
- pressure from a denture — the mental foramen is close beneath a lower denture and there is the anaesthesia of the lower lip on the affected side.

TABLE 47.1   Main Orofacial Neuropathies

Features	V	VII
Major	Sensory loss in the face	Weak muscles of facial expression
Minor	Jaw movements impaired	Reduced sense of taste in anterior ⅔ of tongue

- Trauma to the lingual nerve can arise especially during resections or removal of lower third molars, particularly when the lingual split technique is used.
- Trauma to branches of the maxillary division of the trigeminal nerve may be caused by direct trauma or fractures (usually Le Fort II or III middle-third facial fractures) or surgery.

Bone Disease

- Osteomyelitis in the mandible may affect the inferior alveolar nerve to cause labial anaesthesia.
- Osteochemonecrosis.

- Paget disease.
- Osteopetrosis.

Neuropathies

- Drugs occasionally produce hypoaesthesia (see Box 47.1).
- Multiple sclerosis may cause sensory loss.
- Diabetes may produce a neuropathy.
- Infections such as syphilis, leprosy, Lyme disease or herpesviruses are rare causes.

Neoplastic Disease

- Oral carcinomas may invade the jaws to cause anaesthesia.
- Skull base or central malignancies such as osteosarcoma may produce a similar pattern.
- Nasopharyngeal carcinomas may invade the pharyngeal wall to infiltrate the mandibular division of the trigeminal nerve, causing pain and sensory loss in the region of the inferior alveolar, lingual and auriculotemporal nerve distributions; invade the levator palati to cause soft palate immobility;

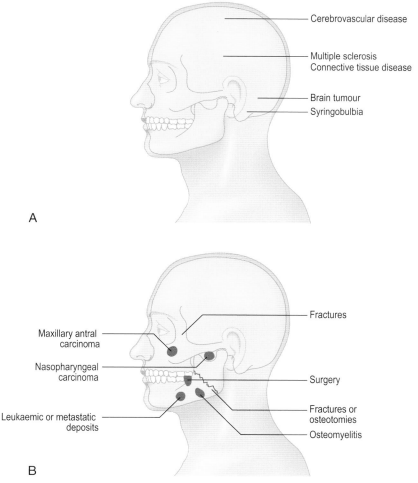

Fig. 47.1 Causes of sensory loss: (A) intracranial; (B) extracranial.

BOX 47.1 Causes of Facial Sensory Loss

Extracranial
- Trauma (e.g. surgical, fractures) to inferior dental, lingual, mental or infraorbital nerves
- Inflammatory:
  - osteomyelitis
  - infections — neurosyphilis, HIV infection, herpesviruses, tuberculosis, leprosy, diphtheria, Lyme disease
  - Vasculitis
- Neoplastic:
  - carcinoma of antrum or nasopharynx
  - metastatic tumours
  - leukaemic deposits
  - paraneoplastic syndrome

Intracranial
- Trauma (e.g. surgical treatment of trigeminal neuralgia)
- Inflammatory:
  - multiple sclerosis/demyelination
  - sarcoidosis
  - connective tissue disorders
  - infections
  - Basilar meningitis
- Neoplastic:
  - cerebral tumours (metastases, glioma, meningioma, acoustic neuroma)
- Vascular:
  - cerebrovascular disease
  - aneurysms
- Syringobulbia
- Drugs (see Table 33.18)
- Others:
  - osteomyelitis
  - Paget disease
  - osteopetrosis
  - benign trigeminal neuropathy
  - idiopathic (connective tissue diseases)
- Psychogenic:
  - hysteria
  - hyperventilation syndrome
- Metabolic and endocrine disease:
  - diabetes
  - chronic kidney disease

- Inflammatory disorders:
  - multiple sclerosis
  - sarcoidosis
  - infections (e.g. HIV, syphilis)
  - connective tissue disorders.
- Neoplasms, such as brain tumours (often metastases).
- Cerebrovascular disease:
  - since other cranial nerves are anatomically close, there may be associated neurological deficits in intracranial causes of facial sensory loss. Thalamic strokes in particular can cause facial sensory loss
  - in posterior cranial fossa lesions, for example, there may be cerebellar features, such as ataxia
  - in middle cranial fossa lesions, there may be associated neurological deficits affecting cranial nerve VI and thus mediolateral eye movements.
- Brainstem lesions that may involve the fifth nuclei and central connections include the brainstem:
  - glioma
  - multiple sclerosis
  - infarction
  - syringobulbia: this leads to sensory loss spreading from the periphery of the face inwards towards the nose, plus a lower motor nerve lesion of the vagus, hypoglossal and accessory nerves, leading to disturbances of speech and swallowing, and bilateral upper motor neurone (UMN) lesions affecting all limbs. A 'syringomyelia-like' syndrome has been infrequently reported in neurological disorders such as Tangiers disease, lepromatous leprosy.
- Cerebellopontine angle lesions that can compress the trigeminal nerve and as they enlarge, affect the neighbouring seventh and eighth nerves, producing facial weakness and deafness include:
  - acoustic neuroma
  - meningioma
  - metastases.
- Petrous temporal bone lesions may cause pain and also affect the sixth nerve (Gradenigo syndrome).
  - Infection spreading from the middle ear
  - Metastases
- Cavernous sinus lesions can compress the trigeminal (Gasserian) ganglion and these include:
  - internal carotid artery aneurysm
  - cavernous sinus thrombosis
  - invasion from a pituitary neoplasm
  - metastasis.
- Benign trigeminal neuropathy is a transient sensory loss in one or more divisions of the trigeminal nerve. It seldom occurs until the second decade or affects the corneal reflex. The aetiology is unknown, though some patients prove to have connective tissue disorder.
- Hysteria, and particularly hyperventilation syndrome, may underlie some causes of facial anaesthesia/hypoaesthesia. Typically, the 'anaesthesia' is bilateral and associated with bizarre neurological complaints.

and, by occluding the eustachian tube, cause deafness (Trotter syndrome).
- Leukaemia, myeloma or metastases (usually from breast, lung, stomach or colon cancer) may cause deposits in the mandible and labial hypoaesthesia.
- Carcinoma of the maxillary antrum may produce ipsilateral upper labial hypoaesthesia or anaesthesia.

Intracranial Lesions

Intracranial lesions affecting the trigeminal nerve or connections are uncommon but often serious. Positive findings in two or more divisions should raise suspicion for a central cause.
Causes include:
- Trauma including surgical treatment of trigeminal neuralgia.

CLINICAL FEATURES

Central (brainstem) lesions of the lower trigeminal nuclei (e.g. in syringobulbia), produce a characteristic circumoral sensory loss. When the spinal tract (or spinal nucleus) alone is involved, the sensory loss is restricted to loss of pain and temperature sensation, but normal touch sensation, i.e. is dissociated. A complete fifth nerve lesion causes unilateral sensory loss on the face, tongue and buccal mucosa. Diminution of the corneal reflex is an early, and sometimes isolated, sign of a fifth nerve lesion.

DIAGNOSIS

Obtain a thorough medical history (to exclude diabetes, renal disease, thyroid disease, connective tissue disorders, surgical history), medication history to exclude drug-induced neuropathy, psychiatric history, family history (inherited neuropathy), social history (alcoholic neuropathy, vitamin deficiency) and occupational history for exposure to toxins. Trigeminal functions that should be tested include the following:

- Skin sensation testing is subjective but done simply by having the patient close their eyes and respond affirmatively to touch with a light wisp of cotton over the three divisions of the trigeminal nerve, the patient is asked to compare the perception on the two sides. It is important to define the pattern and distribution of sensory alteration, using various stimuli:
  - light touch (cotton wool)
  - pinpoint (sterile needle)
  - temperature
  - vibration
  - two-point discrimination.
- Corneal reflex testing is much more objective (this tests the fifth and seventh cranial nerves); touching the cornea gently with sterile cotton wool should produce a blink. Asymmetries of this reflex are a good sign of sensory impairment in the distribution of the trigeminal ophthalmic division.

If there is objective facial sensory and corneal reflex loss, a full neurological assessment must be undertaken, unless the loss is unequivocally related to local trauma (Algorithm 47.1). Spreading numbness is of particular significance. Occasional patients feign sensory loss, and this often has a bizarre distribution such as a hairline or perfect midline demarcation.

Trigeminal motor function is to the muscles of mastication (masseters, temporalis, pterygoids). The function is tested by palpating the muscles during function and performing the jaw jerk. The latter may be impaired if there is a trigeminal nerve lesion or increased if there is a lesion above the pons nucleus, and weak in lesions of the brainstem or cortex. Unilateral cerebral lesions do not affect jaw movements. In trigeminal lesions, there may be atrophy of the masseter and/or temporalis muscles.

Possible investigations in patients with facial sensory loss include (Table 47.2):

- imaging (panoramic, occipitomental, lateral and postero-anterior skull and MRI/CT). Diffusion-weighted MRI can be especially helpful
- a full blood count, ESR; random blood sugar level; syphilis and Lyme disease serology and possibly viral serology (e.g. herpesviruses or HIV); autoantibodies to exclude connective tissue diseases
- quantitative sensory testing (QST) through the use of devices that generate specific physical vibratory or thermal stimuli and those that deliver electrical impulses at specific frequencies.

TABLE 47.2 Aids That Might Be Helpful in Diagnosis/Prognosis/Management in Some Patients With Sensory and Motor Changes[a]	
In All Cases	**In Some Cases**
Neurological testing	Blood pressure
	Full blood picture
	Serum ferritin, vitamin B_{12} and corrected whole blood folate levels
	ESR
	Blood glucose/HbA1c
	SACE
	Serology (HIV, HTLV-1, HSV, VZV, HCV, Lyme disease, syphilis)
	ANA/ENA
	RF
	Nasendoscopy
	Audiometry
	Radiography (panoramic, occipitomental, lateral and postero-anterior skull)
	CT/MRI
	Lumbar puncture
	Psychological assessment

[a]See text for details and glossary for abbreviations.

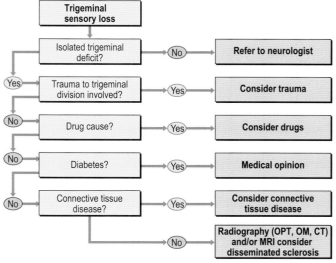

Algorithm 47.1 Sensory loss.

TREATMENT

Most nerve injuries have the greatest chance of recovery in the first 6 months following the trauma. If there has been neurotmesis, early surgical correction can achieve good results. In benign, potentially reversible causes of sensory loss, the underlying cause should be corrected. Various medications including gabapentin, pregabalin and antidepressants (e.g. venlafaxine and amitriptyline) may be trialled to control symptoms of burning or tingling.

Facial hypoaesthesia or anaesthesia results in the loss of protective reflexes and a trigeminal trophic syndrome with facial ulceration can follow. If the cornea is anaesthetic or hypoaesthetic, an eye pad must be worn over the closed eyelids, since the protective corneal reflex is lost, and the cornea may be damaged.

MOTOR CHANGES

The facial nerve (seventh cranial) is the motor nerve to the muscles of facial expression, and facial nerve lesions cause paralysis of the muscles of facial expression, including the orbicularis oculi, orbicularis oris, buccinator, platysma, scalp and auricle muscles.

The facial nerve supplies the stylohyoid and stapedius muscles and has, besides these motor components:
- secretomotor fibres — tearing — lacrimal gland
- saliva production — sublingual, submandibular, nasal and palatine glands
- nervus intermedius, associated with taste perception in anterior two-thirds of the tongue
- sensory component to the external ear.

Facial paralysis (palsy) can be very disfiguring since the ability to smile is impaired, the eye cannot close and the patient may drool.

AETIOLOGY AND PATHOGENESIS

Lesions of the facial nerve central connections (supranuclear or UMN lesions) or the facial nerve itself (nuclear and infranuclear or lower motor neurone (LMN) lesions), or muscle disease, can lead to facial weakness.

Upper Motor Neurone Lesions (Supranuclear Lesions)

UMN lesions may be due to (Box 47.2 and Fig. 47.2):
- stroke (cerebrovascular events), commonly due to haemorrhage or thrombosis in or around the internal capsule, seen mainly in older patients
- a focal brain lesion which may be moderately selective or cause a cerebral palsy
- rarely, a brain cortical lesion affecting the cerebral hemispheres.

Lower Motor Neurone Lesions (Infranuclear Lesions)

- Bell palsy: seen mainly in younger patients and is mainly related to infection and swelling within the confines of the stylomastoid canal, usually due to the herpes simplex virus.

BOX 47.2 Causes of Facial Palsy (Paralysis)

- Upper motor neurone lesion:
  - cerebrovascular event
  - trauma
  - tumour
  - infection
  - multiple sclerosis
  - Moebius syndrome
  - connective tissue disease
- Lower motor neurone lesion:
  - Bell palsy (herpes simplex virus usually)
  - varicella-zoster virus infection (± Ramsay—Hunt syndrome)
  - Lyme disease (Borrelia burgdorferi)
  - HIV infection
  - HTLV-1 infection
  - cytomegalovirus, Epstein—Barr virus and influenza viruses
  - other infections, e.g. leprosy, Guillain—Barré syndrome, Kawasaki disease
  - diabetes
  - middle-ear disease: otitis media, cholesteatoma
  - lesion of skull base: fracture, infection, sarcoidosis
  - parotid lesion, e.g. adenoid cystic carcinoma
  - trauma to a branch of the facial nerve
  - inferior dental regional anaesthetic affecting the facial nerve
  - barotrauma
  - Melkersson—Rosenthal syndrome
  - drugs (e.g. Vinca alkaloids)

- Parotid lesions: benign tumours in the main displace the facial nerve, but malignant tumours infiltrate the nerve and cause paralysis.
  - Ramsay—Hunt syndrome, caused by the varicella-zoster virus infection, which allegedly involves the facial nerve at the geniculate ganglion
  - multiple sclerosis
  - pseudobulbar palsy
  - neoplasm (acoustic neuroma, metastases, glioma or even more rarely a meningioma)
  - lesions affecting the distal facial nerve (e.g. assault with a knife or bottle, malignant tumours in, or surgery on, the parotid or submandibular region).
- Trauma: barotrauma or use of forceps in delivery, stab wounds and facial lacerations. Fracture of the temporal bone can involve the nerve anywhere in the bony canal.
- Occasionally, a temporary facial palsy follows the (mal) administration of an inferior alveolar local analgesic, if the anaesthetic diffuses from the pterygomandibular space distally through the parotid gland, when it can reach and temporarily paralyse the facial nerve.
- Meningitis
- Facial nucleus; such as poliomyelitis, rarely.
- Pontine or posterior cranial fossa. As there are a large number of tracts in close approximation in the pons, the features may be diffuse with frequent bilateral or

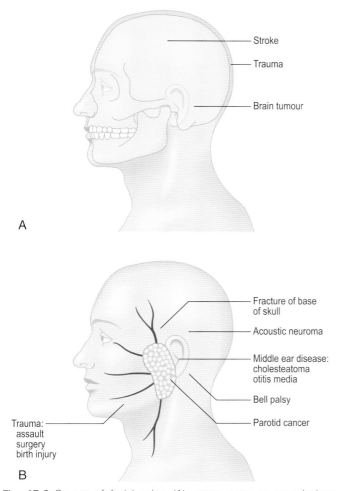

A

B

Fig. 47.2 Causes of facial palsy: (A) upper motor neurone lesions; (B) lower motor neurone lesions of the seventh nerve.

- haemorrhage may occur in the canal in hypertension
- glomus tumour, leukaemic and other malignant deposits or sarcoidosis are rare causes.
- Middle-ear, which includes:
  - chronic otitis media
  - cholesteatoma
  - ear surgery, especially mastoidectomy.
- Sarcoidosis of the parotid gland (as part of uveoparotitis), Crohn disease and related conditions are rare causes.
- Leprosy. It may be possible to palpate the nerve as a cord which can be rolled under the skin.

CLINICAL FEATURES

In facial palsy, the patient typically complains of an impaired smile, speech and ability to whistle. Dysgeusia, subjective change in facial sensation and hyperacusis may be reported.

In addition, on the affected side:
- the forehead is unfurrowed
- the patient is unable to close the eye
- the eye rolls upward (Bell sign) on attempted closure
- tears tend to overflow onto the cheek (epiphora)
- the nasolabial fold is obliterated
- the corner of the mouth droops
- saliva may drool from the commissure
- food collects in the vestibule
- plaque accumulates on the teeth.
  - Lesion laterality and level are important in determining the specific clinical features.
  - UMN lesions produce lower facial weakness and hemiparesis. The neurological lesion is contralateral to the lower facial weakness. The facial weakness does not affect the forehead, since the neurones to the upper face receive bilateral UMN innervation. UMN facial palsy is usually caused by damage in the middle capsule of the brain. The damage thus extends to include hemiplegia and sometimes affects speech, but extrapyramidal influences remain and thus there can still be involuntary facial movements, for example, in laughing because of the bilateral cortical representation. A UMN lesion, therefore, is characterised by:
- contralateral facial palsy
- some sparing of the frontalis and orbicularis oculi muscles
- spontaneous facial movements with emotional responses.
  - There may also be aphasia and, on the side of facial palsy:
- paresis of the arm (monoparesis)
- paresis of the arm and leg (hemiparesis).
  - LMN lesions produce full ipsilateral hemifacial weakness, including the forehead. The facial nucleus itself is affected unilaterally or bilaterally in poliomyelitis and motor neurone disease — the latter usually bilaterally. Lesions at lower levels than the facial nucleus are recognised by the association of LMN facial weakness with other signs.
  - Pontine lesions. The sixth (abducens) nerve nucleus is often also involved, manifesting with a convergent squint (lateral rectus palsy) as well as unilateral facial weakness.

contralateral involvement. The sixth and eighth cranial nerves are often involved along with the seventh nerve and serve as a good localising feature in facial palsy. The causes may include:
- vascular disease (basilar artery aneurysm)
- intrathecal drug injections (e.g. methotrexate for leukaemia).
- Temporal bony canal. The level of involvement can be estimated in three ways: (1) below the geniculate ganglion where lacrimation will be spared; (2) below the chorda tympani where taste from the anterior two-thirds of the tongue is spared; or (3) below the nerve to stapedius which, if involved, may give rise to hyperacusis due to fixation of the stapedius muscle. The causes can be from ganglion peripherally:
  - acute infective polyneuritis (Guillain—Barré syndrome) is a peripheral nervous system affliction often following a viral infection and manifesting mainly with weakness or tingling sensations in the legs. In many instances, the weakness and abnormal sensations spread to the arms and upper body

When the neighbouring paramedian pontine reticular formation and corticospinal tracts are involved, there is a combination of:

- LMN facial weakness
- failure of conjugate lateral gaze (towards the lesion)
- contralateral hemiparesis.
  - Cerebellopontine angle lesions. The fifth, sixth and eighth nerves are affected along with the seventh.
  - Petrous temporal lesions. Facial nerve lesions within the petrous temporal bone result in a combination of a loss of taste on the anterior two-thirds of the tongue and hyperacusis (unpleasantly loud noise distortion) caused by paralysis of the nerve to stapedius.
  - Skull base, parotid gland and in the face itself. This produces an LMN facial palsy characterised only by:
- total unilateral paralysis of all muscles of facial expression
- absence of voluntary and emotional facial responses
- no hemiparesis or aphasia.

DIAGNOSIS

The history should be directed to elicit features suggestive of stroke and trauma, including underwater diving (barotrauma), camping or walking in areas that may contain ticks (Lyme disease), the possibility of HIV infection and, in Afro-Caribbeans, the possibility of HTLV-1 infection. A facial paresis, which is slowly evolving, associated with other focal neurology, facial twitching, multiple cranial nerve deficits or chronic eustachian tube dysfunction suggests a possible malignant cause. A neck or parotid mass or history of previous head or neck malignancy is suspicious (Algorithm 47.2).

- Differentiating supranuclear from infranuclear lesions depends on the presence of other neurological signs.
- Contralateral limb weakness suggests a pontine level lesion and therefore a nuclear facial nerve lesion.
- Cerebellopontine angle lesions typically affect multiple cranial nerves as well as produce hyperacusis and disturbances of lacrimation, taste and salivation.
- Salivation and taste are affected by all facial canal lesions. Lacrimation is affected in a proximal lesion of the facial canal but is spared in a more distal lesion.
- Facial level lesions affect only muscle function, leaving lacrimation, salivation and taste intact.
  The examination should include the following:
- Ear and mouth examination to exclude Ramsay–Hunt syndrome (herpes zoster of the facial nerve ganglion which causes lesions in the palate and ipsilateral ear, and facial palsy).
- Ear examination to look for discharge and other signs of middle-ear disease.
- A full neurological examination, especially to exclude lesions of other cranial nerves, and to exclude a stroke. Test for the facial nerve weakness by asking the patient to:
  - close the eyes against resistance
  - raise the eyebrows

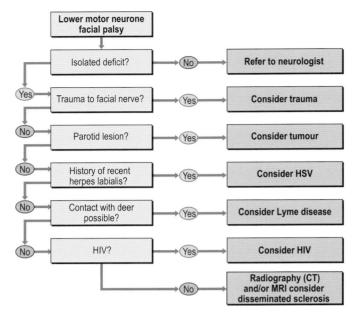

Algorithm 47.2 Lower motor neurone facial palsy.

- raise the lips to show the teeth
- try to whistle.
- A test for loss of hearing should be performed.
- A test for taste loss should be performed.
Investigations that may be indicated include the following (see Table 47.2):
- A study of evoked potentials to assess the degree of nerve damage. Facial nerve stimulation or needle electromyography may be useful, as may electrogustometry.
- Imaging with CT/MRI, and chest and skull radiography to look particularly for central lesions.
- Blood pressure measurement to exclude hypertension.
- Fasting blood sugar levels to exclude diabetes.
- Test for Lyme disease (tick-borne infection with *Borrelia burgdorferi*) by enzyme-linked immunosorbent assay (ELISA) or C6 peptide antibodies, confirming equivocal and positive results with Western blot.
- Tests for virus infections, such as HSV, VZV, HIV or HTLV-1.
- Serum angiotensin-converting enzyme (ACE) levels to exclude sarcoidosis.
- Lumbar puncture is needed occasionally.

TREATMENT

Management is of the underlying condition. Most patients with Bell palsy are otherwise healthy and present no other management difficulties, but there are occasional associations with diabetes mellitus, hypertension and lymphoma.

AUTONOMIC NEUROPATHIES

Autonomic neuropathies are uncommon, diverse and rarely affect the orofacial region. Autonomic cephalgias and sialosis are attributed to autonomic dysfunction. Autonomic neuropathies may cause insensitivity to pain, resulting in oral self-mutilation, such as biting injuries and scarring (of the tongue, lip and buccal mucosa). Familial dysautonomia (Riley—Day syndrome) may manifest with self-mutilation and also sialorrhoea, while cholinergic dysautonomia may cause hyposalivation. Hereditary sensory and autonomic neuropathy type IV causes congenital insensitivity to pain plus anhidrosis (inability to sweat normally, which may cause heat intolerance). Other autonomic neuropathies can also cause loss of bladder control; and postural or orthostatic hypotension. Gastrointestinal symptoms frequently accompany autonomic neuropathy.

Autonomic neuropathies may become life-threatening, as they can affect cardiorespiratory function.

RECOMMENDED READING

Cowart, B.J., 2011. Taste dysfunction: a practical guide for oral medicine. Oral Dis. 17 (1), 2—6.

DeVere, R., 2017. Disorders of Taste and Smell. Continuum (Minneap Minn). 23(2), 421—446. Selected Topics in Outpatient Neurology.

Kumbargere Nagraj, S., George, R.P., Shetty, N., Levenson, D., Ferraiolo, D.M., Shrestha, A., 2017. Interventions for managing taste disturbances. Cochrane Database Syst. Rev. 12 (12), CD010470.

48

Bell's Palsy

> **KEY POINTS**
> - Bell's palsy is an acute lower motor neurone face palsy where there is inflammation with demyelination in the stylomastoid canal.
> - It is characterised by acute spontaneous onset (72 hours or less) of unilateral peripheral facial palsy.
> - Most cases are related to viral infections — mainly herpes simplex virus
> - Management is with corticosteroids and antivirals.

INTRODUCTION

Bell's palsy is an acute lower motor neurone palsy that affects the seventh cranial nerve or facial nerve. There is inflammation of the facial nerve with demyelination, usually in the stylomastoid canal, and oedema further hazarding the blood supply to the nerve interrupting neural transmission. Clinically, 70% of patients with Bell's palsy have complete paralysis and 30% have incomplete paralysis. Herpes simplex virus activation is the likely cause in most cases, although there is no established method of confirming a viral mechanism.

EPIDEMIOLOGY

- Bell's palsy represents about 50% of all facial palsies but is rare at possibly around 10 to 40 cases per 100,000 population. Bilateral paralysis is rare and occurs in 0.3% of patients.
- Bell's palsy can affect any age group but has a slightly higher incidence in mid and later life.
- Both sexes are equally affected.
- No geographic factors are known.

PREDISPOSING FACTORS

Greater incidence of Bell's palsy in patients with:
- Diabetes
- Hypertension
- Immunocompromised status
- Post-upper respiratory viral infection
- Pregnancy

- Chronic granulomatous disorder, such as Crohn's disease or orofacial granulomatosis, when the association is often termed Melkersson—Rosenthal syndrome or sarcoidosis
- Lymphoma

AETIOLOGY AND PATHOGENESIS

The aetiology of Bell's palsy is unknown. The most likely cause in most cases includes reactivation of herpes simplex virus (HSV-1) infection around the geniculate ganglion. Infection, nerve compression and autoimmunity may all play a role.

Histopathology of the facial nerve in patients with Bell's palsy demonstrates a thickened, oedematous perineurium with a diffuse infiltrate of inflammatory cells between nerve bundles and around intraneural blood vessels. Myelin sheaths also undergo degeneration. These changes are seen throughout the course of the nerve, though the damage is maximal in the labyrinthine part of the facial canal.

Facial palsy may be seen in (Table 48.1):
- Herpesviruses
  - usually associated with HSV
  - rarely associated with:
    - varicella-zoster virus (VZV) infection
    - Epstein—Barr virus (EBV) infection
    - cytomegalovirus (CMV) infection
    - human herpesvirus-6 infection
- Retroviruses:
  - human immunodeficiency virus (HIV) infection
  - human T-cell lymphotropic virus (HTLV)-1 infection
- Bacteria:
  - otitis media
  - infections around stylomastoid foramen region
  - *Borrelia burgdorferi* infection (Lyme disease; neuroborreliosis)
  - Syphilis
  - Kawasaki disease
- Heerfordt syndrome (sarcoidosis)
- Melkersson—Rosenthal syndrome
- Disseminated sclerosis

TABLE 48.1 Localisation of Site of Lesion in, and Causes of, Unilateral Facial Palsy

Muscles Paralysed Unilaterally	Lacrimation	Hyperacusis	Sense of Taste	Other Features	Probable Site of Lesion	Type of Lesion
Lower face	N	–	N	Emotional movement retained ± monoparesis or hemiparesis ± aphasia	Upper motor neurone	Stroke, brain tumour, trauma, human immuno-deficiency virus (HIV) infection
All facial muscles	↓	+	↓	± Sixth nerve damage	Lower motor neurone Facial nucleus	Disseminated sclerosis
All facial muscles	↓	+	↓	± Eighth nerve damage	Between nucleus and geniculate ganglion	The fractured base of the skull, posterior cranial fossa tumours, sarcoidosis
All facial muscles	N	±	N or ↓	–	Between geniculate ganglion and stylomastoid canal	Otitis media, cholesteatoma, mastoiditis
All facial muscles	N	–	N	–	In stylomastoid canal or extracranially	Bell's palsy, trauma, local analgesia (e.g. misplaced inferior dental block), Lyme disease, parotid malignant neoplasm, Guillain–Barré syndrome
Isolated facial muscles	N	–	N	–	Branch of facial nerve extracranially	Trauma, local analgesia

N, Normal; +, present; ↓, reduced.

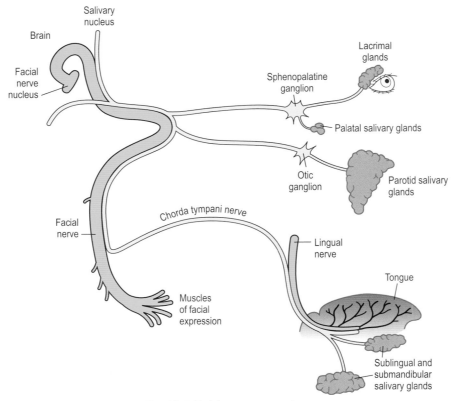

Fig. 48.1 Facial nerve connections.

CLINICAL FEATURES

The facial nerve carries:

- motor nerve impulses to the muscles of the face, and facial expression, and to the stapedius muscle of the stapes in the middle ear
- secretomotor fibres to the lacrimal (tear) glands, and to the submandibular and sublingual salivary glands
- taste from the anterior tongue (Fig. 48.1) via the chorda tympani.

  Since the function of the facial nerve is so complex, many symptoms may occur. Bell's palsy may result in:

- acute onset of unilateral facial weakness or paralysis over a few hours, maximal within 48 hours (Fig. 48.2) with

accompanying symptoms of postauricular pain, dysgeusia, subjective facial numbness (but sensation appears intact on testing) and hyperacusis (heightened sense of hearing)
- reduced lacrimation and salivation secondary to parasympathetic effects.

  Occasionally there may be:

- pain in the region of the ear or the jaw may precede the palsy by a day or two
- a positive family history in up to 10%
- recurrent episodes of palsy in up to 10%.

DIAGNOSIS

Bell's palsy is a diagnosis of exclusion. A thorough history and clinical examination including a cranial nerve exam are necessary. The history should ascertain the following:

- onset and progression of the palsy, precipitating factors
- fever, general malaise, myalgia, arthralgia, headache, rash, recalled tick-bite
- previous episodes of facial palsy, lip or parotid swelling, or uveitis
- ear symptoms (hypo/hyperacusis, tinnitus, vertigo, imbalance, pain)
- evidence of other cranial nerve involvement, e.g. diplopia, hoarseness
- background of autoimmune, granulomatous or metabolic diseases
- use of neurotoxic medications

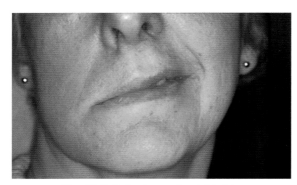

Fig. 48.2 Bell palsy on the right side.

- prior or current malignancy
- pregnancy or recent delivery
- immunosuppression, HIV.

The history should be directed to exclude facial palsy caused by other factors, such as:
- stroke
- trauma including surgery (parotidectomy) and lacerations physically affecting the facial nerve (e.g. in the parotid region or base of the skull), or by underwater diving (barotrauma)
- tumours affecting the facial nerve (e.g. acoustic neuroma or cholesteatoma)
- non-infective inflammatory disorders affecting the facial nerve:
  - disseminated sclerosis
  - connective tissue disease
  - sarcoidosis
  - Melkersson–Rosenthal syndrome
- infections affecting the facial nerve:
  - viral infections (HSV, VZV, EBV, CMV, HIV, HTLV-1)
  - bacterial infections (middle ear infections [e.g. otitis media], Lyme disease [camping or walking in areas that may contain deer ticks]).

Bell's palsy is less likely to be the diagnosis if:
- the paralysis is slowly progressive or chronic
- trauma has occurred
- multiple cranial nerves are involved
- there are other neurological features
- there are signs of neoplasia.

The examination should include the following:
- A full neurological examination, especially to exclude a stroke, and exclude lesions involving other cranial nerves (especially the abducens and vestibulocochlear nerves).
- Examination of the cranial nerves; weakness is demonstrated by testing the corneal reflex and asking the patient to close the eyes against resistance, raise the eyebrows, raise the lips to show the teeth and try to whistle.
- Ear and mouth examination to exclude Ramsay–Hunt syndrome (herpes zoster of the geniculate ganglion, which causes lesions in the palate and ipsilateral ear, and facial palsy).
- Ear examination for discharge and other signs of middle ear disease.

Investigations that may be indicated include the following (Table 48.2):
- Magnetic resonance imaging (MRI) or computed tomography (CT) imaging of the internal auditory meatus, cerebellopontine angle and mastoid may be required to exclude intracranial pathologies such as tumours — particularly in progressive facial palsy.
- A test for tear production (Schirmer's test), in which a strip of filter paper is placed in the lower conjunctival fornix and the amount of tear production is measured.
- Blood pressure measurement to exclude hypertension.
- Blood tests may include:
  - fasting blood sugar levels (to exclude diabetes)

TABLE 48.2 Aids That Might be Helpful in Diagnosis/Prognosis/Management in Some Patients Suspected of Having Bell's Palsy[a]

In Most Cases	In Some Cases
Neurological opinion	Full blood picture
ENT examination	Serum ferritin, vitamin B$_{12}$ and corrected whole blood folate levels
ESR	Blood glucose
Blood pressure	Serology (HSV, VZV, EBV, CMV, HIV, HTLV-1, Lyme disease, syphilis)
	SACE
	ANA
	Audiometry
	Facial nerve tests (stimulation, needle electromyography, electrogustometry, nerve excitability tests, electromyography, electroneuronography)
	Lumbar puncture

[a]See text for details and glossary for abbreviations.
ANA, Antinuclear antibody; *CMV*, cytomegalovirus; *EBV*, Epstein–Barr virus; *ENT*, ear, nose and throat; *ESR*, erythrocyte sedimentation rate; *HIV*, human immunodeficiency virus; *HSV*, herpes simplex virus; *VZV*, varicella-zoster virus.

- serum angiotensin-converting enzyme levels to exclude sarcoidosis
- serum antinuclear antibodies to exclude connective tissue disease
- serological tests for HSV or other viral infections, such as HIV, may need to be considered and, in some areas, Lyme disease (tick-borne infection with *Borrelia burgdorferi*) should be excluded by enzyme-linked immunosorbent assay (ELISA) and western blot assay.
- A test for the degree of nerve damage; facial nerve stimulation or needle electromyography may be useful, as may nerve excitability tests, electromyography and electroneuronography.
- A test for loss of hearing; pure tone audiometry is often used.
- A test for taste loss: electrogustometry.
- A test for balance.
- Occasionally, a lumbar puncture is required.

TREATMENT

Without treatment, 70% of Bell's palsy cases will recover to completely normal function within 4 to 6 months of symptom onset. However, the after-effects in the remaining 15% to 30% can be so severe and distressing, that active treatment is warranted (Table 48.3). A neurological opinion may be in order.

Patient information is an important aspect of management. Oral corticosteroids are the mainstay of acute treatment, ideally within 72 hours of symptom onset. One suggested regimen is prednisolone 60 mg orally once daily for 5 days, followed by a

TABLE 48.3 Regimens That Might Be Helpful in Management of Patients Suspected of Having Bell's Palsy

Treatment	Use in Primary or Secondary Care
1st line	Prednisolone Eye protection
Adjunct	Valaciclovir or aciclovir Facial nerve decompression
Emerging	Botulinum toxin Acupuncture Physiotherapy Hyperbaric oxygen

5-day taper by 10 mg/day. Strong evidence recommends against antiviral monotherapy. Antiviral therapy (valaciclovir or aciclovir) combined with corticosteroids in the acute phase of Bell's palsy may add clinical benefit. Assuming the inciting event is herpes simplex reactivation, the early use of antiviral drugs may decrease the viral load and axonal and Schwann's cell injury.

Complications include the following:

- The commonest complication of Bell's palsy is corneal dryness and scarring due to inadequate eyelid closure. The affected eye should be protected by glasses during the day, and artificial tears used as needed. Overnight, the lid may be taped closed.
- Synkinesis: involuntary movements such as eyelid movements accompanying voluntary movements, such as smiling.
- If paralysis persists and function remains incomplete, the palpebral fissure may narrow, the nasolabial fold deepens and there may be leakage of saliva from the commissure.

FOLLOW-UP OF PATIENTS

The prognosis can be assessed on several factors:
- Favourable prognostic signs include:
  - incomplete paralysis in the first week (94% will fully recover)
  - persistence of the stapedial reflex, measured by electroneurography.
- Poor prognostic signs include:
  - an initially complete paralysis (only 60% recover completely)
  - hyperacusis
  - severe taste impairment on presentation
  - older, diabetic or hypertensive patients.

Long-term follow-up is rarely required as most patients recover.

RECOMMENDED READING

Engström, M., Berg, T., Stjernquist-Desatnik, A., et al., 2008. Prednisolone and valaciclovir in Bell's palsy: a randomised, double-blind, placebo-controlled, multicentre trial. Lancet Neurol. 7, 993.

Gagyor, I., Madhok, V.B., Daly, F., Sullivan, F., 2019. Antiviral treatment for Bell's palsy (idiopathic facial paralysis). Cochrane Database Syst. Rev. 9, CD001869.

Gronseth, G.S., Paduga, R., American Academy of Neurology, 2012. Evidence-based guideline update: steroids and antivirals for Bell palsy: report of the Guideline Development Subcommittee of the American Academy of Neurology. Neurology. 79, 2209–2213.

Holland, N.J., Bernstein, J.M., 2014. Bell's palsy. BMJ Clin. Evid. pii: 1204. Review.

Madhok, V.B., Gagyor, I., Daly, F., et al., 2016. Corticosteroids for Bell's palsy (idiopathic facial paralysis). Cochrane Database Syst. Rev. 7, CD001942.

Potential Malignant Disorders and Cancer

Potentially Malignant Disorders

KEY POINTS
- Potentially malignant disorders (sometimes termed potentially premalignant oral epithelial lesions) encountered during a routine oral mucosal examination represent one of the most significant clinical findings in dental practice. Early diagnosis, referral and appropriate interventions may reduce the rate of progression.
- Potentially malignant clinically obvious disorders include leukoplakia, erythroplakia, proliferative verrucous leukoplakia, submucous fibrosis, actinic cheilitis, oral lichen planus (Chapter 8), lichenoid lesions and graft-versus-host disease (Chapter 34). The rates of transformation differ between these conditions.
- Risk factors for erythroplakia and leukoplakia include tobacco use, alcohol use, betel nut chewing and sunlight exposure.
- Diagnosis and prognosis are aided by a biopsy of the lesion.
- Factors predictive of future malignant transformation may include lesion size, colour, site, age, habits, dysplasia grade, history of cancer in the upper aerodigestive tract, changes in expression of P53 tumour suppressor protein, DNA content (aneuploidy) and loss of heterozygosity.
- Treatment involves the removal of risk factors and excision of dysplastic lesions.

INTRODUCTION

Most mouth cancers are oral squamous cell carcinomas (OSCC) and appear to arise in apparently normal mucosa, in apparently otherwise healthy people but some are preceded by clinically obvious oral potentially malignant disorders (PMDs) (also termed *potentially premalignant oral epithelial lesions*). The 2017 World Health Organization (WHO) definition of oral PMD is 'clinical presentations that carry a risk of cancer development in the oral cavity, whether in a clinically definable precursor lesion or in clinically normal mucosa'.

OSCC is also increased in patients who:
- have had previous oral malignancy

- have had previous malignancy in the upper aerodigestive tract (nose, pharynx, trachea, lungs, oesophagus)
- are immunosuppressed (e.g. in graft-versus-host disease and HIV infection).
  PMD include (Table 49.1):
- Erythroplakia (Fig. 49.1): Defined as a bright red velvety patch which cannot be characterised clinically or pathologically as any other definable disease. Rare but has a very high malignant potential and many cases are already a carcinoma on microscopic examination.
- Leukoplakia (white patch) (Chapter 50): The 2017 WHO definition of leukoplakia is 'white plaques of questionable risk, once other specific conditions and other oral PMDs have been ruled out'. Leukoplakia is a clinical diagnosis only and can only be made by exclusion. Leukoplakias can have malignant potential.
- Proliferative verrucous leucoplakia (PVL): Any leukoplakic lesion that becomes warty, exophytic and widespread and has recurred after treatment should arouse suspicion for PVL. May involve multiple sites in the oral cavity but primarily affects the gingiva, alveolar mucosa, tongue and buccal mucosa.
- Erythroleukoplakia (speckled leucoplakia) (Fig. 49.2): Mixed red-and-white lesions with irregular margins.
- Oral lichen planus/oral lichenoid lesions (Chapter 8): In many geographic areas, these are the most common oral PMDs but have a much lower transformation rate than leukoplakia.
- Oral submucous fibrosis (Chapter 52).
- Graft-versus-host disease (GVHD) (Chapter 34: A complication arising in recipients of allogeneic haematopoietic stem cell or bone marrow transplants. Presents intraorally with striations, white plaques or erosive areas.
- Discoid lupus erythematosus: Malignant transformation is extremely rare.

TABLE 49.1   Oral Potentially Malignant Disorders

Disorder		Predisposing Factors	Features
Actinic cheilitis (solar elastosis)		Sunlight	White plaque/erosions
Erythroplakia		Tobacco/alcohol/betel	Flat red plaque
Leukoplakia	Homogeneous	Tobacco/alcohol/betel, human papillomavirus	White plaque
Leukoplakia	Speckled (erythroleukoplakia)	Tobacco/alcohol/betel, human papillomavirus	Speckled plaque
	Nodular/verrucous	Tobacco/alcohol/betel, human papillomavirus	Nodular white plaque
	Proliferative verrucous leukoplakia	Tobacco/alcohol	White or speckled nodular plaque
	Sublingual leukoplakia/keratosis	Tobacco/alcohol	White plaque
	Candidal leukoplakia	*Candida albicans*	White or speckled plaque
	Syphilitic leukoplakia	Syphilis	White plaque
Lichen planus		Idiopathic	White plaque/erosions
Submucous fibrosis		Areca nut/betel	Immobile mucosa, white plaque
Palatal lesions in reverse smokers		Tobacco	White or speckled plaque
Immunocompromised patients		Papillomaviruses Candidosis	White or speckled plaques
Discoid lupus erythematosus		Idiopathic	White plaque/erosions
Dyskeratosis congenita		Genetic	White plaques
Epidermolysis bullosa		Genetic	Scarring
Fanconi anaemia		Genetic	White plaques Periodontal disease
Paterson—Kelly syndrome (sideropenic dysphagia; Plummer—Vinson syndrome)		Iron deficiency	Postcricoid web
Xeroderma pigmentosum		Genetic	White plaque/erosions

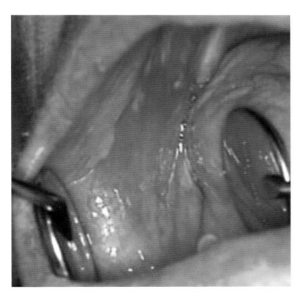

Fig. 49.1 Erythroplakia: usually a potentially malignant disorder or carcinoma.

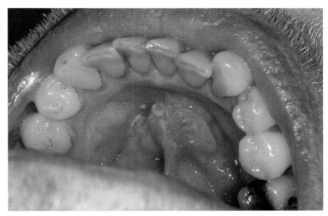

Fig. 49.2 Speckled leukoplakia: often a potentially malignant lesion.

- Paterson—Kelly syndrome (sideropenic dysphagia; Plummer—Vinson syndrome)
- Xeroderma pigmentosum.

AETIOLOGY AND PATHOGENESIS

Oral carcinogenesis is typified by a series of molecular and cellular events that end in neoplasia. Although genetics clearly predispose to PMD in some cases (such as in dyskeratosis congenita, Fanconi anaemia and xeroderma pigmentosum),

Apart from the conditions noted above, rare conditions that predispose to OSCC include:
- dyskeratosis congenita
- epidermolysis bullosa
- Fanconi anaemia

there is substantial evidence that lifestyle factors are often implicated, and most of these have psychotropic actions and are habit-forming or addictive. Those habits that are known to predispose to potential malignancy include:

- tobacco use (Fig. 49.3)
- alcohol use
- betel nut chewing and related products
- sunlight exposure.

Oncogenic human papillomavirus (HPV) types may also be implicated as discussed below.

RISK FACTORS

Tobacco

Many studies have shown an association between tobacco use and oral PMD and OSCC. The relative risk of having an oral dysplastic lesion for smokers compared with non-smokers has been estimated at 7.0. The risk of oral leukoplakia becoming malignant can be strongly related to tobacco use, with the number of cigarettes smoked per day closely associated. Tobacco users are also predisposed to a number of other cancers and potentially malignant conditions (oesophageal, breast, stomach, colorectal, bladder, lung and hepatocellular cancer), and other systemic and oral health issues.

Tobacco contains at least 50 compounds including polycyclic aromatic hydrocarbons such as benzpyrene, nitrosamines, aldehydes and aromatic amines. The precise role of tobacco, however, is surprisingly difficult to define, not least because many heavy smokers also drink alcohol – which is carcinogenic. Different tobacco habits have varied effects:

- In one study, the odds ratio for consumption of greater than 20 cigarettes/day was double that of smokers consuming less than 20 cigarettes/day. Compared with non-smokers, the risk of OSCC in low/medium cigarette smokers was 8.5 and for high tar cigarette smokers was significantly greater at x16.4 in one European study. Smoking cessation seems to produce beneficial effects by reducing the prevalence of oral leukoplakia and the incidence of oral cancer. Ten years

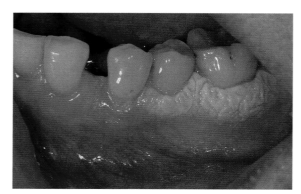

Fig. 49.3 Leukoplakia in a person who for most of his adult life drank a bottle of vodka and smoked 20 cigarettes daily.

after smoking cessation, the risk of oral cancer seems to be similar to that of a never-smoker.

- Reverse smoking is an unusual form of smoking., The lighted end of a cigar, chutta (an Indian smoking product) or cigarette, is placed inside the mouth. Reverse smoking is strongly associated with inducing a 'smokers' leukoplakia and oral cancer. The habit is widely prevalent in south Asia (mainly India, Taiwan and the Philippines) and South America.
- Cigar smoking may predispose to OSCC, and some studies have shown an association with the floor of mouth leukoplakia in women smokers.
- Pipe smoking is most often associated with nicotinic stomatitis, but there is also evidence that pipe smoking may be associated with a predisposition to OSCC.
- The use of smokeless tobacco products has increased considerably across the globe. Smokeless tobacco (ST), for example, snuff-dipping (placing snuff in the buccal sulcus) in women in the south-eastern USA, has been shown to predispose to gingival and alveolar carcinoma close to the area snuff is placed. ST predisposes to OSCC and the products include paan, chaalia, gutka and naswar, and are used in all sections of South Asian society. In India, different forms of chewing tobacco are used such as betel, khaini, pattiwala tobacco, maiwpuri tobacco, zarda, kiwam and gadakhu.
- Tobacco chewing, along with a variety of ingredients in a 'betel quid' (betel vine leaf, betel [areca] nut, catechu and slaked lime, often together with tobacco) appears to predispose to OSCC, particularly when started early in life and used frequently and for prolonged periods. Many migrants to the West and other countries also continue to use ST products even several decades after migration. Asian ethnic migrants to the UK have a significantly higher incidence of oral cancer compared with the native UK populations presumably related to ST use. The combined effect of alcohol and tobacco is far greater than the sum of the two effects and is multiplicative.

Alcohol

Increased consumption of any alcohol-containing beverages is associated with a risk of oral PMD and OSCC. The risk seems to be related to overall alcohol consumption (drink-years) and not to a number of drinks per day. The type of alcoholic beverage also appears to influence the risk – spirits confer higher risks than wine or beer. Ecological studies suggest that the impact of alcohol on oral cancer deaths has increased in recent years. Alcoholic beverages may contain carcinogens or procarcinogens, including ethanol; this is metabolised by alcohol dehydrogenase (ADH) and to some extent by cytochrome p450 (CYP) to acetaldehyde, which may be carcinogenic. Acetaldehyde is degraded by aldehyde dehydrogenases (ALDH) to acetic acid. Genetic variations in the activities of ADH and ALDH (and other enzymes) may influence the outcome of exposure to alcohol, and thus its carcinogenicity in any individual. Many alcoholic drinks also contain congeners and some local brews may contain carcinogens such as nitrosamines or urethane contaminants. Furthermore, alcohol users are also predisposed to a number of other cancers and potentially malignant conditions, and other systemic and oral health issues.

The risk of OSCC decreases after stopping alcohol use but the effects appear to persist for several years. The carcinogenic potential of proprietary alcohol-containing mouthwashes remains controversial.

Chewing Habits

Betel quid is widely used across the world, in south Asian communities particularly, though contents vary in different parts of the world and cultures. The betel quid contents are betel leaf, tobacco, areca nut, spices and sometimes slaked lime. A large variety of additives may be incorporated. Betel (paan; the leaf, stem or inflorescence of *Piper betel*) leaves are from the betel vine, a relative of the pepper family. The leaf contains allylbenzene compounds such as chavibetol, chavicol, estragole, eugenol and methyl eugenol. Areca nut, sometimes referred to as betel nut (although it is from a different plant than the betel leaf) is the seed of *Areca catechu* — the areca palm. Betel quid can be made up at home or purchased as ready to chew.

The betel quid is placed in the mouth, usually the cheek, and gently chewed and sucked sometimes for hours. Betel use not only causes discolouration of the oral mucosa and teeth but can also predispose to oral PMD such as submucous fibrosis, erythroplakia and leukoplakia, and also to OSCC.

Furthermore, betel users are also predisposed to a number of other cancers and potentially malignant conditions (oesophageal, pancreatic and hepatocellular cancer), and other systemic health issues, including;

- cancers: oral, oesophageal, pancreatic, hepatocellular
- hypertension
- metabolic syndrome
- adverse birth outcomes
- liver cirrhosis
- chronic kidney disease
- contact dermatitis
- periodontitis.

Other chewing habits, usually involving tobacco and stimulants, are used in different cultures (e.g. Qat [Khat], Shammah, Toombak).

Sunlight

Actinic radiation may predispose to lip cancer. Facts that support such a relationship include:
- lip cancer involves the more exposed lower lip, rather than the upper lip
- higher incidence of lip cancer in outdoor workers and rural populations than in office workers or urban populations
- fair-skinned people in sunny climates tend to develop lip cancer more than dark-skinned people (as well as skin cancer and melanoma).

Sunlight contains visible light, infrared radiation and ultraviolet (UV) radiation. It is the UV radiation that can cause harmful effects on the skin and lips. There are three basic types of UV: UVA (long-wave UV), UVB (sunburn UV), UVC (short-wave UV). UVB appears to be the most carcinogenic. Tanning beds typically emit about 97% UVA and 3% UVB.

Diet

Charcoal-grilled red meat and fried foods have been implicated as risk factors. Plummer Vinson syndrome (characterised by dysphagia, iron deficiency and oesophageal webbing) can give rise to post-cricoid or oesophageal SCC). An increased consumption of fruits and vegetables is associated with a lower risk of oral cancer.

Other Causes

The carcinogenicity of other psychotropic products such as cannabis remains controversial. The concurrent use of alcohol and tobacco makes it difficult to be certain if cannabis alone is a risk factor for oral cancer. Immune deficiency may predispose to OSCC, especially lip cancer. This is increased in, for example, immunosuppressed renal transplant recipients. Oncogenic HPV subtype is now linked to the rise in oropharyngeal cancer in young people. The oncogenic types, particularly HPV-16 and HPV-18, are the most likely causes of oral mucosal carcinogenesis. It has long been proposed that candidal infection may be a cause of dysplasia. Patients with chronic mucocutaneous candidiasis may be at risk of OSCC and oesophageal malignancy.

Natural History and Malignant Transformation

The natural history of oral PMDs is not absolutely clear (Table 49.2). Cessation of smoking habits appears to result in some lesions regressing or resolving. The risk of malignant transformation is greatest in:
- leukoplakia that exceeds 200 mm^2 non-homogeneous PMD
- red (or speckled) lesions
- Site: PMD on the lateral and ventral tongue, the floor of the mouth and retromolar/soft palate complex
- females
- age above 50 years
- tobacco, alcohol, betel quid and areca nut use
- lesions in non-smokers seem to be at a higher risk of progression to cancer and may involve an underlying genetic predisposition
- dysplasia (severe)
- history of cancer in the upper aerodigestive tract
- expression of P53 tumour suppressor protein
- changes involving chromosomes 3p or 9p; these are termed loss of heterozygosity (LOH)
- DNA content (aneuploidy).

Epithelial dysplasia (from Greek dys = poor and plasia = a moulding) is a term describing the combination of disorderly maturation and disturbed cell proliferation (Box 49.1) seen in OSCC and some oral PMD. Although not all clinically PMD show dysplasia on biopsy examination (Fig. 49.4), most do show dysplasia, and this is one of the main histological features that appears to precede the onset of malignancy and it appears

TABLE 49.2   Malignant Potential in the Most Important Oral Potentially Malignant Disorders

| | Malignant Potential | | |
	High (>60%)	Medium (<30%)	Low (<10%)
Main entities	Erythroplakia	Leukoplakia (non-homogeneous) Candidal leukoplakia	Leukoplakia (homogeneous) Lichen planus/lichenoid lesions
Uncommon entities	Proliferative verrucous leucoplakia	Actinic cheilitis Submucous fibrosis	Discoid lupus erythematosus
Rare entities	Dyskeratosis congenita[a]	Fanconi anaemia[a]	

[a]Malignant potential unclear but involves OSCC (mainly tongue) and other neoplasms, especially acute myeloid leukaemia.

BOX 49.1   Features of Epithelial Dysplasia

- Drop-shaped rete processes
- Basal cell hyperplasia
- Irregular epithelial stratification
- Nuclear hyperchromatism
- Increased nuclear-cytoplasmic ratio
- Increased normal and abnormal mitosis
- Enlarged nucleoli
- Individual cell keratinisation
- Loss or reduction of cellular cohesion
- Cellular pleomorphism
- Loss of basal cell polarity

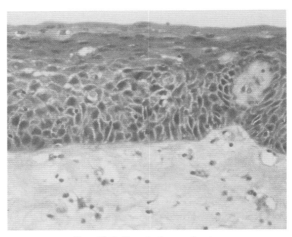

Fig. 49.5 Dysplasia: moderate.

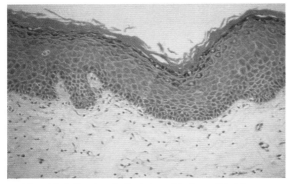

Fig. 49.4 No dysplasia detectable from this biopsy.

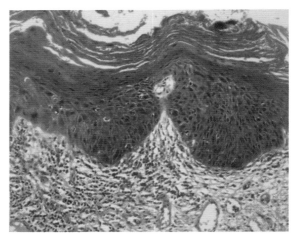

Fig. 49.6 Dysplasia: severe and suggestive of a potentially malignant disorder.

to be the most predictive marker for malignant potential in current use. Cellular atypia is the main feature of dysplasia.

Dysplasia is graded as:

- Mild dysplasia: atypical and immature basal cells extend above the basal layers into the lower third of the epithelium.
- Moderate dysplasia: atypical and immature basal cells extend above the basal layers into the middle third of the epithelium.
- Severe dysplasia: atypical and immature basal cells extend throughout the epithelium.
- Carcinoma in situ: atypical and immature basal cells extend throughout the epithelium together with invasion of the lamina propria.

Dysplasia thus varies in severity from mild to moderate dysplasia — where few of the features of dysplasia are present and the epithelium is reasonably well organised (Fig. 49.5), to the more severe grades where the epithelial organisation is disrupted and many cellular abnormalities present (Fig. 49.6),

the epithelial basement membrane is not seen to be breached but there is a malignant potential. Dysplasia, however, does not always indicate a malignant potential, since mild dysplasia can also be seen in regenerating tissue and some non-precancerous lesions such as some:

- ulcers
- viral infections

- candidal infections
- granular cell tumours.

Nevertheless, many now believe that seeing severe dysplasia is often tantamount to a diagnosis of early carcinoma — since the epithelial basement membrane may well be breached though not detected in the biopsy specimen.

DIAGNOSIS

Performing a biopsy to establish dysplasia is the diagnostic gold standard. The specimen should be taken from the most clinically suspicious area, such as redness, an area of surface thickening or a symptomatic area. To improve the sensitivity and specificity of identification of an area for biopsy, diagnostic adjuncts may be used, such as vital staining with toluidine (tolonium) blue — an acidophilic metachromatic thiazine dye that selectively stains tissue acids, particularly DNA and RNA. Vital staining is based on the fact that dysplastic cells usually contain more nucleic acid than normal cells. Vital staining is not totally specific or sensitive but can assist in deciding where to perform a biopsy. In vivo microscopy technologies, such as high-resolution microendoscopy, optical coherence tomography and reflectance confocal microscopy, allow clinicians to visualise many of the same microscopic features used for histopathologic assessment at the point of care. A negative biopsy cannot reliably exclude the presence of carcinoma or dysplastic foci within a lesion.

TREATMENT

Management of patients with PMD is a controversial issue (Algorithm 49.1 and Algorithm 49.2). A specialist opinion is advised. Fully informed consent is crucial, all the uncertainties being discussed with the patient.

Some oral PMD may be managed conservatively by observation alone. Surgery may have a beneficial effect, but there is no evidence that this will reliably reduce the risk of later recurrence, or malignant transformation of PMD, at the same or another site. Options include traditional excision, cryosurgery and carbon dioxide (CO_2) laser ablation. Factors that influence the type of therapy include patient-related risk factors for malignancy (age, gender and habits) and lesion risk factors (size, location, morphology, malignant transformation rate). Medical measures, such as chemoprevention, that lessen the size, extent or histopathological features of dysplasia within PMD are associated with a risk of adverse effects, particularly with systemic agents (which themselves may be contraindicated in some individuals), and relapse or later malignant transformation can still occur.

FOLLOW-UP

There is neither an evidence base nor absolute consensus as to the optimum review interval or protocol. Since there is no hard evidence as to the ideal frequency of follow-up, it has been suggested that patients with PMD be re-examined by a health professional depending on the degree of dysplasia:
- Mild dysplasia: Review every 6 months for 1 year, then yearly.
- Moderate dysplasia: Review every 6 months for the first 2 years, then yearly.
- Severe dysplasia: Every 3 months for the first 2 years, then every 6 months.

Any changes in clinical features, especially the appearance of a lump or ulcer, merit a repeat specialist opinion and usually a biopsy.

PREVENTION AND DETECTION OF POTENTIALLY MALIGNANT DISORDERS AND CANCER

Unfortunately, many of the population — especially those at highest risk, such as older men who smoke and drink — rarely seek regular dental care or examination. Having a regular dentist is a protective factor. Patients often present late to physicians and with advanced cancers, and furthermore, most physicians and surgeons have often received little or no training in the examination of the mouth. It should be noted also that clinically differentiating oral PMD and OSCC from lesions that are benign can be difficult even for highly trained professionals because these lesions do not always display well-defined clinical features. Not uncommonly, oral PMD and OSCC are asymptomatic, appear innocuous and can be overlooked.

Clinicians should be aware that single ulcers, lumps, red patches or white patches, particularly if any of these are persisting for greater than 3 weeks, may also be manifestations of frank malignancy: biopsy is invariably indicated. Even common, benign-looking oral lesions attributed to friction or

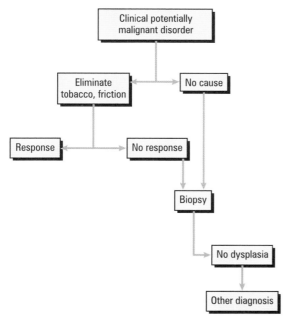

Algorithm 49.1 Treatment of suspected dysplastic lesions.

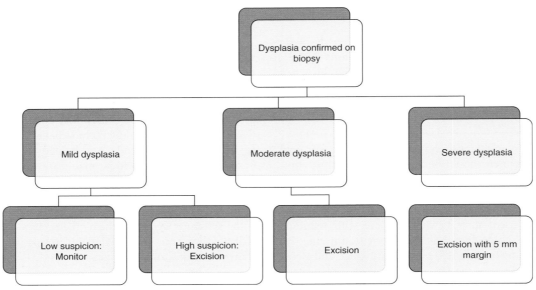

Algorithm 49.2 Treatment of dysplastic lesions.

trauma require evaluation when they persist. Late cancer diagnosis results in treatment that is usually more mutilating, with higher morbidity and costs, and a worse prognosis.

www.OPMDcare.com

RECOMMENDED READING

Joshi, S., Ashley, M., 2016. Cannabis: a joint problem for patients and the dental profession. Br. Dent. J. 220, 597—601.

Mello, F.W., Melo, G., Guerra, E.N.S., Warnakulasuriya, S., Garnis, C., Rivero, E.R.C., 2020. Oral potentially malignant disorders: a scoping review of prognostic biomarkers. Crit. Rev. Oncol. Hematol. 153, 102986.

Porter, S., Gueiros, L.A., Leão, J.C., Fedele, S., 2018. Risk factors and etiopathogenesis of potentially premalignant oral epithelial lesions. Oral Surg. Oral Med. Oral Pathol. Oral Radiol. 125 (6), 603—611.

Speight, P.M., Khurram, S.A., Kujan, O., 2018. Oral potentially malignant disorders: risk of progression to malignancy. Oral Surg. Oral Med. Oral Pathol. Oral Radiol. 125 (6), 612—627.

Syrjänen, S., Lodi, G., von Bültzingslöwen, I., et al., 2011. Human papillomaviruses in oral carcinoma and oral potentially malignant disorders: a systematic review. Oral Dis. 17 (Suppl. 1), 58—72.

Warnakulasuriya, S., 2020. Oral potentially malignant disorders: a comprehensive review on clinical aspects and management. Oral Oncol. 102, 104550.

Warnakulasuriya, S., Kujan, O., Aguirre-Urizar, J.M., et al., 2020. Oral potentially malignant disorders: a consensus report from an international seminar on nomenclature and classification, convened by the WHO Collaborating Centre for Oral Cancer. Oral Dis. 27 (8), 1862—1880.

Leukoplakia

INTRODUCTION

Many white lesions were formerly known as 'leukoplakia' (from the Greek *leukos* = white and *plakia* = patch), a term causing misunderstanding and confusion. Leukoplakia is a clinical diagnosis defined by the World Health Organization as 'a white plaque of questionable risk having excluded (other) known diseases or disorders that carry no increased risk for oral cancer'. It is the most common potentially premalignant condition of the oral cavity. The diagnosis can only be made by exclusion. Approximately 40% of true leukoplakias show histologic evidence of dysplasia, carcinoma in situ or invasive squamous cell carcinoma (SCC), therefore a biopsy is required for definitive diagnosis. Frictional keratosis and specific tobacco-induced lesions, such as smoker's keratosis, are now termed 'keratoses' (*not* 'leukoplakias') and are not considered premalignant disorders (PMDs).

EPIDEMIOLOGY

- Occurs in about 0.1% of the population. Global prevalence of 2% to 4%.
- Occurs predominantly in middle-aged and older patients, increasing prevalence with increasing age.
- Occurs more in men than women.
- It has no known special geographic incidence.

AETIOLOGY AND PATHOGENESIS

Predisposing factors include:
- tobacco use
- excessive alcohol
- betel or areca nut use
- personal or familial history of cancer or cancer therapy
- chronic immunosuppression, age, syndromes such as dyskeratosis congenita
- ultraviolet light damage for lesions of the vermilion
- human papillomavirus in a small number of cases
- sanguinarine (pseudochelerythrine) use. This is a quaternary benzophenanthridine alkaloid extracted from some plants and is used in some oral healthcare products. Sanguinarine is a potent suppressor of NF-κβ activation
- loss of heterozygosity at 3p and/or 9p, aneuploidy, loss or overexpression of p53.

Leukoplakias show, to a varying degree, three main microscopic features:
- Increased keratin production: increased keratin produces the white clinical appearance of keratosis. If nuclei persist into the superficial cell layers, the term 'hyperparakeratosis' is used, whereas if there is excessive mature keratin, with a prominent granular cell layer, the term 'hyperorthokeratosis' is applied. Neither is an index of premalignancy.
- Change in epithelial thickness: thinning (hypoplasia) or thickening (hyperplasia) may be present and, although neither are indices of premalignancy, malignant change is more likely in a hypoplastic epithelium.
- Disordered epithelial maturation: although clinical features, such as the admixture of red lesions, may suggest the degree of malignant potential of a lesion, histological assessment of the degree of disordered proliferation, maturation and organisation of the epithelium (i.e. the degree of dysplasia) continues to provide the best guide. Leukoplakias, even when clinically homogeneous may contain areas of dysplasia, and some studies have even shown carcinoma *in situ* or invasive carcinoma.

CLINICAL FEATURES

Leukoplakias vary in size: the majority are solitary, small and focal white plaques, others more widespread, occasionally involving very large areas of the oral mucosa. In other patients, several discrete separate areas of leukoplakia can be seen. Leukoplakia has a wide range of clinical presentations, from homogeneous white plaques, which can be faintly white or very thick and opaque, to nodular white lesions, or lesions admixed with red lesions. It is generally asymptomatic. The tongue, gingiva, buccal mucosa and palatal mucosa are the most commonly affected sites. High-risk sites for malignant trans-formation (MT) include the soft palate complex, ventrolateral tongue and floor of the mouth (Fig. 50.1).

Leukoplakia is classified as follows (Box 50.1):

- Homogenous leukoplakia: the most common type, well-demarcated, uniform white plaque, usually of *low* malignant potential (Figs 50.2 and 50.3).
- Non-homogenous leukoplakia: *high* risk of MT and, there-fore, are far more serious.
  - Verrucous leukoplakia, which has a well-demarcated border and often occurs on the gingiva.
  - Nodular leukoplakia, which has a nodular surface and is also well demarcated. It may be difficult to distinguish from, or coexist with, verrucous leukoplakia.
  - Erythroleukoplakia, which has areas of erythema within the leukoplakia that may be patchy or speckled (speckled leukoplakia); the erythematous component is generally not well-demarcated (Fig. 50.4).

There are many differences between proliferative verrucous leukoplakia (PVL) and conventional localised leukoplakia. PVL

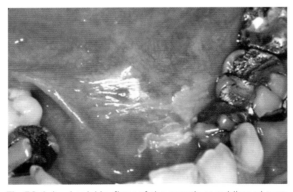

Fig 50.1 Leukoplakia: floor of the mouth or sublingual type.

BOX 50.1   Classification of Leukoplakias

Leukoplakia: Homogeneous
Leukoplakia: Non-homogeneous
- Verrucous
- Nodular
- Erythroleukoplakia (speckled)

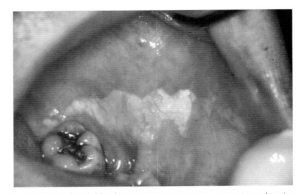

Fig 50.2 Leukoplakia: homogeneous type — most are benign.

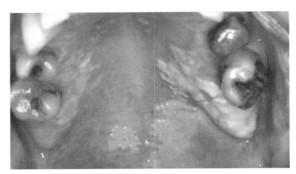

Fig 50.3 Leukoplakia: proliferative verrucous leukoplakia with wide-spread field change over, at least, the palate.

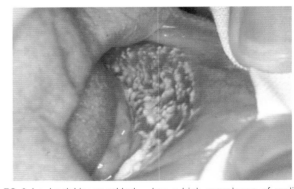

Fig 50.4 Leukoplakia: speckled — has a high prevalence of malignant change.

is characterised by progressive involvement of the oral mucosa by white plaques, often verrucous, at multiple, non-contiguous sites, or it may present as a single large lesion with or without the involvement of contiguous sites. The average age at diag-nosis of PVL is in the seventh decade. In contrast to conven-tional leukoplakia, there is less association with smoking. The most common intraoral sites involved include the gingiva, alveolar mucosa and palatal mucosa. Periodic biopsies are essential for monitoring lesions of PVL as the MT rate is be-tween 40% and 75% over an average follow-up period of seven years.

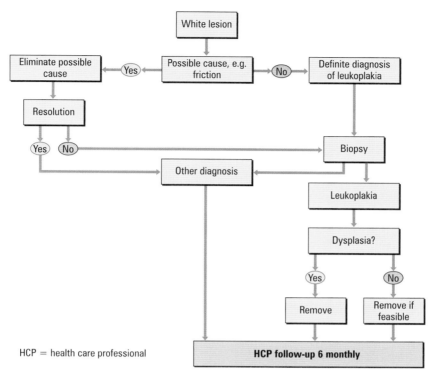

Algorithm 50.1 Management of leukoplakia.

HCP = health care professional

MALIGNANT TRANSFORMATION

The malignant potential of leukoplakia has been reported to be 9.5% (99% CI 5.9% to 14.00%), with an annual transformation rate of 1.56%. Oral erythroplakia has been shown to have a MT rate of 33.1% (99% CI 13.6% to 56.2%). PVL had a high MT rate (49.5%, 99% CI 26.7 to 72.4), with an estimated yearly MT of 9.3%. In general, true leukoplakias do not regress but show progression and enlargement over time. The appearance of the lesion may also change from being homogenous to non-homogenous and from being soft to being firm and indurated. The malignant potential can be estimated from the clinical appearance, site, histology and some aetiological factors.

It is generally accepted that dysplasia may precede malignant change. DNA ploidy studies may become more useful in this respect. Histopathology and the detection of dysplasia alone clearly cannot always reliably identify early malignant changes, since it:

- Is subjective; there is wide inter-examiner and intra-examiner variability.
- Samples are representative of only a small area and, thus, the absence of dysplasia in a biopsy specimen does not necessarily mean that the whole lesion lacks dysplasia.

OTHER LEUKOPLAKIAS

- Chronic hyperplastic candidiasis (CHC, but sometimes known as Candidal leukoplakia) may be associated with an increased risk of malignant change. *Candida albicans* can cause or colonise other keratoses, particularly in smokers, and is especially likely to form speckled leukoplakias at commissures. They may be dysplastic and have higher malignant potential than some other keratoses. CHC leukoplakias may respond to antifungals and cessation of smoking.
- Hairy leukoplakia is caused by Epstein–Barr virus (EBV). It usually has a corrugated surface and affects the margins of the tongue almost exclusively. It is seen in the immunocompromised and is a complication of HIV infection. It is seen in all groups at risk of HIV infection. The condition appears to be benign and self-limiting.
- Syphilitic leukoplakia, especially of the dorsum of the tongue, is a feature of tertiary syphilis and is rarely seen now.

DIAGNOSIS

There are no clinical signs or symptoms that reliably predict whether a leukoplakia will undergo malignant change. The prevalence of MT is highest in lesions with severe dysplasia (Algorithm 50.1). A biopsy is generally indicated and is essential for leukoplakias that are:

- in patients with previous or concurrent head and neck cancer
- non-homogeneous, i.e. have red areas, are verrucous or nodular
- in a high-risk site such as the floor of the mouth or tongue
- focal
- symptomatic

• without obvious aetiological factors.

A biopsy is not always completely diagnostic, partly because dysplastic changes are not always demonstrable in the specimen obtained and there may be skip areas within the dysplastic epithelium. Serial sectioning of removed leukoplakic lesions may reveal a wide range of grades of dysplasia in different parts of a lesion and previously unsuspected carcinoma in up to 5% to 10%. In lesions that are large, multiple biopsies should be performed such as from a white area, from a red area, and an indurated area.

Leukoplakia has an annual MT of 1.56% and 9.3% for PVL. Since it is not at present possible to reliably predict which leukoplakias will progress to carcinoma, much effort has gone into identifying the genetic and other changes that underlie progression to oral squamous cell carcinoma (OSCC), and currently, the most predictive markers of transformation are leukoplakias that are:

• speckled (erythroleukoplakia)
• verrucous
• from high-risk sites, including the soft palate/fauces, the floor of the mouth/ventral tongue
• in a patient with previous cancer in the upper aerodigestive tract
• in non-smoking females
• dysplastic
• DNA polysomic (aneuploidy or tetraploidy)
• positive for genetic markers such as mutated tumour suppressor factor p53, or loss of heterozygosity on chromosomes 3p or 9p.

TREATMENT

Leukoplakia may be potentially malignant (or in a small number may already be carcinomatous) and thus, both behaviour (lifestyle) modification to eliminate risk factors, and active treatment of the lesion are indicated (Table 50.1):

• Patient information is an important aspect of management.

TABLE 50.1 Regimens That Might Be Helpful in Management of Patients Suspected of Having Leukoplakia

Regimen	Use in secondary care
Likely to be beneficial	Excision
Unproven effectiveness	Photodynamic therapy Retinoids Vitamins A, C and E Carotenes Lycopene
Supportive	Cease tobacco, betel or alcohol use

• Removal of known risk factors (tobacco, alcohol, areca nut use) is a mandatory step. Up to 45% of leukoplakias may regress or totally disappear if tobacco use is stopped. Leukoplakias induced by smokeless tobacco may resolve if the habit is ceased.

The current treatment for oral leukoplakia can range from careful observation to surgical intervention. The practice of 'watchful waiting' may be considered in patients with mild dysplasia. Moderate-to-severe dysplasia is more likely to progress and should be excised with clear margins if clinically feasible (such as in young patients with small lesions), and all patients should undergo regular monitoring for recurrence or the development of new leukoplakias.

Surgery

Surgery is the obvious option for the management of leukoplakia with a high predisposition to MT. Resection with a scalpel with a clear margin or laser ablation is probably the most effective and safe means of removing pathologic tissue since — unlike the case with cryosurgery, coagulation or laser vaporisation — a specimen is available for pathologic evaluation. Laser excision seems to have an advantage over the use of a scalpel, as intraoperative bleeding and the need for mucosal or dermoepidermal flaps are reduced. Patients with leukoplakia demonstrating carcinoma in situ and invasive SCC should be referred to a head and neck cancer centre.

Medical Therapies

Since leukoplakias are only potentially malignant, radiotherapy or systemic chemotherapy are inappropriate treatments. Current chemoprevention approaches to prevent MT include retinoids, epidermal growth factor receptor inhibitors/antagonists, cyclooxygenase-2 inhibitors, p53 modulators and topical agents such as bleomycin.

Retinoids (13-*cis*-retinoic acid) can induce regression of leukoplakia. However, adverse effects are severe and many patients do not complete the planned treatment. Chemoprevention with retinoids is not a definitive treatment since there is a high lesion recurrence rate after stopping treatment. Adverse effects are common and most retinoids are teratogenic.

FOLLOW-UP OF PATIENTS

Recurrence has been reported in approximately 7% to 38% of lesions, depending on the selection of leukoplakias and the duration of the follow-up. Regular monitoring, initially every 6 months, is indicated for low-risk lesions. Moderate and severe lesions required more frequent review. Follow-up is usually life-long with clinical photographs. If there is any change causing concern, particularly the development of a lump or ulcer, a specialist opinion should be obtained.

Patients should be regularly checked for any:

- size change
- appearance of red lesions
- ulceration
- recurrences
- new lesions.
  www.opmdcare.com

RECOMMENDED READING

Abadie, W.M., Partington, E.J., Fowler, C.B., Schmalbach, C.E., 2015. Optimal management of proliferative verrucous leukoplakia: a systematic review of the literature. Otolaryngol. Head Neck Surg. 153 (4), 504–511.

Aguirre-Urizar, J.M., Lafuente-Ibáñez de Mendoza, I., Warnakulasuriya, S., 2021. Malignant transformation of oral leukoplakia: systematic review and meta-analysis of the last 5 years. Oral Dis. 27 (8), 1881–1895.

Anderson, A., Ishak, N., 2010. Marked variation in malignant transformation rates of oral leukoplakia. Evid. Based Dent. 16 (4), 102–103.

Bagan, J., Scully, C., Jimenez, Y., Martorell, M., 2010. Proliferative verrucous leukoplakia: a concise update. Oral Dis. 16 (4), 328–332.

Iocca, O., Sollecito, T.P., Alawi, F., et al., 2020. Potentially malignant disorders of the oral cavity and oral dysplasia: a systematic review and meta-analysis of malignant transformation rate by subtype. Head Neck. 42 (3), 539–555.

Kuribayashi, Y., Tsushima, F., Sato, M., Morita, K., Omura, K., 2012. Recurrence patterns of oral leukoplakia after curative surgical resection: important factors that predict the risk of recurrence and malignancy. J. Oral Pathol. Med. 41 (9), 682–688.

Liu, W., Shi, L.J., Wu, L., et al., 2012. Oral cancer development in patients with leukoplakia — clinicopathological factors affecting outcome. PLoS One. 7 (4), e34773.

Ramos-García, P., González-Moles, M.Á., Mello, F.W., Bagan, J.V., Warnakulasuriya, S., 2021. Malignant transformation of oral proliferative verrucous leukoplakia: a systematic review and meta-analysis. Oral Dis. 27 (8), 1896–1907.

Villa, A., Woo, S.B., 2017. Leukoplakia — A diagnostic and management algorithm. J. Oral Maxillofac. Surg. 75, 723.

Woo, S.B., Cashman, E.C., Lerman, M.A., 2013. Human papillomavirus-associated oral intraepithelial neoplasia. Mod. Pathol. 26 (10), 1288–1297.

Erythroplakia (Erythroplasia)

INTRODUCTION

Erythroplakia (from the Greek *erythros* = red and *plakia* = patch) is defined by the World Health Organization as 'any lesion of the oral mucosa that presents as bright red velvety plaques which cannot be characterised clinically or pathologically as any other recognisable condition'. Erythroplakia is regarded as a clinical term with no specific histopathological connotations. Erythroplastic lesions present as well-defined velvety red plaques. Erythroplakia has a high risk of evolution to frank carcinoma. Most already present severe dysplasia or invasive disease at the time of diagnosis: at least 80% are severely dysplastic or frankly malignant, which is why they should be followed at short intervals.

EPIDEMIOLOGY

- Erythroplakia is much less common than leukoplakia. Studies have shown a prevalence rate of 0.02% to 0.1%.
- Occurs in middle-aged and older patients.
- Gender distribution is reported to be equal.
- No known geographic incidence.

AETIOLOGY AND PATHOGENESIS

Aetiology and pathogenesis are similar to that of oral leukoplakia; tobacco chewing, tobacco smoking, betel quid chewing (with or without tobacco) and alcohol. Fruit and vegetable intake may be protective.

CLINICAL FEATURES

Red velvety plaques with generally well-demarcated margins, usually level with or depressed below surrounding mucosa, as commonly seen on:

- soft palate
- floor of mouth
- buccal mucosa (Fig. 51.1).

Lesions are usually asymptomatic. Some erythroplakias are associated with white patches and are then termed speckled leukoplakia or erythroleukoplakia (Table 51.1).

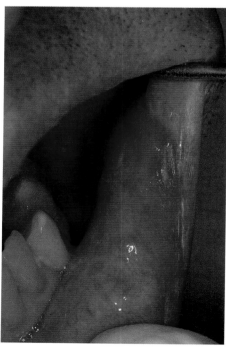

Fig. 51.1 Erythroplakia: usually a potentially malignant lesion. Carcinoma developed in this patient, who actually had long-standing lichen planus with lichenoid dysplasia.

TABLE 51.1 Regimens That Might Be Helpful in Management of Patients Suspected of Having Erythroplakia

Regimen	Use in secondary care
Likely to be beneficial	Excision
Supportive	Cease tobacco, alcohol or betel use

DIAGNOSIS

A biopsy should be undertaken to examine for epithelial dysplasia and carcinoma. The lesion should be differentiated from inflammatory and atrophic red lesions (e.g. in deficiency anaemias, geographic tongue, lichen planus).

TREATMENT

Patient information is an important aspect of management. Any causal factor, such as tobacco, betel and alcohol use should be stopped and the lesion totally excised, when technically feasible.

FOLLOW-UP OF PATIENTS

Erythroplakia or erythroleukoplakia carries a very high potential for malignant development necessitating regular monitoring, which is best carried out by a specialist. It has been reported that 90% of histologically assessed erythroplakia showed invasive carcinoma or carcinoma in situ, and 10% moderate to severe dysplasia. If there is any change causing concern, particularly the development of a lump or ulcer, a further biopsy should be obtained. There is no hard evidence as to the ideal frequency of follow-up, but close follow-ups of the patient for life is recommended.

RECOMMENDED READING

Ferreira, A.M., de Souza Lucena, E.E., de Oliveira, T.C., da Silveira, E., de Oliveira, P.T., de Lima, K.C., 2016. Prevalence and factors associated with oral potentially malignant disorders in Brazil's rural workers. Oral. Dis. 22, 536—542.

Hashibe, M., Mathew, B., Kuruvilla, B., et al., 2000. Chewing tobacco, alcohol, and the risk of erythroplakia. Cancer Epidemiol. Biomarkers Prev. 9 (7), 639—645.

Iocca, O., Sollecito, T.P., Alawi, F., et al., 2020. Potentially malignant disorders of the oral cavity and oral dysplasia: a systematic review and meta-analysis of malignant transformation rate by subtype. Head Neck. 42 (3), 539—555.

Reichart, P.A., Philipsen, H.P., 2005. Oral erythroplakia — a review. Oral Oncol. 41 (6), 551—561.

Shi, L., Jiang, W., Liu, W., 2019. Retrospective analysis of oral erythroplakia focused on multiple and multifocal malignant behavior. Oral Dis. 25 (7), 1829—1830.

Villa, A., Villa, C., Abati, S., 2011. Oral cancer and oral erythroplakia: an update and implication for clinicians. Aust. Dent. J. 56 (3), 253—256.

Wetzel, S.L., Wollenberg, J., 2020. Oral potentially malignant disorders. Dent. Clin. North Am. 64 (1), 25—37.

Oral Submucous Fibrosis

> **KEY POINTS**
> - Oral submucous fibrosis (OSMF) is caused by betel use.
> - It is a potentially malignant disorder.
> - There is no specific therapy for OSMF.

INTRODUCTION

Oral submucous fibrosis (OSMF) is a chronic, potentially premalignant condition seen only in persons who chew betel (*Areca catechu*) nuts, pan masala or gutkha, and it is characterised by tightening of the buccal, and sometimes palatal and lingual mucosae, causing trismus.

EPIDEMIOLOGY

- High frequency in Asian populations, especially in those from the Indian subcontinent. 4/1000 adults in rural India.
- It usually affects persons between the ages of 30 and 65 years. Younger patients (<40 years) have been reported to develop OSMF in response to shorter periods of exposure to betel use.
- The prevalence of OSMF in India has been estimated to range from 0.2% to 2.3% in males and 1.2% to 4.6% in females.
- More than 2.5 million individuals are affected worldwide but it is extremely rare in people not of Asian extraction.

AETIOLOGY AND PATHOGENESIS

The basic issue in OMSF appears to be an increase in submucosal collagen, for which there may be some genetic predisposition. Patients have an increased frequency of human leukocyte antigen (HLA)-A10, HLA-B7 and HLA-DR3. Further, the HLA class I chain-related gene A (MICA), particularly the phenotype frequency of allele A6 of MICA is increased in OSMF, expressed by keratinocytes and other epithelial cells and interacts with gamma/delta T cells in the submucosa. Increased levels of pro-inflammatory cytokines and reduced anti-fibrotic interferon-gamma may be central to the pathogenesis.

Areca nut is the fourth most addictive substance in the world. It contains alkaloids (the most potent of which is arecoline), flavonoids and copper — all of which interfere with collagen metabolism. Arecoline induces the production of:
- collagen
- interleukin 6
- keratinocyte growth factor-1
- insulin-like growth factor-1
- cystatin C (a protein up-regulated in a variety of fibrotic diseases)
- tissue inhibitor of matrix metalloproteinases (TIMP).

Arecoline inhibits matrix metalloproteinases (MMPs — particularly MMP-2) and chewing areca quid may also activate nuclear factor kappa B (NF-κB) expression, thereby further stimulating collagen fibroblasts. Flavonoids, catechin, tannin and possibly copper in betel nuts stabilise collagen molecules and inhibit collagenase.

The carcinogenic properties of areca nut are attributed to polyphenols, alkaloids (most importantly, arecoline), metabolites of alkaloids (e.g. arecoline N-oxide) and areca nut-specific nitrosamines. Chronic exposure to such molecules results in increased oxidative stress and subsequent DNA damage which, when unrepaired, may lead to carcinogenesis.

CLINICAL FEATURES

OSMF can affect the oral and sometimes pharyngeal mucosa. It develops insidiously, usually diffusely, often initially presenting with a burning sensation of the oral mucosa, ulceration, vesicle formation, petechiae, post-inflammatory hypermelanosis and pain. This is followed by symmetrical fibrosis of the cheeks, lips, tongue or soft palate appears as vertical bands running through the mucosa, and oral opening becomes restricted (Table 52.1). In advanced disease, the fibrosis can become so severe that the affected site appears mottled and marble-like, and severely restricts mouth opening and tongue and/or palate

TABLE 52.1 Grading of Oral Submucous Fibrosis severity

Grade	Features
1	Oral opening >35 mm
2	Oral opening 20–35 mm
3	Oral opening <20 mm
4	Oral opening <20 mm + PMD
5	Oral opening <20 mm + OSCC

PMD, Potentially malignant disorder; *OSCC*, oral squamous cell carcinoma.

TABLE 52.2 Regimens That Might Be Helpful in Management of Patient Suspected of Having Submucous Fibrosis

	Regimen
Beneficial	Physiotherapy
Likely to be beneficial	COX-2 inhibitors
	Hyaluronidase
	Intralesional corticosteroids
Unproven effectiveness	Lycopene
	Human placental extract
	Interferon gamma
	Pentoxifylline
	Surgery
Supportive	Physiotherapy (jaw opening exercises)
	Correct any nutritional deficiencies, such as iron and vitamin B complex deficiencies

mobility resulting in difficulty in mastication, speech and swallowing (Fig. 52.1). There is epithelial atrophy and sometimes frank erythroplakia or leukoplakia, with 7% to 13% of cases exhibiting transformation to squamous cell carcinoma (0.5% to 1.1% per year). There may be oesophageal fibrosis and, if the palatal and paratubal muscles are involved, conductive hearing loss may appear because of functional stenosis of the Eustachian tube.

Prognosis

OSMF produces epithelial atrophy, and there is a premalignant potential with 7% to 13% of cases transforming into squamous cell carcinoma.

DIAGNOSIS

The diagnosis is usually clinical, based upon clinical features, history of betel chewing and often of slowly increasing trismus. Diagnosis can be confirmed by biopsy which shows collagen hyalinisation, blood vessel obliteration and extensive fibrosis. Haematology often reveals co-existent anaemia. A biopsy should be undertaken when leukoplakia, erythroplakia or persistent ulceration is noted.

TREATMENT

There is no specific therapy for OSMF and no single treatment modality is effective in the management. Patient information is an important aspect of management. Stopping the consumption of betel products is the mainstay of management (Table 52.2). The condition does not regress with the cessation of the habit. Correct any nutritional deficiencies, such as iron and vitamin B complex deficiencies. Asymptomatic cases should be observed only. Patients with trismus may benefit from physiotherapy to stretch the fibrous bands (Fig. 52.2). Thus, habit cessation and physiotherapy form an indispensable part of the treatment procedure.

Medical therapies range from topical medication (e.g. with cyclooxygenase-2 [COX-2] inhibitors); to intralesionally injected medicaments such as corticosteroids, collagenase or hyaluronidase; to systemic medication with lycopene or pentoxifylline.

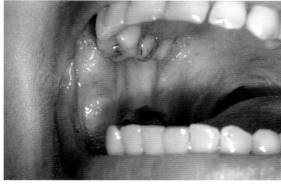

Fig. 52.1 Oral submucous fibrosis.

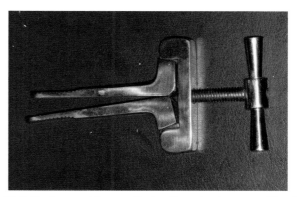

Fig. 52.2 Device used by a patient with oral submucous fibrosis to increase oral opening.

Surgical therapies range from laser release to excision of the fibrotic bands and split skin, radial forearm or other flap repairs.

FOLLOW-UP OF PATIENTS

Close, long-term follow-up is recommended in view of the premalignant potential.

RECOMMENDED READING

Angadi, P.V., Rao, S.S., 2011. Areca nut in pathogenesis of oral submucous fibrosis: revisited. Oral Maxillofac. Surg. 15 (1), 1—9.

Arakeri, G., Brennan, P.A., 2013. Oral submucous fibrosis: an overview of the aetiology, pathogenesis, classification, and principles of management. Br. J. Oral Maxillofac. Surg. 51 (7), 587—593.

Bari, S., Metgud, R., Vyas, Z., Tak, A., 2017. An update on studies on etiological factors, disease progression, and malignant transformation in oral submucous fibrosis. J. Cancer Res. Ther. 13 (3), 399—405.

Kujan, O., Mello, F.W., Warnakulasuriya, S., 2020. Malignant transformation of oral submucous fibrosis: a systematic review and meta-analysis. Oral Dis. 27 (8), 1936—1946.

Kuo, T.M., Luo, S.Y., Chiang, S.L., et al., 2015. Fibrotic effects of arecoline N-oxide in oral potentially malignant disorders. J. Agric. Food Chem. 63 (24), 5787—5794.

More, C.B., Das, S., Patel, H., Adalja, C., Kamatchi, V., Venkatesh, R., 2012. Proposed clinical classification for oral submucous fibrosis. Oral Oncol. 48 (3), 200—202.

More, C.B., Jatti Patil, D., Rao, N.R., 2020. Medicinal management of oral submucous fibrosis in the past decade — a systematic review. J. Oral Biol. Craniofac. Res. 10 (4), 552—568.

Speight, P.M., Khurram, S.A., Kujan, O., 2018. Oral potentially malignant disorders: risk of progression to malignancy. Oral Surg. Oral Med. Oral Pathol. Oral Radiol. 125 (6), 612—627.

Warnakulasuriya, S., Kerr, A.R., 2016. Oral submucous fibrosis: a review of the current management and possible directions for novel therapies. Oral Surg. Oral Med. Oral Pathol. Oral Radiol. 122 (2), 232—241. www.opmdcare.com.

Cancer

KEY POINTS
- The majority of oral cancers are squamous cell carcinomas (SCC).
- Risk factors include sun exposure (lips), tobacco, alcohol and betel use.
- Oropharyngeal carcinoma is increasingly seen in younger people, and has been linked to human papillomaviruses.
- Diagnosis requires biopsy confirmation.
- Surgical resection is the primary modality used to manage most oral cancers.

INTRODUCTION

Oral cancer accounts for a large proportion of cancers in the head and neck region. Cancer of the lip is the most common malignant tumour affecting the head and neck. Oral cavity cancer is classified according to site by the International Classification of Diseases (ICD). In order of decreasing frequency, malignant tumours of the oral cavity affect the anterior two-thirds of the tongue, floor of the mouth, buccal mucosa, retromolar trigone, hard palate and gingivae.

More than 90% of cancers are oral squamous cell carcinomas (OSCC), while the majority of non-squamous cell tumours are of salivary gland origin (Box 53.1). Other malignant oral neoplasms include:
1. Epithelial malignancies:
   - arising from a surface (e.g. melanoma)
   - maxillary antral carcinoma (or other neoplasms)
   - glandular (e.g. salivary gland malignant neoplasms)
   - intrabony epithelial (e.g. malignant odontogenic tumours)

2. Lymphoreticular neoplasms: lymphomas rank second only to carcinoma in frequency of cancers in the head and neck region. The upper jaw, mandible, palate, vestibule and gingiva are, respectively, the most common locations. Swelling, ulceration and radiographic demonstration of bone destruction are the most common signs.
3. Sarcomas: rare but present at any age; have a rapid growth with extensive and ulcerated tumours and may arise:
   - in bone (e.g. osteosarcoma)
   - in connective tissue (e.g. sarcoma)
   - in muscle (e.g. rhabdomyosarcoma)
   - from blood vessels (e.g. Kaposi sarcoma).
4. Metastatic tumours:
   - within a lymph node (e.g. metastases from the oral cavity)
   - within bone (e.g. metastases from lung, breast, kidney, stomach, liver cancer), when most patients complain of swelling, pain and paraesthesia which develop in a relatively short period
   - rarely in the oral soft tissues. Early manifestation of gingival metastases may resemble a hyperplastic or reactive lesion.

ORAL SQUAMOUS CELL CARCINOMA

Introduction

Carcinoma (Fig. 53.1) is an epithelial lesion that grows out of control, as shown by severe dysplasia extending through the full thickness of the epithelium and the rete pegs extending into

BOX 53.1   World Health Organization Classification of Oral Tumours

Tumours of the Oral Cavity and Mobile Tongue
- malignant surface epithelial tumours
  - squamous cell carcinoma
- oral potentially malignant disorders and oral epithelial dysplasia
  - oral potentially malignant disorders
  - oral epithelial dysplasia
  - proliferative verrucous leukoplakia
- papillomas
  - squamous cell papilloma
  - condyloma acuminatum
  - verruca vulgaris
  - multifocal epithelial hyperplasia
- tumours of uncertain histogenesis
  - congenital granular cell epulis
  - ectomesenchymal chondromyxoid tumour
- soft tissue and neural tumours
  - granular cell tumour
  - rhabdomyoma
  - lymphangioma
  - haemangioma
  - schwannoma and neurofibroma
  - Kaposi sarcoma
  - myofibroblastic sarcoma
- oral mucosal melanoma
- salivary type tumours
  - mucoepidermoid carcinoma
  - pleomorphic adenoma
- haematolymphoid tumours
  - CD30-positive T-cell lymphoproliferative disorder
  - plasmablastic lymphoma
  - Langerhans cell histiocytosis
  - extramedullary myeloid sarcoma

Tumours of the Oropharynx (Base of Tongue, Tonsils, Adenoids)
- squamous cell carcinoma
  - squamous cell carcinoma, HPV-positive
  - squamous cell carcinoma, HPV-negative
- salivary gland tumours
  - pleomorphic adenoma
  - adenoid cystic carcinoma
  - polymorphous adenocarcinoma
- haematolymphoid tumours
  - Hodgkin lymphoma
  - Burkitt lymphoma
  - follicular lymphoma
  - mantle cell lymphoma
  - T-lymphoblastic leukaemia/lymphoma
  - follicular dendritic cell sarcoma

Tumours and Tumour-Like Lesions of the Neck and Lymph Nodes
- tumours of unknown origin
  - carcinoma of unknown primary
  - Merkel cell carcinoma
  - heterotopia-associated carcinoma
- haematolymphoid tumours
- cysts and cyst-like lesions
  - branchial cleft cyst
  - thyroglossal duct cyst

- ranula
- dermoid and teratoid cysts

Tumours of Salivary Glands
- malignant tumours
  - mucoepidermoid carcinoma
  - adenoid cystic carcinoma
  - acinic cell carcinoma
  - polymorphous adenocarcinoma
  - clear cell carcinoma
  - basal cell adenocarcinoma
  - intraductal carcinoma
  - adenocarcinoma, not otherwise specified
  - salivary duct carcinoma
  - myoepithelial carcinoma
  - epithelial—myoepithelial carcinoma
  - carcinoma ex pleomorphic adenoma
  - secretory carcinoma
  - sebaceous adenocarcinoma
  - carcinosarcoma
  - poorly differentiated carcinoma
  - lymphoepithelial carcinoma
  - squamous cell carcinoma
  - oncocytic carcinoma
  - sialoblastoma
- benign tumours
  - pleomorphic adenoma
  - myoepithelioma
  - basal cell adenoma
  - Warthin tumour
  - oncocytoma
  - lymphadenoma
  - cystadenoma
  - sialadenoma papilliferum
  - ductal papillomas
  - sebaceous adenoma
  - canalicular adenoma and other ductal adenomas
- non-neoplastic epithelial lesions
  - sclerosing polycystic adenosis
  - nodular oncocytic hyperplasia
  - lymphoepithelial sialadenitis
  - intercalated duct hyperplasia
- benign soft tissue lesions
  - haemangioma
  - lipoma/sialolipoma
  - nodular fasciitis
- haematolymphoid tumours
  - extranodal marginal zone lymphoma of mucosa-associated lymphoid tissue (MALT lymphoma)

Odontogenic and Maxillofacial Bone Tumours
- odontogenic carcinomas
  - ameloblastic carcinoma
  - primary intraosseous carcinoma, not otherwise specified
  - sclerosing odontogenic carcinoma
  - clear cell odontogenic carcinoma
  - ghost cell odontogenic carcinoma
- odontogenic carcinosarcoma
- odontogenic sarcomas

- benign epithelial odontogenic tumours
  - ameloblastoma
  - ameloblastoma, unicystic type
  - ameloblastoma, extraosseous/peripheral type
  - metastasising ameloblastoma
  - squamous odontogenic tumour
  - calcifying epithelial odontogenic tumour
  - adenomatoid odontogenic tumour
- benign mixed epithelial and mesenchymal odontogenic tumours
  - ameloblastic fibroma
  - primordial odontogenic tumour
  - odontoma
  - dentinogenic ghost cell tumour
- benign mesenchymal odontogenic tumours
  - odontogenic fibroma
  - odontogenic myxoma/myxofibroma
  - cementoblastoma
  - cemento-ossifying fibroma
- odontogenic cysts of inflammatory origin
  - radicular cyst
  - inflammatory collateral cysts
- odontogenic and non-odontogenic developmental cysts
  - dentigerous cyst
  - odontogenic keratocyst
  - lateral periodontal cyst and botryoid odontogenic cyst
  - gingival cysts
  - glandular odontogenic cyst
  - calcifying odontogenic cyst
  - orthokeratinised odontogenic cyst
- nasopalatine duct cyst
- malignant maxillofacial bone and cartilage tumours
  - chondrosarcoma
  - mesenchymal chondrosarcoma
  - osteosarcoma
- benign maxillofacial bone and cartilage tumours
  - chondroma
  - osteoma
  - melanotic neuroectodermal tumour of infancy
  - chondroblastoma
  - chondromyxoid fibroma
  - osteoid osteoma
  - osteoblastoma
  - desmoplastic fibroma
- fibro-osseous and osteochondromatous lesions
  - ossifying fibroma
  - familial gigantiform cementoma
  - fibrous dysplasia
  - cemento-osseous dysplasia
  - osteochondroma
- giant cell lesions and simple bone cyst
  - central giant cell granuloma
  - peripheral giant cell granuloma
  - cherubism
  - aneurysmal bone cyst
  - simple bone cyst
- haematolymphoid tumours
  - solitary plasmacytoma of bone

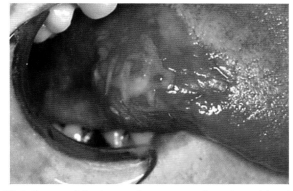

Fig. 53.1 Cancer of the tongue (squamous cell carcinoma) in a typical site.

the underlying lamina propria (i.e. invasion across the epithelial basement membrane). The local invasion and eventual lymphatic and blood spread ultimately lead to metastasis of lymph nodes and organs (mainly the liver, brain and bones). Carcinoma of the oral cavity may develop de novo or from a pre-malignant dysplastic lesion that appears clinically as leukoplakia, erythroplakia or an erythroleukoplakia.

Incidence

OSCC is among the 10 most common cancers worldwide.

Age

OSCC is seen predominantly in older patients (>65 years), but intraoral cancer is increasing, especially in younger adults (<45 years), particularly in the oropharynx.

Gender

OSCC is seen predominantly in males but the male/female differential is decreasing.

Geographic

There is marked inter-country variation in both the incidence of and mortality from OSCC.

There is growing evidence of intra-country differences in OSCC, including ethnic differences in incidence and mortality.

- The incidence of oral cancer is the highest in the world in South-East Asia and Brazil but varies widely in different areas.
- In the developed world, the incidence of OSCC varies between countries, as well as between different regions of the same country. For example, OSCC is more than twice as common in Scotland than in England and Wales; and even within Scotland, there are regional differences.
- Oral cancer is the most common cancer for men and the third most common for women in India, Sri Lanka and

Pakistan; 30% of all new cases of cancer in these countries is oral cancer, whereas only 3% of new cases of cancer in the United Kingdom is oral cancer.

Risk Factors for Oral Squamous Cell Carcinomas

Lifestyle, environment and genetics may play a role, but OSCC appears to be related mainly to a number of lifestyle factors. The association between tobacco use and oral cancer has long been established. Smoking tobacco products (cigarettes, cigars, pipes) is an important risk factor for the development of oral cancer. Smokeless tobacco products (chewing tobacco and snuff) also increase the risk in those who do not smoke tobacco. The association of marijuana use alone, and the development of oral cancer is unclear, but some evidence suggests an increased risk. The risk of developing oral cancer due to alcohol consumption alone appears to be influenced by the type of alcoholic beverage and the frequency of consumption. Concomitant alcohol use and tobacco smoking have a multiplicative effect on the risk of developing OSCC.

While tobacco and alcohol are the main carcinogens implicated in oral cavity cancer, increased OSCC is also seen in the following groups:

- betel quid users (some 20% of the world's population use betel)
- resource-poor groups
- ethnic minority groups.

Dietary, genetic and immunological factors may also play a part, since neither do all tobacco/alcohol users develop cancer, and equally, nor do all patients with cancer have these habits. Ultraviolet radiation is an important etiologic factor for SCC involving the lip. Previous irradiation for either malignant or benign disease, along with infections in the oral cavity such as herpes viruses, chronic candidiasis and syphilis have also been implicated.

Infection with oncogenic human papillomaviruses (HPV), especially HPV-16, are implicated mainly in oropharyngeal cancer (base of tongue, fauces) and does not appear as frequently in the oral cavity. The prevalence rates of HPV positivity were 41% in oropharyngeal cancer and 15% in oral cavity cancers. HPV-associated cancers are:

- often basaloid carcinomas
- associated with HPV-16 (>90%): also types 18, 31, 33
- associated with reduced tumour suppressor gene expression (p53 and Rb genes)
- not linked to alcohol or tobacco use
- associated with a better prognosis than other OSCC.

HPV can be transmitted between the mouth and anogenital region. There are two commercially available prophylactic vaccines against HPV: the bivalent Cervarix® (GlaxoSmithKline), which protects against HPV types 16 and 18 and the tetravalent Gardasil® (Merck) that protects against infection with HPV types 6, 11, 16, 18. A nine-valent HPV vaccine is approved by the US Food and Drug Administration (FDA) for the prevention of HPV-associated head and neck cancers. HPV vaccination is effective in preventing cervical cancer but data regarding the impact on oral disease is limited to studies demonstrating a reduction in oral HPV infection.

Diets rich in fresh fruits and vegetables and of vitamin A may have a protective effect on oral cancer and pre-cancer. No single dietary factor alone appears responsible: antioxidants may be anti-carcinogenic (e.g. in green tea).

Genetics typically play a minor role in OSCC, but there are a few rare cases where patients have a predisposition to develop multiple tumours because they have an inherited condition such as:

- Fanconi anaemia: a recessively inherited disease, characterised by congenital anomalies and bone marrow failure, and a predisposition to develop cancer, particularly SCC in the head and neck and anogenital region, myelodysplastic syndrome and acute myelocytic leukaemia.
- Dyskeratosis congenita: a disease of defective telomere maintenance, characterised by mucocutaneous abnormalities, bone marrow failure and cancer predisposition. Leukoplakias occur in approximately 80% of patients and typically involve the buccal mucosa, tongue and oropharynx. Other sites may be involved (e.g. oesophagus, urethra, lacrimal duct, conjunctiva, anogenital). Patients have an increased prevalence of malignant disease, often SCC within sites of leukoplakia (especially the tongue), or of the skin, Hodgkin lymphoma, gastrointestinal adenocarcinoma, bronchial and laryngeal carcinoma and leukaemia.
- Xeroderma pigmentosum: a rare disease of defective DNA repair mechanisms, predisposing to cancer in light-exposed areas such as skin and lips.
- Rare cases include patients with a mutation in one allele of the tumour suppressor gene p53 locus (Li-Fraumeni syndrome) who have a predisposition not to OSCC but to breast cancer, brain tumours, leukaemia and sarcomas — sometimes in the jaw.

Primary Prevention

Smoking cessation reduces the risk: 10 years after smoking cessation, the risk of oral cancer seems to be similar to that of a someone who has never smoked at all. Treatment of tobacco dependence is therefore important and can be addressed in primary care and smoking cessation clinics. Protection against solar irradiation and photosensitisers could further reduce lip cancers.

Secondary Prevention

Early detection of oral cancer is the key issue to reduce cancer mortality. There is insufficient evidence to recommend screening of the general population for OSCC either by using visual examination or adjunctive tools (e.g. toluidine blue, brush biopsy, fluorescence imaging) to decrease mortality. Screening by visual inspection by qualified healthcare providers for *high-risk* groups has the potential to reduce cancer mortality and contribute to downstaging oral cancers.

Aetiology and Pathogenesis

Potentially malignant (precancerous) disorders that can progress to OSCC are discussed elsewhere and include, especially:

- erythroplakia
- leukoplakia
- oral submucous fibrosis
- actinic cheilitis
- lichen planus/lichenoid lesions.

Carcinogenesis is a multistep process that involves overexpression of oncogenes and inactivation of tumour suppressor genes. OSCC arises because of deoxyribonucleic acid (DNA) mutations caused mainly by free radicals and oxidants. DNA mutations change various crucial genes and other nucleic acid components involved in cell growth and control (and are potential targets for anti-cancer therapies), such as:

- Tumour suppressor genes: such as p16 and p53 — control the fate of chromosomally damaged cells and the cell growth cycle. P53 has been identified as being important in oral cavity carcinomas in smokers.
- Oncogenes: such as the epidermal growth factor receptor (*EGFR*) gene, PRAD-1, Int-2, hst-1, bcl-1 and *ras* — involved in cell signalling. Telomerase genes control telomerases, enzymes involved in chromosome shortening.
- MicroRNAs (mRNA): non-coding pieces of ribonucleic acid (RNA) which are incorporated into the RNA-induced silencing complex, which binds to mRNA to mediate gene expression.

The accumulation of genetic changes can lead to cell dysregulation to the extent that growth becomes autonomous and invasive mechanisms develop; this is carcinoma. The neoplastic process first manifests intraepithelially (oral intraepithelial neoplasia) near the basement membrane as a focal, clonal overgrowth of altered keratinocyte stem cells, which expand upward and laterally, replacing normal epithelium. After some time, invasion of the epithelial basement membrane signifies the start of invasive cancer (Box 53.2). Epithelial cells then proliferate into and invade the underlying tissues (Fig. 53.2). Cancer spread locally may cause pain and other symptoms including dysarthria, dysphagia, tooth mobility and halitosis. Ultimately, cancer spreads (metastasises) via lymphatics to regional lymph nodes, later by the bloodstream to vital organs such as the lungs, brain, liver, bone and elsewhere.

Clinical Features

The majority of OSCCs (>95%) present as ulcers or masses. Early lesions may present as a leukoplakia or erythroplakia. A solitary non-healing ulcer persisting for more than 3 weeks is the most common presentation (Table 53.1). More advanced tumours may invade neighbouring structures causing tooth mobility, trismus, sensory change, referred otalgia, dysphagia, odynophagia, dysarthria and neck masses.

Lip Cancer

Cancer of the lip is the most common malignant tumour affecting the head and neck. Lip cancer may follow chronic

---

BOX 53.2   Microscopic Features of Carcinoma

Disordered Cell Maturation
- Irregular hyperplasia and/or atrophy
- Keratosis/parakeratosis
- Drop-shaped rete processes
- Irregular stratification
- Disturbed cell polarity
- Premature and individual cell keratinisation
- Reduced cell cohesion
- Cell pleomorphism

Disturbed Cell Proliferation
- Loss of basal cell polarity
- Basal cell hyperplasia
- Increased nuclear/cytoplasmic ratio
- Enlarged nucleoli
- Nuclear hyperchromatism
- Increased mitoses
- Anisonucleosis
- Abnormal mitoses
- Mitoses in stratum spinosum

Tissue Changes
- Loss of regular epithelial stratification
- Reduced cell-to-cell cohesion
- Bullous or drop-shaped rete pegs
- Keratin or epithelial pearls
- Invasion of the basement membrane

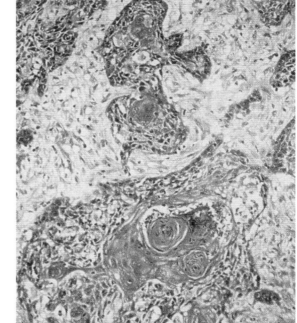

Fig. 53.2 Histopathology of squamous cell carcinoma showing islets of dysplastic epithelium and cell nests in lamina propria.

TABLE 53.1   Features Suggestive of Oral Squamous Cell Carcinomas

Features	Comment
Red lesion	Erythroplakia may be associated
Mixed red/white lesion	Erythroleukoplakia may be associated
Irregular white lesion	Verrucous or nodular leukoplakia may be associated
Lump	Especially if enlarging and/or hard
Ulcer	Especially if persistent, or with fissuring or raised exophytic margins
Pain or numbness	May be a late feature
Abnormal blood vessels supplying a lump	
Tooth mobility	Destruction of the periodontium by malignant cells
Extraction socket not healing	
Induration beneath a lesion	Firm infiltration beneath the mucosa
Fixation of lesion	To deeper tissues or to overlying skin or mucosa
Lymph node enlargement	Especially if there is hardness in a lymph node or fixation
	Enlarged cervical nodes in a patient with OSCC may be caused by infection, reactive hyperplasia, secondary or metastatic disease
Dysphagia	
Weight loss	

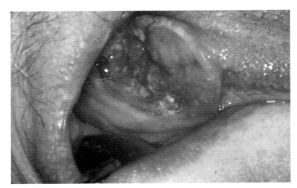

Fig. 53.3 Cancer of the tongue, an ulcerated indurated swelling.

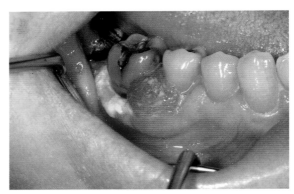

Fig. 53.4 Carcinoma on the gingiva.

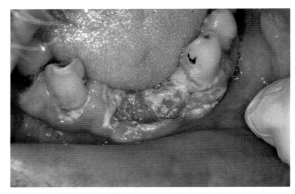

Fig. 53.5 Carcinoma on the alveolus.

actinic cheilitis, induced by sunlight irradiation. About 90% of tumours arise in the lower lip, 7% in the upper lip and 3% at the oral commissure. Lip cancer has a far better prognosis than intraoral cancers.

Intraoral Cancer

Most OSCC involve the lateral border of the tongue (Fig. 53.3) and/or the floor of the mouth (Figs 53.4 and 53.5). Unfortunately, most OSCC are detected only when present for some weeks or months: most intraoral tumours are larger than 2 cm in diameter at presentation.

Carcinomas in the anterior mouth are usually detected at an earlier stage than OSCC of the posterior oral cavity. In the developing world, OSCC is most common in the buccal mucosa and arises mainly from betel use.

Second Primary Tumours

Although a primary OSCC usually presents as a single persistent lesion, patients with OSCC may develop other primary cancers in the upper aerodigestive tract (this includes the mouth, nose, pharynx, larynx, bronchi and lungs and oesophagus). These second primary tumours (SPTs) usually arise because smoking tobacco exposes the whole of the aerodigestive tract to carcinogens. SPTs appear either at the same time (synchronously — within six months of the diagnosis of the primary tumour), or later (metachronously, i.e. at least six months after the primary tumour). SPTs may be seen over three years in 15% to 25% (overall about 3% per year), of patients. The most common sites are the head and neck, followed by the lungs and oesophagus.

Other Medical Problems

Most patients with OSCC are older adults, many have been exposed to tobacco, betel, alcohol or a combination, and they are often also of resource-poor groups. Co-morbidities, such as cardiovascular (e.g. hypertension and ischaemic heart disease), respiratory (e.g. chronic obstructive airways disease) and hepatic (e.g. cirrhosis), are therefore common.

Diagnosis

Early diagnosis is important, since it is generally accepted that prognosis is best in early carcinomas, especially those that are well-differentiated (Box 53.3) and treatment of an early OSCC is likely to be less invasive.

Clinical examination is useful in identifying new tumours. The examination should be preceded by a focused medical history to establish any co-morbidities and risk factors. A systematic approach must be adopted. The whole oral mucosa should be examined as there may be widespread dysplastic mucosa ('field change'), or SPTs, and the cervical lymph nodes must always be examined.

Single ulcers, lumps, red patches or white patches, particularly if any of these persist for more than 3 weeks, may be manifestations of frank malignancy and thus a biopsy is invariably indicated. Frank tumours should be inspected and palpated to determine the extent of spread.

Examination under general anaesthesia (EUA) may be indicated, particularly for patients with:

- tumours in the posterior tongue
- tumours where the margins cannot be readily defined
- an enlarged cervical node but no visible primary neoplasm. Positron emission tomography (PET) may be helpful to identify latent primary neoplasms
- any suggestion of an SPT, as patients may then need a pan-endoscopy of the larynx, pharynx and oesophagus, and/or PET. Fluorodeoxyglucose PET (FDG-PET) will also help detect distant metastases.

OSCC should be staged according to the tumour, node, metastases (TNM) classification of the Union for International Cancer Control (UICC) — according to tumour size, nodal metastases and distant metastases (Tables 53.2 and table 53.3) — since this classification relates well to overall survival rate (i.e. the earlier the stage of the tumour, the better the prognosis and the less complicated and mutilating the treatment will be). The current TNM staging system now incorporates maximum depth of invasion. Patients with greater than 5 mm depth of invasion have a minimum tumour stage of T2; patients with greater than 10 mm depth of invasion have a minimum tumour stage of T3.

BOX 53.3   Grades of Carcinoma

Well-Differentiated
Elongated rete pegs invading lamina propria, with keratin pearls

Moderately Differentiated
Irregular invading rete pegs; loss of cellular cohesion

Poorly Differentiated
Sheets of invading epithelium with no obvious architecture, but severe cellular abnormalities such as pleomorphism and hyperchromatism

---

Clinical palpation of the cervical lymph nodes is necessary but generally regarded as inaccurate as non-palpable micrometastases may be present. To describe the lymph nodes of the neck (for neck dissection to remove nodes with metastases), the neck is

---

TABLE 53.2   Tumour, Node, Metastases Classification of Cancer of the Lip and Oral Cavity

T — Primary Tumour	
TX	Primary tumour cannot be assessed
T0	No evidence of primary tumour
Tis	Carcinoma in situ
T1	Tumour ≤ 2 cm with depth of invasion (DOI) ≤ 5 mm
T2	Tumour ≤ 2 cm, with DOI >5 mm and ≤ 10 mm; or Tumour >2 cm and ≤ 4 cm, with DOI ≤ 10 mm
T3	Tumour >2 cm and ≤ 4 cm with DOI >10 mm; or Tumour >4 cm with DOI ≤ 10 mm
T4a (lip)	Tumour invades through cortical bone, inferior alveolar nerve, floor of mouth or skin (chin or nose)
T4a (oral cavity)	Moderately advanced local disease. Tumour >4 cm with DOI >10 mm; or tumour invades adjacent structures only (e.g. through cortical bone of the mandible or maxilla, or involves the maxillary sinus or skin of the face)
T4b (lip and oral cavity)	Very advanced local disease. Tumour invades masticator space, pterygoid plates or skull base and/or encases the internal carotid artery
N — Regional Lymph Nodes	
NX	Regional lymph nodes cannot be assessed
N0	No regional lymph node metastasis
N1	Metastasis in a single ipsilateral lymph node, 3 cm or less in greatest dimension
N2	Metastasis as specified in N2a, 2b, 2c below
N2a	Metastasis in a single ipsilateral lymph node, more than 3 cm but not more than 6 cm in greatest dimension
N2b	Metastasis in multiple ipsilateral lymph nodes, none more than 6 cm in greatest dimension
N2c	Metastasis in bilateral or contralateral lymph nodes, none more than 6 cm in greatest dimension
N3	Metastasis in a lymph node more than 6 cm in greatest dimension
M — Distant Metastasis	
M0	No distant metastasis
M1	Distant metastasis

divided into six areas called levels, identified by Roman numerals, increasing towards the chest (Table 53.4).

Investigations are indicated with the aim to:

- Confirm the cancer diagnosis histopathologically.
- Determine if there is malignant disease elsewhere:
  - local invasion (e.g. bone, muscles or cervical regional lymph nodes)
  - metastases, which initially are to lymph nodes and later to liver, bone and brain.
- SPTs.
- Ensure the patient is prepared for major surgery, particularly in terms of their understanding and informed consent, general anaesthesia, potential blood loss and ability to metabolise drugs.
- Address potential dental or oral problems pre-operatively, to minimise or avoid later complications.

These principles almost invariably mandate the following investigations:

Lesional Biopsy

An incisional biopsy is invariably required. An excisional biopsy should be avoided since this is unlikely to have excised an adequately wide margin of tissue if the lesion is malignant and will have destroyed clinical evidence of the site and character of the lesion. The biopsy should be sufficiently large to include enough suspect and apparently normal tissue to give the pathologist a chance to make a diagnosis and not to have to request a further specimen. Most biopsy wounds, whether 0.5 cm (too small) or 1.5 cm long (usually adequate) heal within 7 to 10 days. Therefore, it is better to take at least one ample specimen. If the pathology report denies malignancy, yet cancer is still the clinical diagnosis, then the pathology should be re-checked, and a re-biopsy may be indicated.

Radiography

- Jaw (orthopantomogram [OP]), which might demonstrate bone invasion.
- Chest computed tomography (CT) as a pre-anaesthetic check, especially in patients with known respiratory disease, and to demonstrate SPTs or metastases to lungs or hilar lymph nodes, ribs or vertebrae.

TABLE 53.4 Nomenclature of Anatomical Site of Cervical Lymph Nodes

Level	Contents
I	Submental and submandibular triangles bounded by the posterior belly of the digastric muscle, the hyoid bone inferiorly and the body of the mandible superiorly
II	Upper jugular lymph nodes and extends from the level of the hyoid bone inferiorly to the skull base superiorly
III	Middle jugular lymph nodes from the hyoid bone superiorly to the cricothyroid membrane inferiorly
IV	Lower jugular lymph nodes from the cricothyroid membrane superiorly to the clavicle inferiorly
V	Posterior triangle lymph nodes bounded by the anterior border of the trapezius posteriorly, the posterior border of the sternocleidomastoid muscle anteriorly and the clavicle inferiorly
VI	Anterior compartment lymph nodes from the hyoid bone superiorly to the suprasternal notch inferiorly. On each side the lateral border is formed by the medial border of the carotid sheath

- MRI of the primary tumour site, of the head and neck, and of suspected sites of distant metastases, and of the neck to delineate the extent of cervical node metastases. MRI provides superior soft tissue definition compared with CT.
- PET/CT scans combine the advantages of CT for anatomy and PET for function, potentially producing an earlier diagnosis and more accurate staging. FDG-PET scan uses fluorodeoxyglucose, a modified sugar that is absorbed by cancer cells.
- Ultrasound and biopsy or fine needle aspiration of neck lymph nodes that may contain metastases. It has high sensitivity and specificity and a diagnostic accuracy ranging from 89%–98%.
- CT of the neck has a higher sensitivity in detecting metastatic disease in lymph nodes than physical examination.
- sentinel node lymph node biopsy has been shown to be an effective method of assessment of the neck in early-stage oral cancers.
- In selected cases, other investigations that may be indicated, including:

TABLE 53.3 Two-Year Crude Survival Rates

Stage	Tumour, Node, Metastases			Approximate Survival at 5 Years (%)
0	Tis	N0	M0	
I	T1	N0	M0	80
II	T2	N0	M0	75
III	T1, T2	N1	M0	50
	T3	N0, N1	M0	
IVa	T1, T2, T3	N2	M0	10
	T4a	N0, N1, N2	M0	
IVb	Any T	N3	M0	
	T4b	Any N	M0	
IVc	Any T	Any N	M1	

- bronchoscopy if chest radiography reveals any lesions
- endoscopy of the upper aerodigestive tract, especially if there is a history of tobacco use
- gastroscopy if a per-endoscopic gastrostomy (PEG) is to be used for feeding
- liver ultrasound if there is hepatomegaly or abnormal liver function
- doppler duplex flow studies, in planning radial free forearm flaps
- angiography, in planning lower limb free flaps
- electrocardiography
- blood tests:
  - full blood picture and haemoglobin
  - blood for grouping and cross-matching
  - urea and electrolytes
  - liver function tests.

Treatment

Patient Communication

Patient communication and information are crucial aspects in management. Communication, especially breaking bad news such as about cancer well, can help all involved, and reduce the inevitable distress experienced. Management must include paying special attention to psychological reactions. Denial is common. Patients may or may not know or may not want to know that they have cancer and, even if they are aware of it, may not appreciate or be willing to accept the prognosis. The patient should be kept aware of the intended outcomes, prognosis and the potentially adverse effects of treatment.

Quality of Life Issues

Cancer survival rates have been and continue to improve so more patients are living with cancer but also having to cope with the adverse effects of cancer and its treatment. OSCC and its management are associated with more physical, emotional and psychosocial disruption than is the case with some other tumours. This affects patients' quality of life (QoL) and, while the aim of cancer treatment must ideally be to remove or destroy the tumour entirely, the outcome is a balance between this and adverse effects (of treatment and psychological sequelae). Patients with OSCC may be aware that they will almost certainly face pain and swelling and at least some difficulties in eating, chewing, drinking, breathing, speaking, as well as possible changes in appearance. Another common concern is fear of recurrence. Psychosocial dysfunction is virtually invariably to be anticipated, and interventions needed.

If you are concerned, phone a specialist, e-mail or write for an urgent opinion. If a cancer diagnosis has been established, it is reasonable to discuss that:

- tumours differ in their degree of malignancy
- their tumour has been detected at an early stage (hopefully)
- treatment is continually improving
- you have referred them to the best possible centre for treatment
- the oncological multidisciplinary team (MDT) will provide fuller details of treatment options.

Discussion of actual treatment and prognosis should be left to the surgeon/oncologist concerned, as only they are in a position to give accurate facts to the patient.

Multidisciplinary Cancer Care

Cancer care planning is based upon an MDT offering:
- medicine, cardiology, respiratory, dental, psychological, anaesthetic and, palliative advice
- speech and language therapy advice: for pre-operative counselling regarding potential speech and swallowing rehabilitation
- dietary advice: to assess nutritional status and need for feeding by percutaneous gastrostomy (PEG).

The MDT plans the cancer treatment, including avoidance of post-operative complications — this includes planned oral and dental care such as discussions regarding restorative and surgical interventions required before cancer treatment. Oral care is especially important when radiotherapy is to be given or bisphosphonates are used, since there is a risk of osteonecrosis — the initiating factor which is often trauma, such as tooth extraction, or ulceration from an appliance, or oral infection. As much dental treatment as is possible should be completed **before** starting cancer treatment.

Cancer treatment planning is based on:
- tumour size, nodal status and metastases
- balance of benefit of a particular treatment and its potential adverse reactions
- co-existent medical conditions
- social circumstances
- most importantly, patient wishes.

Generally speaking, surgery alone or with post-operative radiotherapy remains the main treatment for OSCC since the adverse effects of therapeutic radiotherapy (RT) and chemotherapy (CTX), are generally greater. OSCC is thus treated largely by surgery and/or RT to control the primary tumour and metastases in the draining cervical lymph nodes with a considered balance between length of survival and the quality of remaining life.

Surgery

Surgical resection is the mainstay of management for most oral cancers. Tumour resection should be performed with a clear margin of 1 cm (vital structures permitting). 'Close' margins (defined as a histopathological margin of <5 mm) mean further surgery or adjuvant RT.

Advantages of surgery include complete tumour and lymph node excision with full histological examination, removal of involved bone and its use for radio-resistant tumours. Disadvantages of surgery are mainly that it is mutilating for very large tumours. To permit normal breathing, a tracheostomy (Fig. 53.6) may be necessary. To support alimentation (feeding), a nasogastric tube or a PEG (Fig. 53.7) may be required.

Surgery attempts to achieve one or more of the following goals:
- **Cure:** the excision of a tumour confined to one area. Surgery may be used along with RT and/or CTX given before, during or after surgery. Neck dissection to clear the neck of cancer containing lymph nodes is often also needed in addition to

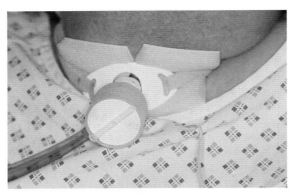

Fig. 53.6 Tracheostomy.

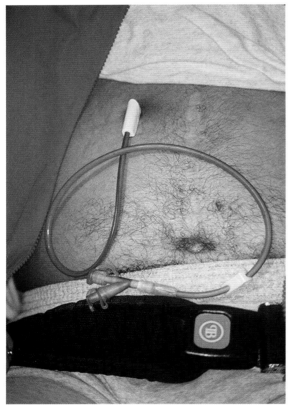

Fig. 53.7 PEG (per-endoscopic gastrostomy).

the excision of the primary tumour. Elective neck management is indicated for any tumour when the risk of occult nodal involvement is greater than 20%. The types of neck dissection are:

- radical neck dissection (RND): removal of all ipsilateral cervical lymph node groups from levels I through V, together with spinal accessory nerve (SAN), sternocleidomastoid muscle (SCM) and internal jugular vein (IJV).
- modified radical neck dissection (MRND): removal of all lymph node groups routinely removed in an RND, but with preservation of one or more non-lymphatic structures (SAN, SCM and IJV).

- selective neck dissection (SND): cervical lymphadenectomy with preservation of one or more lymph node groups that are routinely removed in an RND. Thus, for OSCC, SND (I–III) is commonly performed.
- extended neck dissection: removal of one or more additional lymph node groups or non-lymphatic structures, or both, not encompassed by the RND.
- sentinel lymph node biopsy has been shown to be an effective method of assessment of the neck in early-stage oral cancers to establish whether neck dissection is required.
- **Reconstruction:** Crucially important to restore the appearance and/or function (e.g. the use of tissue flaps, bone grafts or prosthetic materials). Reconstruction is best performed at the time of initial surgery. For soft tissue reconstruction, local flaps (e.g. nasolabial flaps) can repair small defects. Distant flaps are required to repair larger defects; these include:
  - free flaps: microvascular surgery facilitates excellent reconstruction at a single operation using, for example, forearm flaps based on radial vessels, which are particularly useful to replace soft tissue, or those based on the fibula where bone is required.
  - pedicle flaps: myocutaneous or osteomyocutaneous flaps based on a feeding vessel to muscle and perforators to the skin paddle, e.g. flaps based on the pectoralis major, latissimus dorsi or trapezius are now used in a one-stage operation to replace skin and, since they also contain muscle, they have adequate bulk to repair defects and may also be used to import bone (usually rib).
  - hard tissue: mandibular defects are reconstructed with implants to maintain aesthetics and anatomy temporarily until the patient is tumour-free and bone grafting possible. Bone is traditionally taken as free non-vascularised bone grafts from the iliac crest or rib, but these often show poor survival in a contaminated area like the mouth, or in a relatively avascular field after irradiation. An osteomyocutaneous flap, such as a fibula graft, greatly improves the vascular bed for the graft, but requires considerable expertise. Maxillary defects are reconstructed with an obturator (bung), which has the advantage that the cavity can be readily inspected.
- **Debulking:** used when removing a tumour entirely would cause too much damage to an organ or vital structures.
- **Palliation:** used to treat complications of advanced disease, not to cure.

CANCER SURGERY COMPLICATIONS

See Table 53.5.

- **Pain:** Post-operative pain is usually present for at least 24 hours. Severe pain may need to be controlled with opioids.
- **Oedema**
- **Trismus**
- **Infection:** The diagnosis of infection is usually as, at about three to seven days after operation, the wound appears inflamed, swollen and tender. There may be pus and pyrexia. Infection under neck flaps is particularly dangerous

TABLE 53.5 Orofacial Complications of Cancer Therapy

Therapy	Oral Complications
Radiotherapy	Pain, mucositis, hyposalivation, candidosis, caries, sialadenitis, osteoradionecrosis, fibrosis
Chemotherapy	Pain, mucositis, hyposalivation, candidosis, herpesviruses, neuropathy
Surgery	Pain, neuropathy, disfigurement, impaired speech and swallowing Scarring Carotid blow-out (haemorrhage), chyle leakage, salivary leakage

as the internal carotid artery may be eroded (see below 'carotid blow-out'). Infections may settle spontaneously within a few days, but pus or a swab should be taken to identify the organism and test sensitivity to antibiotics. If the wound is not draining but is fluctuant, one or more sutures should be removed, sinus forceps inserted and gently opened to allow pus drainage antibiotics.

- **Flap Complications**
- **Eating Problems:** Nutrition may need to be supplemented enterally by nasogastric (NG) or orogastric tube, (PEG or radiologicallyinserted gastrostomy (RIG).
- **Vascular complications:** Carotid blow-out is more likely where the patient has had radiotherapy, damage to the artery during surgery and salivary fistulae and is associated with over 60% morbidity and 50% mortality.
- **Seroma:** Seroma is the accumulation of serous fluid under large flaps and appears as a large fluctuant swelling that is neither warm nor tender.
- **Sialocele:** Sialocele is a swelling due to leakage of saliva occasionally appearing over the area of the parotid following partial parotidectomy.
- **Frey syndrome:** This may follow damage in the parotid region by trauma, submandibular gland surgery, neck dissection or carotid endarterectomy, and is characterised by skin redness and sweating after eating or thinking or talking about food. Testing with lemon or a positive starch-iodine test can be diagnostic.
- **Chyle leak:** Chyle leak arises from damage to the chyle duct.
- **Nerve damage:** If damaged, the SAN to the trapezius muscle can cause significant shoulder disability. Other nerves also at risk include the vagus, lingual, hypoglossal and marginal mandibular branch of the facial nerves.
- **Radiation toxicities (RT):** RT can cause a range of adverse effects (Table 53.7). Some — notably mucositis and hyposalivation — arise almost immediately and are predictable, whilst others appear later and unpredictably. Mucositis, dysphagia, xerostomia, loss of taste, dermatitis and pain significantly impair QoL, as do hyposalivation (up to 90% incidence) and grade 3 (severe) dysphagia (up to 30%).
- Late RT toxicity is permanent and may also include jaw osteoradionecrosis, sensori-neural hearing loss and skin fibrosis.

RADIOTHERAPY

Adjuvant post-operative RT to the primary site and neck, with or without concurrent chemotherapy, is indicated for patients who have positive or close final resection margins, those who have bone invasion and patients with pathologically positive lymph nodes or to treat the neck prophylactically without a neck dissection. External beam radiotherapy is not recommended as the primary curative treatment in OSCC because the morbidity of treatment limits radiation dose and cure rates. For advanced disease (stages III and IV), the usual management includes surgical resection of the primary tumour, neck dissection, reconstruction and post-operative radiotherapy. Radiotherapy should optimally start within 6 weeks of surgery. The daily dose must be enough to destroy cancer cells while sparing normal tissues of excessive radiation: Typically 2 Gy is delivered daily to a 60 to 70 Gy total dose (Gray (Gy) = energy absorption of 1 joule/kg (1 Gy = 100 rads).

Planning before RT includes CT scan and measurements of the area to be treated, as well as skin markings to help treatment positioning. A mask immobilises the patient's head so that RT will only be delivered to specifically designated areas. Most of this time is spent ensuring that blocking devices, which restrict the RT to the appropriate area, are properly located, and patient and machine properly positioned. Advantages of RT include normal anatomy and function being maintained, general anaesthesia is not needed and salvage surgery is still available if radiotherapy fails. Disadvantages include subsequent surgery being more difficult and hazardous and survival further reduced; failure is probably due to cancer cell repopulation and hypoxia, as well as a cure being uncommon for large cancers. Adverse effects are common with conventional RT, which causes significant acute (during and up to 3 months post-radiation) sequelae, including severe mucositis, and late toxicities (skin and soft tissue atrophy and fibrosis, osteoradionecrosis (ORN), lymphoedema, xerostomia and trismus).

Treatment can be given by different techniques (Table 53.6):
1. INTENSITY MODULATED RADIOTHERAPY (CONFORMATIONAL OR 3D RADIATION)

Intensity modulated radiotherapy (IMRT) uses 3D computerised treatment planning and conformal therapy with x-ray accelerators to deliver radical RT to the target while sparing most normal tissue, thereby reducing toxicities and improving outcomes in patients with OSCC, and their QoL. IMRT irradiates irregularly shaped volumes and can produce concavities in treatment volumes, thus permitting more precision and greater sparing of normal structures, including:
- salivary glands, showing a significant reduction in hyposalivation
- pharyngeal constrictor muscles, therefore potentially reducing radiation-induced dysphagia
- mucosa, thus reducing mucositis
- cochlea, with potential to reduce radiation-induced hearing loss
- optic nerves, brain stem and spinal cord.

IMRT can be optimised further using advances in the imaging techniques, i.e. image-guided radiotherapy.

TABLE 53.6 **Types of Radiation Treatment**

Type	Definition	Sub-Types
External beam	Focus radiation (e.g. x-rays) on cancer. Gamma rays are another form of photon radiation produced as elements (such as radium, uranium and cobalt 60) decay	Linear accelerators produce x-rays of increasingly greater energy. Intensity modulated radiotherapy (IMRT). Intensity graded radiotherapy (IGRT)
Particle beam radiation therapy	Fast-moving subatomic particles (neutrons, pions and heavy ions) deposit more energy (high linear energy transfer or high LET) than do x-rays or gamma rays, causing more damage to targeted cells	Intensity modulated proton therapy (IMPT)
Internal radiotherapy	Radioactive implants placed directly into tumour (less radiation exposure to other body parts)	Brachytherapy, interstitial irradiation

2. IMAGE GUIDED RADIOTHERAPY

Image guided radiotherapy (IGRT) uses adaptive RT based on regular scanning and planning to reduce dosimetric uncertainties associated with the volume changes in tumours and organs at risk. FDG-PET is used to highlight proliferating areas of a tumour and can guide dose escalation using IMRT.

3. VOLUMATED INTENSITY MODULATED ARC THERAPY

Volumated intensity modulated arc therapy (VMAT) delivers IMRT-like distributions in a single rotation of the gantry (e.g. RapidArc), potentially offering shorter planning and treatment time, better dose homogeneity and better sparing of normal tissue.

4. INTENSITY MODULATED PROTON THERAPY

Intensity modulated proton therapy (IMPT) permits 3D dose distributions using charged particles like protons, which deposit little energy until they reach the end of their range when most of their energy is deposited in a small area. The advantages are of low radiation dose to normal tissue with tissue sparing, and better dose homogeneity.

CHEMOTHERAPY

CTX use in OSCC has been restricted by adverse effects. If the cancer is advanced (stage III or IV), however, RT schedules sometimes include CTX, most commonly using cisplatin and cetuximab (a monoclonal antibody against epidermal growth factor receptor). Occasionally, other drugs used may include fluorouracil (5-FU), carboplatin and paclitaxel.

Systemic CTX administered with RT (termed chemoradiotherapy; CRT) is given either:
- before (induction or neo-adjuvant chemotherapy)
- during (concomitant chemotherapy) or
- after (adjuvant chemotherapy).

Concomitant CRT in cases of advanced neck disease, positive margins or extracapsular spread improves control rates. The most recognised concurrent chemotherapy regimen is cisplatin, or substitution by carboplatin. Drugs may act as radiosensitisers and increase the mucositis produced by RT.

Targeted Cancer Therapies

Therapies are being developed to target specific molecules and pathways. Targeted therapies have less severe adverse effects than conventional CTX but if combined with conventional CTX, adverse effects (such as oral ulceration) may actually be increased.

EGFR inhibitors (EGFRI) affect signal transduction pathways, thereby inhibiting cell proliferation. The main EGFRI are cetuximab and panitumumab. Erlotinib is a small molecule inhibitor of the tyrosine kinase domain of EGFR. Lapatinib is a tyrosine kinase inhibitor active against EGFR and Her-2. Cetuximab combined with RT versus RT alone, showed comparable toxicities, except for higher incidences of acneiform rashes, mucosal toxicity and infusion reactions. Panitumumab can induce stomatitis. Combining CTX with TKIs makes scientific sense as both agents are active in head and neck cancer and have different mechanisms of action, but gefitinib in combination with CTX (docetaxel and carboplatin), produces mucositis and myelosuppression in many patients.

Anti-angiogenic approaches with mTOR (mammalian target of rapamycin (sirolimus) inhibitors such as everolimus, temsirolimus and deforolimus or anti-vascular endothelial growth factor (VEGF) antibodies, which inhibit VEGF, also show some promise. Aphthous-like ulcers are their most common adverse effects. Bevacizumab is a monoclonal antibody against VEGF, which can cause stomatitis and impaired wound healing. Sunitinib maleate is a Tyrosine kinase inhibitor of VEGF and platelet- derived growth factor (PDGF), which may induce stomatitis or dysgeusia, or dry mouth. Trastuzumab, a monoclonal antibody against human epidermal growth factor receptor 2 can cause mucositis and neuropathy. Imatinib and sorafenib can cause pigmentation or taste changes.

Rehabilitation

Feeding can be a problem and it may be necessary to feed via PEG or an indwelling central venous (Hickmann) line. Attention is also required to speech, swallowing, oral hygiene and appearance, with prostheses, implants or camouflage in some cases. Physiotherapy is often required.

Prognosis

Two-year crude survival rates are around 85% for stage I disease, 70% for stage II disease, 50% for stage III disease and 10% for stage IV disease (Table 53.3).

Factors influencing prognosis include:

1. Tumour factors:
   - grade: well-differentiated OSCC have better prognosis
   - stage and depth of infiltration, size of tumour and presence of metastases adversely affect prognosis. The prognosis for stage I tumours is thus around 85% 5-year survival, but this figure plummets to 10% in stage IV tumours. Most patients present at a stage (stage II) when tumours are relatively advanced in size (T2 or more)
   - thickness: deep tumours have a worse prognosis
   - site: prognosis is better where the cancer does not involve the floor of mouth, posterior tongue or maxilla.
2. Lymph node factors (invasion, capsular rupture, nodal site, number of involved nodes). Nodal involvement decreases cure rates by around 50%.
3. Patient factors. The prognosis is usually worse for:
   - male gender: possibly because of the somewhat later presentation of males for treatment, or because of associated medical problems
   - age: the poor general health of some aged patients may limit their resistance to the disease or its treatment.
4. Treatment factors: quality of surgical margins: if excision margins are tumour-free, prognosis is better.

Surveillance

Patients should be educated about signs and symptoms of tumour recurrence, including hoarseness, pain, dysphagia, odynophagia, unintentional weight loss and enlarged lymph nodes. Approximately, 80% to 90% of recurrences occur within the first 2 to 4 years.

RADIOTHERAPY TOXICITIES

RT damages only cells undergoing mitosis, such as epithelium. RT can cause a range of adverse effects (see Table 53.7). Some, notably mucositis and hyposalivation, arise almost immediately and are predictable, whilst others appear later and unpredictably. Mucositis, dysphagia, xerostomia, dermatitis and pain significantly impair QoL, as do hyposalivation (up to 90% incidence) and grade 3 (severe) dysphagia (up to 30%).

Late RT toxicity is permanent and may also include:

- jaw ORN
- sensori-neural hearing loss
- skin fibrosis
- laryngeal cartilage necrosis
- cervical atherosclerosis.

Loss of taste is due to taste bud damage or hyposalivation.

Caries can rapidly progress and affect areas usually not predisposed, such as incisal edges, smooth surfaces and the lower incisor as well as other areas.

Candidiasis is an issue for oral cancer patients because of hyposalivation, treatment-related immunosuppression, frequent use of antibiotics and sometimes of cytotoxic drugs. The diet may also favour *Candida* colonisation if fermentable carbohydrates are frequently consumed. The wearing of dental prostheses or obturators also predisposes to oral candidiasis.

Sialadenitis may follow irradiation and cytostatic drugs and, in turn, may lead to irreversible hyposalivation which, with poor general health, renders cancer patients liable to ascending infective (bacterial) sialadenitis, mainly involving *Streptococcus viridans* and *Staphylococcus aureus* (often penicillin-resistant),

TABLE 53.7   Oral complications of Radiotherapy and Management

Complication	Management
Candidosis	Nystatin suspension 100,000 IU/mL as mouthwash four times daily Fluconazole suspension, itraconazole liquid or posaconazole suspension if immunocompromised
Caries	Daily topical fluoride applications; high fluoride toothpastes; ACP Avoid sugary diet
Dental hypersensitivity	Fluoride applications/mouthwashes
Hyposalivation	Saliva substitute (mouth wetting agents)[a] Frequent ice cubes, popsicles or sips of water Sialogogues, e.g. pilocarpine or cevimeline
Mucositis	Prophylaxis: Amifostine 200 mg/m^2/day Betamethasone mouthwash four times daily from the day before radiotherapy, throughout the course Opiates such as buprenorphine for analgesia
Osteoradionecrosis	Avoid by atraumatic extractions under antibiotic cover, with primary wound closure Planned pre-radiotherapy extractions or extractions within 3 months of radiotherapy
Sialadenitis	Antimicrobials
Taste loss	Consider zinc sulphate
Tooth and jaw maldevelopment	—
Trismus	Jaw-opening exercises three times daily

[a]Artificial saliva (e.g. methylcellulose) or mucin.
ACP, Amorphous calcium phosphate.

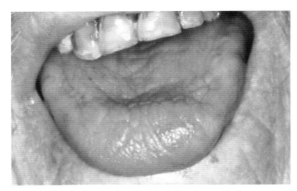

Fig. 53.8 Acute sialadenitis following radiotherapy.

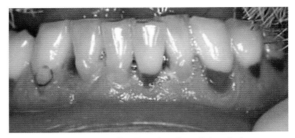

Fig. 53.9 Hyposalivation after head and neck irradiation treatment.

ascending from the oral cavity (Fig. 53.8). The management of sialadenitis often leads to hospitalisation of the patient and includes:

- analgesia and prompt treatment with amoxicillin (flucloxacillin or amoxicillin/clavulanate if staphylococci and not allergic to penicillin; erythromycin or azithromycin in penicillin allergy)
- surgical drainage if there is fluctuation
- hydration
- salivation stimulation by use of chewing gum or sialogogues.

Hyposalivation

Hyposalivation predisposes to caries (Fig. 53.9), candidiasis and bacterial acute ascending sialadenitis (Fig. 53.10). Changes may be quantitative (dry mouth or hyposalivation) or qualitative (pH falls; buffering capacity decreases; electrolytes change).

Factors predisposing to salivary changes include:

- radiation
- dose
- fraction size and number of exposures
- type
- salivary gland
- function before RT
- volume irradiated
  Hyposalivation can be reduced by (Table 53.8):
- minimising doses and field of radiation
- using parotid-sparing techniques such as IMRT
- using amifostine or pilocarpine before therapy and
- avoiding chemo-radiotherapy.

Mucositis

RT it is most often administered in small fractions over several weeks to a localised area. Radiation-induced mucositis is invariable within the radiated field of mucosa and typically begins at cumulative doses of about 15 Gy (i.e. after around 10 days) and reaches full severity at 30 Gy, persisting for weeks or months. Tissues such as the soft palate and the lateral borders and ventral surface of the tongue and floor of the mouth, which have a good vascular supply or a higher cell turnover rate, are more susceptible to radiation mucositis (Fig. 53.11). Risk factors for radiation mucositis include concurrent chemotherapy, younger age,

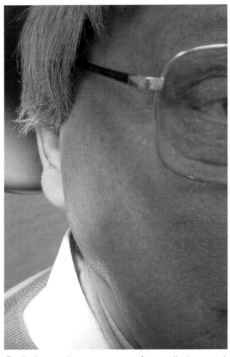

Fig. 53.10 Radiation caries, common after radiotherapy involving the salivary glands.

alcohol, poor oral hygiene, dental disease. Mucositis can lead to a number of problems, including significantly interfering with QoL, acting as a portal for septicaemia, extending hospitalisation and increasing costs of care.

Mucositis can be reduced by (see Table 53.8):

- minimising doses and field of radiation
- using mucosa-sparing blocks
- using amifostine before therapy
- avoiding chemo-radiotherapy
- betamethasone mouthwashes
- using new radiation techniques.

The healing time depends on the radiation dose intensity but is usually complete within three weeks after the end of treatment. Tobacco smoking delays resolution.

Treatment includes:

- opioids, such as morphine and hydromorphone
- avoiding irritants (smoking, spirits or spicy foods)
- good oral hygiene

TABLE 53.8 Minimising Oral Complications of Radiotherapy

Method	Regime	Comments
Minimise radiation dose	Ipsilateral irradiation	
	Positioning devices	
	Shielding	
	Conformational field planning	Intensity modulated radiotherapy (IMRT) or image guided radiotherapy (IGRT)
	Helical tomotherapy	Hi-art
	Gland repositioning	Invasive
Medical protection	Sialoprotective agents	Pilocarpine
		Amifostine
Emergent therapies	Salivary gland transplantation	Minimally invasive salivary gland transfer (MIST)
	Salivary gland cell replacement	Stem cell or bone marrow cell transplantation

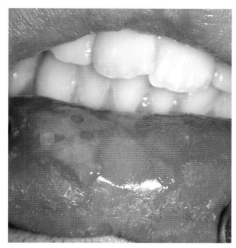

Fig. 53.11 Mucositis presents with widespread erosions in cancer therapy.

- topical analgesics used prior to meals to help combat pain and dysphagia, such as:
  - benzydamine hydrochloride
  - 2% lidocaine (lignocaine) gel.

There are many other preparations used, often variants of the 'magic mouthwash' (viscous lidocaine, diphenhydramine, bismuth salicylate and a corticosteroid).

Trismus

Trismus usually arises because of reduced vascularity from the endarteritis obliterans following radiotherapy that leads to fibrosis in the muscles of mastication and surrounding tissues. The trismus may also result from scar tissue from surgery, nerve damage, tumour infiltration or a combination of factors. RT that affects the TMJ, or the masticatory muscles, is most likely to cause trismus. Tumours related to this type of radiation include nasopharyngeal, base of tongue, salivary gland and cancers of the maxilla or mandible. Trismus is most likely when the RT is in excess of 60 Gy. Radiation-induced trismus may begin towards

the end of RT, or at any time during the subsequent 12 months, and tends to increase slowly over several weeks or months.

Osteoradionecrosis

Osteoradionecrosis follows endarteritis obliterans from RT in high doses involving the oral cavity, maxilla, mandible and salivary glands. ORN is defined as exposed irradiated bone tissue that fails to heal over a period of 3 months.

The mandible, a compact bone with high density and poor vascularity, is more prone than the maxilla to ORN. ORN risk is greatest:

- when radiation dose exceeds 60 Gy
- from 10 days before, to several years after radiotherapy, maximal at 3 to 12 months
- in the malnourished or immunocompromised.

The initiating factor is often trauma, such as tooth extraction, or oral infection or ulceration from a dental appliance. The pathogenesis of ORN is not completely understood but it appears in hypoxic, hypovascular and hypocellular tissue, where there is tissue breakdown leading to a non-healing wound. ORN as a radiation-induced fibroatrophic mechanism, involves free radical formation, endothelial dysfunction, inflammation, microvascular thrombosis, fibrosis and remodelling and, finally, bone and tissue necrosis.

Risk factors for ORN include:

- Radiation related factors: (e.g. total dose, photon energy, brachytherapy, field size, fractionation). With IMRT, only small partial volumes of the jaw are exposed to high radiation doses, so this may translate into a reduction of ORN.
- Trauma and surgery: risk is increased when tooth extractions are performed *after* RT, but there appears little increased risk when extractions are performed before. There is no infection, but teeth in the field of irradiation might be the portal of entry for microorganisms. About 50% of ORN are 'spontaneous' and appear without a history of previous tooth removal. The single most important factor associated with ORN development is mandibular surgery.

- Drug use: alcohol and tobacco are risk factors for ORN. In contrast, corticosteroids or anticoagulants used before or after RT reduce the risk of ORN.
- Genetics: the development of ORN may be related to the presence of the T variant allele at -509 within the transforming growth factor (TGF-β1) gene.

Clinical Features

Presentation of ORN is of exposed bone in an irradiated mouth, with or without external sinuses, pain and pathological fracture.

Management

Treatment is by long-term antimicrobials, especially tetracycline (which has high bone penetration), and local cleansing. Conservative management is preferred, not least since most patients have undergone major surgery before ORN arises and, therefore usually wish to avoid additional jaw surgery. Up to 60% of early and localised cases of ORN resolve with medication and wound care alone. Pentoxifylline (PTX), an antioxidant methylxanthine derivative with an anti-tumour necrosis factor α effect, administered for six months or a combination of PTX and alpha-tocopherol (vitamin E), another antioxidant, accelerates healing. Myocutaneous flaps and microvascular free bone flaps can be used to restore mandibular continuity and bring non-irradiated soft tissue coverage with an intact blood supply.

The role of hyperbaric oxygen (HBO) therapy is controversial.

Prevention of Osteoradionecrosis

ORN is three times higher in dentate than in edentulous patients, which has led to a strategy of preventive extractions of all decayed and periodontally compromised teeth before jaw RT. However, since caries and periodontal disease are so common, there is controversy regarding whether such teeth should *always* be removed. Patients about to be treated with RT do need intensive preventive dental treatment but it is now generally accepted that teeth that really need to be extracted before RT only include those within the high-dose field that are unrestorable or have advanced periodontal involvement. The extractions must be done *before* RT, and patients who required multiple dental extractions or extensive surgical extractions, or both, can be given eight weeks of pentoxifylline 400 mg twice daily with tocopherol 1000 IU, starting a week before the procedure, as prophylaxis.

CHEMOTHERAPY TOXICITIES

The oral adverse effects of CTX can include (Table 53.9):
- mucositis: which may affect some two-thirds of patients. Injury to mucosae tends to be acute but affects the whole gastrointestinal tract. CTX appears to cause injury to the mucosal barrier, with activation of the nuclear factor-κB (NF-κB) pathway and release of cytokines such as tumour necrosis factor (TNF) alpha, IL-1 and IL-6. Most patients

TABLE 53.9 Oral Complications of Chemotherapy and Management	
Complication	**Management**
Bleeding	Local haemostasis
Mucositis	Prophylaxis
	Oral cooling using ice chips
	30 min for 5-fluorouracil
	20 min for edatrexate
Pain	Opioids, e.g. buprenorphine
	Benzydamine hydrochloride used prior to meals
	2% lidocaine (lignocaine) solution mouthwash
Tooth maldevelopment	—
Taste disturbances	See Chapter 18
Candidosis	Nystatin suspension 100,000 IU/mL as mouth wash four times daily
	Fluconazole if immunocompromised

on high-dose CTX develop severe oral mucositis, which usually appears within 4 to 7 days after initiation of treatment and peaks within 2 weeks
- infections: especially candidal, herpesviruses and human papillomaviruses
- pain: related to mucositis or infections
- bleeding: thrombocytopenia
- hyposalivation
- taste disturbances
- tooth maldevelopment.

Mucositis

Unlike the case with radiotherapy, chemotherapy is usually administered over a short time, so the injury to mucosae tends to be acute but affects the whole gastrointestinal tract. The damage induced by CTX is a complex phenomenon that affects both epithelium and lamina propria. There are several stages in mucositis:
- initiation: the production of reactive oxygen species, direct cellular damage.
- activation of transcription factors (e.g. NF-κB) leading to a local increase in pro-inflammatory cytokines (e.g. interleukin [IL]-6, and TNF);
- Feedback mechanisms result in amplification and acceleration of the process, which finally leads to ulceration;
- There is healing following cessation of the process.

The oral microflora is considered to play only a secondary role in the pathogenesis of mucositis.

Risk factors for CTX mucositis include:
- age
- body mass index
- female gender
- salivary function
- poor oral health
- mucosal trauma
- co-morbidities (e.g. diabetes mellitus, impaired renal function).

Clinical Features

Mucositis typically presents as widespread erythema, ulceration, swelling and atrophy. Since CTX-induced damage affects the entire alimentary tract mucosae, terms such as alimentary mucositis and mucosal barrier injury are also then appropriately used. Mucositis presents with:

- pain
- erythema
- ulceration
- sometimes bleeding.

Diagnosis

Diagnosis of mucositis is clinical, and it is helpful to score the degree in order to monitor progression and therapy (Table 53.10).

Quality of Life

Many patients report oral mucositis as the most debilitating and troublesome adverse effect of cancer therapy, and that opioid analgesics do not always adequately relieve pain, but instead lead to other issues such as dry mouth and constipation. Mucositis is also associated with poorer treatment outcomes and increased financial burdens, a longer hospital stay, as well as an increased use of narcotics and nutritional support. In some patients, mainly those undergoing myeloablative haematopoietic stem cell transplant (HSCT), or bone marrow transplant, mucositis predisposes to fever and infections, and occasionally mortality.

Treatment

Fortunately, although there are few randomised controlled studies, and the available prophylactic and therapeutic strategies are limited, discomfort from mucositis can be reduced.

Since infections may be associated, appropriate diagnosis and antimicrobial agents must be considered. Fungal or bacterial infections may be seen particularly in either CTX- (or RT-) induced mucositis.

Interventions that have some proven success with some evidence base include:

- excellent oral care, including pre-treatment dental evaluation
- oral cryotherapy using ice popsicles
- exposure to soft laser
- systemic administration of keratinocyte growth factor (palifermin), FDA-approved for use in patients with haematologic malignancies receiving myelotoxic therapy requiring haematopoietic stem cell support.

Interventions that show some statistically significant evidence of a benefit also include aloe vera, amifostine, granulocyte-colony stimulating factor (G-CSF), intravenous glutamine, honey, sucralfate and polymyxin/tobramycin/amphotericin (PTA) antibiotic pastille/paste. There are many other preparations used, often variants on the 'magic mouthwash' (viscous lidocaine, diphenhydramine, bismuth salicylate and a corticosteroid). The Multinational Association of Supportive Care in Cancer and International Society of Oral Oncology (MASCC/ISOO) Clinical Practice Guidelines for the management of mucositis includes the following interventions: (1) anti-inflammatory agents, (2) photobiomodulation therapy, (3) protocols categorised as basic oral care, (4) growth factors and cytokines, (5) antimicrobials, mucosal coating agents, anaesthetics and analgesics, (6) cryotherapy, (7) vitamins, minerals and nutritional supplements, (8) natural and miscellaneous agents.

RECOMMENDED READING

Brocklehurst, P., Kujan, O., O'Malley, L.A., Ogden, G., Shepherd, S., Glenny, A.M., 2013. Screening programmes for the early detection and prevention of oral cancer. Cochrane Database Syst. Rev. 11, CD004150.

Chaitanya, N.C., Allam, N.S., Gandhi Babu, D.B., Waghray, S., Badam, R.K., Lavanya, R., 2016. Systematic meta-analysis on association of human papilloma virus and oral cancer. J. Cancer Res. Ther. 12 (2), 969–674.

Dhanda, J., Rennie, L., Shaw, R., 2018. Current trends in the medical management of osteoradionecrosis using triple therapy. Br. J. Oral Maxillofac. Surg. 56 (5), 401–405.

El-Rabbany, M., Duchnay, M., Raziee, H.R., et al., 2019. Interventions for preventing osteoradionecrosis of the jaws in adults receiving head and neck radiotherapy. Cochrane Database Syst. Rev. 2019 (11), CD011559.

Elad, S., Cheng, K.K.F., Lalla, R.V., et al., Mucositis Guidelines Leadership Group of the Multinational Association of Supportive Care in Cancer and International Society of Oral Oncology (MASCC/ISOO), 2020. MASCC/ISOO clinical practice guidelines for the management of mucositis secondary to cancer therapy. Cancer. 126 (19), 4423–4431.

Heifetz-Li, J.J., Abdelsamie, S., Campbell, C.B., Roth, S., Fielding, A.F., Mulligan, J.P., 2019. Systematic review of the use of pentoxifylline and tocopherol for the treatment of medication-related osteonecrosis of the jaw. Oral Surg. Oral Med. Oral Pathol. Oral Radiol. 128 (5), 491–497.e2.

Kerawala, C., Roques, T., Jeannon, J.P., Bisase, B., 2016. Oral cavity and lip cancer: United Kingdom national multidisciplinary guidelines. J. Laryngol. Otol. 130 (S2), S83–S89.

Ndiaye, C., Mena, M., Alemany, L., et al., 2014. HPV DNA, E6/E7 mRNA, and p16INK4a detection in head and neck cancers: a systematic review and meta-analysis. Lancet Oncol. 15, 1319.

Raggio, B.S., Winters, R., 2018. Modern management of osteoradionecrosis. Curr. Opin. Otolaryngol. Head Neck Surg. 26 (4), 254–259.

Walsh, T., Macey, R., Kerr, A.R., Lingen, M.W., Ogden, G.R., Warnakulasuriya, S., 2021. Diagnostic tests for oral cancer and potentially malignant disorders in patients presenting with clinically evident lesions. Cochrane Database Syst. Rev. 20 (7), CD010276.

TABLE 53.10	World Health Organization Mucositis Scale	
Grade	**Clinical features**
0	None
I	Oral soreness, erythema
II	Erythema and ulcers, but able to eat solids
III	Ulcers, but requires liquid diet
IV	Oral alimentation not possible

Eponymous and Other Conditions

54

Eponymous Conditions

This chapter includes synopses of several eponymous conditions relevant to oral medicine, presented alphabetically.

Abrikossof tumour Granular cell myoblastoma (tumour).

Addison disease (hypoadrenocorticism) Adrenocortical destruction, reduced cortisol and subsequent increased release of pituitary adrenocorticotrophic hormone (ACTH). A rare disease of young or middle-aged females, the usual cause is autoimmune hypoadrenalism, rarely, tuberculosis, histoplasmosis (sometimes in HIV/AIDS) or carcinomatosis. Weight loss, weakness and hypotension, with brown hyperpigmentation, especially in sites usually pigmented (areolae and genitals) or traumatised, in flexures, on the gingiva, and at the occlusal line are seen. Diagnosis is from low blood pressure, low plasma electrolyte and cortisol levels and impaired response to ACTH stimulation (Synacthen test). Management is fludrocortisone plus corticosteroids.

Adies (Holmes—Adie) pupil A benign condition. One pupil is dilated and reacts only very slowly to light or convergence together with loss of knee or ankle jerks.

Albers-Schonberg disease Osteopetrosis.

Albright syndrome (McCune—Albright syndrome) Polyostotic fibrous dysplasia with skin pigmentation and an endocrine abnormality (usually precocious puberty in girls).

Allgrove syndrome — Triple-A syndrome (AAA), or Achalasia—Addisonianism—Alacrimia syndrome A genetic defect due to mutations in the *AAAS* gene, which codes for a WD-repeat protein termed ALADIN which may cause hyposalivation but the main problems are progressive adrenocortico-hypofunction, lack of tears, achalasia, hypotension and hyperpigmentation.

Alstrom syndrome Congenital nerve deafness and retinitis pigmentosa.

Apert syndrome Autosomal dominant craniofacial synostosis, which includes facial dysmorphology, limb (hands and feet) defects and learning disability.

Argyll—Robinson pupils Small, irregular, unequal pupils which fail to react to light, but do react to accommodation. Characteristically caused by neurosyphilis, may also be seen in diabetes, disseminated sclerosis or other conditions.

Arnold—Chiari syndrome A congenital malformation in which the brainstem and cerebellum are longer than normal and protrude into the spinal canal.

Ascher syndrome (Ascher—Laffer syndrome) Congenital double lip with blepharoclasia and thyroid goitre.

Avellis syndrome A unilateral paralysis of the larynx and palate.

Bannayan—Riley—Ruvalcaba syndrome A rare autosomal dominant disorder related to Cowden syndrome, affecting chromosome 10q and the PTEN (phosphatase and tensin homologue) gene, characterised by excessive growth before and after birth. The head is large (macrocephaly) and often long and narrow (scaphocephaly); normal intelligence or mild learning disability; pigmented macules on the penis, tongue polyps and/or subcutaneous hamartomas.

Battle sign Bruising over the mastoid bone — a sign of a basilar skull fracture.

Becker syndrome Severe muscular dystrophy that results in progressive weakness of limb and breathing muscles.

Beckwith—Wiedemann syndrome Congenital gigantism, and omphalocoele or umbilical hernia.

Beeson sign Myalgia, facial oedema and fever in trichinosis.

Behçet syndrome 'Adamantiades syndrome'. Aphthous ulceration with skin, genital and other lesions (see Chapter 27).

Bell palsy The common lower motor neurone facial palsy (see Chapter 48).

Bell sign Seen in lower motor neurone facial palsy when the eye rolls upward on attempted closure.

Bence—Jones protein Immunoglobulin light chains which spill over into the urine (Bence—Jones proteinuria) when there is overproduction of γ-globulins in myelomatosis.

Biemond syndrome Congenital obesity and hypogonadism.

Binder syndrome Congenital maxillonasal dysplasia, and absent or hypoplastic frontal sinuses.

Blackfan—Diamond syndrome Congenital red cell aplasia.

Block—Sulzberger disease (incontinentia pigmenti) Congenital hyperpigmented skin lesions, skeletal defects, learning disability and hypodontia.

Bloom syndrome Congenital telangiectasia, depigmentation and short stature.

Bohn nodules Keratin-filled cysts derived from palatal salivary gland structures scattered all over the palate, especially at the junction of the hard and soft palate.

Book syndrome Autosomal dominant condition of palm and sole hyperhidrosis, hypodontia and premature whitening of hair.

Bourneville disease (epiloia, tuberous sclerosis) Autosomal dominant; two loci — one on 9q34 and one on 16p13. A phakomatosis, there are fibromas at the nail bases (subungual fibromas); hamartomas in the brain, kidneys and heart; and nodules in the nasolabial fold (adenoma sebaceum), plus pitting enamel hypoplasia.

Bruton syndrome Sex-linked hypoimmunoglobulinaemia, cervical lymph node enlargement, oral ulceration, recurrent sinusitis, absent tonsils.

Burkitt lymphoma Caused by Epstein—Barr virus, most common in children in sub-Saharan African endemic malaria areas, especially Uganda and Kenya, characterised by lymphomatous deposits in many tissues, especially the jaws (in 50% of patients). Responds well to chemotherapy.

Byar—Jurkiewicz syndrome Gingival fibromatosis, hypertrichosis, giant fibroadenomas of the breast, and kyphosis.

Cannon disease Congenital white sponge naevus.

Carabelli cusp Congenital additional palatal cusp on upper molars.

Carney syndrome Autosomal dominant syndrome of myxomas, spotty lip pigmentation and endocrine overactivity (often Cushing syndrome). Cardiac myxomas cause death or serious disability in a quarter of affected patients.

Castleman disease A rare disorder characterised by benign tumours in lymph node tissue throughout the body (i.e. systemic disease [plasma cell type]).

Challacombe scale: a scale to assess clinical oral dryness (see Chapter 20).

Chediak—Higashi syndrome A congenital immune defect in which neutrophils have large inclusions. Juvenile periodontitis and early tooth loss, plus oral ulceration.

Christmas disease Blood clotting factor IX defect.

Chvostek sign Tapping the skin over the facial nerve elicits involuntary twitching of the muscles of the upper lip or ipsilateral side of the face — a sign of hypocalcaemia.

Clutton joints Symmetrical hydrarthrosis of knees in congenital syphilis, appearing around puberty.

Cockayne syndrome Premature ageing, dwarfism, deafness and neuropathy.

Coffin—Lawry syndrome Congenital osteocartilaginous anomalies and learning disability.

Coffin—Siris syndrome Congenital defective neutrophil function, susceptibility to infection and skin pigmentation.

Cohen syndrome Autosomal recessive syndrome of alveolar bone loss, neutropenia, learning disability and obesity.

Costen syndrome Outmoded term relating to facial pain, otalgia and occlusal abnormalities, replaced by 'temporomandibular pain — dysfunction syndrome'.

Cowden syndrome Autosomal dominant disorder affecting PTEN (phosphatase and tensin homologue) gene, congenital multiple hamartomas with oral papillomatosis and risk of breast and thyroid cancer.

Coxsackie virus Named after a town in New York state, coxsackie viruses are many and can cause herpangina, hand, foot and mouth disease, and other illnesses.

CREST syndrome Calcinosis, Raynaud disease, oesophageal involvement, sclerodactyly and telangiectasia (see scleroderma).

Crohn disease (See orofacial granulomatosis: OFG) A chronic inflammatory idiopathic granulomatous disorder that may be caused by *Mycobacterium avium* subspecies *paratuberculosis*. Mutations in the *CARD15* gene (*NOD2* gene) are also implicated. About 20% have a blood relative with some form of inflammatory bowel disease.

Cronkhite—Canada syndrome Hypogeusia followed by diarrhoea, and ectodermal changes including alopecia, nail dystrophy and skin and buccal melanotic hyperpigmentation. Colonic polyps may be present.

Cross syndrome Athetosis, learning disability, gingival fibromatosis and hypopigmentation.

Crouzon syndrome Autosomal-dominant premature fusion of cranial sutures, midface hypoplasia and proptosis.

Curry—Jones syndrome Unilateral coronal synostosis and microphthalmia, plagiocephaly, craniofacial asymmetry, iris coloboma, broad thumbs, hand syndactyly, foot polydactyly, skin lesions, gastrointestinal abnormalities and developmental delay.

Cushing syndrome Moon face with buffalo hump, hirsutism and hypertension due to an ACTH-producing pituitary adenoma.

Darier disease (Darier—White disease) An autosomal-dominant skin disorder with follicular hyperkeratosis, and sometimes white oral papules.

Destombes—Rosai—Dorfman syndrome Rosai—Dorfman syndrome.

Di George syndrome A third branchial arch defect related to a chromosome 22 anomaly (CATCH22 syndrome) causing immunodeficiency; cardiac, thyroid and parathyroid defects.

Down syndrome (trisomy 21) The commonest recognisable congenital chromosomal anomaly. Patients are of short stature with characteristic brachycephaly, midface retrusion and upward sloping palpebral fissures (Mongoloid slant). Learning disabilities and dental anomalies and periodontitis are common.

Duhring disease Dermatitis herpetiformis.

Eagle syndrome An elongated styloid process associated with dysphagia and pain on chewing, and on turning the head towards the affected side.

ECHO viruses Enteric cytopathogenic human orphan viruses.

Ehlers—Danlos syndrome A group of congenital collagen disorders (autosomal dominant, autosomal recessive or X-linked), with altered mechanical properties of skin, joints, ligaments and blood vessels. Phenotypes vary depending upon which collagen type is affected. EDS is characterised by hyperflexible joints, hyperextensible skin, bleeding and bruising, and mitral incompetence. Patients can bend the thumb right back (Fig. 54.1) and may be able to touch the tip of their nose with their tongue. Recurrent dislocation of the temporomandibular joint may be seen. Dental anomalies include deep-fissured premolars and molars, dentinal abnormalities, such as shortened deformed roots, and multiple

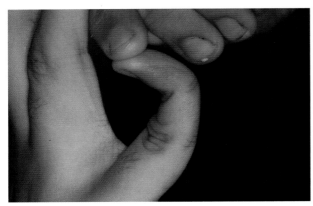

Fig. 54.1 Ehlers-Danlos syndrome showing hyperflexibility of joints.

large pulp stones. Ten types were described: in types IV, VIII and IX there is severe early-onset periodontal disease with loss of permanent teeth. Type III genotypes show resistance to local analgesia.

Ellis–van Creveld syndrome Also known as 'chondroectodermal dysplasia'. This syndrome mapped to chromosome 4p consists of congenital polydactyly, dwarfism, ectodermal dysplasia, hypodontia and hypoplastic teeth and multiple fraenae.

Epstein–Barr virus A herpesvirus implicated in infectious mononucleosis, hairy leukoplakia, nasopharyngeal carcinoma and some lymphomas.

Epstein pearls Cystic keratin-filled nodules derived from entrapped epithelial remnants along the line of fusion along the midpalatine raphe.

Ewing tumour A primary malignant neoplasm of undifferentiated bone mesenchymal cells, extremely aggressive, expands rapidly, invades the soft tissues, and metastasises early. Characteristically affects children and young adults, particularly males, but is rare in the jaws. Radiographically it has either a sunray or an onion-peel appearance due to the deposition of new bone in layers. Microscopy shows sheets of uniform small round cells, with scanty, indistinct cytoplasm which contain glycogen. Treatment is chemo-radiotherapy, with a 5-year survival rate of over 50%.

Fabry disease Angiokeratoma corporis diffusum universale. An X-linked recessive error of glycosphingolipid metabolism with angiokeratomas on the scrotum, hypertension, fever, renal disease and risk of myocardial infarction.

Fallot tetralogy The combination of a ventricular septal defect (VSD) with pulmonary stenosis, the aorta 'overriding' the VSD and right ventricular hypertrophy.

Fanconi anaemia Congenital anaemia, abnormal radii and risk of oral carcinoma and leukaemia.

Felty syndrome Rheumatoid arthritis and neutropenia.

Filatov disease Infectious mononucleosis.

Fitzgerald–Gardner syndrome Gardner syndrome

Foix–Chavany–Marie syndrome Bilateral anterior opercular syndrome, is a paralysis of the face and pharynx with anarthria, drooling and general weakness in the face, caused by bilateral damage to the brain operculum, usually from a stroke, trauma or infection, and causing no limb paralysis and not interfering with involuntary movement such as smiling, chewing or blinking eyes.

Fordyce disease (Fordyce spots) See Chapter 23.

Frey syndrome Gustatory sweating and flushing after trauma to the skin overlying a salivary gland due to crossover of sympathetic and parasympathetic innervation to the gland and skin.

Froehlich syndrome Congenital obesity, hypogonadism and risk of learning disability and open bite.

Gardner syndrome Familial adenomatous polyposis (FAP), formerly termed familial polyposis coli (FPC). An autosomal dominant condition caused by a mutation in *APC* tumour suppressor gene on chromosome 5. Intestinal polyps have a 100% risk of undergoing malignant transformation, so early identification of disease is critical. Gardner described the occurrence of FAP with extracolonic manifestations of desmoids, osteomas and epidermoid cysts. Unerupted and supernumerary teeth may be present. Multifocal pigmented lesions of the fundus of the eye are seen in 80%.

Garré osteomyelitis This is proliferative periostitis.

Gasserian ganglion The trigeminal ganglion.

Gaucher disease The most common genetic disease affecting Ashkenazi Jewish people of Eastern European ancestry, leading to a specific deficiency of the enzyme glucocerebrosidase and lipid-storage disorder. It may cause dry mouth.

Gilles de la Tourette syndrome Coprolalia (utterance of obscenities).

Goldenhar syndrome A variant of congenital hemifacial microsomia, presenting with microtia (small ears), agenesis of the mandibular ramus and condyle, vertebral abnormalities and epibulbar dermoids.

Goltz syndrome (focal dermal hypoplasia) An X-linked disorder with multiple mesenchymal defects, skin lesions, oral warts and dental defects.

Gorlin–Goltz syndrome (Gorlin syndrome; multiple basal cell naevi syndrome; naevoid basal cell carcinoma syndrome [NBCCS]). An autosomal-dominant trait related to chromosome 9q22.3-q31 and associated with *patch* gene mutations and deletions. The syndrome consists of multiple basal cell carcinomas (BCC), keratocystic odontogenic tumours (KCOTs), vertebral and rib anomalies and temporoparietal bossing with broad nasal roots, calcification of the falx cerebri and abnormal sella turcica. Jaw cysts are indistinguishable from other KCOTs and are treated similarly. Diagnosis is suggested by major criteria – positive family history; more than one BCC; KCOTs (first sign in 75%); palmar or plantar pits; or calcified falx cerebri. Minor criteria include congenital skeletal anomalies: bifid, fused, splayed or missing ribs; or bifid, wedged or fused vertebrae; occipitofrontal circumference over 97th percentile, with frontal bossing; cardiac or ovarian fibromas; medulloblastoma; lymphomesenteric cysts; and congenital malformations, such as cleft lip and/or palate, polydactyly, congenital ocular anomaly (cataract, microphthalmos, coloboma).

Graves disease Hyperthyroidism with ophthalmopathy and exophthalmos.

Grinspan syndrome Lichen planus, diabetes and hypertension (probably actually due to lichenoid reactions to antihypertensive and antidiabetic drugs).

Guillain—Barré syndrome Acute infective polyneuritis; facial palsy may be seen.

Hailey—Hailey disease Autosomal-dominant, benign familial pemphigus presenting in the second or third decade with skin and oral blisters and vegetations.

Haim—Munk syndrome Similar to Papillon—Lefevre syndrome, plus pyogenic skin infections, arachnodactyly, acro-osteolysis, onychogryphosis and pes planus.

Hajdu—Cheney syndrome Rare connective tissue disorder, featuring ulcerating lesions on the palms and soles, accompanied by softening and destruction of bones (acro-osteolysis). Abnormal development of bones, joints and teeth also occurs.

Hallerman—Streiff syndrome Congenital cranial anomalies, micro-ophthalmia, cataracts, mandibular hypoplasia and abnormal temporomandibular joint.

Hand—Schüller—Christian disease Langerhans histiocytosis.

Hansen disease Leprosy.

Heck disease (focal epithelial hyperplasia) Papillomas caused by human papillomaviruses 13 or 32, seen especially in ethnic groups such as American Indians and Inuits.

Heefordt syndrome Sarcoidosis associated with lacrimal and salivary swelling, uveitis and fever (uveoparotid fever) and facial palsy.

Henoch—Schonlein purpura IgA vasculitis is a purpuric disease of the skin, mucous membranes and sometimes other organs that most commonly affects children and which may cause oral petechiae.

Hermansky—Pudlak syndrome Congenital albinism and bleeding tendency.

Hodgkin disease Lymphoma that affects particularly males in middle age. Progressive lymphoid tissue involvement often begins in the neck with enlarged, discrete and rubbery lymph nodes. Drinking alcohol may cause pain in affected lymph nodes. Pain, fever, night sweats, weight loss, malaise, bone pain and pruritus are common. Treatment by chemotherapy and radiotherapy is remarkably successful.

Horner syndrome This is caused by interruption of sympathetic nerve fibres peripherally as a result, for example, of trauma to the neck, or lung cancer infiltrating the superior cervical sympathetic ganglion, and comprises, usually, unilateral:
- miosis (pupil constriction)
- ptosis (drooping of the upper eyelid)
- loss of sweating of the ipsilateral face
- apparent enophthalmos (retruded eyeball).

Horton cephalgia Migrainous neuralgia.

Hughes syndrome Anti-phospholipid syndrome: blood hypercoagulability leads to deep vein thrombosis, stroke (CVEs), coronary thrombosis and pregnancy complications.

Hunterian chancre Syphilitic primary chancre.

Hurler syndrome Congenital mucopolysaccharidosis causing growth failure, learning disability, large head, frontal bossing, hypertelorism, coarse facial features (gargoylism) macroglossia (Fig. 54.2) and mandibular radiolucencies.

Hutchinson—Gilford syndrome Progeria (see Werner syndrome).

Hutchinson teeth Screwdriver-shaped incisor teeth in congenital syphilis.

Hutchinson triad Hutchinson teeth, interstitial keratitis and deafness.

Imerslund—Grasbeck syndrome Juvenile pernicious anaemia.

Jackson—Lawler syndrome A type of pachyonychia congenita with no oral leukoplakia, but neonatal teeth and early loss of secondary teeth.

Jadarsohn—Lewandowski syndrome Pachyonychia congenita.

Job syndrome Hyper-IgE syndrome.

Jones syndrome Curry—Jones syndrome.

Kaposi sarcoma (KS) A malignant neoplasm of endothelial cells caused by human herpesvirus 8, seen especially in HIV/AIDS or immunosuppressed patients. Can present orally.

Kartagener syndrome Primary ciliary dyskinesia (PCD). Congenital dextrocardia, immunodeficiency, sinusitis and recurrent respiratory infections (and male infertility).

Kawasaki disease (mucocutaneous lymph node syndrome) Fever, cheilitis, lymphadenopathy, desquamation of hands and feet, and cardiac lesions in periodic epidemics with geographic spread, suggest an infectious aetiology. Management includes gamma globulin and aspirin and long-term anticoagulation.

Kikuchi—Fujimoto disease A self-limiting idiopathic illness of pyrexia, neutropenia and cervical lymphadenopathy in young Asian women. Can be confused histologically and clinically with lymphoma or systemic lupus erythematosus.

Kimura disease A chronic idiopathic inflammatory condition presenting with a painless, slowly enlarging soft tissue mass

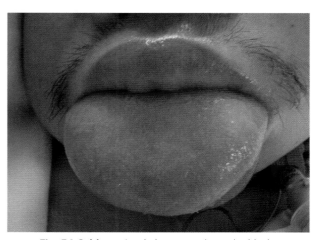

Fig. 54.2 Macroglossia in mucopolysaccharidosis.

(or masses), associated lymphadenopathy and peripheral eosinophilia; 85% of cases are seen in males.

Klinefelter syndrome A chromosome abnormality in men, causing hypogonadism.

Klippel—Feil anomaly Congenital association of cervical vertebrae fusion and short neck, low-lying posterior hairline, syringomyelia and other neurological anomalies, and sometimes unilateral renal agenesis and cardiac anomalies.

Koplik spots Small white spots on the buccal mucosa during measles prodrome.

Kuttner tumour Salivary swelling in IgG4 syndrome.

Kveim test An outdated skin test for sarcoidosis.

Laband syndrome (Zimmerman—Laband syndrome) A form of hereditary gingival fibromatosis with skeletal anomalies and large digits.

Langerhans cell histiocytoses (histiocytosis X) Rare neoplasms arising from Langerhans cells (dendritic intraepithelial macrophage-like cells). Swelling and gingival ulceration, particularly in the molar region, are common and teeth may loosen and exfoliate. Failure of healing of a socket, or the appearance of a pathological fracture may be presenting features. The spectrum includes the following:

- Solitary eosinophilic granuloma of bone: usually benign with osteolytic lesion only and seen in adults. There is sometimes gross periodontal destruction.
- Multifocal eosinophilic granuloma (Hand—Schuller—Christian disease): a more malignant form in children and young adults characterised by osteolytic lesions and sometimes diabetes insipidus and proptosis.
- Letterer—Siwe disease: the most malignant form; seen in infants and characterised by failure to thrive, fever, hepatosplenomegaly and skeletal osteolytic lesions that may cause pain, swelling and loosening of teeth.
- Differentiate from other osteolytic disorders, especially carcinomatosis and myelomatosis. Diagnose by radiography and biopsy: foamy macrophages (Birbeck granules may be seen by EM), eosinophils and bone destruction. Surgery is used to manage solitary lesions; radiotherapy/chemotherapy for the multifocal disease.

Larsen syndrome A mainly autosomal recessive condition, consisting of cleft palate, flattened facies, multiple congenital dislocations and deformities of the feet.

Laurence—Moon—Biedl syndrome Congenital retinitis pigmentosa, obesity, polydactyly, learning disability and blindness.

Laugier—Hunziker syndrome (Laugier—Hunziker—Baran syndrome) Labial and oral mucosal brown to black pigmented macules and nail hyperpigmentation.

Lemierre syndrome Throat infection is followed by identified potentially lethal anaerobic septicaemia — postanginal septicaemia with metastatic abscesses — most commonly in the lung, due to the anaerobe *Fusobacterium necrophorum*.

Leopard syndrome (cardiocutaneous lentiginosis syndrome) Leopard syndrome and Noonan syndrome are allelic disorders caused by different mutations in *PTPN11*, a gene encoding the protein tyrosine phosphatase SHP-2 located at chromosome 12q24.1. It consists of:

- lentigines (multiple)
- electrocardiographic conduction abnormalities
- ocular hypertelorism
- pulmonary stenosis
- abnormalities of genitalia
- retardation of growth
- deafness.

Lesch—Nyhan syndrome Congenital defect of purine metabolism causing learning disability, choreoathetoid cerebral palsy and aggressive self-mutilation.

Letterer—Siwe disease Langerhans histiocytosis.

Lewar—disease (pulse granuloma) A hard mass in the lower buccal sulcus indented or ulcerated by a denture flange. Hyaline bodies seen subperiosteally on histology are vegetable leguminous pulses, which provoke a foreign body reaction. Vegetable matter becomes embedded under the mucosa following tooth extraction or from denture pressure. Treatment is by curettage.

Loeys—Dietz syndrome A recently discovered AD syndrome features similar to Marfan syndrome with bifid uvula but related to transforming growth factor gene.

Lowe syndrome (cerebrohepatorenal syndrome) Congenital hypotonia and flexion contractures.

Ludwig angina Infection of sublingual and submandibular fascial spaces.

Lyell disease (toxic epidermal necrolysis) Originally described in relation to staphylococcal infection (see Chapter 29).

Lyme disease Infection with *Borrelia burgdorferi* from deer ticks, causing rashes, fever, arthropathy and facial palsy. First recognised in the town of Lyme, Connecticut, USA, but prevalent worldwide. CDC recommendations for serologic diagnosis are to screen with a polyvalent ELISA test or C6 peptide antibodies and confirm equivocal and positive results with a western blot assay.

Maffucci syndrome Multiple enchondromas, haemangiomas (often in the tongue), and risk of malignant chondrosarcomas.

MAGIC syndrome **M**outh **a**nd **g**enital ulcers and **i**nterstitial **c**hondritis. A variant of Behçet syndrome.

Mantoux test Skin test for delayed-type hypersensitivity reaction to **b**acillus **C**almette **G**uerin (BCG; for tuberculosis).

Marcus Gunn syndrome Jaw-winking syndrome (eyelid winks during chewing), with ptosis.

Marfan syndrome An autosomal-dominant condition linked to chromosome 15 in *FBN1* gene, which codes for fibrillin-1, essential for the formation of elastic fibres. Reduced levels of fibrillin-1 allow transforming growth factor (TGFβ) to damage the heart and lungs. Prevalent among basketball and volleyball players, patients are tall, thin and with arachnodactyly (long, thin spider-like hands). There may be spontaneous pneumothorax, lens dislocation, aortic regurgitation or dissecting aneurysms, mitral valve prolapse, and palate is occasionally cleft or with bifid uvula. Joint laxity is common and TMJ may dislocate. Multiple dental cysts are less common oral complications. Can be confused with Loeys—Dietz syndrome, caused by mutations in the TGFβ receptor genes TGFβR1 and TGFβR2.

Marie—Sainton syndrome Cleidocranial dysplasia.

Melkersson—Rosenthal syndrome The rare association of facial swelling (usually granulomatous cheilitis), with facial palsy and fissured tongue.

Miescher cheilitis Oligosymptomatic labial granulomatosis or Crohn disease.

Mikulicz disease Salivary gland and lacrimal gland swelling, often related to IgG4 syndrome.

Mikulicz syndrome Salivary gland and lacrimal gland swelling related to malignant disease.

Mikulicz ulcer Minor aphthous ulceration.

Moebius syndrome A complex congenital anomaly involving multiple cranial nerves, affecting mainly the abducens and facial nerves, and often associated with limb anomalies. Muscle transplantation has been used to address the lack of facial animation, lack of lower lip support and speech difficulties.

Moon molars Hypoplastic molars from congenital syphilis.

Munchausen syndrome The fabrication of stories by the patient, aimed at the patient receiving operative intervention.

Murray—Puretic—Drescher syndrome (juvenile hyaline fibromatosis) A rare autosomal recessive disease characterised by cutaneous nodules, especially around the head and neck and often involving the lips. The effects increase with age and also include joint contractures, gingival swelling and osteolytic lesions.

Murray syndrome Multiple hyaline dermal tumours, gingival fibromatosis and recurrent infections.

Nelson syndrome A rare condition with hyperpigmentation caused by ACTH overproduction in response to adrenalectomy, used for breast cancer.

Neumann bipolar aphthosis The association of recurrent aphthae with genital ulceration; probably this is a stage in the development of Behçet syndrome.

Nikolsky sign A term meaning blistering, or the extension of a blister, on gentle pressure (seen mainly in pemphigus and pemphigoid).

Non-Hodgkin lymphomas (NHL) More common than Hodgkin disease and generally with a poorer prognosis, and a predilection for the gastrointestinal tract and central nervous system. Enlargement of cervical lymph nodes is often the first sign, but NHL may occur in the gingivae or faucial region; a recognised complication of HIV/AIDS and may be Epstein—Barr virus related.

Noonan syndrome (see also Leopard syndrome) Congenital short stature and webbed neck, sometimes with cardiac anomalies, pulmonary stenosis and cherubism.

Ollier syndrome Multiple enchondromas.

Osler—Rendu—Weber disease (hereditary haemorrhagic telangiectasia; HHT) An autosomal-dominant disorder where telangiectases are present orally, periorally and in the nose, gastrointestinal tract and occasionally on the palms. Telangiectases may bleed, and cryosurgery or laser treatment may be needed (Fig. 54.3).

Paget disease of bone A bone disorder characterised by the total disorganisation of bone remodelling.

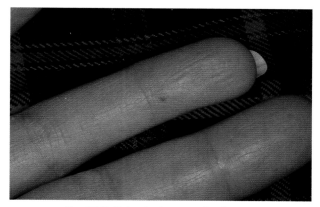

Fig. 54.3 Telangiectases on the fingers.

Papillon—Lefevre syndrome A congenital condition mapped to chromosome 11q with a defect in the polymorphonuclear leukocyte lysosomal enzyme cathepsin c, causing palmoplantar hyperkeratosis and juvenile periodontitis, which affects both dentitions, and immunodeficiency. Acitretin may correct the defective CD3-induced T lymphocyte activation.

Parrot nodes Frontal bossing in congenital syphilis.

Parry—Romberg syndrome Progressive hemifacial atrophy.

Paterson—Kelly—Brown syndrome (Plummer—Vinson syndrome) The association of dysphagia (due to a post-cricoid web of *Candida* which is premalignant), microcytic hypochromic anaemia, koilonychia (spoon-shaped nails) and angular cheilitis (secondary to the anaemia).

Paul—Bunell test (Paul—Bunell—Davidson or Forssman antibody test) A serological test for heterophile antibodies in infectious mononucleosis (glandular fever).

Peutz—Jeghers syndrome An autosomal-dominant condition due to a chromosome 19p *STK11/LKB1* (serine/threonine kinase 11) often associated with gene mutation mutations in LKB1. It consists of circumoral melanosis and intestinal polyposis. Oral brown or black macules appear in infancy and affect especially the lips and buccal mucosa and may be seen on extremities and abdomen. The intestinal polyposis may cause intussusception or other types of obstruction. Almost 50% of patients develop and die from some type of cancer by age 57 years — often extra-intestinal cancers.

Pfeiffer disease Infectious mononucleosis.

Pierre—Robin syndrome Congenital micrognathia, cleft palate and glossoptosis.

Pindborg tumour Calcifying epithelial odontogenic tumour.

Plummer—Vinson syndrome Patterson—Kelly—Brown syndrome.

Popischill—Feyrter aphthae A term used for palatal ulceration in neonates.

Prader—Willi syndrome Congenital obesity, hypogonadism, learning disability, diabetes and dental defects.

Quincke oedema Angioedema.

Ramon syndrome Cherubism, arthritis, epilepsy, gingival fibromatosis, hypertrichosis and learning disability.

Ramsay—Hunt syndrome A lower motor neurone facial palsy due to herpes zoster of the geniculate ganglion of the seventh nerve. Presents with vesicles in the ipsilateral pharynx, external auditory canal and on the face.

Rapp—Hodgkin syndrome Ectodermal dysplasia, kinky hair, cleft lip/palate, popliteal pterygium and ectrodactyly.

Raynaud syndrome A vascular spasm in response to cooling, seen in the digits in connective tissue disorders.

Reiter syndrome The association of arthritis, urethritis and balanitis, and conjunctivitis, found mainly in men with HLA-B27 and a high incidence of sexually transmitted infections (mainly Chlamydia). Reiter syndrome is the most common cause of arthritis in young men. A postdysenteric form is more common in women, often after infection with *Shigella flexneri*, *Salmonella typhimurium*, *Yersinia enterocolitica*, *Campylobacter jejuni* or *Chlamydia trachomatis*. Oral lesions are circinate papules on the palate and elsewhere. Skin lesions resemble psoriasis on the palms and soles (keratoderma blennorrhagica). Treatment is with NSAIDs.

Rett syndrome Congenital bruxism and hand-wringing, often with a learning disability.

Reye's (Reye) syndrome is a rare but serious condition that causes swelling in the liver and brain. Reye's syndrome most often affects children and teenagers recovering from a viral infection, most commonly the flu or chickenpox. Signs and symptoms: confusion, seizures and loss of consciousness require emergency treatment. Early diagnosis and treatment of Reye's syndrome can save a child's life. Aspirin has been linked with Reye's syndrome. Though aspirin is approved for use in children older than age 3, children and teenagers recovering from chickenpox or flu-like symptoms should never take aspirin.

Rieger syndrome Congenital ocular anomalies, iridal hypoplasia, glaucoma and blindness, maxillary hypoplasia and dental hypoplasia with oligo- and microdontia.

Riga—Fede disease TUGSE (traumatic ulcerative granuloma with stromal eosinophilia).

Riley—Day syndrome Inherited familial dysautonomia; sympathetic dysfunction, salivary swelling, sialorrhoea and self-mutilation, seen particularly in Ashkenazi Jews.

Romberg syndrome (hemifacial atrophy) Progressive atrophy of the soft tissues usually of half the face, associated with contralateral Jacksonian epilepsy and trigeminal neuralgia. It starts in the first decade and lasts about 3 years before it becomes quiescent.

Rosai—Dorfmann syndrome Sinus histiocytosis with massive lymphadenopathy. A benign, non-Langerhans cell, histiocytic proliferative disorder that primarily affects lymph nodes.

Rothmund—Thomson syndrome Congenital poikiloderma, hypogonadism, dwarfism, cataracts and microdontia.

Rubinstein—Taybi syndrome (broad thumb—great toe syndrome) Short stature with small head size, and developmental delay. The most striking physical feature is broad, sometimes angulated thumbs and first toes. Facial features include a prominent beaked nose and down-slanting eyes. Undescended testes occur in males.

Rutherfurd syndrome Corneal dystrophy, neurosensory hearing loss, gingival fibromatosis and delayed tooth eruption.

Ruvalcaba—Myrhe—Smith syndrome Bannayan—Riley—Ruvalcaba syndrome.

Sabin—Feldmann test Serological test for toxoplasmosis.

Saethre—Chotzen syndrome An autosomal-dominant craniosynostosis associated with cleft palate as well as other disturbances of the facial skeleton and extremities.

Saxon test A simple, reproducible, cheap test for hyposalivation, which involves chewing on a weighed sterile sponge for 2 and then re-weighing the sponge. Normal subjects produce at least 2.75 g of saliva in 2 minutes.

Schmidt syndrome Autoimmune polyendocrinopathy; congenital hypoadrenocorticism, hypoparathyroidism, diabetes and malabsorption, with candidosis.

Schmincke—Regaud tumour A lymphoepithelial carcinoma usually at the base of the tongue.

Seckel syndrome Congenital microcephaly, learning disability, zygomatic and mandibular hypoplasia.

Simpson—Golabi—Behmel syndrome X-linked dysplasia gigantism, with tissue overgrowth leading to coarse ('bulldog-like') face with protruding jaw and tongue, and wide nasal bridge, and an increased risk of Wilm tumour and neuroblastoma.

Sipple syndrome Multiple endocrine neoplasia (MEN) type 3 (MEN 3; sometimes called 2b) affecting several endocrine glands with multiple mucosal neuromas, phaeochromocytoma and medullary thyroid carcinoma (calcitonin levels raised).

Sjögren—Larsson syndrome Congenital ichthyosis, learning disability, cerebral palsy and indifference to pain.

Sjögren syndrome See Chapter 26.

Sluder syndrome Migrainous neuralgia.

Smith—Lemli—Opitz syndrome Congenital short stature, learning disability, syndactyly, urogenital and maxillary anomalies.

Stafne bone cavity An ectopic inclusion of salivary tissue in the mandible, often from the submandibular gland. Radiography shows cystic radiolucency. No treatment is indicated, but if a diagnosis cannot be confirmed by sialography, or if serial radiographs show an increase in cavity size, exploratory surgery is indicated.

Stevens—Johnson syndrome See Chapter 29.

Still syndrome Juvenile rheumatoid arthritis.

Sturge—Weber syndrome (encephalotrigeminal angiomatosis) A congenital hamartomatous angioma of the upper face (naevus flammeus), oral mucosa and underlying bone (with hemihypertrophy of bone and accelerated eruption of associated teeth), extending intracranially to cause convulsions, and contralateral hemiplegia and intracerebral calcifications, and sometimes learning disability.

Sutton ulcers Major recurrent aphthae (see Chapter 7).

Sweet syndrome Acute neutrophilic dermatosis with erythematous, well-demarcated skin papules and plaques; red mucosal lesions and ulcers, often associated with a malignant disease or induced by drugs. Treatment is with systemic corticosteroids.

Takayasu disease Pulseless aorta and large arteries.

Thibierge—Weissenbach syndrome The CREST syndrome.

TORCH syndrome Toxoplasmosis, other infections, rubella, cytomegalovirus, herpes simplex induced foetal abnormalities.

Treacher—Collins syndrome (mandibulofacial dysostosis) Autosomal-dominant first branchial arch defect with downward sloping (anti-mongoloid slant) palpebral fissures, hypoplastic malar complexes, mandibular retrognathia, deformed pinnas, hypoplastic sinuses, eye colobomas and middle and inner ear hypoplasia (deafness).

Trotter syndrome Acquired unilateral deafness, pain in the mandibular (third) division of the trigeminal nerve, ipsilateral palatal immobility and trismus due to invasion of the nasopharynx and the trigeminal nerve by a malignant tumour. *Pterygopalatine fossa syndrome* is a similar condition, where the first and second divisions of the trigeminal nerve are affected.

Turner syndrome Complete or partial deletion of the X chromosome. Affects females only, with short stature, low hairline, web neck, broad chest and widely spaced nipples, increased carrying angle of the elbows and non-functioning ovaries. Occasionally cherubism is found.

Turner tooth Hypoplastic tooth due to damage to the developing tooth germ.

Tzanck cells Abnormal epithelial squames in pemphigus or herpetic infections.

Urbach—Wiethe disease Lipoid proteinosis and hyalinosis cutis et mucosae.

Von Recklinghausen disease Multiple neurofibromas with skin pigmentation, skeletal abnormalities and central nervous system involvement.

Von Willebrand disease Common bleeding disorder caused by defective blood clotting factor VIII and platelet dysfunction.

Waardenburg syndrome Congenital heterochromia iridis (different coloured eyes), deafness and white forelock, with prognathism.

Waldeyer ring Lymphoid tissue surrounding the entrance to the oropharynx (tonsils and adenoids).

Wallenberg syndrome Posterior inferior cerebellar artery occlusion leading to the lateral medullary syndrome.

Warthin tumour Benign salivary gland neoplasm — adenolymphoma or papillary cystadenoma lymphomatosum.

Wegener granulomatosis Idiopathic disseminated malignant granulomatosis. A rare, idiopathic disorder of necrotising granulomatosis. Initially affecting the respiratory tract, arteritis affects small vessels in the lungs, kidneys, eyes, skin,

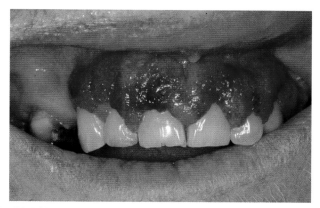
Fig. 54.4 Wegener granulomatosis showing strawberry-like swelling on the gingiva.

muscles, joints and mouth and is potentially lethal. A painless progressive swelling of the gingiva in a previously healthy mouth, particularly associated with swollen inflamed papillae with a fairly characteristic 'strawberry-like' appearance, should arouse suspicion (Fig. 54.4). Diagnosis is supported by biopsy, imaging and anti-neutrophil cytoplasmic antigens (ANCA), anaemia, elevated ESR, CRP or PV and white blood cell and platelet counts. Management is antimicrobials, cytotoxic agents or radiotherapy.

Werner syndrome Congenital alopecia, dwarfism, senility, early atherosclerosis, delayed tooth eruption and mandibular hypoplasia.

Whipple disease A rare potentially lethal bacterial infection with *Tropheryma whippelii* that infects the small bowel to cause malabsorption, but may affect the immune system, heart, lungs, brain, joints and eyes.

William syndrome Genetic disorder characterised by mild learning disability, unique personality characteristics, distinctive facial features and cardiovascular disease (elastin arteriopathy). A range of connective tissue abnormalities is observed and hypercalcaemia and/or hypercalciuria are common.

Wilson syndrome (hepatolenticular degeneration) Disorder of copper metabolism leading to hepatic disease; renal disease; spasticity; tremor and mental problems.

Wiskott—Aldrich syndrome X-linked recessive immunodeficiency with thrombocytopenia, infections, eczema (TIE syndrome) and lymphoreticular malignancies.

Witkop disease Hereditary benign intraepithelial dyskeratosis — seen mainly in parts of the USA.

Zimmerman—Laband syndrome Laband syndrome.

Zinsser—Cole—Engelmann syndrome Dyskeratosis congenita.

55

Other Conditions

This chapter includes synopses of a number of conditions relevant to oral medicine, not appearing elsewhere. These are presented alphabetically. If a specific condition is not found here, please refer to the index, since it may well be located elsewhere in the book.

Acanthosis nigricans A rare paraneoplastic condition where papillomatous oral lesions are seen often in patients with internal malignancy.

Acatalasia Autosomal recessive defect in the enzyme catalase, which normally removes reactive oxygen species, such as hydrogen peroxide, from tissues. Severe periodontal destruction and oral ulceration can result.

Achondroplasia (chondrodystrophia fetalis) An autosomal dominant condition in which endochondral ossification is reduced. The most common form of short-limbed dwarfism — patients have disproportionately short limbs, bowed legs, kyphosis, prominent buttocks and abdomen, and trident hands with short fingers. The skull is relatively large, having prominent frontal, occipital and parietal bones. The middle third of the face can be hypoplastic with the nasal bridge depressed and a class III type malocclusion. The foramen magnum is often narrow and spinal cord compression can occur. Joints can be of limited mobility and the pelvic inlet narrow.

Acrodermatitis enteropathica A rare genetic disorder of zinc metabolism causing mouth ulceration and candidosis, rash around orifices, and alopecia.

Actinic prurigo (AP) A chronic, pruritic skin disease caused by an abnormal reaction to sunlight.

Actinomycosis An uncommon infection with *Actinomyces israelii*, below the mandibular angle (not lymph nodes) that may follow jaw fracture or tooth extraction. Prolonged therapy, usually with penicillin, is indicated.

Acute necrotising ulcerative gingivitis A non-contagious anaerobic gingival infection associated with overwhelming proliferation of *Borrelia vincentii* and fusiform bacteria.

Adenomas. An adenoma is a benign tumour of epithelial tissue with glandular origin, glandular characteristics, or both. Adenomas can grow from many glandular organs.

Adenomatosis. A form of cancer characterized by multiple adenomas within an organ or system. Represents some 35% of adenomas.

Amelogenesis imperfecta A rare genetic defect of enamel formation due to mutations in AMELX, ENAM and MMP20 genes, with a wide variety of patterns. All teeth are equally affected, as are other family members. Diagnosis is from clinical features (Fig. 55.1 and Table 55.1). Fluorosis, tetracycline staining, dentinogenesis imperfecta and oculo-dentodigital dysplasia may need to be differentiated. Management requires restorative dental care.

Amyloidosis The deposition in tissues of amyloid — an eosinophilic hyaline material, with a fibrillar structure on ultramicroscopy. Amyloid can be identified via Congo red stain under fluorescent or polarised light, thioflavine T stain under fluorescent light or immunoreactivity with antibodies for immunoglobulin light chains.

Primary (including myeloma-associated) amyloidosis: associated with deposits of immunoglobulin light chains. Manifestations include macroglossia and oral petechiae or blood-filled bullae (secondary purpura).

Secondary amyloidosis: seen mainly in rheumatoid arthritis (RA) and ulcerative colitis, rarely affects the mouth and is associated with deposits of AA proteins.

Diagnose from a biopsy; blood picture; raised ESR, CRP or PV and marrow biopsy; serum proteins and electrophoresis; urinalysis (Bence–Jones proteinuria); skeletal survey for myeloma. Manage by chemotherapy (melphalan, corticosteroids or fluoxymesterone).

Angina bullosa haemorrhagica (localised oral purpura) Blood blisters in the mouth or pharynx, mainly on the soft palate, seen in the absence of any immunological or platelet-associated cause. Seen mainly in older people, the aetiology is unclear, though there are occasional associations with the use of steroid inhalers. There is rapid onset, with the breakdown of the blister in a day or two to an ulcer. Diagnose from clinical features, although it may be necessary to confirm haemostasis is normal; and rarely to biopsy to exclude pemphigoid. Manage by reassurance. Topical analgesics may provide symptomatic relief.

Angiomas See haemangiomas.

Angiomyoma A rare benign hamartoma involving blood vessels and muscle.

Ankyloglossia (tongue-tie) An uncommon genetic condition which results in the lingual fraenum anchoring the tongue tip, restricting tongue protrusion and lateral movements. Oral cleansing (but not speech) is impaired. Differentiate from tethering by scarring. Management is surgery (fraenectomy) if severe.

Aspergillosis *Aspergillus* spp. may infect the paranasal sinuses, palate or other sites by direct extension and haematogenously,

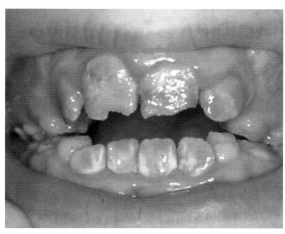

Fig. 55.1 Amelogenesis imperfecta.

especially in the immunocompromised. Diagnosis is by demonstration of hyphae in a smear, serology and biopsy. Intravenous amphotericin may be effective

Branchial cyst A lymphoepithelial cyst that may arise from the enclavement of salivary tissue in a lymph node, or the cervical sinus. It usually becomes apparent in the third decade. It requires excision.

Bullous pemphigoid An autoimmune disease usually with widespread crops of tense, fluid-filled blisters on the skin. The diagnosis is confirmed by biopsy. Bullous pemphigoid is treated with prednisolone (enteric-coated). For Mucous membrane pemphigoid, see Chapter 30.

Caries Dental caries can occur on any tooth surface exposed to the oral environment, but not surfaces retained within the bone. There are four factors in the aetiology: a tooth surface (enamel or dentine); cariogenic (or potentially caries-causing) bacteria in dental plaque; fermentable carbohydrates; and time. The specific bacterial species believed to cause caries include *Streptococcus mutans* and *Lactobacilli*. Particularly for root caries, the most closely associated bacteria are *Lactobacillus acidophilus*, *Actinomyces viscosus*, *Nocardia* spp. and *S. mutans*. Sugars (sucrose, glucose, fructose) are metabolised to acetic, lactic, formic and succinic acids. Different individuals are susceptible to different degrees depending on the tooth shape, oral hygiene and the flow and buffering capacity of their saliva.

Carotid body tumour A slow-growing, but malignant neoplasm of chromaffin cells that both invades locally and metastasises. It presents as a mass over the internal carotid artery and transmits the carotid pulsation. It must be resected.

CATCH22 Stands for **c**ardiac abnormality, **a**bnormal facies, **T**-cell deficit due to thymic hypoplasia, **c**left palate and **h**ypocalcaemia due to hypoparathyroidism, caused by a chromosome **22** defect.

Cheek biting (morsicatio buccarum) (see Chapter 23) Common seen in adults mainly, especially anxious patients, and those with other psychological related disorders. Abrasion of the superficial epithelium leaves whitish fragments on a reddish background. The lesions are invariably restricted to the lower labial mucosa and/or buccal mucosa near the occlusal line on one or both sides.

Chemical burns Can be caused by various chemicals or drugs; notably, aspirin put in the sulcus to try to relieve toothache, or cocaine. A white lesion with sloughing mucosa is seen. Diagnosis is by history and clinical features.

Chikungunya fever A mosquito-borne arboviral illness similar to dengue fever; causes arthralgia and mouth ulceration.

Chondroma A benign tumour, rare in the jaws. The anterior maxilla, mandibular symphysis and the coronoid and condylar processes are the most common sites. Chondromas are typically found in older patients and form slow-growing, painless masses. Provided surgical excision of these masses is complete, recurrence is unlikely.

Chondrosarcomas These tend to affect the older patient and, although isolated cases arise from chondromas, most arise *de novo*. The behaviour is very unpredictable, but many grow rapidly and produce extensive local destruction. Radical surgery, the only means of eradicating the tumour, can be difficult as the edges may not be apparent clinically or radiographically. Multiple local recurrences are common, and the prognosis is worse than for osteosarcoma.

Chorea Consists of a writhing movement of continuous abrupt and intermittent movements that flow randomly from one

TABLE 55.1	Amelogenesis Imperfecta			
Type	**1**	**2**	**3**	**4**
Name	Hypoplastic	Hypocalcified	Hypomaturation	Hypomaturation with taurodontism
Defect	Matrix	Calcification	Maturation	Mixed — between types 1 and 3
Enamel thickness and colour	Thin, hard, pitted or grooved	Normal thickness, softer and liable to attrition Discoloured white to brownish-yellow, and darkening with age	Normal thickness, softer and liable to attrition	Variable
Radiographic features	Normal enamel density	Enamel similar to dentine		
Inheritance	AD, AR or x	AD or AR	AD, AR or x	AD

AD, Autosomal dominant; *AR*, autosomal recessive; *X*, X-linked.

part of the body to another. Chorea may affect the head and neck, especially in tardive dyskinesia. This is usually a late (hence tardive) complication manifesting as non-random, focal patterned or stereotyped movement induced by dopamine receptor blocking drugs, such as metoclopramide, phenothiazines or butyrophenones, and is somewhat similar to oromandibular dystonia. Senile chorea, including edentulous dyskinesia or orodyskinesia, is found in 16% of the edentulous.

Chronic ulcerative stomatitis This is similar to erosive lichen planus, with ulcers and erosions affecting mainly the buccal or lingual mucosae, but sometimes the gingivae. The lesions and clinically normal mucosa have a distinct pattern of a particulate stratified squamous-epithelium-specific (SES) antinuclear antibody (ANA) on direct immunofluorescent examination of perilesional tissue, and patients can have circulating ANA. Hydroxychloroquine is an effective therapy.

Cleidocranial dysplasia (dysostosis) A rare autosomal dominant condition, or mutation. Clinical features include an exaggerated transverse diameter of the cranium, delayed fontanelle closure, multiple wormian bones, frontal and parietal bossing, depressed nasal bridge, maxillary hypoplasia, underdeveloped paranasal sinuses, high arched palate (? cleft), delayed or failed tooth eruption, multiple supernumerary teeth, dentigerous cysts, aplastic or hypoplastic clavicles (shoulders can be approximated), short stature and other skeletal anomalies.

Diagnosis is from the family history and ability to bring together the shoulders; jaw, skull and skeletal radiography. Management is to leave unerupted teeth alone unless there are complications. Eruption of permanent teeth is retarded and dentigerous cysts are frequently found. Supernumerary teeth are common in cleidocranial dysplasia, especially in the anterior mandible. The crowns of the teeth are normal, but the roots can be short, thin and lack acellular cement. Surgery is often necessary.

Coeliac disease Coeliac disease is a reaction to gluten, ingestion of which activates immune cells in the small intestine, which trigger inflammation and local damage, disrupting food absorption. Untreated coeliac patients lose weight, develop deficiency syndromes such as anaemia, and experience symptoms such as diarrhoea. Dental hypoplasia and oral ulceration may result. Diagnosis is confirmed by malabsorption, blood tissue transglutaminase antibodies and villous atrophy on jejunal biopsy. Gluten is found in wheat, barley and rye, which means that many dietary staples, such as bread, many breakfast cereals and foods like pizza and pasta, can no longer be eaten.

Congenital epulis A rare reactive process seen on the alveolus of a neonate.

Constricted pupils Constricted pupils (miosis) can be caused by sympathetic nerve lesions, cholinergic drugs (e.g. pilocarpine or neostigmine) or opiates (heroin, etc.). Thus, heroin addicts may be recognised by 'pin-point pupils'. Raised intracranial pressure is the most important cause of pupil constriction and is noted when the pupil also

becomes non-reactive owing to pressure on the oculomotor nerve. It may occur after a head injury, intracranial haemorrhage or brain tumour.

CREST syndrome Calcinosis, Raynaud disease, oesophageal involvement, sclerodactyly and telangiectasia (see scleroderma).

Creutzfeldt—Jakob disease (CJD) is a rapidly progressive, invariably fatal neurodegenerative disorder believed to be caused by an abnormal isoform of a cellular glycoprotein known as the prion protein. CJD occurs worldwide and the estimated annual incidence in many countries, including the United States and the United Kingdom, has been reported to be about one case per million population (see Prion Diseases).

Cri-du-chat syndrome Short arm of chromosome 5 deletion, resulting in microcephaly, hypertelorism and laryngeal hypoplasia causing a characteristic shrill cry.

Crystal deposition diseases ('gout') A term used to encompass diseases that produce crystals in joints (e.g. gout, chondrocalcinosis, secondary gout caused by cytotoxic therapy) including the temporomandibular joint (TMJ). Gout itself is an uncommon disorder of metabolism in which excessive levels of uric acid in the blood and other body fluids crystallise out in synovial fluid causing acute inflammation. The patient complains of a painful, swollen joint and 'panmeniscal crepitation' is elicited on movement. Acute attacks are often preceded by a 'binge' of dietary or alcohol excess or 'starvation', trauma or unusual physical exercise, surgery or systemic illness. In chronic gout, tophi are frequently felt in the cartilage of the pinna of the ear. Diagnosis is clinical, but usually confirmed by a leucocytosis, raised ESR, CRP or PV raised serum urate level and aspiration biopsy for examination under polarising light for crystals of urate (or pyrophosphate in pseudo-gout). Imaging is not often particularly helpful, since the appearance resembles osteoarthritis. Treatment must not be restricted just to the local treatment of the TMJ. NSAIDs should be started. Colchicine is effective. Gout is usually treated prophylactically with allopurinol. Dietary advice and weight control are also important.

Cyst A pathological cavity having liquid, semi-liquid or gaseous contents. It is frequently, but not always, lined with epithelium. Cysts of the jaws mostly arise from the odontogenic epithelium and are relatively common lesions (Chapter 14). Non-odontogenic developmental cysts are uncommon and were said to form from entrapment of epithelium during the fusion of embryological processes, but this embryological concept has now been discarded. The lining of these cysts is either stratified squamous epithelium or pseudostratified ciliated columnar (respiratory) epithelium. Non-odontogenic cysts include the following:
- *Nasopalatine or incisive canal cysts:* derived from the vestigial oronasal ducts. They may occur either within the nasopalatine canal, or in the soft tissues of the palate at the opening of the canal, grow slowly and may discharge into the mouth giving a salty taste. Radiological

examination shows a well-defined, rounded ovoid or occasionally heart-shaped defect in the anterior maxilla. Nasopalatine cysts must be distinguished from a normal large anterior palatine fossa which may be up to 7 mm in diameter, and from radicular cysts associated with the maxillary incisors. These cysts should be enucleated and seldom recur.

- *Nasolabial cysts:* soft tissue cysts found within the nasolabial fold. They are lined by respiratory epithelium, and if allowed to grow may distort the upper lip and alar base. Treatment is by simple excision.

Cystic hygroma A developmental anomaly of lymphatics presenting as a swelling of the neck seen before the age of 2 years. It may extend into the mediastinum and/or tongue. Cystic hygroma is usually surgically removed.

Dentinogenesis imperfecta A rare autosomal-dominant disorder in which the dentine is abnormal in structure and, hence, translucent (Fig. 55.2), and poorly attached to the enamel. All teeth are affected, but primary teeth are more severely affected than permanent teeth. In the permanent dentition, the teeth that develop first are generally more severely affected than those that develop later. The teeth:

- are translucent
- may vary in colour from grey to blue or brown
- enamel is poorly adherent to the abnormal underlying dentine and easily chips and wears
- crowns are bulbous with pronounced cervical constriction and the roots are short
- fracture easily (there is progressive obliteration of pulp chambers and root canals with secondary dentine)
- periapical radiolucencies are not uncommon.

There are three types of dentinogenesis imperfecta:

- Type I (associated with osteogenesis imperfecta): most severe in deciduous dentition; bone fractures; blue sclerae; progressive deafness; caused by mutations in one of several genes.
- Type II (hereditary opalescent dentine): defect equal in both dentitions; caused by mutations in the DSPP gene. A few families with type II have progressive hearing loss in addition to dental abnormalities.
- Type III (Brandywine type — first identified in Brandywine, Maryland, USA): associated with occasional shell teeth and multiple pulpal exposures; caused by mutations in the DSPP gene.

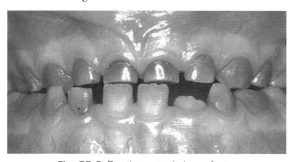

Fig. 55.2 Dentinogenesis imperfecta.

Differentiate mainly from amelogenesis imperfecta, tetracycline staining and dentine dysplasia. Management is by restorative dental care.

Dermatitis herpetiformis An uncommon chronic skin disorder associated often with gluten-sensitive enteropathy, affecting mainly middle-aged males. Symmetrical papulovesicular eruptions on extensor surfaces. Oral lesions of vesicles and/or desquamative gingivitis, similar to pemphigoid typically follow skin lesions. Biopsy of perilesional tissue, with histological and immunostaining examination, are essential to diagnosis, showing IgA deposits at the papillae. Jejunal biopsy is often indicated. Dapsone is the main therapy — sulphamethoxypyridazine and sulphasalazine are alternatives. A gluten-free diet can minimise disease activity and can reduce or avoid the need for drugs.

Dermatomyositis A rare autoimmune disorder that occasionally presents with oral ulcers and erythema of the tongue, palate or gingivae.

Dermoid cyst A rare developmental cyst that presents as a doughy painless swelling in the midline floor of the mouth and needs to be differentiated from ranula and cystic hygroma. Diagnosis is by aspiration, but there is a risk of infection. Management is by surgical removal.

Desquamative gingivitis A fairly common problem in which the gingivae show chronic desquamation and is a term that denotes a particular clinical picture and not a diagnosis in itself. Many of the patients are middle-aged women. Desquamative gingivitis is mainly a manifestation of:

- mucocutaneous disorders, usually. Most gingival involvement in the vesiculobullous or skin diseases (dermatoses) is related to lichen planus or pemphigoid, but pemphigus, dermatitis herpetiformis, linear IgA disease, chronic ulcerative stomatitis and other conditions may need to be excluded. Most of these conditions are acquired, but a few are congenital with a strong hereditary predisposition, such as epidermolysis bullosa
- chemical damage, such as reactions to sodium lauryl sulphate in toothpastes
- allergic responses
- drugs
- psoriasis
- pyostomatitis vegetans.

Some patients make no complaint, but others complain of persistent gingival soreness, worse when eating spices or acidic foods, such as tomatoes or citrus fruits. Most patients are seen only when vesicles and bullae have broken down to leave desquamation, and the clinical appearance is thus of erythematous gingivae, mainly labially, the erythema and loss of stippling extending apically from the gingival margins to the alveolar mucosae. The desquamation may vary from mild almost insignificant small patches to widespread erythema with a glazed appearance. In addition to a full history and examination, biopsy examination and histopathological and immunological investigations are frequently indicated. Conditions which should be excluded include:

- reactions to mouthwashes, chewing gum, medications and dental materials
- candidosis
- lupus erythematosus
- plasma cell gingivitis
- Crohn disease, sarcoidosis and orofacial granulomatosis
- leukaemias
- factitial (self-induced) lesions.

The treatment of desquamative gingivitis consists of:
- improving the oral hygiene
- minimising irritation of the lesions
- specific therapies for the underlying disease where available
- local or systemic immunosuppressive or dapsone therapy, notably corticosteroids.

Corticosteroid creams used overnight in a soft polythene splint may help.

Dilated pupils (mydriasis) Can be caused by parasympathetic lesions affecting the third nerve, Holmes—Adie syndrome, Horner syndrome, anticholinergic drugs (e.g. atropine or similar drugs), sympathomimetic drugs (e.g. adrenaline, cocaine). Users of cocaine or crack cocaine may thus have dilated pupils.

Drug addiction (illegal drug use) This is increasingly common, particularly in urban areas. Addicts in need of a 'fix' will often falsely complain of severe pain or injury. Disturbed behaviour in a drug addict may be caused by withdrawal symptoms and the patient may need compulsory detention. If an addict is admitted to the ward, contact a licensed psychiatrist for heroin or cocaine to be given for addicts. The most serious problems in the management of addicts include:
- overdose
- withdrawal effects
- behavioural problems (including theft)
- violence
- hepatitis
- HIV infection
- other infections
- hyposalivation
- oral lesions typically are those of these conditions or neglect of hygiene.

Dysarthria (disordered speech) Normal speech involves a complex series of muscles, particularly the muscles of respiration, larynx, pharynx, palate, tongue and lips and, like all voluntary muscle activity, is under control from higher centres, both pyramidal and extrapyramidal. The act of speaking is a highly coordinated sequence involving articulation and phonation under the direct control of the vagus, glossopharyngeal, hypoglossal and facial nerves. Conditions affecting the tongue, palate, pharynx, larynx or these nerves or their central connections, or sensory nerves, can lead to disturbed speech. However, speech also involves a wide range of acquired skills, deficiencies of which impede interpersonal communication irrespective of any other impairment in language usage.

Deranged speech can be due commonly to drugs (including alcohol), central nervous system (CNS) disorders such as learning disabilities, cerebral palsy, parkinsonism, delirium or dementia; loss of voice due to laryngeal disease or paralysis (dysphonia); or defects in articulation because of paralysis, rigidity, tissue loss or scarring, or involuntary movements of tongue or palate. The most common oral cause of dysarthria is immobility of the tongue after a lingual block local analgesic injection, trauma to the tongue, scarring, diseases affecting the tongue (such as carcinoma) or foreign bodies (such as in oral piercing). Spastic dysarthria is usually caused by cerebrovascular disease affecting the motor cortex (causing pseudobulbar palsy), extrapyramidal disease, such as parkinsonism, or drugs, such as phenothiazines; basal ganglia disease causes choreic dysarthria; cerebellar disease causes ataxic dysarthria. Alcohol also has this effect. Paralytic dysarthria is less common but may be caused by medulla oblongata disease (bulbar palsy), cranial nerve lesions affecting nerves VII, IX, X, XI or XII, myopathies, such as myasthenia gravis. Patients with persistent dysarthria should be referred for a neurological opinion.

Dyskinesias Abnormal movements of the tongue or facial muscles, sometimes with abnormal jaw movements, bruxism or dysphagia. Involuntary tongue protrusion and retraction, and facial grimacing are common dyskinesias. They differ from dystonias mainly in that muscle spasm is less prominent, but they may be difficult to differentiate clinically. They are usually caused by extrapyramidal diseases, such as athetosis, or drugs. Most dyskinesias resolve within 4 weeks of stopping any causal medication. If not, treat with anti-parkinsonian drugs (e.g. benzhexol), baclofen, benzodiazepines, dopamine depletors (reserpine or tetrabenazine), calcium channel blockers, clozapine, buspirone, α-adrenergic agonists, vitamin E or botulinum toxoid.

Dysphasias Disturbances of language use (or aphasias), and may be caused by brain disease, such as stroke or after a head injury, in which there is a loss of production and comprehension of speech and language.

Dystonias A group of uncommon neurological diseases characterised by abnormal movements, such as sustained and patterned contractions producing abnormal postures, repetitive twisting or squeezing.

Epidermolysis bullosa A rare genetically determined disorder related to a defect in the epidermolysis bullosa antigen in the epithelial basal lamina, leading to blistering after trauma, and scarring, which may cause severe disability, such as limb deformities, microstomia, ankyloglossia and trismus. Enamel hypoplasia may be seen. Diagnosis is from the family history and a biopsy to exclude other blistering diseases. Management includes careful attention to oral hygiene. Trauma should be minimised, and drugs such as phenytoin may help reduce blistering.

Epidermolysis bullosa acquisita A rare non-inherited chronic mechano-bullous disease characterised by autoantibodies directed against type VII collagen. Clinically, bullae are frequently induced after mechanical irritation. The diagnosis should be made on the history, clinical features, histopathological, direct and indirect immunofluorescent examination. Biopsy of perilesional tissue, with histological and immunostaining examination, is essential to the diagnosis. Topical corticosteroids effectively control gingival lesions. Systemic corticosteroids alone or in association with immunosuppressive agents and dapsone are suggested treatments.

Exfoliative cheilitis (tic de levres) (see Chapter 25) Characterised by continuous production and desquamation of unsightly, keratin scales which, when removed, leave a normal lip beneath (Fig. 55.3). Can become infected, which greatly exacerbates the condition (infected exfoliative cheilitis).

Familial holoprosencephaly Congenital malformation of the forebrain and midface: microphthalmia, hypopituitarism and hypertelorism.

Fibro-osseous lesions A group of disorders of unknown aetiology, composed of fibrous and ossified tissue. The main disorders include Paget disease of bone, fibrous dysplasia and cherubism and the ossifying fibroma.

Fissured lip Lip fissures may appear especially where there is exposure to adverse environments (Fig. 55.4), or where the lip swells as in Down syndrome or cheilitis granulomatosa.

Fissured (plicated or scrotal) tongue An extremely common genetic condition, the dorsum has deep irregular fissures but is normally papillated (Fig. 55.5). A fissured tongue may also be seen in Down syndrome or Melkersson–Rosenthal syndrome. There are associations with erythema migrans in particular. The diagnosis is usually clear cut. The lobulated tongue of Sjögren syndrome must be differentiated.

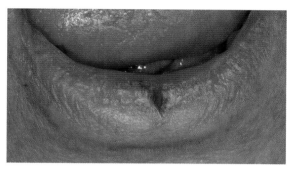
Fig. 55.4 Fissured lip.

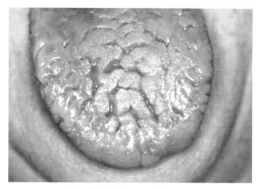
Fig. 55.5 Fissured tongue.

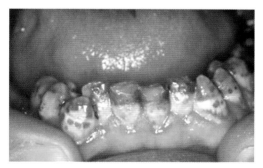
Fig. 55.6 Severe fluorosis.

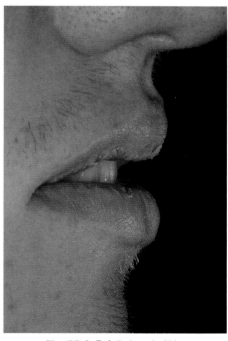
Fig. 55.3 Exfoliative cheilitis.

Fluorosis The condition of enamel defects caused by high levels of fluoride. High levels of drinking water are uncommon in the developed world but are particularly common in parts of the Middle East, India and Africa. Fluorosis affects many teeth:

- *Mildest form:* white flecks or spotting or diffuse cloudiness.
- *More severe form:* yellow-brown or darker patches.
- *Most severe form:* yellow-brown or darker patches, sometimes with pitting (Fig. 55.6).

Diagnosis is from history, clinical appearance and data about the fluoride content of drinking water. It is necessary to differentiate between amelogenesis imperfecta and tetracycline staining. Management of severe forms is by the use of veneers or crowns.

Foliate papillitis The foliate papillae are found on the posterolateral border of the tongue, at the junction of the anterior two-thirds with the posterior third. The size and shape of the foliate papillae are variable and occasionally they swell if irritated mechanically or if there is an upper respiratory infection, and this is termed 'foliate papillitis'. Located at a site of high predilection for lingual cancer, they may give rise to unnecessary concern about cancer.

Furred tongue Coating of the tongue is quite commonly seen in healthy adults, particularly in edentulous patients, those who are on a soft, non-abrasive diet, those with poor oral hygiene or those who are fasting. The coating in these instances appears to be of epithelial, food and microbial debris, which collects since it is not mechanically removed. Indeed, the tongue is the main reservoir of some microorganisms, such as *Candida albicans* and some *Streptococci*. The tongue may be coated with off-white debris in many illnesses, particularly febrile diseases, hyposalivation and ill patients — especially those with poor oral hygiene or who are dehydrated. The history is important to exclude a congenital or hereditary cause of a white lesion or candidosis. The clinical appearances may strongly suggest the diagnosis, but investigations are often required if the white lesion does not scrape away from the mucosa with a gauze. A biopsy may then rarely be indicated. Treatment is of the underlying cause.

Geotrichosis An uncommon opportunistic oral infection caused by *Geotrichum candidum*. Oral geotrichosis shows three clinical varieties: pseudomembranous (75%), hyperplastic and palatine ulcer. It is treated as oral candidosis.

Gingival bleeding This is usually explained by the presence of gingivitis. However, unexplained bleeding can be due to thrombocytopenia (e.g. in leukaemia, HIV disease, idiopathic thrombocytopenic purpura, myelodysplastic syndromes) or occasionally warfarin, other drugs or blood clotting defects.

Glossitis The term given when the tongue is sore or, more appropriately, when the dorsum of the tongue becomes depapillated and red. Causes include anaemia, vitamin or iron (haematinic) deficiency, chemotherapy or radiation therapy, or infection, such as candidosis. Glossitis in haematinic deficiency states is seen mainly in:

- malabsorption states
- pernicious anaemia
- chronic bleeding from the gastrointestinal or genitourinary tract
- vegans
- dietary faddists
- resource-poor circumstances (deficiencies of vitamins of the B group other than B_{12} are an occasional cause of glossitis, mainly seen in chronic alcoholics or those with malabsorption or starvation).

The tongue may appear completely normal or there may be:

- linear or patchy red lesions: especially in vitamin B_{12} deficiency
- depapillation with erythema: in deficiencies of iron, folic acid or B vitamins lingual depapillation begins at the tip and margins of the dorsum, but later involves the whole dorsum (bald tongue).

Various other patterns are described, in deficiencies of:

- riboflavin: papillae enlarge initially, but are later lost
- niacin: red, swollen, enlarged 'beefy' tongue
- pyridoxine: swollen, purplish tongue.

There may also be:

- pallor
- burning mouth syndrome
- ulceration
- angular stomatitis.

Differentiate from erythema migrans, lichen planus and acute candidosis. A sore tongue can be the initial symptom of iron, folate or vitamin B_{12} deficiency and can precede any haemoglobin fall, a full blood picture with assays of iron (serum ferritin), vitamin B and folate are essential. A biopsy is rarely indicated. Replacement therapy should be instituted after the underlying cause is established and rectified.

Glossopharyngeal neuralgia. A rare condition in which pain with all the characteristics of trigeminal neuralgia is experienced in the posterior tongue, fauces, pharynx and sometimes beneath the angle of the mandible. Treatment is with carbamazepine or, in intractable cases, posterior fossa neurosurgery.

Glycogen storage diseases Inborn errors of metabolism. Type 1B results in neutropenia and periodontal destruction.

Gonorrhoea Infection with *Neisseria gonorrhoea* in the mouth is uncommon or rarely recognised. Pharyngitis may occur after orogenital or oroanal contact. Treat with amoxicillin or ciprofloxacin.

Gout See Crystal deposition diseases.

Granular cell myoblastoma (granular cell tumour) A fairly common hamartoma, the origin of which is unclear. Presents as a pedunculated or occasionally sessile swelling on the gingivae, tongue, buccal mucosa or lip. It should be excised. Histology shows a pseudo-epitheliomatous appearance, but it is benign.

Haemangioma. A benign tumour of blood vessels. On the skin may appear as a birthmark, the strawberry naevus.

Haemangiopericytoma A rare tumour arising from pericytes; there are benign and malignant forms.

Haemochromatosis An inborn error of iron overload which may cause diabetes, cardiomyopathy and mucocutaneous brown pigmentation or salivary swelling, one of the most common metabolic errors, manifesting mainly in males, iron is excessively absorbed and deposits in tissues, causing hyperpigmentation, diabetes, hypogonadism, cirrhosis and cardiomyopathy.

Haemophilia Haemophilia A: deficiency of blood clotting factor VIII. Haemophilia B: Christmas disease. Haemophilia C: von Willebrand disease.

Hairy leukoplakia Epstein-Barr virus-induced bilateral leucoplakia of the tongue in HIV disease (see Chapter 39).

Hand, foot and mouth disease A common Coxsackie virus infection (usually A16) occurring in small epidemics in children. Manifests with erythematous papules on buccal mucosa, palms of hands and soles of feet (see Chapter 37).

Hemifacial spasm A spasm of the angle of the mouth or the eyelid, worse towards evening. Usually idiopathic, it may be caused by a vascular anomaly affecting the vertebrobasilar vessels (dolichoectasia) causing pressure on the facial nerve. Some cases herald a cerebellopontine angle lesion or other lesion irritating the facial nerve. CT or MRI are indicated. Botulinum toxin injections into the affected muscles may give relief. Anticholinergics, phenytoin, carbamazepine or benzodiazepines may help. Rarely are myectomy or microvascular decompression indicated. Hemimasticatory spasm is similar but affects the masticatory muscles and may be associated with progressive hemifacial atrophy. It also often responds to botulinum toxin.

Herpangina A Coxsackie virus infection (usually A7, A9, A16; B1, B2, B3, B4 or B5) or enterovirus (17). Clinical features include oropharyngeal ulcers, no gingivitis, cervical lymphadenitis (moderate), fever, malaise, irritability, anorexia, but no rash.

Holoprosencephaly A common developmental defect affecting the neural crest cells populating the frontonasal mass and the forebrain, with the associated appearance of midface defects.

Hypercementosis This may be idiopathic or arise in:
- occlusal trauma
- an over erupted non-opposed tooth
- periapical infection
- Paget disease
- acromegaly.

Hypereosinophilic syndrome A multisystem disorder in which there can be oral ulceration and sinusitis, characterised by a high blood eosinophil count ($>1.5 \times 10^9$/L) for greater than 6 months. Categorised under the idiopathic group of eosinophilias, the lymphocytic form is characterised by T-lymphocyte clonality, IL-5 production and a possible progression to T-cell lymphoma. Oral lesions are more frequently associated with the myeloproliferative form, characterised by an increased risk of developing myeloid malignancies. Patients may be asymptomatic or severely unwell and can present with generalised non-specific features such as fatigue, night sweats and pruritus; diarrhoea; urticaria; thrombocytopenia; cardiomyopathy and a range of other complications. Diagnosis is supported by raised ESR, abnormal LFTs, abnormal ECG and chest radiography showing pleural effusions. Treatment is with corticosteroids, interferon or emergent monoclonals such as imatinib.

Hyperparathyroidism *Primary hyperparathyroidism* — usually due to a parathyroid adenoma, carcinoma or hyperplasia of parathyroid tissue or ectopic production of parathyroid hormone (PTH) (e.g. by tumours of lung or kidney). May also rarely occur in association with adenomas of other endocrine glands (the multiple endocrine adenoma syndromes). Serum calcium levels are raised, as usually is the alkaline phosphatase. Phosphate levels are reduced. The clinical features are the direct result of either excess PTH or calcium, and particularly include renal stones, bone lesions, polyuria and abdominal pain ('stones, bones and abdominal groans'). Anorexia and psychoses are not uncommon:
- *Secondary hyperparathyroidism:* usually the consequence of renal disease in which low serum calcium as a consequence of impaired renal production of dihydroxycholecalciferol induces increased parathyroid activity, and eventually hyperplasia of the parathyroid glands. Secondary hyperparathyroidism may also follow malabsorption syndromes. Calcium levels are usually normal or low.
- *Tertiary hyperparathyroidism:* a consequence of chronic overstimulation of the gland in secondary hyperparathyroidism, which rarely leads to the neoplastic change in the parathyroids, which then escape the normal control of serum calcium.

Oral manifestations of hyperparathyroidism include reduced bone density (the outlines of the maxillary antrum, inferior dental canal and inferior border of the mandible can become less distinct), loss of the lamina dura, root resorption and radiolucencies (particularly of the mandible). The radiolucent lesions are either areas of high osteoclastic activity or giant cell lesions. The giant cell lesions can present intraorally as epulides. Hyperparathyroidism is managed by excision of the neoplastic or hyperplastic parathyroid tissue. In the secondary and tertiary disorders, treatment of the underlying disorder is also required.

Hypodontia A reduction in the number of teeth. The teeth most commonly missing are third molars and maxillary lateral incisors, followed by mandibular and maxillary second premolars. It may be associated with microdontia. If greater than 6 teeth missing, the term oligodontia is sometimes used. Anodontia is the total absence of the dentition. A genetic trait, ectodermal dysplasia should be considered.

Hypoglossal nerve lesions LMN lesions of the twelfth cranial nerve lead to unilateral tongue weakness, wasting and fasciculation. When protruded, the tongue deviates towards the weaker side. Bilateral supranuclear (UMN) twelfth nerve lesions produce slow, limited tongue movements; the tongue is stiff and cannot be protruded far, and fasciculation is absent. Causes of lesions may be within the brainstem (infarction, syringobulbia, motor neurone disease or poliomyelitis; at the skull base (jugular and anterior condylar foramina) causes include trauma and tumours (nasopharyngeal carcinoma, glomus tumour or neurofibroma) and within the neck and nasopharynx trauma or tumours (nasopharyngeal carcinoma, metastases) or polyneuropathy.

Hypoparathyroidism Usually caused by damage to, or loss of, parathyroid tissue during neck surgery (e.g. thyroidectomy). It may also arise rarely as a familial disorder (idiopathic hypoparathyroidism) or very rarely as a consequence of *in* *utero* damage when it is associated with cellular immuno-deficiency (CATCH 22 syndrome). The major clinical features are related to the low serum calcium levels. Tetany (hyperexcitability of muscles) is the most obvious and disturbing feature and can lead to a laryngeal spasm. Hypoparathyroidism frequently causes paraesthesia in the mouth. Tapping the skin over the facial nerve can elicit involuntary twitching of the muscles of the upper lip or ipsilateral side of the face (Chvostek sign). Hypoparathyroidism can cause enamel hypoplasia of developing teeth and delayed tooth eruption. Treat with hydroxycholecalciferol.

Hypophosphatasia A rare genetic defect in alkaline phosphatase, causing cemental aplasia or hypoplasia and tooth mobility and early loss. Serum alkaline phosphatase is decreased with increased vitamin B_6 and increased urinary phosphoethanolamine.

Hypoplasminogenaemia A rare genetic defect in plasminogen. Manifestations include swollen, painless, nodular and ulcerated gingivae covered with a yellowish-pink pseudo-membrane, and ligneous conjunctivitis.

Idiopathic bone necrosis An unusual disorder in which a small portion of bone, typically of the mylohyoid ridge, undergoes spontaneous necrosis and sequestration with pain and ulceration.

Impetigo contagiosa A highly contagious skin infection with streptococci (group A). Uncommon, and seen mainly in children aged 2 to 6 years. Clinical features include papules which change into vesicles surrounded by erythema, then multiple pustules with golden crusts (see Chapter 40).

Isolated mucocutaneous melanotic pigmentation (IMMP) is a distinct condition similar to Peutz—Jegher syndrome but with no mutations in LKB1 though associated with various malignant neoplasms in women.

Juvenile hyaline fibromatosis A hereditary condition which may involve the gingiva, with swelling and a prominent PAS-positive matrix of chondroitin sulphate.

Leiomyoma A rare benign tumour from smooth muscle.

Leukaemia A malignant proliferation of leukocytes. Common oral manifestations of leukaemia include lymphadenopathy, bleeding, petechiae, gingival swelling and ulceration. Other findings include sensory changes (particularly of the lower lip), extrusion of teeth, painful swellings over the mandible, parotid swelling (Mikulicz syndrome, fungal infections and predisposition to herpesvirus lesions. Diagnose by a blood film, white cell count (raised), differential count (shows blasts), platelet count (reduced) and bone marrow biopsy. Treat mainly by chemotherapy. Oral hygiene should be carefully maintained with chlorhexidine mouth rinses and a soft toothbrush. Prophylactic antifungal and antiviral therapy are also indicated. Many chemotherapeutic agents can cause oral ulceration. Methotrexate is a major offender, but ulceration may be prevented or ameliorated by concomitant intravenous administration of folinic acid ('leucovorin rescue') or topical folinic acid. There are several types of leukaemia:

- *Acute lymphoblastic leukaemia* (ALL). The most common leukaemia of childhood, it has a peak incidence at 3 to 5 years of age. Malignant lymphoblasts proliferate and infiltrate the viscera, skin and CNS. Marrow infiltration causes granulocytopenia (predisposing to infections), thrombocytopenia (causing a bleeding tendency) and anaemia ('there is no leukaemia without anaemia').
- *Acute myeloblastic leukaemia* (AML). The most common acute leukaemia in adults. Features are similar to ALL, but central nervous system involvement is rare.
- *Chronic lymphocytic leukaemia* (CLL). The most common chronic leukaemia. It mainly affects the older patient. Some patients are asymptomatic, while in others there is fever, weight loss, anorexia, haemorrhage and infections. Lymph node enlargement is early and may be detected in the neck. CLL may need no treatment.
- *Chronic myeloid leukaemia* (CML). This is characterised by the proliferation of myeloid cells in the bone marrow, peripheral blood and other tissues, and mainly affects those over 40 years of age. Splenomegaly and hepatomegaly are common. Anaemia, weight loss and joint pains are not uncommon. The prognosis is variable, but sooner or later, there is a transformation into an acute phase similar to AML (blast crisis).

Leukocyte adhesion deficiency (LAD) Autosomal recessive defect in beta integrins (Mac-1 or P150,95), impeding polymorphonuclear leukocyte adhesion and migration. Presents with infections and juvenile periodontitis.

Leukopenia This may result from viral infections (especially HIV), drugs, irradiation or can be idiopathic. There is a predisposition to infections, and persistent ulcers lacking an inflammatory halo. Diagnose by a full blood picture and bone marrow biopsy. Manage by improving oral hygiene; antimicrobials as necessary.

Linear IgA disease and chronic bullous dermatosis of childhood. These are subepithelial immune blistering diseases in which there is a linear deposition of IgA autoantibodies at the epithelial basement membrane zone:

- *Linear IgA disease* (adults): oral lesions that mimic mucous membrane pemphigus, in particular oral vesicles and ulcers.
- *Chronic bullous dermatosis* (childhood): similar oral lesions and sometimes scarring.

Diagnosis is by biopsy of perilesional tissue, with histological and immunostaining. Most patients respond to high-dose prednisolone (enteric-coated), dapsone or sulphonamides.

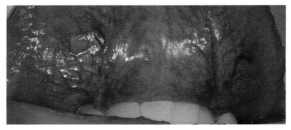

Fig. 55.7 Lingual (sub-lingual) varices.

Lingual varicosities A fairly common condition of older people in which distended blood vessels are seen on the tongue ventrum (Fig. 55.7). No treatment is necessary.

Lipoma A rare benign tumour of adipose tissue, presenting as a slow-growing, yellowish, soft, semifluctuant, painless mass usually in the buccal mucosa. Diagnose by biopsy; manage by excision.

'Loose bodies' Hydroxyapatite crystal deposits within the temporomandibular joint space may be seen in osteochondritis dissecans (1 to 3 'loose bodies'); osteoarthritis (1 to 10 'loose bodies'); chip fracture of the articular surface (1 to 3 'loose bodies'); or synovial chondromatosis (50 to 500 'loose bodies'); and can cause pain. If the pain does not respond to conservative treatment, joint exploration may be needed.

Lupus erythematosus A rare autoimmune disease seen usually in females. The aetiology is unclear, but drugs, hormones and viruses may contribute to genetically predisposed persons:
- Discoid lupus erythematosus (DLE): oral lesions are seen in up to 25% of those with cutaneous DLE, mainly in the buccal mucosa, gingiva and lip. Characteristic features include central erythema, white spots or papules, radiating white striae at margins and peripheral telangiectasia.
- Systemic lupus erythematosus (SLE): oral lesions like those in DLE, but usually more severe ulceration. SLE may also be associated with Sjögren syndrome and, rarely, temporomandibular joint arthritis.
- Diagnose by biopsy, blood picture and autoantibodies, especially crithidial (double-stranded DNA). Antinuclear factors are present in SLE, not in DLE. Biopsy shows the lupus band test with basement membrane zone deposits of IgG/IgM. Differentiate from lichen planus, leukoplakia (keratosis), galvanic-induced white lesions and carcinoma. Management includes:
- DLE: topical corticosteroids, cryosurgery or excision of localised lesions; there is a small predisposition to carcinoma.
- SLE: systemic corticosteroids, azathioprine, chloroquine or gold.

Lymphangioma. A localised collection of distended lymphatic vessels. Can result in a large cyst in the neck or armpit.

Lymphomas (See also Burkitt lymphoma, Hodgkin disease and non-Hodgkin lymphoma). Malignant tumours originate in lymph nodes and lymphoid tissue.

Malignant melanoma A malignant tumour of melanocytes usually presenting as a heavily pigmented (occasionally non-pigmented) macule or, later, a nodule or ulcer. It may spread across several cm. The palate is most frequently affected, with spread to regional lymph nodes and then the bloodstream. To differentiate naevi and other pigmented lesions, diagnosis is by wide excision biopsy. However, if melanoma clinically is a significant possibility, the patient should be referred for immediate surgery.

Masseteric hypertrophy May result from repeated jaw clenching or bruxism.

Measles A common childhood exanthem, caused by the measles virus. Features include Koplik spots rash (maculopapular), conjunctivitis, runny nose, cough, fever, malaise and anorexia (see Chapter 37).

Meth mouth A term that applies to teeth affected by problems that can include caries, attrition, cracks and erosion attributed to heavy methamphetamine use caused by a combination of drug-induced hyposalivation, poor oral hygiene, frequent consumption of carbonated beverages, and tooth grinding and clenching.

Mixed connective tissue disease (MCTD) Characterised by anti-RNP autoantibodies, this may present with hyposalivation, trigeminal neuropathy, oral ulceration or Sjögren syndrome.

Multiple endocrine adenoma (MEN) syndrome There are three main types:
- MEN 1: parathyroid tumours, pancreatic tumours and pituitary tumours.
- MEN 2a: medullary thyroid cancers (MTC), phaeochromocytoma and parathyroid tumours.
- MEN 2b: MTCs, phaeochromocytoma and neuromas.

There are specific genetic causes for each of the three types and any particular MEN family will have only one type of MEN.

Mucormycosis (zygomycosis: phycomycosis) is infection by *Mucor* or *Rhizopus* spp., mainly of the paranasal sinuses and nose of immunosuppressed or poorly controlled diabetic or leukaemic patients. Diagnosis is by biopsy and culture: treatment is by control of underlying disease, debridement and intravenous amphotericin.

Muscular dystrophies Genetic myopathies which may cause facial muscle weakness:
- Facioscapular humeral muscular dystrophy: an autosomal-dominant condition, which progresses slowly. A dull-looking face which has no expression in conversation and can only just straighten the lips for a smile is characteristic, especially if seen with the absence of blinking. As the name implies, the shoulders and upper part of the arms are also involved.
- Dystrophia myotonica: an autosomal-dominant condition. The first muscles involved are the sternomastoids and facial muscles, but the muscles of mastication may also become involved, with progress to other muscle groups. Myotonic features are seen early and followed by muscle wasting. Other features are premature baldness, cataracts, testicular atrophy and cardiomyopathy.

Myasthenia gravis An autoimmune disorder with defective neuromuscular transmission, which may first present as weakness of ocular movement or even facial movement.

Myelodysplastic syndrome A spectrum of essentially pre-leukaemic states. Can cause oral ulceration.

Myeloma A plasma cell tumour. Typically progresses to myelomatosis, but can present as:
- soft-tissue myeloma
- solitary osseous myeloma
- multiple myeloma (myelomatosis) — a disease mainly of middle-aged and older people and is sometimes related to exposure to ionising radiation or petroleum products. The initial feature is abnormal serum immunoglobulins, occasionally detectable by chance, raised ESR, rouleaux formation or high PV, or serum protein investigations. Years may elapse before discrete, punched-out radiolucent

osteolytic lesions appear, especially in the skull and jaws. When the jaws are involved, there may be pain, paraesthesia or anaesthesia, loosening of teeth and pathological fracture. Anaemia, weakness and weight loss are manifestations of advanced disease. A few patients also develop amyloidosis. The neoplastic proliferation of plasma cells in the bone marrow and their release of cytokines, such as interleukin-1, ultimately causes hypercalcaemia, renal failure, suppression of haemopoiesis and many other secondary effects. The abnormal immunoglobulins have defective antibody activity, and thus infections occur, and there may be plasma hyperviscosity with a clotting or bleeding tendency and neurological sequelae.

Diagnosis depends on showing:
- a monoclonal immunoglobulin peak on serum electrophoresis
- spillover of light chains into the urine (Bence—Jones proteinuria)
- plasma cell neoplasia on marrow biopsy
- osteolytic lesions on skeletal radiographs or by bone scanning.

Management is by radiotherapy and cytotoxic chemotherapy.

Myositis ossificans A rare idiopathic condition in which muscles ossify. Occasionally the same reaction follows trauma to the muscle. Radiographs tend to show the calcifications and alkaline phosphatase levels are markedly raised.

Myxoma Rare in the oral cavity, this can arise in bone or soft tissue and, although benign, is aggressive and difficult to eradicate because it tends to infiltrate normal tissue.

Nasopharyngeal carcinoma Appears to be EBV-related, is common in Inuits and Chinese. The commonest features are a blocked nose, unilateral deafness and cervical lymphadenopathy. Trotter syndrome may occur. Treatment is usually chemo-radiotherapy.

Necrotising sialometaplasia A rare condition in which there is ulceration, usually in a smoker in the palate, which heals spontaneously over several weeks. Associated with salivary gland infarction, histology can be confusing, since it has an appearance resembling neoplasia (pseudoepitheliomatous hyperplasia).

Nerve sheath tumours Neoplasms arising from a nerve or showing nerve sheath differentiation. Benign and malignant variants. Several distinct benign subtypes are recognised, including Schwannoma (neurilemoma, neurinoma), neurofibroma and perineurioma:
- *Schwannomas:* (see below).
- *Neurofibromas:* unencapsulated tumours composed of spindle cells in a fibromyxoid stroma.
- *Perineuriomas:* arise in soft tissues or nerves and are composed of cells with elongated bipolar cytoplasmic processes arranged in whorls or a storiform pattern. The neoplastic cells express vimentin and epithelial membrane antigen but are negative for S-100 protein, desmin, muscle-specific actin and CD34.
- Most malignant NSTs arise from Schwann cells, and approximately two-thirds are associated with neurofibromas.

Neurilemmoma (Schwannoma) A rare benign encapsulated neoplasm of neurilemmal cells of the nerve axonal sheath with distinct Antoni A and B components, hyaline vessel walls, and nuclear palisading. Tumour cells are strongly immunopositive for S-100 protein. Presents as a slowly enlarging painless mass, usually in the tongue, sometimes with facial pain and/or atrophy of the muscles of mastication. Facial nerve Schwannomas can cause facial palsy or compressive hearing loss resulting from ossicular interference and sensorineural hearing loss due to effects on the cochlear nerve in the internal auditory canal. Can present with vestibular symptoms resulting from compression of the vestibular nerve; sensorineural hearing loss, tinnitus and disequilibrium. Schwannomas that arise from the glossopharyngeal, vagus or accessory nerves can be in the jugular foramen and present with variable cerebellar and acoustic symptoms or can cause glossopharyngeal dysfunction (e.g. hoarseness, difficulty swallowing) and/or spinal accessory symptoms (e.g. trapezius atrophy). Schwannomas involving the oculomotor, trochlear and abducens nerves are rare but can include palsy of the affected muscle and ipsilateral cavernous sinus symptoms if the mass is in the sinus. Hypoglossal Schwannomas can present with ipsilateral deviation of the tongue, possibly with associated hemiatrophy.

Neurofibromas (See Von Recklinghausen disease) Neurofibromas occasionally undergo sarcomatous change. Mucosal 'neurofibromas' (plexiform neuromas) may be seen in multiple endocrine neoplasia type III syndrome (with medullary carcinoma of the thyroid). Management is by excision. Neurofibromatosis type 2 (NF2) is also called the multiple inherited Schwannomas, meningiomas and ependymomas (MISME) syndrome. Diagnosis is by biopsy.

Noma (cancrum oris; gangrenous stomatitis) A severe fascial necrosis that may follow acute ulcerative gingivitis in malnourished, debilitated or severely immunocompromised patients, especially in Africa (see Chapter 40). Spreading necrosis penetrates the buccal mucosa, leading to gangrene, orocutaneous fistulae and scarring. Anaerobes and bone viruses have been implicated.

Orofacial—digital syndromes A group of inherited conditions manifesting with cleft lip and other facial anomalies, tongue clefts and multiple fraenae. Various dental defects, lingual and gingival nodules may be seen.

Ossifying fibroma This has features both of a developmental anomaly and a neoplasm. It presents as a painless, localised slow-growing, hard swelling of the jaw which radiographically is a well-defined radiolucency with a thin sclerotic margin containing irregular opaque masses. Histological examination shows little or no distinction between ossifying fibroma and fibrous dysplasia, except perhaps that a cellular, homogeneous calcified material is usually more obvious in ossifying fibroma. The distinction between ossifying fibroma and fibrous dysplasia, therefore, relies heavily on the localised nature and slow growth pattern of the ossifying fibroma. Surgical enucleation is curative.

Osteitis deformans Paget disease.

Osteochondroma (osteocartilaginous exostosis) Arises from the epiphyseal region of bone as cartilage-capped bony outgrowths, usually in children. Lesions may be solitary, or multiple in the syndrome of hereditary multiple exostoses. In the jaws, the most common site is the coronoid process. Solitary lesions are entirely benign, but in patients with multiple osteochondromas, there is a significant risk of malignant change.

Osteogenesis imperfecta (brittle bone syndrome; fragilitas ossium) A group of at least four types of inherited bone disorder characterised by excessive bone fragility and a number of extra-skeletal connective tissue disorders. Affected children may have multiple rib fractures (giving a 'beaded' radiographic appearance) and shortened concertina-like long bones. The skull is soft, with multiple wormian bones. Fracture of limb bones following mild injury is the most common skeletal problem. Patients are usually of short stature, with grossly deformed limbs and deformities of the spine and trunk and often cannot walk. Some have dentinogenesis imperfecta.

Blue sclera occurs in up to 90% of all patients. Deafness is common due to defective sound conduction through the external and middle ear. Hormones (calcitonin), vitamins (e.g. vitamin C or D), fluoride and flavonoids are of little value and surgical intervention for skeletal deformities is usually needed.

Osteomyelitis This literally means 'inflammation of the bone marrow', although sometimes the subperiosteal bone is mainly affected. Acute osteomyelitis primarily affects the mandible, usually affects adults and is essentially an osteolytic, destructive process, but an osteoblastic response is typical of sclerosing osteomyelitis. In children, proliferative periostitis may occur. Bacteria can spread to the bone:

- from local odontogenic infections (the commonest cause)
- from other adjacent structures (e.g. otitis media, tonsillitis, suppurative sialadenitis)
- haematogenous spread of organisms (this is rare in relation to the jaws).

When osteomyelitis of the mandible does occur, it may be a sign of an underlying debilitating disease, such as diabetes mellitus, an immune defect, or the effects of alcoholism: alternatively, it may be related to reduced vascularity, such as after irradiation or in rare conditions like Paget disease or osteopetrosis. *Staphylococcus aureus* is the commonest organism causing osteomyelitis in the jaws, but streptococci (both α- and β-haemolytic) and anaerobic organisms (e.g. *Bacteroides* and *Peptostreptococci* species) are occasionally implicated.

In acute osteomyelitis the organisms excite acute inflammation in the medullary bone and the consequent oedema and exudation cause pus to be forced under pressure through the medullary bone. The pressure causes thrombosis of intrabony vessels (i.e. the inferior dental artery), reducing the vascular supply to the bone, which then necroses. Eventually, pus bursts through the cortical plate to drain via sinuses in the skin or mucosa. Where pus penetrates the cortex, it may spread subperiosteally, stripping the periosteum and, thus, further reducing the blood supply. Necrotic bone becomes sequestrae surrounded by pus and these either spontaneously discharge or remain and perpetuate infection. The periosteum lays down new bone to form an involucrum encasing the infected and sequestrated bone. The involucrum, although perforated by sinuses, may prevent sequestra from being shed. Finally, if little new bone is formed, a pathological fracture may occur. Mandibular osteomyelitis presents with a deep-seated, boring pain and swelling. Teeth in the affected segment are mobile and tender to percussion, and pus oozes from the gingival crevices. Once pus penetrates the cortical plate, the pain improves and discharge appears. Labial anaesthesia is a characteristic feature because of pressure on the inferior alveolar nerve. The patient is often febrile and toxic with enlarged regional lymph nodes. Diagnosis is clinical, supported by imaging which, in established cases, shows marked bony destruction and sequestration but, since the changes are seen only after there has been significant decalcification of bone, early cases may not be detected and, in these, isotope bone scanning using technetium diphosphonate may show increased uptake. There is a leucocytosis with neutrophilia, and a raised ESR, CRP or PV. Treatment is by antibiotic therapy and usually drainage. Penicillin is the drug of choice, but many staphylococci are now penicillin-resistant, and for these infections, flucloxacillin or fusidic acid may be used. Lincomycin and clindamycin also give high bone levels, but, because of a high incidence of pseudo membranous colitis, are now regarded as second-line drugs. Metronidazole gives good bone levels and is indicated where an anaerobic infection is suspected. Drainage of established pus follows the same guidelines used for other infections. When dead bone is exposed in the mouth, it can often be left to sequestrate without surgical interference, but sequestrectomy should be undertaken if the separated dead bone fails to discharge and decortication of the mandible may be needed in order to allow this and drainage.

Hyperbaric oxygen is an effective adjunct for recalcitrant osteomyelitis, especially where anaerobic organisms are involved:

- *Acute maxillary osteomyelitis:* this is seen rarely, and usually in infants, presumably because the lack of development of the antrum at this age makes the maxilla a dense bone.
- *Chronic osteomyelitis:* this presents with intermittent pain and swelling, relieved by the discharge of pus through longstanding sinuses. Bone destruction is localised and often a single sequestrum may be the source of chronic infection. Removal of the sequestrum and curettage of the associated granulation tissue usually produces complete resolution.
- *Focal sclerosing osteomyelitis:* this is usually asymptomatic and is revealed as an incidental radiographic finding. Most common in young adults, it is usually associated with apical infection of a mandibular molar. Radiographically there is a dense, radio-opaque area of sclerotic bone related to the tooth apical area, caused by the formation of endosteal bone. This appears to be a response to low-grade infection

in a highly immune host. Following tooth extraction, the infection usually resolves (but the area of sclerotic bone often remains).

- *Diffuse sclerosing osteomyelitis:* a sclerotic endosteal reaction that, like focal sclerosing osteomyelitis, appears to be a response to low-grade infection. However, the area of bone involved is widespread and it sometimes involves most of the mandible or occasionally the maxilla. Sometimes the infection arises in an abnormally osteosclerotic mandible, such as in Paget disease, osteopetrosis or fibrous dysplasia. Intermittent swelling, pain and discharge of pus may persist for years. Management is difficult because of the extensive nature of the disease process. Long-term antibiotics, curettage and limited sequestrectomy all have their place.
- *Proliferative periostitis (Garré osteomyelitis):* This is more common in children than adults. The cellular osteogenic periosteum of the child responds to low-grade infection, such as apical infection of a lower first molar tooth, by proliferation and deposition of subperiosteal new bone. The subperiosteal bone may be deposited in layers, producing an onion-skin appearance radiologically, which can simulate Ewing sarcoma. The endosteal bone, however, may appear to be completely normal, but in severe cases also appears moth-eaten radiologically. Removal of the infective source is usually followed by complete resolution, although subsequent bone remodelling can take a considerable time.

Osteonecrosis of jaws (ONJ) ONJ, or osteochemonecrosis, can arise in people who have used bisphosphonates. Intravenous bisphosphonates, such as Pamidronate (Aredia) and Zoledronate (Zometa), are a particularly high risk, but even oral bisphosphonates used for greater than 3 years are a risk. ONJ usually presents after dental treatment, especially surgery, with painful, exposed and necrotic bone, primarily of the alveolar bone of the mandible. Therefore, it is best to avoid elective oral surgery, including endosseous implant placement, or the treatment should be carried out well before commencing bisphosphonates. Therapy is primarily supportive, involving nutritional support along with superficial debridement and oral saline irrigation. Antibiotics are indicated only for definite secondary infection. Necrotic bone requires resection. Vascularised free tissue transfer provides an immediate reconstruction option with a shortened treatment course.

Osteopetrosis (marble bone disease; Albers—Schonberg disease) Bone disease characterised by increased bone density with replacement of normal medullary bone by irregular avascular bone. Marrow is replaced by bone, and thus extramedullary sites such as the liver, spleen and lymph nodes develop haemopoietic function. Osteopetrosis is inherited in an autosomal-dominant or recessive manner. Patients with the autosomal-dominant form of osteopetrosis have good general health and a normal lifespan. There is no effective treatment for the recessive form: regular blood transfusions, corticosteroids and splenectomy may correct the anaemia; cranial nerve decompression may be necessary

and, if hydrocephalus develops, ventricular shunts may be required. However, most affected children die in the first decade of life, usually as a consequence of overwhelming infection or haemorrhage. The jaws, particularly the maxillae, are thickened and sclerotic and the paranasal sinuses are often reduced in size. Recurrent sinusitis and cranial nerve palsies (especially II, III, V, VII and VIII) are other orofacial problems of osteopetrosis. Children with the recessive form of osteopetrosis may have teeth with hypoplastic enamel, shortened roots and increased susceptibility to caries. Eruption of teeth can be delayed or absent. Pathological fracture is common. As a consequence of the sclerotic bone, dental extractions can be difficult and the mandible is also liable to fracture. The reduced vascularity of bone predisposes to postextraction osteomyelitis.

Osteoporosis A fairly common condition, characterised by the loss of both the organic matrix and the mineralised components of bone, although serum biochemistry is normal. The most common cause of osteoporosis is ageing, especially in females (hormonal), but drugs (especially corticosteroids) and several other disorders can also increase the rate of bone loss. The main clinical problem of osteoporosis is a fracture of either the neck or the femur or collapse of vertebral bodies. Osteoporosis has no notable oral manifestations but may affect the jaws and predispose to fracture or periodontal bone loss. Osteoporosis is managed by treatment of the underlying disorder (where possible) and by use of stimulators of osteogenesis (fluoride, phosphate, sex hormones or PTH) or inhibitors of bone resorption (e.g. calcium, vitamin D, bisphosphonates). The bisphosphonates predispose to osteonecrosis of the jaws.

Osteoradionecrosis (ORN) This can arise in people who have been irradiated in the region of the jaws (Chapter 53). It presents similarly to ONJ. It can be spontaneous, but it most commonly results from tissue injury, especially surgery. Therapy is as for ONJ, plus hyperbaric oxygen.

Osteosarcoma An aggressive malignant neoplasm which typically affects young patients. Males are affected twice as frequently as females. Only rarely are the mandible or maxilla affected. The aetiology is largely unknown, although about 3% of patients with osteosarcomas have a history of irradiation for other lesions. It should be noted that there is another peak incidence of osteosarcoma in the over-50s, which probably represents the small but significant malignant change in patients with pre-existing Paget disease. Osteosarcomas are classified as either sclerosing or osteolytic, depending on the degree of bone formation or destruction, and may be predominantly medullary or subperiosteal. A rare subtype called a *parosteal or juxtacortical osteosarcoma*, grows from the superficial surface of the bone and is relatively well differentiated. This variant grows much more slowly than the conventional osteosarcoma and metastasises late. A characteristic feature of osteosarcoma is the 'sunray' appearance on radiography. In the jaws, symmetrical widening of the periodontal ligament in associated teeth may be an early sign. Although the prognosis for osteosarcomas of the jaws is marginally better than for those of the long bones, the outlook is usually poor.

Pachyderma oralis White sponge naevus.

Pachyonychia congenita A rare, usually autosomal-dominant syndrome, in which the main clinical sign is onychodystrophy of all finger and toenails. There may be oral white lesions.

Papillomas The most common benign soft-tissue neoplasms; usually caused by human papillomavirus (HPV) infections. Commonly asymptomatic, a papilloma is a pedunculated lesion, either pink or white if hyperkeratinised, on the palate, tongue or other sites. Diagnosis is confirmed by biopsy (Fig. 55.8). Management is with topical podophyllin or intralesional α-interferon, imiquimod or surgery.

Paraneoplastic pemphigus This is associated mainly with non-Hodgkin lymphoma, chronic lymphoid leukaemia, sarcomas, thymomas or Castleman disease. There are serum autoantibodies reacting with transitional epithelium, and lichenoid features on biopsy, with intra- and subepithelial clefting, and IgG and C3 deposits. Antibodies are directed against desmosomes and hemidesmosomes, especially against desmoplakin or BP1. Clinical features include severe stomatitis and cheilitis in all cases, conjunctival lesions, genital lesions, and polymorphous skin eruption on the trunk, palms and soles.

Periodic fever, aphthae, pharyngitis and adenopathy (PFAPA) An unusual cause of mouth ulceration (with the other features) in children, which appears to respond to cimetidine and colchicine. There is a disorder of innate immunity with environmentally triggered activation of complement and IL-1β/-18.

Phakomatoses The term given to a range of disorders affecting ectoderm, with neurological manifestations and sometimes with a learning disability, which include: Sturge–Weber syndrome, Von Recklinghausen neurofibromatosis, ataxia telangiectasia and tuberous sclerosis (epiloia; Bourneville disease).

Pharyngeal pouch A rare pulsion diverticulum that appears because of a potential weakness in the pharyngeal muscles. Dysphagia is characterised by regurgitation of food results and may cause aspiration into the lungs.

Porphyrias A group of rare disorders of porphyrin metabolism:

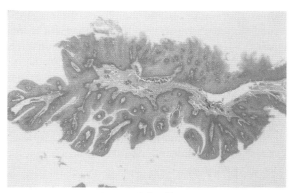

Fig. 55.8 Papilloma.

- *Erythropoietic porphyria* may cause reddish discolouration of both dentitions, hirsutism and skin blisters.
- *Hepatic porphyria* predisposes to mouth blisters (and is a contraindication to the use of intravenous barbiturates).

Pregnancy gingivitis An exacerbation of chronic gingivitis by pregnancy. Common mainly after the second month of pregnancy, pregnancy gingivitis presents with erythema, swelling and liability to bleed. Occasionally, a proliferative response at the site of a particularly dense plaque accumulation leads to a pregnancy epulis (pyogenic granuloma). This is a soft, red or occasionally firm swelling of the dental papilla. It may be asymptomatic unless traumatised by biting or toothbrushing. Oral hygiene should be improved. If asymptomatic, an epulis should be left alone — it may regress after parturition. If symptomatic, an excision biopsy is indicated.

Prion Diseases A group of rare, uniformly fatal neurodegenerative diseases. They occur in three forms: sporadic (85% to 90% of cases), genetic (10% to 15%) and acquired (<1%). Prions or proteinaceous infectious particles are the misshaped proteins responsible for causing transmissible spongiform encephalopathies, or prion diseases. Clinical presentation is a very rapidly progressive dementias. Symptoms may include behavioural/psychiatric changes, memory impairment, visual disturbances, myoclonus, ataxia, language and hearing problems, and movement dysfunction. Diagnosed by pathology See Creutzfeldt-Jakob disease (CJD).

Progeria (Werner syndrome) A collagen abnormality causing dwarfism, premature ageing and a characteristic facial appearance due to a disproportionately small face with mandibular retrognathia and a beak-like nose. Death occurs usually in the mid-teens.

Pseudohypoparathyroidism is a rare condition in which PTH is secreted normally, but the tissue receptors are unresponsive. The features are similar to those of hypoparathyroidism, plus a tendency to short stature and small fingers, but no dental manifestations.

Pseudoxanthoma elasticum An autosomal-recessive condition of progressive calcification of elastic tissue in the retina, skin, cardiovascular system and oral lesions of yellow plaques, somewhat resembling Fordyce spots.

Psoriasis Psoriasis of the oral mucosa is rare and is characterised by erythema, white or greyish plaques and lesions similar to erythema migrans. Gingival involvement in the form of desquamative gingivitis may rarely be seen. Biopsy, with histological and immunostaining are essential to the diagnosis. Topical corticosteroids may be helpful in these cases.

Pyostomatitis vegetans Oral condition characterised by miliary pustules and ulcers or erosions affecting the gingivae, particularly labially, and the buccal, labial, lingual or palatal mucosae, typically associated with, and following the onset of, inflammatory bowel disease. Biopsy of perilesional tissue, with histological and immunostaining examination is essential to the diagnosis. The oral lesions may respond at least partially to topical corticosteroids. The underlying disease should be treated, typically with dapsone, systemic corticosteroids, sulphasalazine, azathioprine or sulphamethoxypyridazine. Some patients report benefits from zinc supplementation. Lesions may resolve the following colectomy.

Radiolucencies Radiolucent lesions in the jaws may be due to cysts, infection, neoplasms arising in bone and metastatic neoplasms, bone disease (hyperparathyroidism, hypophosphatasia, cherubism; fibrous dysplasia; osteoporosis; osteonecrosis) and bone marrow expansion (haemolytic anaemias) or odontogenic cysts or tumours.

Radio-opacities Radio-opaque lesions in the jaws may be due to unexpected teeth, foreign bodies, bone disease (osteomyelitis; fibrous dysplasia; Paget disease; Gardner syndrome; osteopetrosis; neoplasms arising in bone and metastatic neoplasms especially from the prostate) or odontogenic lesions such as odontomes, hypercementosis and calcifying odontogenic tumour.

Rickets and osteomalacia Bone diseases are characterised by a decrease in the mineral, but not the organic content of bone. Unmineralised osteoid is present in large amounts, but there is a deficiency of mature mineralised bone. The term 'rickets' is used when the disorder affects children (when bones are still growing), the term 'osteomalacia' when adults are affected. The most common cause of rickets and osteomalacia in the western world is a deficiency of vitamin D, which can arise from a dietary deficiency of vitamin D, gastrointestinal disease or disorders of vitamin D metabolism. Dietary deficiency of vitamin D is still seen in older reclusive patients and in Asians living in Northern Europe on a poor diet which also contains phytates (such as in chapatis), since these inhibit calcium absorption from the gut, especially if they have little sun exposure in purdah. Vitamin D is normally synthesised in skin stimulated by sunlight. Renal disease impairs the conversion of vitamin D to dihydroxycholecalciferol and consequently can lead to 'renal rickets'. Rickets is clinically characterised by a spectrum of bony deformities, which range from mild bowing of the long bones of the legs to gross skeletal deformity and dwarfism. Osteomalacia causes generalised bone pain and tenderness, vertebral collapse, pelvic deformities and myopathy. Correction of any underlying clinical disorder is required and supplements of one of the metabolites of cholecalciferol are the usual lines of therapy for osteomalacia and rickets.

Rubella A highly infectious viral disease (Rubeola) that causes cervical lymphadenopathy, a macular rash starting on the face and behind the ears, mild fever, sore throat and, occasionally, palatal petechiae. Transplacental infection of the foetus may cause high-tone deafness, learning disability, blindness, cardiac defects or death (see Chapter 37).

Salivary fistula An abnormal communication between the gland or ducts and skin or mucous membrane. Internal fistulae are uncommon and asymptomatic. Trauma to the major glands or duct may (rarely) cause a persistent external fistula that is unpleasant and may lead to infection. Surgical repair is then indicated.

Scleroderma An uncommon idiopathic connective tissue disease seen mainly in middle-aged females. Clinical features include oral telangiectases, restricted mouth opening with microstomia, pale fibrotic 'chicken' tongue and a widened periodontal space on radiography, but the teeth are not mobile. Diffuse scleroderma is clinically characterised by skin thickening involving the face, neck, trunk and proximal upper and lower extremities, as well as significant internal organ involvement, including the lungs, heart, gastrointestinal tract and kidney, and is classically associated with antitopoisomerase-I antibodies (anti-topo-I or anti-Scl-70) and the absence of anticentromere antibodies (ACA). Limited scleroderma involves skin thickening in the face, neck and distal extremities, with frequent development of isolated pulmonary hypertension and ischaemic digital loss, characterised by ACA. The CREST syndrome (calcinosis, Raynaud syndrome, oesophageal lesions, sclerodactyly, telangiectasia) is a rare variant. Overlap syndromes, such as MCTD, with features of SLE, polymyositis (PM), RA and scleroderma are associated with anti-U1-small nuclear ribonucleoprotein particle (U1-snRNP) antibodies. Diagnosis is from clinical features, histopathology and autoantibodies. Management is often with penicillamine.

Scurvy Vitamin C (ascorbic acid) deficiency. Arises when no fresh fruit or vegetables are eaten for a long period. Diffusely swollen, boggy and purplish gingivae with purpura and haemorrhage are seen. Diagnosis is from leukaemia mainly from the dietary history, clinical features, blood film and white cell ascorbic acid. Management is with vitamin C.

Solitary bone cysts Lesions that occur most commonly in the long bones, they may also be found occasionally in the jaws. Their cause is speculative, but they may arise after trauma to the bone when an intramedullary haematoma forms and then degenerates rather than healing. Haemorrhagic bone cysts are generally painless and expansion is uncommon, the lesions usually being coincidentally discovered during radiographic examination. They are seen most often in the posterior body of the mandible in young persons. Clear or blood-stained fluid may be found within the bony cavity, but preoperative aspiration may at times not yield any product. Radiologically there is a well-defined translucency with a scalloped appearance around the apices of the teeth, which are vital. Surgery is undertaken in order to make a definitive diagnosis. There is no detectable cyst lining and sometimes only a thin fibrous membrane. Curettage produces bone fragments and connective tissue sometimes with granulation tissue. However, such surgical opening of the cavity usually leads to spontaneous resolution.

Subepithelial immune blistering diseases These include pemphigoid variants, dermatitis herpetiformis, acquired epidermolysis bullosa, linear IgA disease and chronic bullous disease of childhood.

Superior vena cava obstruction Obstruction of cardiac venous return, usually by lung cancer, may produce oedema and cyanosis of the face, neck and arms.

Surgical emphysema Escape of air into the tissues, usually after using an air rotor to section a tooth for removal, may give rise to diffuse swelling, which characteristically is painless, but gives rise to crepitus on palpation.

Syphilis (see Chapter 40) A sexually transmitted infection caused by *Treponema pallidum*. Other treponematoses, including yaws, bejel and pinta, are rare in the developed world: Forms of syphilis include:

- *Congenital syphilis:* infection passed across the placenta from the infected mother.
- *Acquired syphilis:* predominantly an infection of the sexually promiscuous.
- *Primary syphilis (Hunterian or hard chancre):* this is a small papule which develops into a large painless indurated ulcer, with regional lymphadenitis.
- *Secondary syphilis:* oral lesions include mucous patches, split papules or snail-track ulcers, which are highly infectious.
- *Tertiary syphilis:* this may cause glossitis (leukoplakia) and gumma (usually midline in the palate or tongue). These are non-infectious.

Teething Teething is the name sometimes given to children who are irritable, febrile and drooling, sometimes with a rash, but tooth eruption per se may cause a little discomfort but is not associated with fever or a rash, and most examples of 'teething' are probably infections such as herpetic stomatitis, pharyngitis or tonsillitis. Paracetamol is of value and the most important measure is to ensure hydration. Teething gels containing lidocaine, tannic acid, glycerol or essential oils (e.g. menthol, thymol) may be of some benefit but those containing salicylates or alcohol are best avoided.

Temporomandibular joint dislocation Occurs if the condyle moves too far forwards and over the articular eminence. The jaw locks in an open position with intense pain (see Chapter 42).

Thyroglossal cyst Arises from remnants of the thyroglossal duct and is midline at any point between the tongue and thyroid gland, and moves up on protrusion of the tongue. The cyst may cause dysphagia or become infected. It should be surgically removed.

Tobacco Use can cause a range of oral conditions from staining, to malodour, candidosis, dry mouth, taste disturbances, dry socket, implant failure, ANUG, periodontitis, keratosis, leukoplakia, to oral cancer.

Tooth root resorption Can arise because of:

- chronic infection
- chronic trauma
- impactions
- cysts and tumours
- tooth subluxation, luxation or radiotherapy
- systemic disease (Paget disease; hypo- or hyperparathyroidism; Turner syndrome; Gaucher disease or calcinosis).

Tooth surface loss Tooth surface loss includes attrition (Fig. 55.9), abrasion and erosion (and possibly abfraction).

TORCH syndrome or complex Foetal anomalies involving the heart, skin, eye and CNS, caused by perinatal infections with toxoplasmosis; other infections (hepatitis B, Coxsackie, syphilis, VZV, HIV, parvovirus B19) rubella; cytomegalovirus; or herpes simplex virus.

Toxic epidermal necrolysis (TEN; Lyell disease) A rare clinicopathological entity, with high mortality, characterised by extensive detachment of full-thickness epithelium. The distinction from erythema multiforme is unclear, but most cases of TEN are drug-induced and the lesions are extremely widespread. Drugs appear to trigger what appears to be an immunologically related reaction with sub- and intra-epithelial vesiculation. An increased number of cases in HIV/AIDS patients has been recorded. TEN presents with a cough, sore throat, burning eyes, malaise and low fever, followed after about 1 to 2 days by the skin and mucous membrane lesions. The entire skin surface and oral mucosa may be involved, with up to 100% sloughing off. Oral mucosae are involved in almost all cases. Gingival lesions are common and clinically are inflamed, with blister formation leading to painful widespread erosions.

Sheet-like loss of the epithelium and a positive Nikolsky sign are characteristic. Biopsy of perilesional tissue, with histological and immunostaining examination, is essential to the diagnosis. Histopathological examination is characteristic, showing necrosis of the whole epithelium detached from the lamina propria. Patients with TEN must be admitted to a hospital intensive care unit as soon as possible for management.

Toxoplasmosis Infection by the parasite *Toxoplasma gondii*, which infests members of the cat family who excrete it in faeces. *T. gondii* survives in soil for up to 1 year, and infection is generally by ingestion of cysts or oocysts, which are present in up to 10% of lamb and 25% of pork used for human consumption. In normal healthy patients, symptomatic toxoplasmosis manifests as:

- glandular fever syndrome, with a negative Paul–Bunell test
- ocular toxoplasmosis with chorioretinitis.

Transplacental transmission may result in foetal defects. In immunocompromised patients such as those with HIV/AIDS, *T. gondii* may produce CNS involvement.

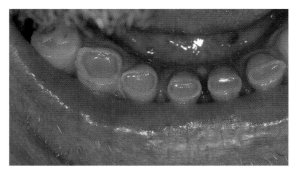

Fig. 55.9 Attrition, showing exposure of dentine and formation of secondary dentine.

Toxoplasmosis is diagnosed by detection of serum antibodies by the Sabin—Feldmann dye test, indirect haemagglutination or IgM fluorescent antibody tests, and isolation of *T. gondii* or histological demonstration of trophozoites. Toxoplasmosis is treated with pyrimethamine and sulphadiazine.

Trichodento-osseous syndrome Autosomal dominant; kinky hair, amelogenesis imperfecta; taurodont molars and brittle nails.

Tuberculosis Infection with mycobacteria, usually *Mycobacterium tuberculosis*. A common global bacterial infection. TB is usually pulmonary and seen especially in immunocompromised people). Solitary chronic oral ulcers, frequently of the tongue (see Chapter 40).

TUGSE (traumatic ulcerative granuloma with stromal eosinophilia) Also known as traumatic granuloma, eosinophilic ulcer and eosinophilic granuloma, this is not related to eosinophilic granuloma of bone as in Langerhans cell histiocytosis. TUGSE may affect patients of all ages, including neonates, when it is known as Riga—Fede disease. TUGSE is a reactive condition seen most commonly on the dorsal and lateral tongue, followed by the lips and buccal mucosa as a deep, rolled bordered and indurated ulcer to exophytic and lobular looking like a pyogenic granuloma. It probably is initiated by trauma, resolves spontaneously slowly over many weeks and may recur. The clinical features may mimic squamous cell carcinoma (SCC). A biopsy is indicated if the ulcer persists greater than 3 weeks and shows eosinophils in areas of muscle damage. The treatment is surgery; intralesional corticosteroids if it recurs.

Tularaemia Infection by the coccobacillus *Francisella tularensis*. The epidemics are thought to be waterborne. Most patients are young and female. In most of the cases, the disease presents itself in oropharyngeal form, with fever and tonsillopharyngitis and cervical lymphadenopathy. Streptomycin is given to most patients in combination with tetracycline, doxycycline or chloramphenicol.

Ulcerative colitis Inflammatory bowel disease, which may present with persistent diarrhoea and is frequently painless, with the passage of blood and mucus in severe cases, iron deficiency anaemia, weight loss, and mucosal pustules (pyostomatitis vegetans), irregular chronic ulcers and aphthae. Diagnosis is by biopsy, full blood picture, sigmoidoscopy and barium enema. Management is with haematinics for any secondary deficiencies; topical corticosteroids may be helpful; as may sulphasalazine, or corticosteroid enemas.

White sponge naevus (Cannon disease, pachyderma oralis, white folded gingivostomatitis). Rare autosomal-dominant defect of keratin causing a benign familial disorder with shaggy bilateral white leukoplakic type lesions (see Chapter 23). Usually in the buccal mucosa.

GLOSSARY

A

AC angular cheilitis
ACA anti-centromere antibodies
ACE angiotensin-converting enzyme
ACE2 receptor the main receptor for SARS-CoV-2 virus
ACTH adrenocorticotrophic hormone
ALU aphthous-like ulcers
ANA anti-nuclear antibodies
ANCA anti-neutrophil cytoplasmic antigen
ANUG acute necrotising ulcerative gingivitis
ART anti-retroviral therapy
ATA anti-topoisomerase antibodies

B

BANA benzoyl-arginine-naphthyl-amide
BARK bilateral alveolar ridge keratosis
bid or bd twice a day
BMS burning mouth syndrome
BNF *British National Formulary*
BP blood pressure
BRONJ bisphosphonate-related osteonecrosis
BS Behçet syndrome

C

CAT computed tomography
CATCH 22 cardiac defects, abnormal facies, thymic hypoplasia, cleft palate and hypocalcaemia resulting from chromosome 22 deletions
CBCT cone beam CT
CBT cognitive behavioural therapy
CD cluster of differentiation 4 (a type of helper T lymphocyte)
CDC Centers for Disease Control and Prevention (USA)
CMC chronic mucocutaneous candidosis
CMV cytomegalovirus
CNS central nervous system
CO complaining of
COPD chronic obstructive pulmonary disease
COVID19 the systemic disease caused by SARS-CoV-2 virus
COX-2 cyclooxygenase-2
CPITN community periodontal index of treatment needs
CRP C-reactive protein
CSF cerebrospinal fluid
CT computed tomography
CTR chemoradiotherapy
CTX chemotherapy
CVA cerebrovascular accident
CVE cerebrovascular event
CXR chest x-ray

D

DEXA dual-energy x-ray absorptiometry
DIF direct immunofluorescence
DIGO drug-induced gingival overgrowth
DIHS drug-induced hypersensitivity syndrome
DLE disseminated lupus erythematosus
DPF *Dental Practitioners Formulary*

DRESS drug rash with eosinophilia and systemic symptoms
Ds DNA double strand deoxyribonucleic acid
Dsg desmoglein
DXR radiotherapy

E

EB epidermolysis bullosa
EBV Epstein—Barr virus
ECG electrocardiogram
EGFR epidermal growth factor receptor
ELISA enzyme-linked immunosorbent assay
EM erythema multiforme
EMA European Medicines Agency
ENA extractable nuclear antigen
ENT ears, nose and throat (otorhinolaryngology)
ESR erythrocyte sedimentation rate
EUA examination under (general) anaesthetic

F

FBC full blood count
FBP full blood picture
FDA Food and Drug Administration (USA)
FH family history
FNA fine needle aspiration
FNAB fine needle aspiration biopsy

G

G6PD glucose 6 phosphate dehydrogenase
GA general anaesthesia
GI gastrointestinal
GDP general dental practitioner
GIT gastrointestinal tract
GMH general medical history
GMP general medical practitioner
GORD gastro-oesophageal reflux disease
GP general practitioner
GU genitourinary
GVHD graft-versus-host disease

H

HAART highly active antiretroviral therapy
HBV hepatitis B virus
HCV hepatitis C virus
HHV human herpesviruses
HIV human immunodeficiency virus(es)
HL Hodgkin lymphoma
HLA human leukocyte antigen
HMG-CoA 3-hydroxy-3-methyl-glutaryl-coenzyme A reductase
HPA Health Protection Agency (UK)
HPA hypothalamo-pituitary-adrenal
HPC history of the present complaint
HPV human papillomaviruses
HRQoL health-related quality of life
HSCT haematopoietic stem cell transplantation
HSV herpes simplex virus
HTLV human lymphotropic virus

I

IFN interferon
IgG immunoglobulin G

IIF indirect immunofluorescence
IL interleukin
IRIS immune reconstitution inflammatory syndrome

K

KCOT keratocystic odontogenic tumour
KS Kaposi sarcoma
KSHV Kaposi sarcoma herpesvirus (HHV-8)

L

LA local anaesthesia
La — (also SS-B) autoantibody in Sjögren syndrome
LFT liver function tests
LMS locomotor system
LP lichen planus

M

MALT mucosa-associated lymphoid tissue
MDR-TB multidrug-resistant tuberculosis
MDT multidisciplinary team
MEN multiple endocrine neoplasia
mg milligram
MMP mucous membrane pemphigoid
MRG median rhomboid glossitis
MRI magnetic resonance imaging
MRS Melkersson-Rosenthal syndrome
MRSA methicillin-resistant *Staphylococcus aureus*
MS multiple (disseminated) sclerosis

N

NAAT nucleic acid amplification test
NHL non-Hodgkin lymphoma
NICE National Institute for Health and Clinical Excellence (UK)
NIHR National Institute for Health Research
NSAID nonsteroidal anti-inflammatory drugs
NSM necrotising sialometaplasia

O

OFG orofacial granulomatosis
OLP oral lichen planus
ORN osteoradionecrosis
OTC over the counter

P

PAS periodic acid Schiff
PCR polymerase chain reaction
PET positron emission tomography
PFAPA periodic fever, adenitis, pharyngitis, aphthae
PI protease inhibitor
PMH past medical history
POM prescription-only medicine
PPI proton pump inhibitor
PRN as necessary
PV pemphigus vulgaris; plasma viscosity

Q

QoL quality of life

R

RANKL   receptor activator of nuclear factor kappa-β ligand
RAS   recurrent aphthous stomatitis
RAST   radioallergosorbent test
RF   rheumatoid factor
RMH   relevant medical history
Ro   (also SS-A) autoantibody in Sjögren syndrome
ROM   range-of-movement
RS   respiratory system
RT   radiotherapy

S

SACE   serum angiotensin-converting enzyme
SCID   severe combined immune deficiency
SH   social history
SJS   Stevens-Johnson syndrome
SLE   systemic lupus erythematosus
SLN   sentinel lymph node
SNRI   serotonin—norepinephrine reuptake inhibitor
SPT   second primary tumour

SS   Sjögren syndrome
SS-A   auto antibodies in Sjögren syndrome (also Ro)
SS-B   auto antibodies in Sjögren syndrome (also La)
SSI   sexually-shared infections
SSRI   selective serotonin re-uptake inhibitor
STI   sexually transmitted infections
SUNCT   severe unilateral neuralgia with conjunctivitis and tearing

T

TAC   trigeminal autonomic cephalgia
TB   tuberculosis
TEN   toxic epidermal necrolysis
TMJ   temporomandibular joint
TMPD   temporomandibular pain dysfunction
TORCH   toxoplasmosis; rubella; cytomegalovirus; herpes
TN   trigeminal neuralgia
TNF   tumour necrosis factor
TPMT   thiopurine methyl transferase

TUGSE   traumatic ulcerative granuloma with stromal eosinophilia

U

U&E   urea and electrolytes
UADT   upper aerodigestive tract
URTI   upper respiratory tract infection
US   ultrasound
UTI   urinary tract infection

V

VRSA   vancomycin-resistant *Staphylococcus aureus*
VZV   varicella zoster virus

W

WBC   white blood cell count
WCC   white cell count

X

XTR-TB   extended drug—resistant tuberculosis